Comparative Reproductive Biology

Comparative Reproductive Biology

Edited by

Heide Schatten, PhD
Gheorghe M. Constantinescu, DVM, PhD, Drhc

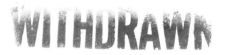

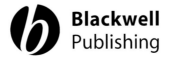
Blackwell
Publishing

Heide Schatten, PhD, is an Associate Professor at the University of Missouri, Columbia. She is well published in the areas of cytoskeletal regulation in somatic and reproductive cells and on cytoskeletal abnormalities in cells affected by disease, cellular and molecular biology, cancer biology, reproductive biology, developmental biology, microbiology, space biology, and microscopy. A member of the American Society for Cell Biology, American Association for the Advancement of Science, Microscopy Society of America, and American Society for Gravitational and Space Biology, she has received numerous awards including grant awards from NSF, NIH, and NASA.

Gheorghe M. Constantinescu, DVM, PhD, Drhc, is a Professor of Veterinary Anatomy and Medical Illustrator at the College of Veterinary Medicine of the University of Missouri-Columbia. He is a member of the American, European and World Associations of Veterinary Anatomists and also author of more than 380 publications, including *Clinical Anatomy for Small Animal Practitioners* (Blackwell, 2002) translated in three languages. During his career of more than 50 years, he has been honored by numerous invited presentations, awards, diplomas, and certificates of recognition.

©2007 Blackwell Publishing

Blackwell Publishing Professional
2121 State Avenue, Ames, Iowa 50014, USA

Orders: 1-800-862-6657
Office: 1-515-292-0140
Fax: 1-515-292-3348
Web site: www.blackwellprofessional.com

Blackwell Publishing Ltd
9600 Garsington Road, Oxford OX4 2DQ, UK
Tel.: +44 (0)1865 776868

Blackwell Publishing Asia
550 Swanston Street, Carlton, Victoria 3053, Australia
Tel.: +61 (0)3 8359 1011

Authorization to photocopy items for internal or personal use, or the internal or personal use of specific clients, is granted by Blackwell Publishing, provided that the base fee is paid directly to the Copyright Clearance Center, 222 Rosewood Drive, Danvers, MA 01923. For those organizations that have been granted a photocopy license by CCC, a separate system of payments has been arranged. The fee codes for users of the Transactional Reporting Service is ISBN-13: 978-0-8138-1554-1/2007.

First edition, 2007

Library of Congress Cataloging-in-Publication Data
Comparative reproductive biology / [edited by] Heide Schatten and Gheorghe M. Constantinescu.–1st ed.
p. ; cm.
Includes bibliographical references.
ISBN-13: 978-0-8138-1554-1 (alk. paper)
ISBN-10: 0-8138-1554-1 (alk. paper)
1. Domestic animals–Reproduction 2. Animal breeding. 3. Artificial insemination. 4. Veterinary obstetrics. I. Schatten, Heide. II. Constantinescu, Gheorghe M., 1932–
[DNLM: 1. Reproduction. 2. Anatomy, Comparative. 3. Animals, Domestic–physiology. 4. Physiology, Comparative. 5. Reproductive Techniques–veterinary. SF 887 C737 2007]
SF871.C56 2007
636–dc22

                                                                2006033456

The last digit is the print number: 9 8 7 6 5 4 3 2 1

Table of Contents

Foreword

I was honored when my colleague and friend Dr. Heide Schatten asked me to write a foreword for this book. It is a great pleasure to strongly recommend Drs. Heide Schatten and Gheorghe M. Constantinescu's latest scholarly work *Comparative Reproductive Biology*. Both editors are internationally known scientists and well qualified to oversee and contribute to such a comprehensive task. Furthermore, they have recruited an exceptional group of reproductive biologists to author chapters in their areas of expertise.

When considering the physiological systems of the body, the degree of species variation within the reproductive system compared to other systems is remarkable. Furthermore, it is essential that researchers, educators, and students alike remain acutely aware of the fundamental comparative differences in the reproductive biology of domestic species (carnivores, pigs, ruminants, and horses). As a researcher, understanding the comparative differences in ovarian and uterine function among mammalian species has been essential in helping me develop new approaches to a problem. Too many of us are guilty of basing our understanding of mammalian reproduction on our species of interest. Therefore, this book will be especially helpful in educating a broad audience of readers regarding the important differences in how domestic species reproduce.

As a teacher, I consistently emphasize that "structure dictates function." Therefore, I appreciate the strong morphological approach that the editors have taken in organizing and preparing the chapters. This book does an excellent job of synthesizing the classical information on reproductive biology (anatomy, histology, endocrinology, etc.) with an extensive list of reproductive biotechnologies: transgenic animals, gender selection in mammalian semen and preimplantation embryos, artificial insemination, embryo transfer and *in vitro* fertilization, comparative cryobiology of preimplantation embryos, animal cloning, comparative placentation, and pregnancy diagnostics. Consequently, this book will serve as an excellent reference for those with an interest in the reproductive biology of domestic species.

It is with enthusiasm that I endorse Drs. Schatten and Constantinescu's most recent contribution to the field of reproductive biology.

Michael F. Smith, Ph.D.
Professor of Animal Sciences
University of Missouri-Columbia

Preface

Rapid progress in reproductive biology and the desire of many new and established scientists to find classic as well as contemporary aspects in one comprehensive book has inspired this work. *Comparative Reproductive Biology* offers both broad and specific knowledge in areas that have advanced the field in recent years, including advances in cell and molecular biology applied to reproduction, transgenic animal production, gender selection, artificial insemination, embryo transfer, cryobiology, animal cloning, and many others. It includes topics in animal reproduction that are usually only found as part of other books in animal science such as anatomy, developmental anatomy, developmental biology, histology, cell and molecular biology, physiology, radiology, ultrasonography, and others. We have made an effort to design a book that includes most, if not all, relevant areas of animal reproduction. The book is intended for a large audience as a reference book on the subject, rather than as a handbook or course textbook. It will fill a gap in the literature and is meant to be of interest to scientists in animal science, to teachers in the professional curriculum, to veterinarians, to clinicians, to professional students, to graduate students (PhD and Masters trainees), and others interested in animal reproduction.

There is currently no comparable and competitive book on the market. Most existing books are limited to various aspects of reproductive biology, such as oestrus cycles, pregnancy and parturition, dystocia and other conditions and/or disorders associated with parturition, surgical interventions, infertility, embryo transfer, physiology (the endocrinology of reproduction included), and mating and artificial insemination in domestic animals. An abundance of research papers are published in all fields, including the large field of physiology of reproduction of domestic animals. Many are referred to in the specific chapters of this book. This comprehensive book on various aspects of reproduction is timely due to the growing interest in the field. It provides insights into fascinating new approaches that have grown steadily since the introduction of the now well accepted *in vitro* fertilization and nuclear cloning techniques with applications for human health and agricultural and biomedical research.

The chapters are written by renowned scientists in their respective fields and their presentations include the biological aspects of reproduction in domestic animals such as dogs, cats, pigs, large and small ruminants, and horses. The specific chapters start with the developmental anatomy of reproductive organs, continuing with anatomy, histology, cellular and molecular biology, comparative reproductive physiology, transgenic animals, gender selection in mammalian semen and pre-implantation embryos, artificial insemination, embryo transfer and *in vitro* fertilization, comparative cryobiology of preimplantation embryos, animal cloning, comparative placentation, pregnancy diagnostics in domestic animals, and ultrasonography in small ruminant reproduction.

We are grateful to all of the authors for contributing their unique expertise and we hope the reader will find this book of value.

Heide Schatten
Gheorghe M. Constantinescu
Columbia, Missouri, USA

List of Contributors

Yuksel Agca, DVM, PhD
Assistant Professor
University of Missouri-Columbia
College of Veterinary Medicine
Comparative Medicine Center
W-230 Vet. Med. Bldg.
1600 E. Rollins Street
Columbia, MO 65211
Phone: (573) 884-0311
Fax: (573) 884-7521
E-mail: agcay@missouri.edu

GC Althouse, DVM, MS, PhD
Diplomate of the American College of
   Theriogenologists
Associate Professor
Chief, Section of Reproductive Studies
New Bolton Center
382 West Street Road
University of Pennsylvania
Kennett Square, PA 19348-1692
Phone: (610) 925-6220
Fax: (610) 925-8134
E-mail: gca@vet.upenn.edu

Anthony W.S. Chan, DVM, PhD
Yerkes National Primates Research Center
Emory University School of Medicine
Suite 2212, Neurosciences Research Bldg.
954 Gatewood Rd. N.E.
Atlanta, GA 30329
E-mail: achan@genetics.emory.edu

Ileana A. Constantinescu, DVM, MS,
Clinical Assistant Professor
Department of Biomedical Sciences
W-150 Vet. Med. Bldg.
College of Veterinary Medicine
University of Missouri-Columbia
1600 E. Rollins Street
Columbia, MO 65211
Phone: (573) 882-7228
Fax: (573) 884-6890
E-mail: constantinescui@missouri.edu

Gheorghe M. Constantinescu, DVM, PhD, Drhc
Professor and Medical Illustrator
Department of Biomedical Sciences
W-119 Vet. Med. Bldg.
College of Veterinary Medicine
University of Missouri-Columbia
1600 E. Rollins Street
Columbia, MO 65211
Phone: (573) 882-7249
Fax: (573) 884-6890
E-mail: constantinescug@missouri.edu

Ross P. Cowart, DVM, MS
Diplomate of the American Board of Veterinary
   Practitioners
Food Animal Practice Specialty
Associate Professor
University of Missouri-Columbia
College of Veterinary Medicine
A-308 Clydesdale Hall
379 E. Campus Drive
Columbia, MO 65211
Phone: (573) 882-7821
Fax: (573) 884-5444
E-mail: cowartr@missouri.edu

John K. Critser, PhD
Department of Veterinary Pathobiology
Gilbreath-McLorn Professor of Comparative Medicine
Director, Comparative Medicine Center
College of Veterinary Medicine
University of Missouri
1600 E. Rollins Road, E-109
Columbia, MO 65211
Phone: (573) 884-9469
Fax: (573) 884-7521
E-mail: critserj@missouri.edu

Jonathan A. Green, PhD
Assistant Professor
Division of Animal Sciences
163 ASRC, 920 E. Campus Drive
University of Missouri-Columbia
Columbia, MO 65211
Lab Phone: (573) 882-6532
Office Phone: (573) 884-1697
Fax: (573) 882-6827
E-mail: greenjo@missouri.edu

John F. Hasler, PhD
427 Obenchain Rd.
Bonner Peak Ranch
Laporte, CO 80535
Home Phone: (970) 377-2670
Alternate Phone: (970) 484-9860
Cell: (970) 222-5302
E-mail: jfhasler05@msn.com

Liangxue Lai, PhD
Division of Animal Sciences
163 ASRC, 920 E. Campus Drive
University of Missouri-Columbia
Columbia, MO 65211

Gaurishankar Manandhar
Research Assistant Professor
Department of Animal Sciences
University of Missouri-Columbia
S 141, ASRC, 920 E. Campus Drive
Columbia, MO 65211
Phone: (573) 884-1549
E-mail: manandharg@missouri.edu

Herris Maxwell, DVM
Diplomate of the American College of Theriogenologists
Associate Clinical Professor
Auburn University
College of Veterinary Medicine
JTV Large Animal Teaching Hospital
Auburn, AL 36849-5540
E-mail: maxwehs@vetmed.auburn.edu

Richard Meadows, DVM
Diplomate of the American Board of Veterinary
    Practitioners
Clinical Associate Professor
University of Missouri-Columbia
College of Veterinary Medicine
A-370 Clydesdale Hall
379 E. Campus Drive
Columbia, MO 65211
Phone: (573) 882-7821
Fax: (573) 884-5444
E-mail: meadowsr@missouri.edu

Burkhard Meinecke, DVM
Professor
Department of Reproductive Medicine
School of Veterinary Medicine Hannover
Buenteweg 15
D-30559 Hannover, Germany

Sabine Meinecke-Tillmann, DVM
Professor
Department of Reproductive Medicine
School of Veterinary Medicine Hannover
Buenteweg 15
D-30559 Hannover, Germany
E-mail: Sabine.Meinecke-Tillmann@tiho-hannover.de

Hongshen Men, PhD
University of Missouri-Columbia
College of Veterinary Medicine
Comparative Medicine Center
Vet. Med. Bldg.
1600 E. Rollins Street
Columbia, MO 65211

Steven F. Mullen, PhD
University of Missouri at Columbia
College of Veterinary Medicine
Department of Veterinary Pathobiology
Cryobiology Laboratory
1600 E Rollins St
Columbia, MO 65211
Phone: (573) 884-9523
Fax: (573) 884-7521
E-mail: sfm5ff@missouri.edu

Randall S. Prather, PhD
Curators' Professor
Distinguished Professor of Reproductive Biotechnology
Associate Leader-Food for the 21st Century-Animal
    Reproductive Biology Cluster
Co-Director National Swine Resource and Research
    Center
Division of Animal Science
920 East Campus Drive, E125D ASRC
University of Missouri-Columbia
Columbia, MO 65211-5300, U.S.A.
Phone: (573) 882-6414
Fax: (573) 884-7827
E-mail: PratherR@Missouri.Edu

Cheryl S. Rosenfeld, DVM, PhD
Assistant Professor
Department of Biomedical Sciences
University of Missouri
440F Life Sciences Center
1201 Rollins Road
Columbia, MO 65211
Office Phone: (573) 882-6798
Lab Phone: (573) 882-5132
E-mail: rosenfeldc@missouri.edu

Heide Schatten, PhD
Associate Professor
University of Missouri-Columbia
College of Veterinary Medicine
W-123 Vet. Med. Bldg.
1600 E. Rollins Street
Columbia, MO 65211
Phone: (573) 882-2396
Fax: (573) 884-5414
E-mail: schattenh@missouri.edu

Clifford F. Shipley, DVM
Associate Professor
Diplomate of the American College of Theriogenologists
University of Illinois
College of Veterinary Medicine
1008 West Hazelwood Drive
Urbana, IL 61802
Clinic Phone: (217) 333-2000
Office Phone: (217) 333-2479
Fax: (217) 333-7126
E-mail: cshipley@uiuc.edu

Peter Sutovsky, PhD
Assistant Professor
University of Missouri-Columbia
S141 ASRC
920 East Campus Drive
Columbia, MO 65211-5300
Phone: (573) 882-3329
Fax: (573) 884-5540
E-mail: sutovskyP@missouri.edu

Manoel Tamassia
University of Illinois at Urbana-Champaign
College of Veterinary Medicine
Dept of Veterinary Clinical Medicine
1008 West Hazelwood Dr.
Urbana, IL 61802, USA
E-mail: tamassia@uiuc.edu

Bhanu Prakash Telugu
Division of Animal Sciences
163 ASRC, 920 E. Campus Drive
University of Missouri-Columbia
Columbia, MO 65211

Eric M. Walters, PhD
Research Assistant Professor
Molecular Embryology/Cryobiology Laboratory
National Swine Research and Resource Center
Department of Veterinary Pathobiology
University of Missouri-Columbia
1600 E. Rollins Street E160
Columbia, MO 65211
Phone: (573) 882-7343
Fax: (573) 884-7521
E-mail: walterse@missouri.edu

Suzanne Whitaker, DVM
Former Clinical Instructor at the University of
Missouri-Columbia
Phone: (573) 999-7179
E-mail: coopngraham@hotmail.com

Comparative Reproductive Biology

Chapter 1

Developmental Anatomy of Reproductive Organs

Ileana A. Constantinescu

Male and Female Reproductive Systems

The male and the female reproductive systems consist of the gonads, the reproductive tracts, and the external genitalia (the mammary glands are also included in this section). Although functionally distinct, the urinary and reproductive systems are intimately associated in origin, development, and certain final relationships in the adult anatomy. Common features of the two systems include the following:

- Both systems originate in the intermediate mesoderm.
- The (excretory) ducts of both systems initially share a common cavity—the *urogenital sinus* (a subdivision of the *cloaca*).

The common origin and close spatial association of the urinary and reproductive systems render a rather complicated organization. Some of their common primordia will differentiate in accordance with the established sex of the emerging new individual. Some of the organs are formed by association of structures that arise independently at different times and places. Some structures form and degenerate without ever becoming functional, while others undergo partial degeneration and their remnants are incorporated into a new organ for a new function.

The reproductive organs of both sexes develop from common primordia that follow a similar, consistent pattern of formation well into the fetal period. This development includes transition through an "indifferent" (undifferentiated) stage during which all component structures are present and appear the same in both sexes. When the primordia of the reproductive system are established (before differentiation), all embryos are potentially bisexual. As a result, developmental errors may lead to various degrees of intermediate sex.

Development of Gonads

During their development the gonads pass through two distinct stages: the Indifferent stage and the Differential stage.

Indifferent Stage

The outline of the gonads appears (in most mammals) when the embryo possesses from 38 pairs to 40 pairs of somites (at about 24 days in dogs, 27 days in horses, and 28 days in oxen). The *gonadal primordium* is represented by genital (gonadal) ridges—paired longitudinal condensations of intermediate mesoderm (with contribution from the adjacent coelomic mesothelium) along the axis of, and medial to, the *mesonephros* (the primordium of the excretory system).

The cells of the ridges become aligned to form a number of irregularly shaped cords, the primitive sex cords, which extend into the center (medulla) of the ridge and connect to the surface epithelium. At this stage the embryos exhibit gonads, which show no evidence as to whether they will develop into testes or ovaries (hence, the "indifferent" stage in gonadal development).

Differential Stage

Although genetic sex is established at the time of fertilization, the gonads do not attain morphological sex characteristics until toward the end of the embryonic period. This differentiation is much accelerated (and slightly earlier in males) at the beginning of the fetal period.

Regardless of their future fate, the primordia of all reproductive male and female structures form in both sexes. At this stage in development, the primordia are represented by the undifferentiated gonad and two duct systems—the paired *mesonephric* and *paramesonephric ducts*. It is these primordia that, remodeled by complete or partial regression, addition to, or incorporation into present or later-to-emerge structures, will form the adult, functional reproductive male and female organs.

The mesonephric (Wolffian) duct is the salvaged remnant of the mesonephros (one of the three overlapping kidney systems). In amniotes, the mesonephros regresses by the end of the embryonic period; the exception is the mesonephric duct (and part of its tubules), which is retained and remodeled as genital ducts in the male. The paramesonephric (Müllerian) duct forms as an epithelial invagination ventrolateral to the mesonephros. Cranially, each tube opens into the abdominal cavity; caudally, each fuses with its counterpart to enter the urogenital sinus ventral to the mesonephric duct. In females, the Müllerian duct forms most of the genital duct system.

Testes

Developmental processes represent an extensive panorama of complex, interdependent, precisely sequenced and coordinated interactions of genetic and environmental modulators that work together to create an unique organism. The sexual identity of an individual is established with the process of fertilization; the individual's sexual distinction is the result of exposure to gonadal hormones, which start to be secreted as soon as the gonads emerge from the indifferent stage. The gonadal differentiation reflects morphogenic changes that involve the sex cords and *interstitial cells* (cells between the cords). Toward the end of the third week after fertilization (a few days later in species with longer gestation), primordial germ cells (future gametes) migrate from the endoderm of the yolk sac and become embedded into the indifferent gonad.

In a genetically male embryo, the germ cells carry an XY chromosome. The Y chromosome possesses the SRY gene, which encodes the testis-determining factor (TDF) that directs testicular differentiation, thus establishing the gonadal sex. In the presence of TDF, the sex cords become organized into *s*eminiferous tubules—elongated, tortuous cords that extend into the center (medulla) of the gonad and contain differentiated germ cells, spermatogonia. Seminiferous tubules connect to the retained mesonephric tubules of the mesonephric duct via the rete testis (a network of thin tubules located in the medulla of the testis and originating from sex cords that lack germ cells). The cord cells (which form the walls of the seminiferous tubules) differentiate into Sertoli (sustentacular) cells that secrete a glycoprotein, a Müllerian-inhibiting substance (MIS), which is responsible for the regression of the paramesonephric ducts. The interstitial (Leydig) cells begin secreting testosterone that induces sexual differentiation of the duct system and of the external genitalia.

As the medulla becomes the functional part of the testis, the cortex is reduced and separated from the surrounding surface epithelium by a thick layer of connective tissue—the *tunica albuginea*. The tunica albuginea serves as a pathway for blood vessels.

Ovaries

In the genetic female embryo with an XX chromosome complex, the absence of the Y chromosome redirects differentiation of the indifferent gonad to become an ovary. The cells of cords dissociate into clusters surrounding individual or groups of germ cells, which together form primordial follicles (the proliferation of both types of cells is completed before birth). Within the follicles, germ cells differentiate into primary oocytes that remain arrested in meiosis I until ovulation. The medulla of the gonad is greatly reduced and replaced by vascular stroma. In the absence of a Y chromosome with its supportive contribution, the mesonephric ducts degenerate.

Development of Reproductive Tracts

In mammals, the gonads develop in close association with the two paired duct systems—the mesonephric and paramesonephric ducts, present in both sexes.

Development of Male Reproductive Tracts

Testosterone secretion by fetal testes triggers the morphogenic changes in the duct system and external genitalia (if exposure to testosterone is denied, the embryo, regardless of its genetic sex, will develop as a female).

The cranial portion of the mesonephric duct (and associated tubules) regresses while the reminder undergoes regional differentiation. Its tubules that become connected with the sex cords via rete testis will form the efferent ductules (those left out persist as functionless vestiges, either as the "appendix of epididymis" or as the "paradidymis"). The mesonephric duct in the area of the testis becomes extensively elongated and convoluted to form the epididymis; its caudal end extends to enter the urogenital sinus (the mesoderm of the caudal region of the duct differentiates to form the seminal vesicles).

In amniotes, as a rule, the paramesonephric ducts degenerate completely by the beginning of the fetal period. Vestigial structures are seen either as the "appendix testis"—a tiny portion of its cranial extent, or as the "uterus masculinus"—a small diverticulum wherein the fused ducts open into the urogenital sinus.

Development of Female Reproductive Tract

In females, the mesonephric duct degenerates, leaving the paramesonephric duct system to form the main reproductive tracts. The cranial-most portions of the paired duct remain continuous with the peritoneal cavity, narrow and convoluted to form the *oviducts* (uterine tubes). The degree of fusion of the paramesonephric ducts varies among domestic species, being most extensive in horses and least in carnivores; in rodents and rabbits there are two cervices that open into a single vagina, while in marsupials, the tubes do not fuse to any extent. Therefore, the marsupials are provided with a double vagina. Caudally, the unfused portions form the uterine horns. As the embryo assumes its rounded shape, the caudal portions of the tubes are shifted medially and fuse together to differentiate into the body of the uterus, the cervix, and the cranial one-third part of the vagina. The extent to which the urogenital sinus participates in the formation of the vagina varies with the species. This involvement is demonstrated by the positioning of the urethral and vaginal openings and the length of the vestibule.

Vestigial structures of (particularly) the caudal end of the mesonephric duct are consistently represented by Gärtner's ducts, seen in the cow as small openings into the vestibule; in the sow as tubular cords in the wall's uterine horns or vagina; and in carnivores, in the wall of the vagina.

Development of the Male and Female External Genitalia

In this subsection, the urogenital sinus, the Indifferent stage and the Differential Stage for both male and female will be discussed.

Urogenital Sinus

The urogenital sinus is a developmental structure common to the male and the female.

In early mammalian embryos, the caudal end of the primitive gut (caudal to the origin of the *allantois*—a ventral evagination of hindgut that collects and disposes of fetal urinary wastes) is represented by the wide diverticulum—the cloaca, temporarily closed by the cloacal membrane. Toward the end of the embryonic stage, with the advancement of the tail fold, a mass of mesenchyme—the urorectal septum—extends caudally from the junction with the allantois, dividing the cloaca into a dorsal part, the rectum, and a ventral part, the urogenital sinus. The external surface of the wall in between the two openings becomes the perineum.

Indifferent Stage

At this point in development, the cloacal region and its associated structures represent the indifferent condition, allowing no distinction between sexes. Under the influence of gonadal hormones, the urogenital sinus and its rudiments undergo specific, sex-appropriated changes. External genitalia are derived from a series of mesodermal proliferations (swellings) adjacent to the still-existent cloacal membrane. These proliferations are the following:

- **Cloacal folds**—the paired, elongated proliferations that flank the cloacal membrane.
- **Genital tubercle**—(the primordium of the phallus and the clitoris, respectively); a median outgrowth formed by the fusion of the cranial portions of cloacal folds (cranioventral to the opening of urogenital sinus).
- **Urethral folds**—folds formed caudal to the genital tubercle. When the urogenital septum is completed, the cloacal folds are subdivided into urethral folds and anal folds.
- **Genital (labioscrotal) swellings**—paired proliferations that border the urethral folds. By the end of the embryonic stage and several weeks into the fetal stage, the sex hormones released by the differentiating gonads induce progressive modelings of these primordia and will attain distinct and recognizable male versus female characteristics.

Differential Stage—Male

Androgens secreted by the fetal testes induce rapid elongation of the genital tubercle to form the phallus (a deficiency in or an insensitivity to androgens lead to a predominance of female characteristics under the influence of maternal and placental estrogens). Elongation of the phallus pulls the paired urethral folds forward to form the lateral walls of the urethral groove along the ventral aspect of the phallus. Midline fusion of the folds over the groove establishes the penile urethra. The rapid expansion, paralleled by the cranial shift of the genital tubercle, elongates the genital raphe—the first external indication of a developing male.

In the adult, the phallus forms the body of the penis, and the original swelling, the genital tubercle, becomes the *glans penis*. In domestic mammals (except the cat), the phallus extends cranially, deep to the skin of the ventral body wall, and its free end is encircled by a ring of ectoderm, the *prepuce*. Mesenchyme in the glans and body of the penis of the dog (and other nondomestic mammals) ossifies to form an *os penis* (there is a cartilage in the cat).

The genital swellings (scrotal swellings in male) enlarge, migrate cranially (to a greater or lesser extent depending on the species), and fuse with one another on the midline. The two swellings remain separated by the scrotal septum, and each makes up half of the scrotum. The accessory genital glands are positioned around the pelvic urethra and vary greatly among species. The *prostate* gland (present in all domestic species) and the bulbourethral gland (absent in the dog) form as endodermal evaginations of the urogenital sinus. The vesicular gland arises as a mesodermal evagination from the caudal part of the mesonephric duct.

Differential Stage—Female

In the absence of androgens, feminization of the external genitalia occurs. At first, the phallus elongates rapidly (the genital tubercle in the female is larger than in the male during early stages of development), but its growth gradually slows and it becomes internalized in the floor of the vestibule to form the *clitoris* (in the bitch and mare the clitoris is well-developed, but it is poorly so in the other species).

The urethral folds enlarge to overgrow the genital tubercle. They fuse only partially—at their dorsal and ventral ends. Their unfused portions form the *labia* of the vulva. The labioscrotal swellings (labial swellings in the female) flatten laterally and undergo complete regression in female domestic animals (in humans and rabbits they form the labia majora; the labia minora originate from urethral folds). Mucus-producing vestibular glands (homologues of the bulbourethral glands) are present in cows and cats only (and sometimes in sheep). Accessory genital glands in both sexes reach full development at sexual maturity. The ligamentous attachments of the genital ducts in both sexes originate in the urogenital fold, a remnant of the mesonephros. In the female, this fold forms the suspensory ligament of the ovary, the mesovarium, the mesosalpinx, and the cranial part of the mesometrium. (In the male, it forms the mesorchium and mesoductus deferens.) The caudal extension of the fold forms the proper ligaments of the gonads in both sexes.

Mammary Glands (*Mammae*)

Mammary glands (in both sexes) begin as paired, band-like thickenings of ectoderm—the mammary ridges, on the ventrolateral surface of the body between the bases of the limb buds. The length of the ridges varies with the species: They extend from the axilla to the inguinal region (as in carnivores and swine), are restricted to the axilla (as in elephants) or are restricted to the inguinal region (as in ruminants and horses).

Each mammary gland begins as a mammary bud—a localized condensation of somatic mesoderm and overlying ectoderm at a specific location along the mammary ridge. In many species, more buds form than are retained in the adult; some buds degenerate while others persist and develop as supernumerary teats. The epithelium of each bud branches into the underlying somatic mesenchyme as solid cords. These cords become associated with the glandular tissue and become patent (around the time of birth) to form individual lactiferous ducts. Each duct opens individually on the surface of the teat. The number of ducts in each mammary gland varies with the species, ranging from 1 (in cows and ewes) to 14 (in bitches and sows). Soon after birth, the teat (*papilla*) of each mammary gland forms by proliferation of the mesenchyme surrounding each bud.

Bibliography

Balinsky, B. I. 1970. *An Introduction to Embryology,* 3rd ed. Philadelphia: Saunders.

Barone, R. 1978. *Anatomie Comparée des Mammifères Domestiques, tome troisième, fascicule II,* Appareil Uro-génital. Lyon, France: Laboratoire d'Anatomie École Nationale Vétérinaire.

Dyce, Keith M., Wolfgang O. Sack, and Cornelius J. G. Wensing. 2002. *Textbook of Veterinary Anatomy,* 3rd ed. Philadelphia: Saunders.

Fletcher, Thomas F., and Alvin F. Weber. 2004. *Veterinary Developmental Anatomy.* Veterinary Embryology Class Notes.

Latshaw, William K. 1987. *Veterinary Developmental Anatomy. A Clinically Oriented Approach.* Hamilton, Ontario: BC Decker Inc.

Nickel, Richard, August Schummer, Eugen Seiferle, and Wolfgang O. Sack. 1973. *The Viscera of the Domestic Mammals*: Verlag Paul Parey. New York: Springer-Verlag.

Noden, Drew M., and Alexander DeLahunta. 1985. *The Embryology of Domestic Animals.* Philadelphia: Williams & Wilkins.

Sadler, T. W. 2000. *Langman's Medical Embryology,* 8th ed. Philadelphia: Lippincott, William and Wilkins.

Chapter 2

Anatomy of Reproductive Organs

Gheorghe M. Constantinescu

Part 2.1
Male Genital Organs

The male reproductive or genital organs consist in all species of the testicle, epididymis, ductus deferens, spermatic cord, accompanying tunics of spermatic cord and testicle (paired structures), accessory genital glands (paired or single structures), penis, prepuce, and the male urethra.

A general presentation of these structures precedes the species-specific details.

The Testicle

The testicle is the male essential reproductive gland that produces spermatozoa through the process of spermatogenesis, and also produces testosterone, the male hormone. The testicle has an ovoid shape, a head, a tail, a lateral surface, a medial surface, a free border, and an epididymal border where the epididymis is attached.

The testicle is covered by a white fibrous capsule called *tunica albuginea*, which sends, inside of the testicle, interlobular connective tissue walls called *septa*, or *septula* when they are very small. The albuginea consists of collagen fibers and a few elastic fibers. The branches of the testicular artery and vein travel within the albuginea. This tunic also covers the ductus epididymidis. The septa/septula consist of collagen fibers, vessels, and nerves; divide the parenchyma of the testicle in lobules; and build up a loose connective tissue structure called *mediastinum testis*, which also contains vessels and nerves. The lobules contain the *seminiferous tubules*. The peripheral segment of the seminiferous tubules is *convoluted*; the tubules end as *straight* seminiferous tubules, which interconnect with each other inside of the mediastinum testis in a network of ducts called *rete testis*. The rete testis continues as *ductuli efferentes*, which are coiled (see Figure 2.1).

The Epididymis

The *epididymis* (see Figure 2.1) is the first excretory organ of the male genital system. The epididymis is attached to the testicle and consists of the ductuli efferentes and the *ductus epididymidis*, surrounded by the testicular albuginea. The ductus epididymidis is very tortuous and extremely long in all species. On the lateral aspect of the testicle, between it and the epididymis, a large space is outlined under the name of *testicular bursa*. The epididymis has a head, a body, and a tail.

The head contains the ductuli efferentes of the testicle, and the origin of the ductus epididymidis. The body encloses the coiled ductus epididymidis. Both the ductuli efferentes and ductus epididymidis are located within the lobules of the epididymis. The ductus epididymidis continues inside of the tail of the epididymis with the ductus deferens. The tail of the epididymis is anchored to the tail of the testicle by the *proper ligament of the testicle*.

The Ductus Deferens

The *ductus deferens* is the continuation of, and extends from the ductus epididymidis to the urethra. The ductus deferens is held in place by the *mesoductus deferens* while running within the spermatic cord. It then enters the abdominal cavity and, switching the direction, passes within the pelvic cavity over the dorsal aspect of the urinary bladder. It crosses the ipsilateral ureter and opens on the roof of the pelvic urethra, lateral to the *colliculus seminalis*. (The colliculus seminalis is an elevation on the roof of the prostatic segment of the male urethra at the end of the urethral crest; for details, see veterinary anatomy books).

In some species, the last part of the ductus deferens, called the *ampulla*, is thickened due to the abundance of ampullar glands. The inconstant common excretory passage lateral to the colliculus seminalis for the ductus deferens and the vesicular gland in some species is called the *ejaculatory duct*.

The ductus deferens consists of an adventitia, a muscular tunic, and a mucous membrane.

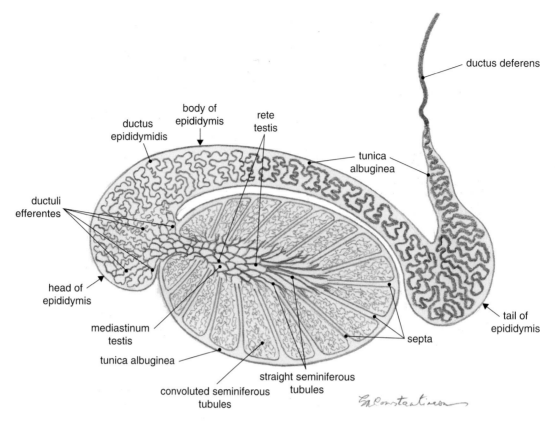

Figure 2.1. Internal organization of testicle and epididymis.

The Spermatic Cord

The *spermatic cord* (see Figure 2.2) consists of the following structures:

- the ductus deferens held by the mesoductus deferens
- the blood and lymphatic vessels and nerves that supply the testicle and the epididymis, surrounded by a peritoneal fold from the *visceral lamina of the vaginal tunic* called the *mesorchium*
- smooth muscle fibers
- visceral lamina of the vaginal tunic

The spermatic cord is located within the vaginal canal and outlined by the *parietal lamina of the vaginal tunic.* The liaison between the parietal and the visceral laminae of the vaginal tunic is called the *mesofuniculus.*

The mesorchium is divided into the *proximal mesorchium,* between the vaginal canal and the epididymis, and the *distal mesorchium,* between the epididymis and the testicle. The limit between the two mesorchia is the

peritoneal fold that holds the epididymis, called the *mesepididymis* (see Figure 2.3).

The Tunics of the Spermatic Cord and the Testicle

There are six tunics surrounding the testicle (see Figures 2.4 and 2.5). Three tunics come from the abdominal cavity during the descent of the testicle; the other three are outside of the abdominal cavity, as part of the body wall. Therefore, the testicular tunics may be divided into two groups of structures: intraabdominal and extraabdominal tunics.

The Intraabdominal Tunics

The *intraabdominal tunics,* those structures brought by the testicle during its descent, are the internal spermatic fascia and the visceral and parietal laminae of the vaginal tunic.

The *internal spermatic fascia* is the continuation of the transverse fascia (the endoabdominal fascia) after it passes through the deep inguinal ring. The *cremaster muscles* protected by the *cremasteric fascia* are associated to the internal spermatic fascia.

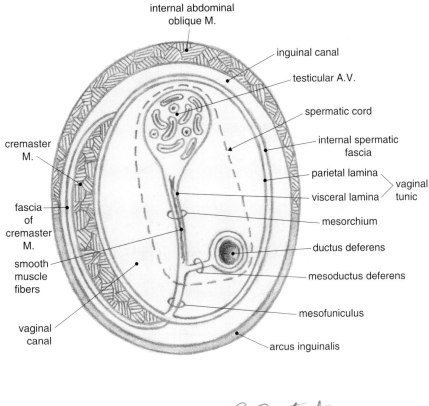

internal abdominal oblique M.

inguinal canal

testicular A.V.

spermatic cord

internal spermatic fascia

cremaster M.

parietal lamina

visceral lamina

vaginal tunic

fascia of cremaster M.

mesorchium

ductus deferens

smooth muscle fibers

mesoductus deferens

mesofuniculus

vaginal canal

arcus inguinalis

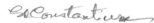

Figure 2.2. Transverse section through the spermatic cord (outlined by the broken line).

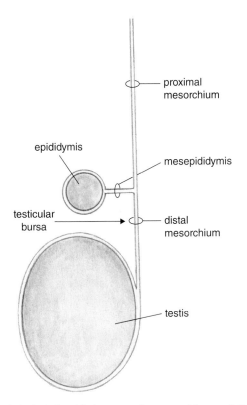

proximal mesorchium

epididymis

mesepididymis

testicular bursa

distal mesorchium

testis

Figure 2.3. Relationship between the mesorchium and the mesepididymis.

Both the visceral and parietal laminae of the vaginal tunic are continuations of the visceral and parietal peritoneum, respectively, after they pass through the *inguinal canal* via the *deep inguinal ring*. (The inguinal canal is outlined cranially by the caudal border of the internal abdominal oblique muscle and caudally by the arcus inguinalis, and between the superficial and deep inguinal rings (for details see veterinary anatomy books). The reflection of the parietal peritoneum within the deep inguinal ring is called the *vaginal ring*. The virtual space between the two laminae around the spermatic cord is called the *vaginal canal*. The *vaginal cavity* is the space between the same two laminae around the testicle.

The Extraabdominal Tunics

The extraabdominal tunics are the external spermatic fascia and the skin. The skin consists of the tunica dartos and the scrotal skin.

The *external spermatic fascia* is the continuation of the superficial fascia that covers the external abdominal oblique muscle, associated with subcutaneous loose connective tissue. The fascia continues in the perineal region under the name of the *deep perineal fascia*.

The *tunica dartos* consists of smooth muscle fibers that surround each testicle and build up together a partition wall between the testicles called the *scrotal*

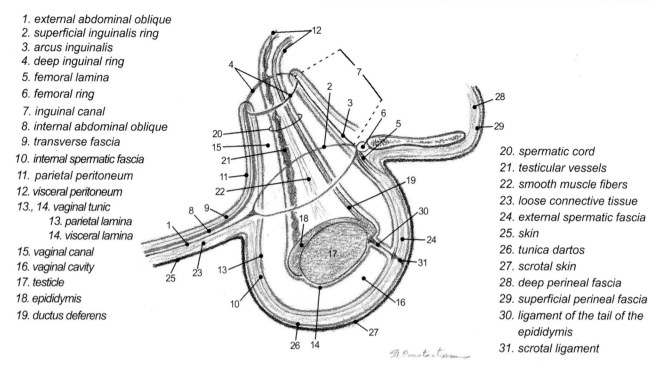

1. external abdominal oblique
2. superficial inguinalis ring
3. arcus inguinalis
4. deep inguinal ring
5. femoral lamina
6. femoral ring
7. inguinal canal
8. internal abdominal oblique
9. transverse fascia
10. internal spermatic fascia
11. parietal peritoneum
12. visceral peritoneum
13., 14. vaginal tunic
    13. parietal lamina
    14. visceral lamina
15. vaginal canal
16. vaginal cavity
17. testicle
18. epididymis
19. ductus deferens

20. spermatic cord
21. testicular vessels
22. smooth muscle fibers
23. loose connective tissue
24. external spermatic fascia
25. skin
26. tunica dartos
27. scrotal skin
28. deep perineal fascia
29. superficial perineal fascia
30. ligament of the tail of the epididymis
31. scrotal ligament

Figure 2.4. Schematic median section through the inguinal region, testicle, and testicular tunics.

(interdartoic) septum. From the scrotal septum the dartos extends dorsally, and surrounds and protects the penis. The dartos continues in the perineal region under the name of *superficial perineal fascia.* The *ligament of the tail of epididymis* joins the tail of the epididymis to the

internal spermatic fascia (in ungulates). In Carnivores the tail of the epididymis is adherent to the internal spermatic fascia; therefore, there is no ligament of the tail of epididymis. The *scrotal ligament* joins the ligament of the tail of epididymis to the dartos in Ugulates, whereas

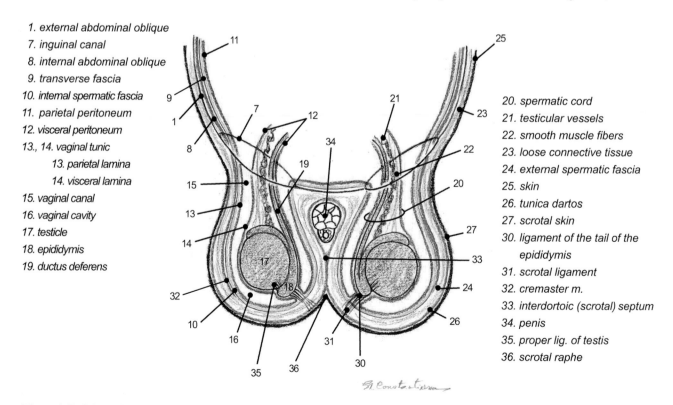

1. external abdominal oblique
7. inguinal canal
8. internal abdominal oblique
9. transverse fascia
10. internal spermatic fascia
11. parietal peritoneum
12. visceral peritoneum
13., 14. vaginal tunic
    13. parietal lamina
    14. visceral lamina
15. vaginal canal
16. vaginal cavity
17. testicle
18. epididymis
19. ductus deferens

20. spermatic cord
21. testicular vessels
22. smooth muscle fibers
23. loose connective tissue
24. external spermatic fascia
25. skin
26. tunica dartos
27. scrotal skin
30. ligament of the tail of the epididymis
31. scrotal ligament
32. cremaster m.
33. interdortoic (scrotal) septum
34. penis
35. proper lig. of testis
36. scrotal raphe

Figure 2.5. Schematic transverse section through the inguinal canals, penis, testicles, and testicular tunics.

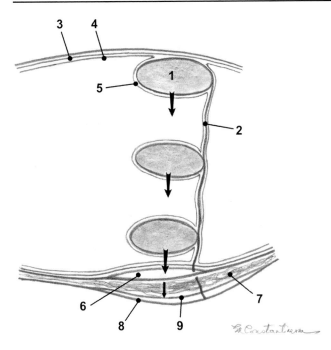

Figure 2.6. The descent of the testicle. 1. Testicle; 2. Gubernaculum testis (which will become the proper lig. of testis, the lig. of the tail of epididymis and the scrotal lig); 3. Transverse fascia (which will become the internal spermatic fascia); 4–5. Peritoneum (which will become the vaginal tunic): 4. Parietal peritoneum (parietal lamina of vaginal tunic), 5. Visceral peritoneum (visceral lamina of vaginal tunic); 6. Inguinal canal; 7. Subcutaneous connective tissue and superficial fascia (which will become the external spermatic fascia); 8–9. The skin (which will become 8. Scrotal skin and 9. Tunical dartos).

in Carnivores it joins the internal spermatic fascia to the dartos.

The *scrotal skin* that supports both testicles is separated by the *scrotal raphe* into two halves, one for each testicle.

The Descent of the Testicle

A simple and helpful description of the descent of the testicle is necessary to better understand the testicular tunics and the relationships among them (see Figure 2.6). In the early stages of the developmental life, the testicle is located on the roof of the future abdominal cavity, between the transverse fascia (on the dorsal surface of the testicle) and the visceral peritoneum (on the ventral surface of the testicle). The caudal extremity of the testicle is anchored to the skin by a mesenchymal structure, the *gubernaculum testis*, which passes through the inguinal canal on its way to the skin.

The transverse fascia is intimately lined by the parietal peritoneum, both of them passing through the inguinal canal under the name of *vaginal process*. The gubernaculum testis regresses gradually and pulls down the testicle. A short period of time before birth, which varies with the species, the testicle lands on the abdominal opening of the inguinal canal (the deep inguinal ring). At this stage of descent, the visceral peritoneum that accompanies the testicle comes in intimate contact with the parietal peritoneum. Shortly before or after birth, depending on species, the testicle passes through the inguinal canal toward the scrotum. It brings with it the visceral and parietal peritoneum and the transverse fascia, whose names will change into the visceral and parietal laminae of the vaginal tunic, and the internal spermatic fascia, respectively. These are the so-called intraabdominal testicular tunics. Outside of the body wall, the testicle finds the external spermatic fascia, the tunica dartos, and scrotal skin, all three extraabdominal testicular tunics. The remnant of the gubernaculum testis following the normal positioning of testicle is a structure divided in three parts: the proper ligament of the testicle, the ligament of the tail of the epididymis, and the scrotal ligament.

The Accessory Genital Glands

The accessory genital glands are the following: the glands of the ampullae of ductus deferentes (singular, ampulla of ductus deferens), the vesicular glands/seminal vesicles, the prostate, and the bulbourethral glands. They differ from species to species and from an intact male to a castrated male.

The *glands of the ampullae of ductus deferentes* are simple, branched tubuloalveolar glands located in the propria-submucosa of each ampulla.

The paired *vesicular glands* are compound tubular or tubuloalveolar glands, lie over the neck of the urinary bladder, and open on the sides of the colliculus seminalis.

The *seminal vesicles* are special vesicular glands found only in the horse.

The *prostate* has two parts: one compact or external part called the body, and a disseminated or internal part. The body overlaps the ampullae of the ductus deferentes and the excretory ducts of the vesicular glands, or it completely surrounds the urethra. In some species, the body is separated into a right and a left *lobe* connected by an *isthmus*. The prostate gland totally or partially surrounds the pelvic urethra, which at the area of contact with the prostate gland has a specific name, the prostatic part of the urethra. The short part of the pelvic urethra, between the neck of the urinary bladder and the prostatic part, is called the preprostatic part of the urethra. The prostate consists of individual tubuloalveolar glands. Numerous *prostate excretory ductules* open into the urethra. The disseminated part of the prostate forms a glandular layer in the wall of the pelvic urethra in some species.

The paired *bulbourethral glands* are located dorsolateral to the last portion of the pelvic urethra called the urethral isthmus. The bulbourethral gland is a compound tubular or tubuloalveolar gland.

The Penis

The *penis* is an external genital organ, the male organ of copulation. It consists of a root, a body, and a free part surrounded by the prepuce.

The *root* of the penis consists of two crura (singular, crus) and the bulbus penis. The paired *crus penis* is the proximal end of the corpus cavernosum penis. This segment is attached to the ischiatic arch and is covered by the ischio-cavernosus muscle. The *bulbus penis* is the caudal extent of the *corpus spongiosum penis*.

The *body* of the penis has a dorsal surface, with a dorsal groove only in the horse, and a ventral (urethral) surface. A urethral groove is sculpted on the ventral surface and protects the penile urethra and the corpus spongiosum penis.

The *free part* of the penis starts from the attachment of the prepuce on the penis and ends as the glans penis. The *glans penis* is the head of the penis, which contains the corpus spongiosum glandis. The glans is a cushion that overlaps the distal end of the albuginea of the corpus cavernosum penis. The dorsal process, the long part, the bulb, the crown, the septum, the neck, and the fossa of the glans penis, as well as the urethral sinus, are species specific and will be described later.

The *prepuce* is the skin that surrounds the free part of the penis like a muff. With the penis in the resting position, the prepuce is a folded skin, with external and internal laminae. The *external lamina* is a typical skin with hair and sebaceous glands, while the *internal lamina* is provided with fine hairs, sebaceous glands, and sweat glands. The internal lamina comes in intimate contact with the fully erect penis. A circular orifice called the *preputial ostium (orifice)* is outlined by the transition between the two preputial laminae. The cavity between the internal lamina and the penis in a resting position is called the *preputial cavity*. The preputial ring, fold, diverticulum, frenulum, raphe, and muscles are species specific and will be described later.

The intimate structure of the penis consists of the following: the corpus cavernosum penis with or without a septum, provided with trabeculae and cavernae, and surrounded by its own tunica albuginea; the corpus spongiosum penis with trabeculae and cavernae, and surrounded by its own tunica albuginea; the corpus spongiosum glandis; the bulbus penis; fasciae; ligaments; arteries; veins; lymph nodes; and nerves.

The paired *corpus cavernosum penis* (plural, corpora cavernosa) originate from the ischiatic arch and join with each other; in most species they are separated by the *septum penis*. The tunica albuginea sends inside the corpora cavernosa many trabeculae that separate several vascular spaces from each other. These spaces are called *cavernae*.

The *corpus spongiosum penis* is a sponge-like, erectile tissue that surrounds the urethra and is covered by its own *tunica albuginea*. *Trabeculae* and *cavernae* are also present in the corpus spongiosum penis. The *corpus spongiosum glandis* is a similar kind of structure that surrounds the glans penis.

The *bulbus penis* is the expanded caudal extent of the corpus spongiosum penis. The bulbus penis is part of the root of the penis (together with the crura of the penis). Two fasciae and two ligaments suspend the penis.

The Male Urethra

The *male urethra* is the common excretory duct for the urine and semen. The urethra consists of a pelvic part and a penile part.

The *pelvic part*, surrounded by a cavernous tissue called the spongy layer (*stratum spongiosum*) is divided into a *preprostatic* part, a *prostatic* part, a *postprostatic* part, and the *urethral isthmus*. The prostatic part is associated with the prostate gland. Inside of the prostatic part and on the roof, in a cranio-caudal order, the following structures can be identified:

- the *urethral crest*, from the *internal urethral orifice* to the colliculus seminalis, or even beyond it
- the *colliculus seminalis*, the prominence bearing on each side the ejaculatory orifice, or the separate openings of the ductus deferentes and the excretory ducts of the vesicular glands
- the *ejaculatory orifice*, the opening of the *ejaculatory duct* on the colliculus seminalis (inconstantly the ductus deferens is associated with the excretory duct of the vesicular gland in the so-called ejaculatory duct)
- the *uterus masculinus*, the rudimentary male uterus, a remnant of the paramesonephric ducts during the intrauterine life; it is also known as the utriculus prostaticus
- the *prostatic sinus*, a symmetrical recess between the urethral crest and the lateral urethral wall, where the prostatic ductules open
- the entire urethral mucosa, provided with longitudinal folds
- the muscular tunic, the smooth muscle of the pelvic urethra that surrounds the disseminated part of the prostate if present, or the spongy layer of the pelvic urethra
- the urethralis muscle, the striated muscle that surrounds the pelvic urethra.

The *urethral isthmus* is the narrow transition between the pelvic urethra and the penile urethra, around the ischiatic arch. The *penile part* of the urethra, surrounded by the corpus spongiosum penis, opens by the *external urethral orifice*.

Major Muscles, Blood Supply, Lymph Drainage, and Nerve Supply for the Male Genitalia

In addition to the cremaster muscle, the major *striated muscles* associated with the male genital organs are the following:

- urethralis
- ischiourethralis
- bulboglandularis
- superficial transverse perineal
- ischiocavernosus
- bulbospongiosus

- retractor penis (predominantly smooth)
  - anal part
  - rectal part
  - penile part
- cranial preputial (absent in the horse)
- caudal preputial (absent in the horse)

For details regarding the origin, insertion, and action of these muscles, see veterinary anatomy books, the *Nomina Anatomica Veterinaria* (*N.A.V.*), and the *Illustrated Veterinary Anatomical Nomenclature*.

The *blood supply* to the male genitalia is as follows:

- The testicle is supplied by the testicular artery and vein with species-specific differences of origin (within the mesorchium, the vein surrounds the testicular artery as a network—the pampiniform plexus, whose role is to cool down the arterial blood before it reaches the testicle). When the artery and vein reach the testicle, they perforate the albuginea, run with a species-specific design, and branch to supply the testicular tissue.
- The epididymis receives epididymal branches from the testicular artery and vein.
- The ductus deferens is supplied either by branches from the testicular artery or the prostatic artery, or by the artery of the ductus deferens from the prostatic artery (in Carnivores).
- The extraabdominal testicular tunics are supplied by the ventral scrotal artery and vein, branches of the external pudendal artery and vein.
- The pelvic urethra is supplied by the urethral artery or branch, originating from the internal pudendal artery. The urethral vein is present only in Carnivores. In the other species, the pelvic urethra is discharged by branches of the obturator and prostatic veins.
- The accessory genital glands are supplied by the prostatic artery and vein, or by branches of these vessels.
- The penis is supplied by the artery of the penis (from the internal pudendal artery), which branches into the artery of the bulbus penis (to the bulbus penis and corpus spongiosum penis), the deep artery of the penis (to the corpus cavernosum penis), and the dorsal artery of the penis. The external pudendal artery may also be involved in supplying blood to the penis. The middle artery of the penis (from the obturator artery) and the cranial artery of the penis (from the external pudendal artery), both in the horse only, contribute to the blood supply of the penis. The veins are satellite to the arteries.

  The deep artery of the penis is coiled in the resting position of the penis, especially in species with a musculomembranous type of penis. The branches of this artery have a helical arrangement and characteristic smooth muscle cells that act during the erection. In the resting position, the smooth muscle cells are organized in ridges or pads that protrude into the lumen of the vessels, causing partial obliteration. As the smooth muscle cells relax, the blood flow into the cavernae increases considerably and causes erection. The cavernae are drained by venules (Dellmann and Brown 1998).

- The prepuce is supplied by the superficial caudal epigastric artery and vein, branches of the external pudendal artery and vein.
- The penile urethra is supplied by the artery and vein of the bulbus penis.

For species-specific differences, see veterinary anatomy books, the *N.A.V.*, and the *Illustrated Veterinary Anatomical Nomenclature*.

Lymph drainage in the male genitalia occurs as follows:

- Lymph from the testicle and epididymis is drained into the lumbo-aortic and renal lymph nodes.
- Lymph from the ductus deferens (the segment included in the spermatic cord) is drained into the lumboaortic and renal lymph nodes. Lymph from the rest of the ductus deferens, the pelvic urethra, the prostate, the vesicular glands, and the bulbourethral glands drains into the medial iliac lymph nodes.
- Lymph from the scrotum is drained into the scrotal lymph nodes.
- Lymph from the penis is drained into the superficial inguinal, deep inguinal, scrotal, and/or medial iliac lymph nodes.

For species-specific differences, see veterinary anatomy books and the *Illustrated Veterinary Anatomical Nomenclature*.

The *nerve supply* for the male genital organs is as follows:

- The testicle and the epididymis are supplied by the testicular plexus, with nerve fibers from the aortic abdominal plexus, caudal mesenteric plexus, lumbar splanchnic nerves and hypogastric nerves (all sympathetic), and the pelvic nerves through the pelvic plexus (parasympathetic).
- The ductus deferens, the vesicular glands, the prostate, the bulbourethral glands, and the pelvic urethra are supplied from the pelvic plexus (sympathetic and parasympathetic fibers) by specific plexuses.
- The penis as a whole is supplied by the pudendal nerve (parasympathetic), which also supplies the scrotum by the dorsal scrotal branches and continues as the dorsal nerve of the penis, and by the nerve of the corpus cavernosum penis from the prostatic plexus (both sympathetic and parasympathetic).

For species-specific differences, see veterinary anatomy books, the *N.A.V.*, and the *Illustrated Veterinary Anatomical Nomenclature*.

Part 2.2
Female Genital Organs

The female genital organs consist of the paired ovary and uterine tube, the uterus, vagina, vestibule, vulva and clitoris, and the female urethra. The female genital organs can be systematized into the reproductive glands (the ovaries), the tubular genital organs (the uterine tubes, the uterus, vagina, vestibule, and vulva), and the clitoris. The female urethra and the vulva are considered as external female genital organs.

The Ovary

The *ovary* is the female essential reproductive gland, which produces ovules (ovocytes, oocytes), the two female hormones progesterone and estradiol, and also oxytocin, relaxin, inhibin, and activin.

Ovoidal-shaped, each ovary has a hilus, a medial surface, a lateral surface, a free border, a mesovarian border, a tubal extremity, and a uterine extremity.

The *hilus* is the area of attachment of the mesovarium and the entrance of ovarian vessels.

The *medial* and *lateral surfaces*, and the *free border* of the ovary are convex and irregular. The orientation of the surfaces is not always medial and lateral. In *the Mare only*, the free border is concave because of the depression called the *ovarian fossa*, where ovulation occurs (some veterinary clinicians prefer to call it the "ovulation fossa").

The *mesovarian border* is opposite to the free border and is the site for attachment of the mesovarium.

The *tubal extremity* is that end of the ovary facing the infundibulum of the uterine tube.

The *uterine extremity* is opposite to the previous and attached to the apex of the uterine horn by the proper ligament of the ovary.

A dense white capsule, the *tunica albuginea* covers the ovary immediately beneath a *cuboidal surface epithelium*. In all species except the horse, a peripheral parenchymatous zone called the *cortex* is located in intimate contact with the albuginea; the cortex contains follicles and corpora lutea. In the center of the ovary, a vascular zone called the *medulla* supports the blood vessels that nourish the ovary, lymphatics, nerves, and smooth muscle fibers (*in the horse the medulla is peripheral, and the cortex is central*). The loose connective tissue in both the cortex and medulla is called *stroma* (Figures 2.7 and 2.8 show the internal organization of the cow's and Mare's ovary, respectively).

Depending upon the evolution of the follicles and the sexual cycle, the following structures may be identified within the ovary:

- The *primordial ovarian follicle* is a small immature ovocyte that has not undergone recruitment and is surrounded by a single layer of flattened follicular cells; it is also called the *unilaminar ovarian follicle*.
- The *primary ovarian follicle* consists of an ovocyte surrounded by one or more layers of cuboidal or columnar follicular cells before the appearance of an antrum filled with follicular liquor; the follicle becomes surrounded by a sheath of stroma, the *follicular theca*.
- The *secondary ovarian follicle* is a growing primary ovocyte surrounded by a stratified follicular epithelium and a developing follicular theca.
- The *tertiary or vesicular ovarian follicle* (antral or graafian follicle) is a large, full-sized primary ovocyte with a central cavity called the antrum that is filled with follicular liquor, contains follicular epithelium and a very developed theca, and is surrounded by the *zona pellucida*.
- The *corpus luteum* is the yellow endocrine body formed in the site of a ruptured ovarian follicle and developed from cells of granulosa and internal theca after ovulation.
- The *corpus albicans* is the remaining structure after the degeneration of the corpus luteum. If pregnancy does not occur, the corpus luteum undergoes regression to the corpus albicans.
- The *atretic ovarian follicle* is an abnormal follicle, which began to mature but did not become a dominant follicle (a dominant ovarian follicle matures completely and forms the corpus luteum); the atretic ovarian follicle degenerates before coming to maturity.

The three ligaments of the ovary are:

- the *suspensory ligament*—joins the ovary to the diaphragm
- the *proper ligament*—joins the ovary to the apex of the uterine horn
- the *mesovarium*—the most cranial segment of the *broad ligament*. The mesovarium is in continuation with the mesometrium (which suspends the uterus) and has two segments: proximal and distal. The *proximal mesovarium* is separated from the *distal mesovarium* by the origin/attachment of the mesosalpinx. The proximal mesovarium extends from the abdominal wall (where

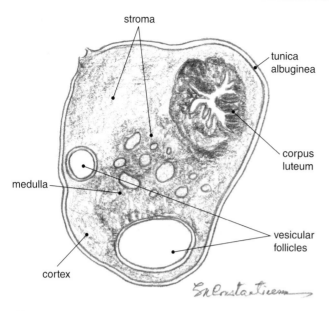

Figure 2.7. Internal organization of the cow's ovary.

the broad ligament originates) to the origin of the mesosalpinx, while the distal mesovarium is very short, from the origin of the mesosalpinx to the ovary.

Two groups of vestigial structures from the developmental life, called *epoöphoron* and *paroöphoron,* may be associated with the ovary:

- structures that originate from the epoöphoron
  - the *duct of the epoöphoron,* the vestige of the cranial part of the mesonephric duct
  - the *transverse ductules,* remnants of the mesonephric tubules, which extend from the duct of the epoöphoron to the hilus of the ovary and pass through the mesovarium and mesosalpinx

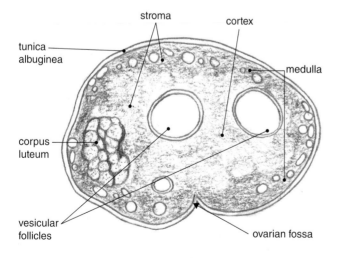

Figure 2.8. Internal organization of the mare's ovary.

- the *vesicular appendages,* which are pedunculated cysts near the infundibulum of the uterine tube
- the paroöphoron, a group of caudal mesonephric tubules in the mesosalpinx, near the uterine extremity of the ovary

The Uterine Tube

The *uterine tube* is a duct that extends from the apex of the uterine horn toward the ovary on the lateral side of the broad ligament. The uterine tube is flexuous to allow distension during pregnancy, and it has an uneven size. The uterine tube, also called the *salpinx or fallopian tube,* consists of a folded mucosa, a smooth muscular coat that is thicker toward the uterus, and a serous layer lined by loose connective tissue. The serous layer is that part of the mesosalpinx that surrounds the tube.

The following structures are parts of the uterine tube: the ovarian end provided with the abdominal opening, the infundibulum, fimbriae of the infundibulum, ovarian fimbria, ampulla, isthmus, and the uterine part provided with the uterine ostium.

- The *abdominal opening/ostium of the uterine tube* is the far most and very narrow opening of the salpinx.
- The ovarian end of the uterine tube is also called the *infundibulum of the uterine tube.* It is funnel-shaped and mobile with regard to the ovary. When the ovulation occurs, the infundibulum embraces the ovary for receiving the ovocyte. The contact between the infundibulum and the ovary is enhanced by the fimbriae.
- The *fimbriae of the infundibulum,* fringe-like processes, are scattered around the border of the opening of the infundibulum and do not allow the ovocytes to drop into the peritoneal cavity. The *ovarian fimbria* is that fringe attached directly to the ovary.
- The *ampulla of the uterine tube* is the relatively wide part of the salpinx, between the abdominal ostium and the isthmus.
- The *isthmus* is the narrow part of the salpinx, in some species without a visible delimitation between it and the ampulla. Also the lumen of the isthmus is not always different from that of the ampulla.
- The *uterine part* is the shortest segment of the uterine tube. The uterine part passes through the wall of the apex of the uterine horn and in some species even ends on a papilla, whereas in other species the salpinx gradually continues with the uterine horn. The *uterine orifice/ostium of the uterine tube* opens at the end of the uterine part of the salpinx.
- The salpinx is held in position by a segment of the broad ligament called the *mesosalpinx.* This is a serous fold that originates from the lateral aspect of the mesovarium. The latter is therefore divided into the proximal and the distal mesovarium. The mesosalpinx surrounds the ovary in a species-specific manner. Between the ovary,

the distal mesovarium, and the mesosalpinx, a cavity called the *ovarian bursa* is outlined. The opening of this bursa is medially oriented.

The Uterus

The *uterus* is the organ of gestation. It has three distinct segments: the horns, body, and cervix. In most animals the uterus has two horns, a body and a cervix, and it is called the *uterus bicornis*. In the Rabbit, for example, the horns, body, and cervix are paired; this type of uterus is called *uterus duplex*. In primates, including humans, and in other species the uterus has only one compartment and the cervix, which is characteristic for the *uterus simplex*.

The uterine horns of the uterus bicornis have mesometrial and free borders, and corresponding cavities. The uterine body has right and left borders, dorsal and ventral surfaces, and a cavity. The uterine velum and fundus are species-specific structures. The endometrium, with species-specific features, the myometrium, and the perimetrium are layers of the constitution of the entire uterus. The cervix has a prevaginal part and a vaginal part, and is centered by a cervical canal. The latter communicates with the uterus cranially, and with the vagina caudally.

The *uterine horns*, right and left, are very different from species to species in terms of the shape, location, and size. The uterine horns are the most cranially extended components of the uterus, and they continue caudally with the body of the uterus. Each uterine horn has two openings/communications: at the apex (tip), it communicates with the uterine tube; the uterine orifice of the uterine tube makes the transition to the salpinx. Caudally the uterine horn opens into the body of the uterus in species-specific different manners. Each uterine horn has a *mesometrial border* where the mesometrium is attached, and a *free border* on the opposite side.

The *body of uterus* is a unique compartment located caudal to the uterine horns, between them and the cervix. The body has *a right and a left border* that continues onto the cervix, sites where the paired mesometrium is attached. The *dorsal* and the *ventral surfaces* complete the external features of the body of the uterus. The *cavity of the uterus* has a different size and shape according to species.

The *cervix*, with very thick muscular walls and rich in elastic fibers, is the neck of the uterus. The *prevaginal part of the cervix* is located cranial to the vagina, while the *vaginal part of the cervix* protrudes into the vagina. The cranial extent of the vagina surrounds the vaginal part of the cervix like a niche; this "niche" is called the fornix. The *cervical canal* is much narrower than the uterine cavity. This canal communicates with the body of the uterus by the *internal orifice of the uterus*, and with the vagina by the *external orifice of the uterus*. *Longitudinal folds* and other species-specific features are characteristic for the cervical mucosa.

The entire uterus has a mucosa called the *endometrium*, a muscular tunic called the *myometrium*, and a serous tunic—the visceral peritoneum—called the *perimetrium*. The mucous membrane of the uterine horns and body in ruminants is provided with specific structures called *caruncles*.

The myometrium consists of a three-layer smooth muscle: circular and oblique inner layers, and a longitudinal outer layer. Under the serous layer a *subserous layer* separates the perimetrium from the myometrium. The *broad ligament* suspends the ovary (mesovarium) and the horns and body of the uterus (*mesometrium*).

Originating from the floor of the pelvic cavity and continuing between the peritoneal laminae of the mesometrium, the connective tissue, smooth muscle, vessels, and nerves are collectively called the *parametrium*. The *round ligament of the uterus* originates from the tip of the uterine horn; this ligament differs widely in size, length, and position from species to species. The round ligament of the uterus extends up to, and even passes through the deep inguinal ring and the inguinal canal, accompanied by the peritoneum and transverse fascia as the *vaginal process*.

The Vagina

The *vagina* is a unique canal located between the cervix and the external urethral orifice, or the hymen. The fornix, ventral and dorsal walls, hymen, vaginal opening into the vestibule, and, in some species, the remnant of the caudal part of the mesonephric duct are the structures of the vagina.

- The *fornix* is the most cranial extent of the vagina, looking like a blind pouch that surrounds the vaginal part of the cervix. In some species the fornix is discontinuous due to the presence of dorsal and/or ventral frenula (singular, frenulum) of the cervix.
- The *ventral* and *dorsal walls* are held in place by the pelvic diaphragm. The pelvic diaphragm consists of the levator ani and coccygeus muscles, and the internal and external fasciae of the pelvic diaphragm in the retroperitoneal space.
- The *hymen*, poorly developed in domestic animals, is a transverse fold of the vaginal mucosa on the floor of the vagina just cranial to the external urethral orifice.
- The *vaginal ostium or orifice* is the communication between the vagina and the vestibule.

The mucous membrane has a distinct appearance in bovine species. The muscular tunic is represented by smooth muscles. Only the cranial end of the vagina is covered by the peritoneum. As in the uterus, a subserous loose connective tissue is present under the serous layer.

The Vestibule

The *vestibule* is the transition between the vagina and the vulva, very long in domestic animals in comparison to humans, but with the exception of the cat, shorter than the vagina. The bulbus vestibuli, and the major and minor vestibular glands are the structures of the vestibule, with species-specific differences.

- The *bulbus vestibuli* is a symmetrical cavernous tissue in the lateral walls of the vestibule.
- The *major vestibular glands*, present in several species, are symmetrical glands that lie on the floor of the vestibule; their ducts open on the lateral walls of the vestibule.
- The *minor vestibular glands* are scattered on the lateral walls and the floor of the vestibule.

The Vulva and the Clitoris

The vulva and the clitoris are considered the external female genitalia. The *vulva* is provided with labia, commissures, and the pudendal fissure.

There are two pairs of *labia: major* and *minor*, that are not distinguishable in domestic animals, with some exceptions. The major labia are lateral to the minor labia.
The *dorsal* and the *ventral commissures of the labia* outline the *pudendal fissure*, the external urogenital fissure.

The *clitoris* is the rudimentary homologue of the penis; the clitoris is located on the floor of the vestibule. The only difference between the male and the female consists in the lack of urethra within the clitoris (there is a penile urethra in the male). The clitoris consists of two crura and the body with the corpus cavernosum, the glans with the corpus spongiosum, and the fascia of the clitoris. There are significant species differences of the clitoris.

- The *right* and *left crura* originate from the ischiatic arch and join into the body of the clitoris.
- The *body of the clitoris* is the result of fusion of the crura.
  - The *corpus cavernosum of the clitoris* is the erectile tissue of the crura and body. There is a partial *septum* of the corpus cavernosum.
  - The *glans* provided with a corpus spongiosum is the free end of the clitoris, protected in the *fossa of the clitoris*, which is similar to the preputial cavity of the male. The fossa of the clitoris is almost obliterated by adhesion of the prepuce to the glans in the cat, sow, and ruminants. The *prepuce of the clitoris* is formed by the ventral commissure of the labia and by a transverse fold of the vestibular mucosa to which the *frenulum* is attached. The frenulum is present only in the dog and the mare.
  - The *fascia of the clitoris* surrounds and protects the organ. It is well developed in the mare.

The Female Urethra

The *female urethra* corresponds to the male preprostatic urethra. The female urethra extends from the *internal urethral ostium* to the *external urethral ostium*.

The urethra consists of a mucosa, a muscular tunic, and the adventitia; it is surrounded by a cavernous tissue called the *corpus spongiosum*. A *urethral crest* similar to that of the male urethra is found starting from the internal urethral ostium and extending up to the middle of the urethra. *Urethral glands* and *lacunae (evaginations)*, *paraurethral glands*, and *ducts* differ from species to species and are associated with the female urethra.

Major Muscles, Blood Supply, Lymph Drainage, and Nerve Supply for the Female Genitalia

The major *striated muscles* associated with the female genital organs are the following:

- urethralis (in the female species the urethralis originates from the vagina and forms a sling ventral to the urethra)
- ischiourethralis
- bulboglandularis (associated with the major vestibular glands)
- ischiocavernosus (rudimentary in the female species)
- bulbospongiosus (because of the elongated vestibule, the bulbospongiosus is divided into:
  - constrictor vestibuli
  - constrictor vulvae
- retractor clitoridis (predominantly smooth)
  - anal part
  - rectal part
  - clitoridean part

For species-specific differences, see veterinary anatomy books and the *Illustrated Veterinary Anatomical Nomenclature*.

The *blood supply* to the female genitalia is as follows:

- The ovary is supplied by the ovarian artery and the ovarian vein with species-specific differences of origin. The ovarian artery also supplies the distal part of the salpinx by the branch of the uterine tube, and the apex of the uterine horn by the uterine branch.
- The whole uterus—with the exception of the apex of the uterine horn—is supplied by the uterine artery, which is a branch of the vaginal artery in carnivores, of the umbilical artery in the pig and ruminants, and of the external iliac artery in the horse. In the horse only, the uterine horns and part of the uterine body are supplied by the uterine artery from the external iliac artery; the rest of the body and the cervix are supplied by the uterine branch of the vaginal artery. In the pig, ruminants, and horse, the cervix is supplied by the uterine branch from the vaginal artery. The uterine vein is a branch of the vaginal vein in carnivores. In the other species, the vaginal vein is joined by the uterine branch. In the pig, the uterine vein is a branch of the ovarian

vein, in the ruminants is a slender and inconstant branch of the internal iliac vein, and in the horse is a branch of the internal iliac vein.

- The vagina is supplied by the vaginal artery and vein.
- The vestibule is supplied by the middle rectal artery, the artery of the bulbus vestibuli and the urethral artery, and also by the corresponding veins.
- The vulva is supplied by dorsal and ventral labial branches of the internal pudendal and external pudendal arteries, respectively.
- The clitoris is supplied by the artery of the clitoris.

For species-specific differences, see veterinary anatomy books, the *N.A.V.,* and the *Illustrated Veterinary Anatomical Nomenclature.*

Lymph drainage in the female genitalia occurs as follows:

- The lymph from the ovary and uterine tube drains into the lumbo-aortic lymph nodes.
- The lymph from the uterus drains in the lumbo-aortic lymph nodes (for the horns), and in the medial sacral lymph nodes (for the body and the cervix).
- The lymph from the vagina drains into the internal iliac, ano-rectal, and sacral lymph nodes.
- The lymph from the vestibule, vulva, and clitoris drains into the ano-rectal lymph nodes.

The *nerve supply* is provided by the following nerves and plexuses:

- The ovary and the uterine tube are supplied by the ovarian plexus, which originates from the cranial mesenteric plexus (both sympathetic and parasympathetic) and the last lumbar sympathetic ganglia.
- The uterus is supplied by the cranial mesenteric plexus via the ovarian plexus and by the uterovaginal plexus (from the pelvic plexus, both sympathetic and parasympathetic).
- The vagina and the vestibule are supplied by the vaginal nerves from the uterovaginal plexus (from the pelvic plexus, both sympathetic and parasympathetic).

- The vulva is supplied by the labial nerves, branches of the superficial perineal nerve (of the pudendal), and by branches of the pelvic plexus, both sympathetic and parasympathetic.
- The clitoris is supplied by the dorsal nerve of the clitoris, the branch of the pudendal nerve, and by branches of the pelvic plexus, both sympathetic and parasympathetic.

The Mammary Gland (*Mamma*)

This is intended to be a unique subsection on the topic for all species. The *mammary gland,* a modified cutaneous (sweat) gland, is by definition one mammary complex that consists of one body and one papilla (see Figure 2.9). In the ruminants and equine species, the mammary glands are collectively called *udder.* The papilla is also called *nipple* in carnivores and sows, or *teat* in ruminants and equine species. In all species, the papilla are paired, but their number differs from species to species. The numbers typically are 10 in dogs, 8 in cats, 14 in pigs, 4 in cows, and 2 in small ruminants and horses. There are normal and abnormal variations in number.

The mammary glands are attached to, and suspended from the ventral body wall. According to the position of the glands, there are species-specific thoracic (in humans, monkeys, and elephants), thoracoabdominal (in cats), thoracoinguinal (in dogs and pigs), or inguinal mammary glands (in all ruminants and horses).

The body, which is conical shaped, consists of skin, glandular tissue, and connective tissue. Adjacent mammae are superficially separated by longitudinal or transversal intermammary grooves in ruminants and equine species.

A single gland consists of glandular tissue and a duct system. The glandular tissue is separated in lobes by connective tissue. Each lobe is divided in lobules, which are clusters of up to 200 alveoli that secrete into a central ductule (the lactiferous alveolar ductule). The lobules are separated from each other by a thin layer

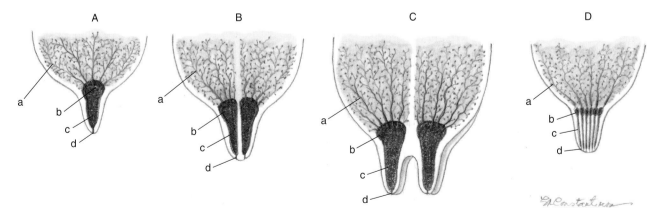

Figure 2.9. The duct system and lactiferous cistern in mammary glands (schematic): **A.** small ruminants; **B.** mare and sow; **C.** cow; **D.** carnivores; **a.** lactiferous ducts; **b.** gland cistern (**b** and **c** form the lactiferous sinus s. cistern); **c.** papillary cistern; **d.** papillary ducts.

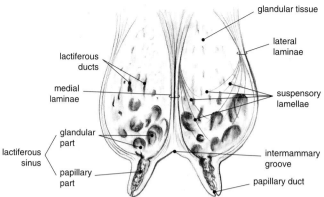

Figure 2.10. Suspensory apparatus of the cow's mammary gland (udder).

of connective tissue. The lactiferous alveolar ductules continue with intralobular and interlobular ductules. All the above-mentioned structures are located within a lobe. At the end of each lobe, the duct system is represented by a lactiferous duct. The lactiferous ducts are the first visible structures of the duct system, and all of them convey the milk to the lactiferous sinus; the ducts become larger and larger as they approach the lactiferous sinus (see Figure 2.10).

The lactiferous sinus or cistern is the dilated part of the duct system and consists of a glandular part (gland cistern) and a papillary part (papillary or teat cistern). The glandular part is located in the ventral end of the mammary gland, whereas the papillary part is located within the papilla. At the base of papilla in the cow the mucosa makes several folds resembling a flower, known as the "rosette of Fürstenberg," with clinical importance. The papillary duct is the narrow passage of the papillary part of the lactiferous sinus at the very end of the papilla and is provided with a sphincter. This duct is also called teat or streak canal in ruminants. Its opening is called the papillary orifice or ostium. In some species, a papilla is perforated by two or more papillary ducts, each of which opens by its own ostium. There are differences among species in terms of the number of glandular complexes that open through one teat. So there are from 5 to 7 glandular complexes per teat in the cat, from 8 to 14 in the dog, from 2 to 3 in the pig, 2 in the horse, and 1 in all ruminants.

The entire mammary gland is covered and protected by a capsule, which is continuous with the interlobar connective tissue. In the large animals, especially in the cow, the udder is suspended by the so-called *mammary suspensory apparatus*. This apparatus consists of lateral laminae and medial laminae, both provided with suspensory lamellae that anchor the laminae into the glandular tissue. The lateral laminae originate from the femoral laminae of the external abdominal oblique muscles. The internal laminae originate from the symphyseal tendon and the abdominal tunic, the latter being the elastic component of the mammary suspensory apparatus. (The symphiseal tendon is the common origin of the symmetrical gracilis and adductor muscles.)

Rudimentary developed and nonfunctional mammary glands also exist in male species. These glands are located in the same place(s) as in the female species and are represented by small teats.

Blood Supply, Lymphatic System, and Nerve Supply for the Mammary Gland

The mammary gland blood supply varies from species to species, and especially during the lactating period. The *arteries* are provided by the cranial epigastric artery through the cranial superficial epigastric artery; by the external pudendal artery through the caudal superficial epigastric artery and the ventral labial branch; and by the internal pudendal artery through the ventral labial and mammary branch. In the Mare and in the cow the caudal superficial epigastric artery is called the *cranial mammary artery*, and in the same species the ventral labial branch is called the *caudal mammary artery*. In the cow the cranial mammary artery (the caudal superficial epigastric artery) anastomoses with the cranial superficial epigastric artery, whereas the caudal mammary artery (the ventral labial branch of the external pudendal artery) anastomoses with the ventral labial and mammary branch of the internal pudendal artery. (Figure 2.11 shows the blood supply to the cow's udder.)

The *veins* in general follow the arteries. In cows with voluminous and very productive udder, the cranial mammary vein (the *milk vein*) is very large and can be seen under the skin. This vein is flexuous and runs in a cranial direction, penetrating a ring in the ventral abdominal wall where the vein joins the cranial epigastric vein. The ring, which is large enough to introduce a finger within, is called the *milk well*. In accordance with the position of the cow lying down and compressing the udder and the vascular supply, the blood returns to the systemic circulation through one of the cranial mammary, caudal mammary, or external pudendal veins.

The *lymphatic system* is mainly represented by the mammary lymph nodes (superficial inguinal lymph nodes). The subiliac, ischial, or deep inguinal (iliacofemoral) lymph nodes may also drain the udder. The afferent lymphatic vessels start from widely spread papillary plexuses.

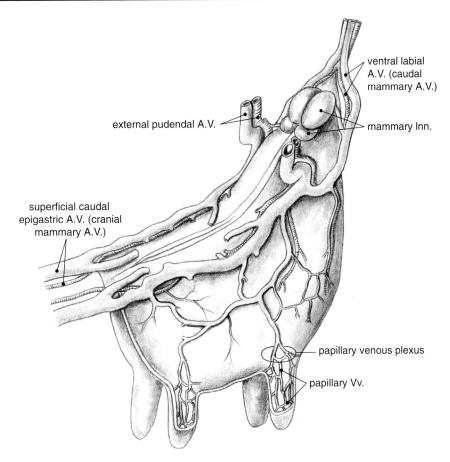

Figure 2.11. Blood supply to the cow's udder (modified and redrawn in pencil from R. Barone, Laboratoire d'Anatomie École Nationale Vétérinaire, Lyon, 1978).

The *nerves* that supply the mammary glands originate from the thoracic, lumbar, and sacral spinal nerves. In the cow, the udder is supplied by the genitofemoral nerve (from the lumbar spinal nerves) and by the mammary branches of the pudendal nerve (from the sacral spinal nerves). The genitofemoral nerve carries efferent and afferent sympathetic fibers. There is no proof of a parasympathetic nerve supply to the mammary gland.

This is, again, a general and acceptable description for all species.

Part 2.3
The Genital Apparatus in the Carnivore

Male Genitalia

The male genitalia in carnivores are presented in four subsections, following the same pattern as was chosen for the general description. Therefore, the first subsection covers the testicle, epididymis, ductus deferens, spermatic cord, and the tunics. The second subsection covers the accessory genital glands, the third subsection the penis, and the last subsection the male urethra.

The Testicle, Epidydimis, Ductus Deferens, Spermatic Cord, and the Tunics

The descent of the testicles occurs very late during the development. The testicles take their normal place within the scrotum between the second and the third week *after* birth.

Globular in shape, the two testicles of carnivores weigh from 1/750 to 1/1850 of the body weight. The long axis of each testicle is obliquely oriented, cranioventrally. The albuginea is thick, and the *mediastinum testis* is located in the middle of the testicle. The *testicular artery*, which runs deep to the albuginea, shows a characteristic design on the surface of the testicle. Small *arterio-venous anastomoses* between the testicular artery and vein were described in the dog.

The *epidydimis* is attached to the dorsolateral border of the testicle. The head of the epididymis starts from the medial surface of the testicle, but it reaches the dorsolateral position to continue with the body and the tail. In the dog, both the head and the tail of the epididymis exceed the head

and the tail of the testicle, whereas in the cat only the head of the epididymis slightly exceeds the head of the testicle. The albuginea of the epidydimis is thinner than that of the testicle. The ductus epididymidis in the dog is between 5 mm and 8 mm long, whereas in the cat it is from 1.5 mm to 3 mm long; it is tortuous in both species. The tail of the epidydimis is attached to the tail of the testicle by a short proper ligament of the testicle, and to the internal spermatic fascia directly (there is no ligament of the tail of the epidydimis in carnivores because the internal spermatic fascia is adherent to the tail of the epididymis). The scrotal ligament joins the internal spermatic fascia to the dartos (see the general description). Figures 2.12 and 2.13 show the testicle of the dog; Figures 2.14 and 2.15 show the testicle of the cat.

The *ductus deferens* begins as a flexuous duct along the epidydimal border of the testicle and medial to the epidydimis in a caudocranial direction because of the position of the testicle. After the ductus deferens passes over the head of the epidydimis, it enters into the spermatic cord and continues up to the vaginal ring. Within the abdominal cavity, the ductus deferens makes a curve in a dorsocaudal direction to enter the pelvic cavity and reach the urethra. In its route from start to finish, the mesoductus deferens, also part of the spermatic cord, is attached to the ductus deferens. Before it reaches the urethra, the ductus deferens crosses the ureter ventrally, then dorsally over the lateral ligament of the urinary bladder. To reach the urethra, the ductus deferentes penetrate the prostate gland and open on the lateral sides of the colliculus seminalis. Before they

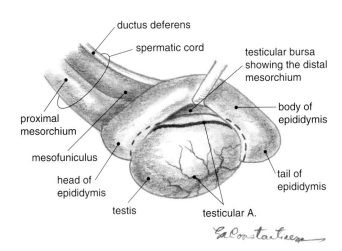

Figure 2.12. Testicle of the dog—lateral aspect.

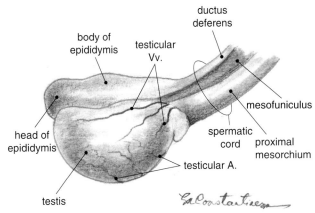

Figure 2.13. Testicle of the dog—medial aspect.

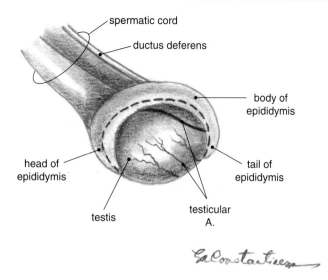

Figure 2.14. Testicle of the cat—lateral aspect.

present. No vesicular glands are present in any of these species (see Figures 2.16 and 2.17).

The *prostate gland* has two parts: the body and the disseminated part. In both species, the body has two lobes, right and left, with an uneven surface. In the dog, the body is spherical and completely surrounds the urethra, whereas in the cat, the prostate is attached only to the roof and the lateral walls of the urethra. The prostate opens on the roof of the prostatic part of the urethra. The disseminated part of the prostate is present as small lobules in both species.

The *bulbourethral glands* (present only in the cat) are very small (up to 5 mm in diameter) and lie in intimate contact with the dorsolateral wall of the urethra, at the level of the ischial arch.

touch the prostate gland, the ductus deferentes and the ureters are held by the genital fold, a visceral peritoneal fold. The uterus masculinus usually can be seen between the two layers of the genital fold. The ampulla of the ductus deferens with the glands is present only in the dog, but it is not too obvious.

The *spermatic cord* and the *tunics of the spermatic cord and testicle* don't differ from the general description, but they differ slightly from the dog to the cat. In the dog, the spermatic cord is from 8 cm to 10 cm long in a middle-sized individual, and it is ventrocaudally obliquely oriented. The scrotum and the testicles are situated distally in the perineal region. In the cat, the spermatic cord is horizontal and proportionally longer in comparison to that of the dog. The scrotum and the testicles are located proximally in the perineal region, in a subanal position.

The Accessory Genital Glands

In the dog, only the *prostate gland* is present, whereas in the cat, the *prostate and the bulbourethral glands* are

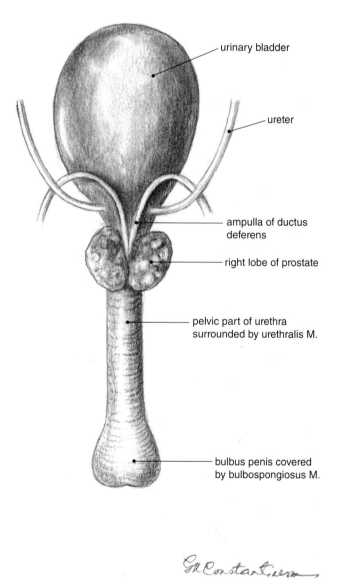

Figure 2.16. Accessory genital glands in the male dog—dorsal view.

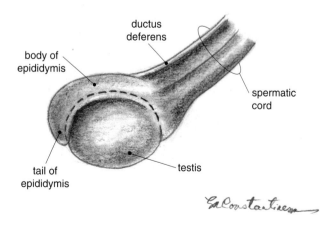

Figure 2.15. Testicle of the cat—medial aspect.

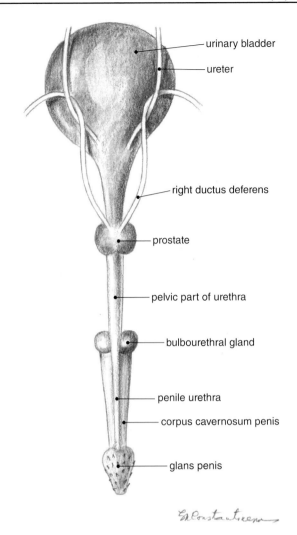

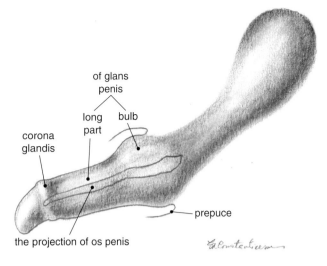

Figure 2.18. Penis of the dog.

Figure 2.17. Accessory genital glands in the male cat—dorsal view.

Blood Supply, Lymph Drainage, and Nerve Supply for the Penis

The blood supply is provided by branches of the internal and external pudendal arteries and veins, with their branches. The lymph is drained into the superficial inguinal lymph nodes. The nerve supply is provided by the pudendal nerve and pelvic plexus (with the pelvic nerves as the parasympathetic component, and the hypogastric nerve as the sympathetic component). (For details, see "Vessels and Nerves of the Penis" in Evans, 1993.)

A corona glandis is present in the dog. The penis of the cat is caudoventrally oriented, so that the urethra looks in a caudoventral direction. In the cat the penis is provided with an indistinct glans penis and small cornified

The Penis

The penis of the dog is very different from all the other species by the following features:

1. It is provided with an *os penis* (a cartilage is found in the cat).
2. The corpus spongiosum penis is twice as thick as the corpus cavernosum penis.
3. It has a very long glans penis, with a *long part* and a *bulb*. "The phenomenon of delayed erection in the dog is due to slow engorgement of the bulbus glandis and the pars longa glandis" (for details, see "Mechanism of Erection" in Evans, 1993).
4. The internal lamina of the prepuce is attached to the bulb of the glans penis; therefore, the fully erect penis is represented only by the glans penis.

Figures 2.18 and 2.19 show the penis of the dog and the penis of the cat, respectively.

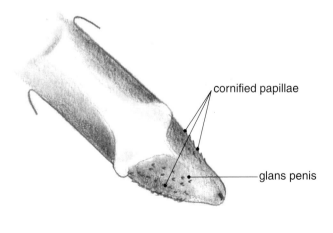

Figure 2.19. Penis of the cat.

papillae. The papillae are considered as a secondary sex characteristic.

The Male Urethra

Specific structures of the pelvic part of the urethra are the very prominent U-shaped urethral crest and the symmetrical openings of the ampullae of the ductus deferentes on both sides of the colliculus seminalis (since there are no vesicular glands in the dog and cat, there is no ejaculatory duct).

The spongy layer of the pelvic urethra consists of vascular erectile tissue and continues with the corpus spongiosum penis. The urethral glands are scattered between the spongy layer and the muscular tunic of the pelvic urethra.

Blood and Nerve Supply for the Male Urethra

The blood suppliers for the urethra are the urethral branch of the prostatic artery and the urethral artery from the internal pudendal artery for the pelvic part of the urethra, the artery of the bulbus penis for the penile part, and the satellite veins. The nerve supply is provided by the pelvic plexus.

Female Genitalia

The female genitalia in Carnivores are discussed in seven subsections, starting with the ovaries and ending with the female urethra.

The Ovary

Located 1 cm to three cm caudal to each kidney, the ovaries of Carnivores are completely surrounded by the ovarian bursae. The ovary is easier to isolate during an ovariectomy in the cat than in the dog. In the dog, the entrance into the ovarian bursa is so narrow that the ovary cannot be exposed unless the orifice is enlarged with scissors. The ovaries are compressed by the abdominal viscera toward the roof of the abdominal cavity, the right ovary dorsal to the pancreas and the descending duodenum, and the left ovary dorsolateral to the descending colon. The suspensory ligament is very long.

In the dog, the ovaries are longer than in the cat, and flat (2 cm in the dog versus 8 mm to 9 mm in the cat), with a shallow hilus, smooth with the exception of the time of sexual cycle, when the surface is irregular (less irregular in the cat). The color is pink-gray in both species.

The Uterine Tube

The uterine tube is 6 cm to 10 cm long in the dog and 4 cm to 6 cm in the cat; each uterine tube is very narrow (from 1 mm to 1.5 mm) and provided inside with a few longitudinal folds. In both species, the uterine part of the salpinx ends on a small papilla. Figure 2.20 shows the cat's ovary, and Figure 2.21 shows the genital apparatus of the female dog.

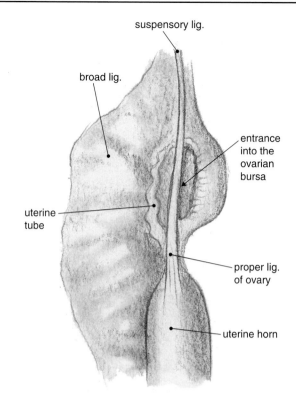

Figure 2.20. The cat's ovary.

The Uterus

The very long and ventrally slightly curved uterine horns in the dog have an average length of 12 cm to 16 cm and a diameter of 8 mm to 9 mm (9 cm to 11 cm and 3 mm to 4 mm, respectively, in the cat) (see Figure 2.21). The uterine velum, which separates the two openings of the uterine horns inside of the uterine body, is very short. The uterine body is from 3 cm to 4 cm long, and the cervix is from 1.5 cm to 2 cm long (2 cm, and from 5 mm to 8 mm, respectively, in the cat), the diameter of both the uterine body and the cervix is 1 cm in the dog and smaller in the cat.

The round ligament of the uterus (the longest is found in the dog and the cat) originates from the lateral surface of the mesometrium, is enclosed in a lateral fold of the broad ligament, and extends from the apex of the uterine horn to the inguinal region, passing through the inguinal canal. On its way through the inguinal canal and even outside of the body wall, the round ligament is accompanied by the vaginal process, up to the lateral sides of the vulva, where it appears as a round, soft prominence. The round ligament of the uterus travels through the inguinal canal, similar to the gubernaculum testis (see "The Descent of the Testicle" earlier in the chapter).

The Vagina

Especially for the dog, the vagina is very long (it averages 12 cm to 15 cm in middle-size individuals, versus 2 cm to

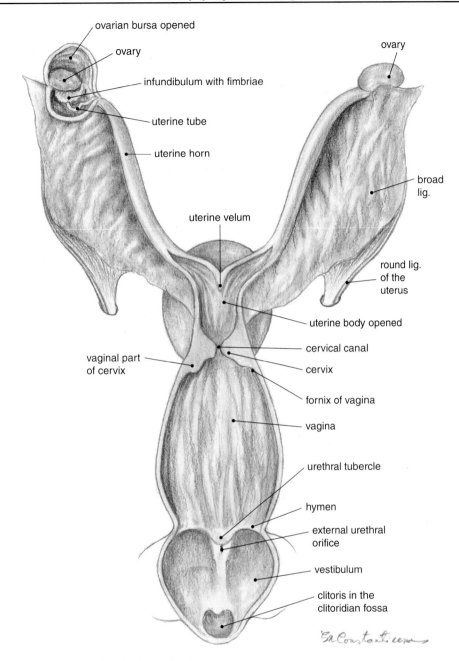

Figure 2.21. Genital apparatus of the female dog—dorsal aspect.

3 cm in the cat) (see Figure 2.21 and Figure 2.22). The fornix is very deep ventrally and provided dorsally with a thick fold that joins the vaginal part of the cervix to the roof of the vagina. The hymen is rudimentary. The external urethral orifice, which opens between the vagina and the vestibule, is provided in the dog only by a *urethral tubercle* at the end of a longitudinal prominence.

The Vestibule

In the dog, the vestibule is from 5 cm to 6 cm long, whereas in the cat, it is approximately as long as the vagina (See Figure 2.21 and Figure 2.22). The vestibular bulb is present only in the dog. Minor vestibular glands are present in both species, but major vestibular glands are present only in the cat.

The Vulva and the Clitoris

Regarding the vulva (see Figures 2.23 and 2.24), the vulvar labiae are thick in both species, and sometimes the major labiae can be differentiated from the minor labiae. The dorsal commissure is round in the dog and pointed in the cat, while the ventral commissure is pointed in the dog and rounded in the cat. The caudal end of the round ligaments and vaginal processes may extend up to the lateral sides of the vulva.

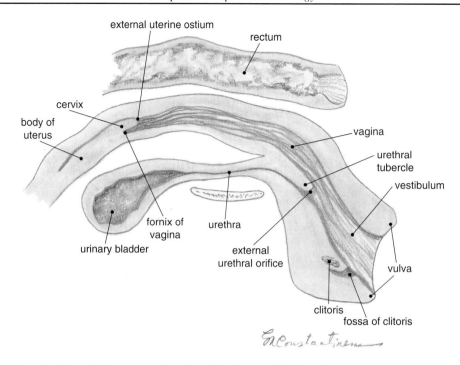

Figure 2.22. Sagittal section through the uterus and vagina of the dog (modified and redrawn in pencil from Evans,1993).

The clitoris is very large in both species, especially in the dog, in which the crura of the clitoris measure between 2 cm and 3 cm, and the body measures approximately 4 cm. The glans is well developed in the dog, and the fossa of the clitoris is deep. The mucosa of this fossa is provided with folds that outline shallow depressions, showing an areolar aspect. In addition, there is a vertical fold within the fossa.

In the cat, the glans is poorly developed, but a small cartilaginous structure resembling the os penis can be found.

The Female Urethra

In the female urethra of carnivores, there are no differences from the general description.

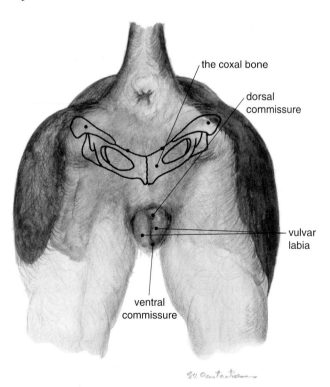

Figure 2.23. Vulva of the female dog.

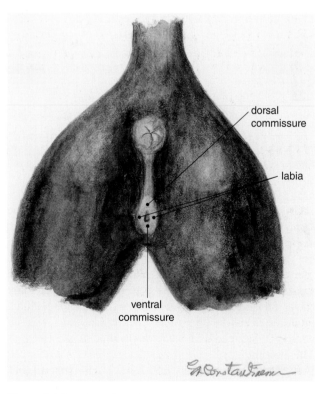

Figure 2.24. Vulva of the female cat.

Part 2.4
The Genital Apparatus in the Pig

Male Genitalia

The male genitalia in the pig are presented in four subsections, following the same pattern as was chosen for the general description. Therefore, the first subsection covers the testicle, epididymis, ductus deferens, spermatic cord, and the tunics. The second subsection covers the accessory genital glands, the third subsection the penis, and the last subsection the male urethra.

The Testicle, Epidydimis, Ductus Deferens, Spermatic Cord, and the Tunics

The descent of the testicles is tardy. They will take their definitive place within the scrotum shortly *before* birth. Relatively frequent cryptorchid individuals are characteristic for this species.

The two testicles represent from 1/200th to 1/300th of the body weight. They are very large and can reach weights of between 200 g and 800 g The testicles are located in a subanal position close to the anus, and their tails are oriented dorsally and slightly caudally. This is the same as the orientation for the tail of the epididymis. Therefore, the voluminous spermatic cord is very long and almost horizontal. The inguinal canal is very oblique caudoventrally, which facilitates the scrotal herniae in this species. The albuginea, and especially the mediastinum testis and the septa, are very thick. The testicular artery has a species-specific design.

The *epididymis* is voluminous. The tail of epididymis is projected far caudally, exceeding the tail of the testicle and looking like an appendix of the testicle. The head of the epididymis exceeds a little the head of the testicle. The ductus epididymidis is from 17 mm to 18 mm long and very tortuous. The proper ligament of the testicle and the ligament of the tail of the epididymis are present.

The *ductus deferens* is very long, up to 30 cm. It is provided *neither* with an ampulla *nor* with glands. The *spermatic cord* and the *tunics of the spermatic cord and testicle* are slightly different from the other species, in that that the spermatic cord is very long and almost horizontal, and the mesofuniculus is attached to the dorsal wall of the vaginal canal. In addition, the scrotum is in a subanal position. Figure 2.25 shows the testicle, epididymis, and spermatic cord, and Figure 2.26 the testicle of the boar.

The Accessory Genital Glands

All three major genital glands are present in the male pig (see Figure 2.27).

The vesicular glands are very large in an adult intact male. On the contrary, the glands are very reduced until puberty and in the castrated males. Pyramidally shaped, each vesicular gland weighs from 75 g to 400 g and reaches from 12 cm to 17 cm in length, from 6 cm to 8 cm in width, and from 3 cm to 5 cm in thickness. The base of the pyramid is cranially oriented and dropped into the abdominal cavity, dorsal to the urinary bladder. The symmetrical glands touch each other in the median plane, covering and hiding the prostate gland. The vesicular glands are located within the genital fold. Their surface is lobulated and pinkish red. The unique excretory canal of each gland opens on the ipsilateral side of the ductus deferens, lateral to the colliculus seminalis. Before puberty or in castrated males early in life, these glands are very small, on each side of the compact part of the prostate gland.

The prostate gland has a very small compact part, and a widely spread disseminated part. The yellowish-pinkish compact part consists of two symmetrical lobes and is overlapped by the vesicular glands, whereas the disseminated part completely surrounds the urethra. Many excretory canals of both parts open into the prostatic urethra. Before puberty and in castrated males early in life, the compact part of the prostate is very small.

The bulbourethral glands are very large, completely covering the urethra from the bulbus penis (at the pelvic outlet) to the cranial border of the pelvic floor. They may reach from 15 cm to 18 cm in length and from 5 cm to 6 cm in width. Completely surrounded by the bulboglandularis muscles, these glands touch each other by the medial borders. Each gland has only one excretory canal, which opens within the urethral recess (this description is specific to the pig and the ruminants), and which is connected to the penile urethra, close to the ischial arch, at the transition between the urethral isthmus and the penile urethra. Before puberty or in castrated males early in life, the bulbourethral glands are very reduced in volume.

The Penis

The penis of the pig has several particular and distinct features, as follows:

1. The penis is very long (60 cm average) and thin (2 cm in diameter).
2. There is a *sigmoid flexure* very close to the origin of the penis, which starts cranial to the attachment of the ischiocavernosus muscle and to the testicles.

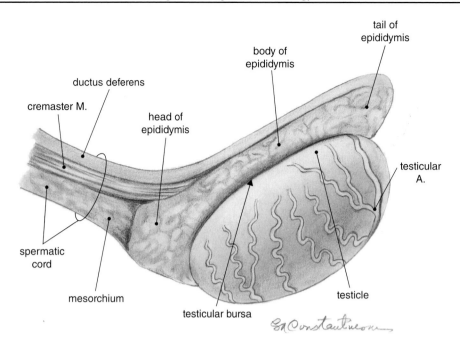

Figure 2.25. Testicle, epididymis, and spermatic cord of the boar—lateral aspect.

3. The albuginea is very thick, and surrounds not only the corpus cavernosum penis, but also the urethra and the corpus spongiosum penis; there is no median septum of the penis between the two corpora cavernosa, but instead a fibrous axis.
4. The bulbus penis is voluminous.
5. With the exception of a small appearance at the level of the bulbus penis, the corpus spongiosum penis is practically absent.
6. The bulbospongiosus muscle is limited to the bulbus penis.
7. The ischiocavernosus muscle is attached to the proximal curve of the sigmoid flexure.
8. The retractor penis muscle extends cranial to the distal curve of the sigmoid flexure.
9. The apex of the penis, provided with a reduced glans penis, is cylindrical in shape and spiraled first to the right, then dorsally, and finally to the left; this spiralization is due to the asymmetry of the corpora cavernosa and the albuginea; a raphe penis joins the glans to the free part of the penis.
10. The glans penis is provided with a venous plexus that joins the venous supply of the corpus spongiosum penis.
11. The prepuce is divided into two uneven compartments by a circular fold of the internal lamina, which separates the cavity into a very long caudal compartment (20 cm to 25 cm) and a very short cranial compartment. The cranial compartment is provided with a *preputial diverticulum*, specific to the pig, a large dorsal bilobed sac (approximately 135 ml capacity), which empties its secretion on the roof of the preputial cavity. The two symmetrical halves of the diverticulum are separated by a median fold attached to the roof of the diverticulum. The internal lamina of the prepuce and the skin covering the free part of the penis contain numerous lymph nodules.
12. The cranial preputial muscles are strong, cover the preputial diverticulum, helping to empty it, and fuse with each other on the ventral aspect of the prepuce.
13. The caudal preputial muscles are thin. They extend from the superficial inguinal rings to the lateral borders of the prepuce; they do not reach the preputial ostium.

Figures 2.28 and 2.29, respectively, show the Pig's penis within the prepuce and the preputial diverticulum.

The Male Urethra

The pelvic part of the urethra measures between 15 cm and 20 cm. A very thin, spongy layer is surrounded by a smooth muscle and the urethralis muscle.

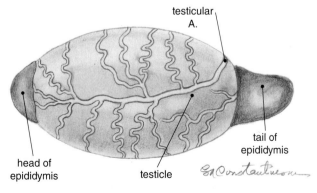

Figure 2.26. Testicle of the boar—the free border.

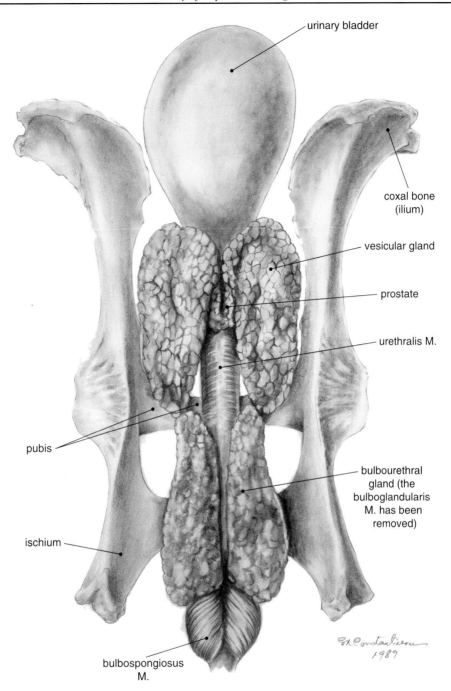

urinary bladder

coxal bone
(ilium)

vesicular gland

prostate

urethralis M.

pubis

bulbourethral
gland (the
bulboglandularis
M. has been
removed)

ischium

bulbospongiosus
M.

Figure 2.27. Accessory genital glands of a mature boar—dorsal aspect.

Before opening on the roof of the prostatic part of the urethra, each ductus deferens is covered by the ipsilateral vesicular gland and travels between the two lobes of the prostate gland. The colliculus seminalis is not prominent and is surrounded by numerous orifices of the prostate gland.

Notice the presence of the urethral recess (*vide supra*), which is described and illustrated later in this chapter in "The Genital Apparatus in the ruminants" section, "The Urethra" subsection (Figure 2.53).

The blood and nerve supplies and the lymph nodes are similar to those described in Chapter 1. In the pig, the penis is supplied only by the artery of the penis, a branch of the internal pudendal artery.

Female Genitalia

The female genitalia in the pig are discussed in seven subsections, starting with the ovaries and ending with the female urethra.

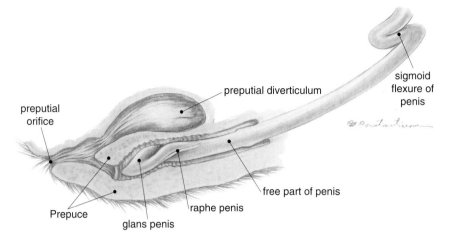

Figure 2.28. The pig's penis within the prepuce—lateral view.

The Ovary

Berry-shaped because of numerous follicles and corpora lutea on their surface, the ovaries (see Figure 2.30) are 4 cm to 5 cm long with a diameter of 2 cm to 3 cm. The follicles are separated by deep grooves. The hilus is obvious and located on the mesovarian border of the ovary. The ovaries exceed the pelvic cavity and are found 5 cm to 6 cm away from the cranial border of the pubic bones in nonpregnant mature sows.

The suspensory ligament and the proximal mesovarium are extremely long, especially in multiparous sows. The ovarian bursa is very large and wide, and oriented ventromedially. The proper ligament of the ovary is muscular and short with a fan-shaped spread into the mesometrium.

The Uterine Tube

Suspended by a short mesosalpinx, the uterine tube travels from the apex of the uterine horn in the lateral wall of the ovarian bursa, then in the medial wall, and opens on the inner surface of the mesosalpinx, facing the ovary.

The infundibulum is very wide and completely surrounds the ovary. It is provided with multiple fimbriae.

The ampulla of the salpinx is three times longer than the isthmus, and very flexuous. The isthmus joins the uterine horn in an oblique position, and the uterine ostium of the tube is surrounded by numerous little endometrial tubercles disposed like a double or triple rosette.

The Uterus

Comparatively, the sow has the longest uterus (see Figure 2.31). The horns can reach from 120 cm to 140 cm in length. They are very flexuous, intermingle with the jejunal loops,

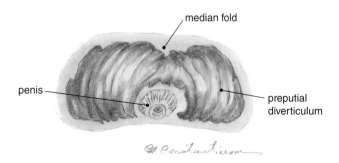

Figure 2.29. The preputial diverticulum in the pig—transverse section.

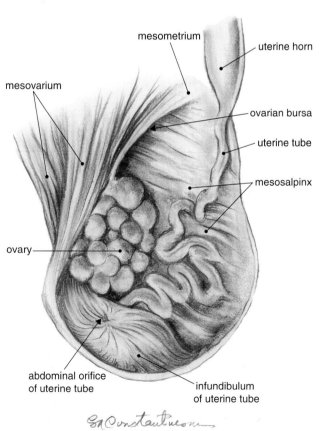

Figure 2.30. The ovary of the sow.

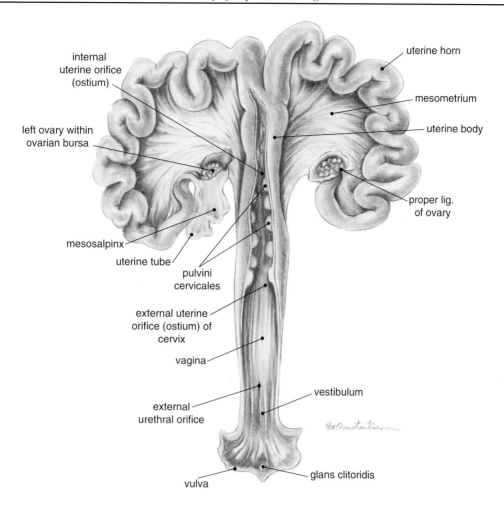

internal
uterine orifice
(ostium)

uterine horn

mesometrium

left ovary within
ovarian bursa

uterine body

proper lig.
of ovary

mesosalpinx

uterine tube

pulvini
cervicales

external uterine
orifice (ostium) of
cervix

vagina

vestibulum

external
urethral orifice

glans clitoridis

vulva

Figure 2.31. The uterus of the sow—dorsal view.

and may spread on the floor of the abdominal cavity. The body of the uterus is short (5 cm to 6 cm long), and the cervix is three times longer than the body (from 15 cm to 25 cm). The cranial extent of the cervix drops within the abdominal cavity.

The transition between the apex of the uterine horn and the corresponding uterine tube is progressive. Each uterine horn opens separately into the uterine body after the horns converge and unite with each other for a short distance. Inside of the uterus, the horns are separated by a short velum. There are many irregular endometrial folds in the uterine horns and body.

The cervix is not well outlined. It lacks the vaginal portion, and the external uterine orifice as well as the transition to the vagina are not well marked. Longitudinal folds and prominences are shown on the endometrium. The prominences, shaped as cushions or processes *(pulvini cervicales),* interdigitate with each other and occlude the cervix.

The broad ligament is very thick, rich in muscular fibers. The round ligament of the uterus is present and extends within the inguinal canal.

The Vagina
There is no fornix in the sow because the cervix doesn't protrude into the vagina. Specific features of the vagina for this species (see figure 2.31) are that it is almost as long as the cervix, and it is provided with thick and prominent longitudinal folds and a hymen in very young animals. The peritoneum covers only the cranial part of the vagina. The rest of the organ is located within the pelvic diaphragm.

The Vestibule
Shorter than the vagina, the vestibule extends from the external urethral ostium to the vulva (see Figure 2.31). Associated to the external urethral ostium is a reduced suburethral diverticulum, which should be taken into consideration during artificial insemination. Several longitudinal folds of the mucosa and two symmetrical rows of the openings of the minor vestibular glands are also exposed. The vestibule is provided with a bulbus vestibuli.

The Vulva and the Clitoris
The two labiae of the vulva are thick, and the ventral commissure is pointed and provided with a few hairs. The

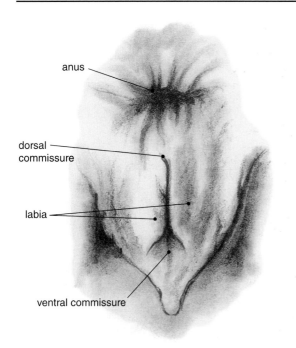

Figure 2.32. The vulva of the sow.

clitoris is very long (from 7 cm to 8 cm), flexuous, and almost lacking the gland. The prepuce is connected to a small gland surrounded by a shallow preputial fossa (see Figure 2.31 and 2.32).

The Female Urethra

The female urethra is not different from the general description. The only exception is the presence of a *suburethral diverticulum*, at the level of the external urethral ostium, similar to that in the ruminants (see the subsection "Female Urethra," under "Female Genitalia" in the chapter section "The Genital Apparatus in the Ruminant").

Blood and Nerve Supply for the Female Genitalia

The blood supply of the female genital organs includes the ovarian artery, the uterine artery, the vaginal artery, and the artery of the clitoris (for the clitoris and the bulbus vestibuli). The nerve supply follows the general description.

Part 2.5
The Genital Apparatus in the Ruminant

Male Genitalia

The bull is considered as the ruminant type for the general description, while the specific characteristics of the ram and buck will be mentioned in each chapter.

The Testicle, Epidydimis, Ductus Deferens, Spermatic Cord, and the Tunics

Oval shaped, each testicle of the bull is between 10 cm and 12 cm long and 6 cm to 8 cm wide, and weighs between 250 g and 300 g. In the small ruminants, the testicles are more spherical. In the ram, the testicles weigh between 200 g and 250 g each, whereas in the buck they weigh between 130 g and 160 g each.

The testicles are located in a vertical position, with the head of the epididymis proximal and the tail of the epididymis distal to the two corresponding poles of the testicles and exceeding these two poles. The epididymal border of the testicle in the bull is oriented medially, while in the small ruminants it is oriented caudomedially. The epididymal canal is as long as 40 mm to 50 mm in the Bull and 40 mm to 60 mm in the small ruminants.

The proper ligament of the testicle and the ligament of the tail of the epididymis are very strong in all ruminants. Refer to Figures 2.33 through 2.41 for diagrams of the testicle, epidydimis, ductus deferens, spermatic cord, and tunics discussed here.

The ductus deferens is provided with a 12 cm to 15 cm ampulla, which travels side by side with the symmetrical structure before it enters below the prostate and opens into the urethra. The excretory duct doesn't join the duct of the vesicular gland; therefore, there is no ejaculatory duct.

The spermatic cord is vertical and 20 cm long. The extraabdominal testicular tunics, including the scrotal septum, are thick, especially in the bull. The scrotal raphe is deep and obvious.

The Accessory Genital Glands

The vesicular glands are elongated and large in the bull, reaching 10 cm in length; they are rounded and much smaller in the small ruminants. The surface of the glands is uneven and lobulated. Each lobule has its excretory canal, which joins the other canals in a common excretory duct. The latter travels deep to the prostate gland before opening into the urethra.

Only in the bull, the prostate has a reduced body located on the dorsal aspect of the urethra. The two lobes and the isthmus are vaguely separated from each other. However, the disseminated part is present in all ruminants. The disseminated part in the bull extends up to the urethral isthmus and totally surrounds the urethra; in the ram, it is present only on the dorsal and lateral walls of the urethra; and in the buck, it completely surrounds the urethra (see Figures 2.42 and 2.43).

The bulbourethral glands are elliptically shaped in the bull, spherical in the small ruminants, and located in all these species dorsal to the urethral isthmus. These glands are covered by the bulboglandularis muscle; therefore, in the bull they cannot be felt by rectal palpation. The excretory duct opens into the urethra via the urethral recess, in a similar manner as shown in the pig (see the subsection "The Accessory Genital Glands" under "Male Genitalia" in "The Genital Apparatus in the Pig" section of this chapter). The urethral recess is illustrated in Figure 2.53.

The Penis

Of fibroelastic type, the penis in ruminants is very long, but with a small diameter. In the bull, the penis can reach from 80 cm to 100 cm in length, with a diameter of 3 cm to 4 cm; while in the small ruminants, the penis is from 30 cm to 50 cm long and with a smaller diameter than that of the Bull. The tunica albuginea is very thick and surrounds the corpus cavernosum, the corpus spongiosum, and the penile urethra all together. There is a vertically oriented fibrous septum inside of the corpus cavernosum penis, from which the trabeculae originate and outline the caverns (see Figure 2.42 and Figures 2.44 through 2.52 for drawings related to this subsection).

The root of the penis is very large, showing a thick and wide bulbus penis and bulbospongiosus muscle. Similar to that of the pig, the bulbospongiosus muscle doesn't continue on the ventral surface of the penis. The crura are strong and covered by the very large ischiocavernosus muscles.

The body of the penis is double flexed before it reaches the level of the spermatic cords. The first flexure is dorsal to the second. Interestingly, the retractor penis muscles don't follow the sigmoid flexure. They travel straight cranially, attach to the ventral flexure, and continue cranially toward the glans penis; they diminish and disappear before they reach the glans. The corpus spongiosum penis continues the bulbus penis for a short distance cranially.

In the bull, the free part of the penis is only 10 cm long in the resting position. The cylindrical shaped penis becomes gradually conical and ends in a glans penis. The free part is slightly twisted counterclockwise, showing an obliquely

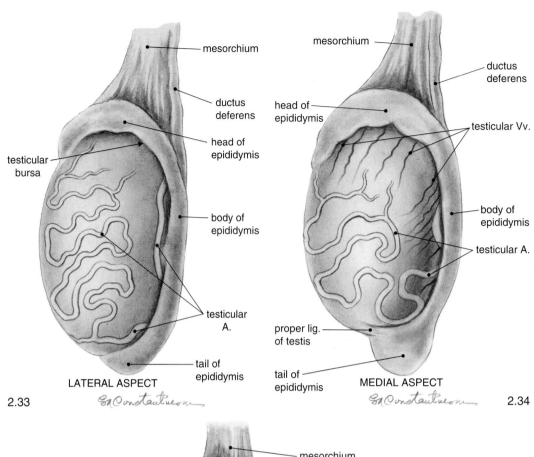

mesorchium

ductus
deferens

head of
epididymis

testicular
bursa

body of
epididymis

testicular
A.

tail of
epididymis

LATERAL ASPECT

2.33

mesorchium

ductus
deferens

head of
epididymis

testicular Vv.

body of
epididymis

testicular A.

proper lig.
of testis

tail of
epididymis

MEDIAL ASPECT

2.34

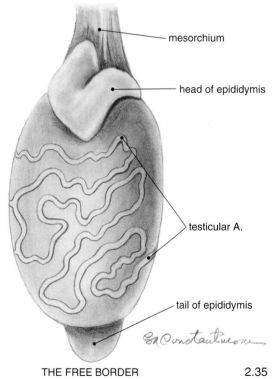

mesorchium

head of epididymis

testicular A.

tail of epididymis

THE FREE BORDER

2.35

Figure 2.33–2.35. The left testicle and epididymis of the bull.

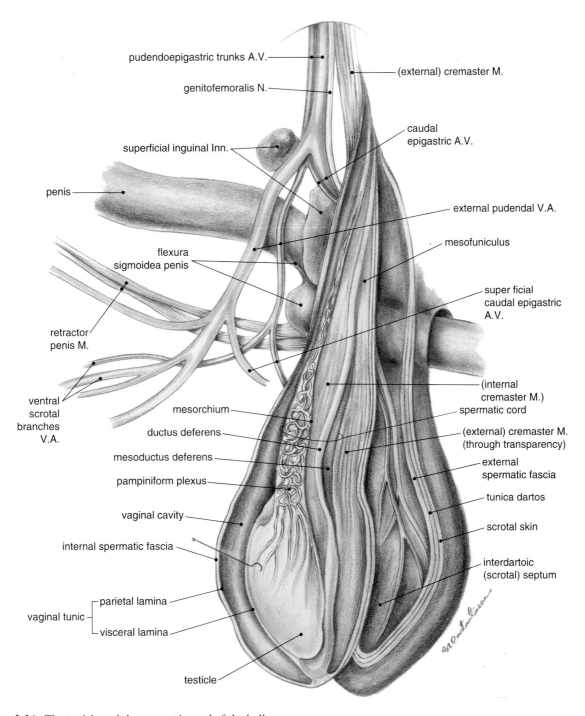

Figure 2.36. The testicle and the spermatic cord of the bull.

pudendoepigastric trunks A.V.

genitofemoralis N.

superficial inguinal Inn.

penis

flexura
sigmoidea penis

retractor
penis M.

ventral
scrotal
branches
V.A.

mesorchium

ductus deferens

mesoductus deferens

pampiniform plexus

vaginal cavity

internal spermatic fascia

parietal lamina

vaginal tunic

visceral lamina

testicle

(external) cremaster M.

caudal
epigastric A.V.

external pudendal V.A.

mesofuniculus

super ficial
caudal epigastric
A.V.

(internal
cremaster M.)
spermatic cord

(external) cremaster M.
(through transparency)

external
spermatic fascia

tunica dartos

scrotal skin

interdartoic
(scrotal) septum

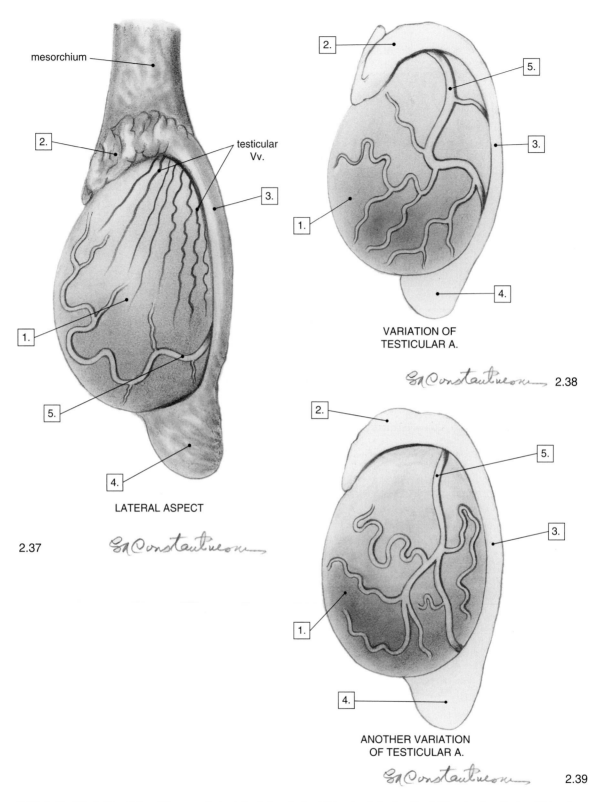

mesorchium

2.

testicular
Vv.

3.

1.

5.

4.

LATERAL ASPECT

2.37

2.

5.

3.

1.

4.

VARIATION OF
TESTICULAR A.

2.38

2.

5.

3.

1.

4.

ANOTHER VARIATION
OF TESTICULAR A.

2.39

Figure 2.37–2.39. The left testicle of the ram: **1**. testicle; **2**. head of epididymis; **3**. body of epididymis; **4**. tail of epididymis; **5**. testicular artery.

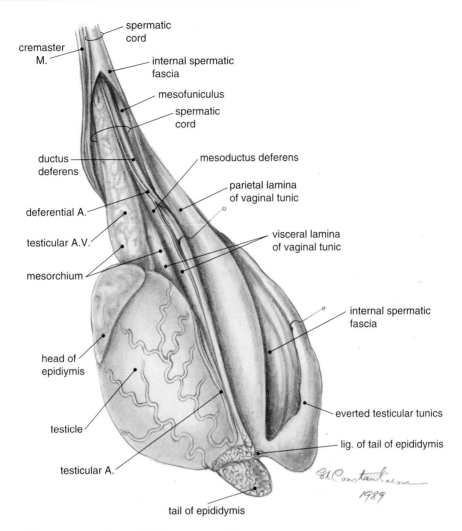

Figure 2.40. Right testicle and spermatic cord of the buck—medial aspect.

oriented raphe penis at the end of the preputial frenulum. In the bull and the buck only, an apical ligament is present on the dorsal aspect of the albuginea. The fibers of the ligament are unevenly dispersed, and they differ in thickness and elasticity. This fact, added to the presence of helicoid fibers within the albuginea, explains the twisted shape of the free part of the penis in the bull. Characteristic for the ram is the presence of an erectile tubercle (tuberculum spongiosum) on the left side of the free part of the penis. The raphe penis is also present in the small ruminants.

The glans penis differs in shape from species to species and is accompanied by the apparent urethral process. In the bull, the glans is rounded, elongated, and ends by bending over the external urethral process. In the small ruminants, the glans is sharply separated from the free part of the penis by a recess. In the ram, a tubercle is present at the caudal end of the glans penis, in a position opposite to the tuberculum spongiosum.

The prepuce is long and narrow. It is provided by longitudinal and some transverse folds. The preputial frenulum continues with the raphe penis. The preputial orifice is also narrow and protected by long hairs. Both cranial and caudal preputial muscles are present, with the caudal muscles longer than the cranial muscles.

The Male Urethra
Except for the urethral recess (common to ruminants and the pig) and the terminal part of the penile urethra, the urethra in ruminants is similar to that in the general description (see Figure 2.53; also refer to Figures 2.45, 2.47, 2.48, 2.49, 2.50, 2.51, and 5.52).

In ruminants, the male urethra is different from other species as far as the urethral process is concerned. In the bull, the urethral process becomes apparent at the ventral aspect of the glans penis and doesn't exceed the cranial limit of the glans. In small ruminants, the urethral process is 4 cm long in the ram and 2.5 cm long in the buck, and it exceeds the limit of the glans. The urethral process in small ruminants contains erectile tissue, which shows during the erection.

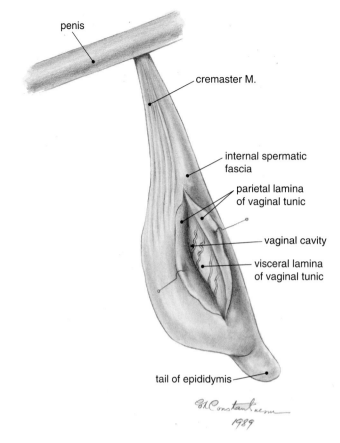

Figure 2.41. Right testicle and spermatic cord of the buck with testicular tunics—medial aspect.

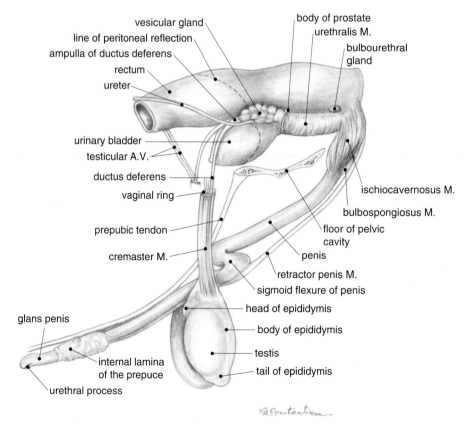

Figure 2.42. Genital apparatus in the bull—left lateral aspect (modified and redrawn in pencil from R. Barone, Laboratoire d'Anatomie École Nationale Vétérinaire, Lyon, 1978).

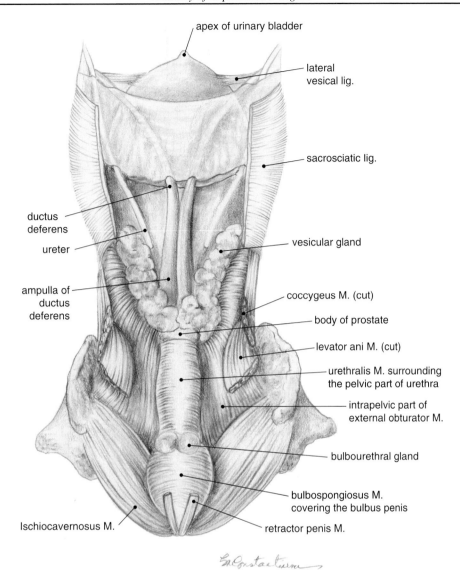

apex of urinary bladder

lateral
vesical lig.

sacrosciatic lig.

ductus
deferens

ureter

vesicular gland

ampulla of
ductus
deferens

coccygeus M. (cut)

body of prostate

levator ani M. (cut)

urethralis M. surrounding
the pelvic part of urethra

intrapelvic part of
external obturator M.

bulbourethral gland

bulbospongiosus M.
covering the bulbus penis

Ischiocavernosus M.

retractor penis M.

Figure 2.43. Genital apparatus in the bull—dorsal view (modified and redrawn in pencil from R. Barone, 1978; Nickel, Schummer, and Seiferle, 1979–1981; and Sack, 1991).

Blood and Nerve Supply for the Male Genitalia

The blood and nerve supply are similar to those of the pig. Inspection of the penis in the bull and the stallion alike before starting sexual activity, and before collecting semen for artificial insemination is mandatory. To accomplish that, the penis should be examined outside of the prepuce; this can be done by regional anesthesia of the pudendal and caudal rectal nerves (see Figure 2.54).

Here is the easiest technique for blocking these nerves (from Popescu, Paraipan and Nicolescu, 1958, "Subsacral anaesthesia in the bull and the horse," in Westhues and Fritsch, 1964):

Instruments. Needle, length 23 cm, diameter 2.5 mm; 20 ml syringe.

Technique. With the tail held high, the left hand locates the sacral promontory per rectum. The hand is drawn back along the sacrum 2–3 cm from the midline to locate the ventral sacral foramina. By counting back, the third ventral foramen (exit of the pudendal nerve) is found. The index or middle finger remains on this point. With the right hand a needle with a short beveled point is inserted in the midline third of the distance from anus to tail base, and pushed through the connective tissue between rectum and pelvis (the pelvic diaphragm – N.R.), directed cranially and slightly paramedially, so that the point finally rests at the foramen palpated by the left hand. An assistant attaches the syringe to the needle and injects about 20 ml solution (3–5% procaine). Alternatively the assistant may hold the needle while the operator injects.

The syringe is removed and the needle withdrawn 5–6 cm under rectal control until the point reaches the fourth sacral foramen (exit of the hemorrhoidal nerve—actual name caudal rectal). 20 ml solution is likewise injected. The whole procedure is repeated on the other side, so that

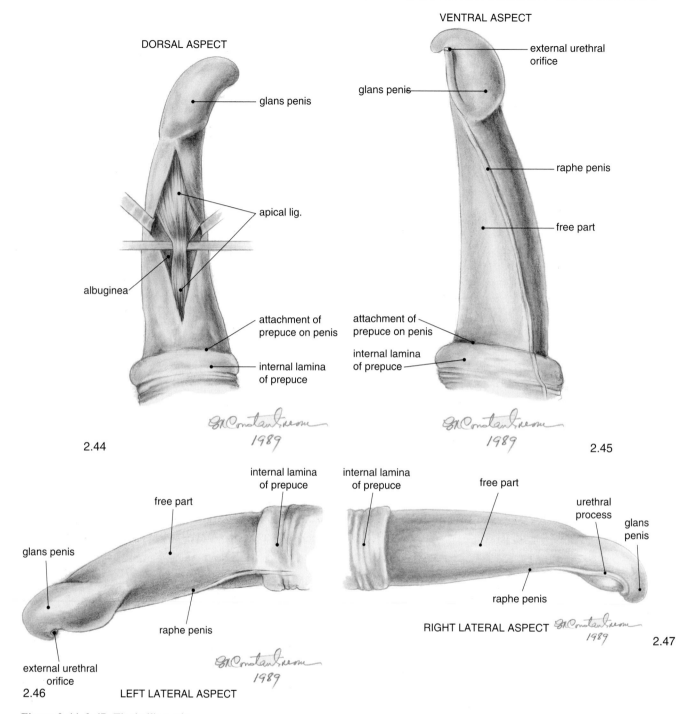

DORSAL ASPECT

glans penis

apical lig.

albuginea

attachment of
prepuce on penis

internal lamina
of prepuce

2.44

VENTRAL ASPECT

external urethral
orifice

glans penis

raphe penis

free part

attachment of
prepuce on penis

internal lamina
of prepuce

2.45

free part

internal lamina
of prepuce

glans penis

raphe penis

external urethral
orifice

2.46   LEFT LATERAL ASPECT

internal lamina
of prepuce

free part

urethral
process

glans
penis

raphe penis

RIGHT LATERAL ASPECT

2.47

Figure 2.44–2.47. The bull's penis.

a total of 80 ml anesthetic is required. On completion, gentle massage with the left (inside rectum) hand ensures better dispersal of the solution. Within 5–20 minutes prolapse of the penis occurs as well as anaesthesia of the perineum and penis. In some cases vasopuncture (A. sacralis medialis, A. sacralis lateralis and veins) accidentally occurs during insertion of the needle. This is obvious as blood leaves the needle, which must be withdrawn immediately and the direction altered.

Wethues and Fritsch comment on the subsacral anaesthesia that "the infiltration of the pudendal and hemorrhoidal (caudal rectal) nerves as they leave the sacrum in the third and fourth ventral sacral foramina appears technically easier than LARSEN's method."

Several other methods were tried to anesthetize the penis and the perineum in the bull and the stallion (and internal genitalia in the cow and the mare), with lower results, and

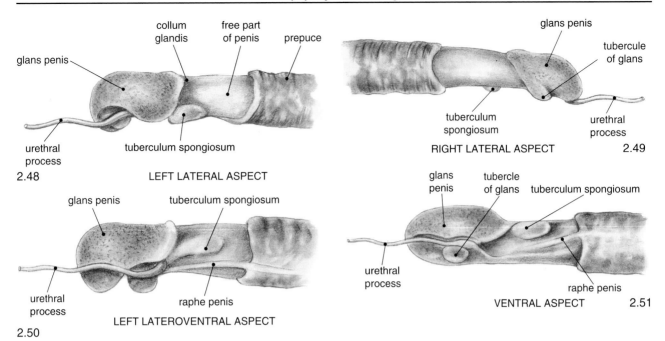

Figure 2.48–2.51. The ram's penis.

the methods were technically very difficult to perform. The subsacral anaesthesia remains the easiest and most precise method to anesthetize the perineum and the penis (and the internal genitalia, as well).

Female Genitalia

The female genitalia in ruminants are discussed in seven subsections, starting with the ovaries and ending with the female urethra.

The Ovary

Relatively small for the size of the species, the ovaries in the cow are each about 3.5 cm to 4 cm long, 2 cm wide, and 1 cm to 2 cm thick; while in the small ruminants they are each about 1.5 cm to 2 cm long, and 1 cm to 1.5 cm wide. In all ruminants, around the attachment of the mesovarium the surface of the ovary is smooth, while the rest of the surface is uneven as the result of numerous follicles and corpora lutea in various stages of development. The follicles and corpora lutea are as big as to be easily palpable by rectal

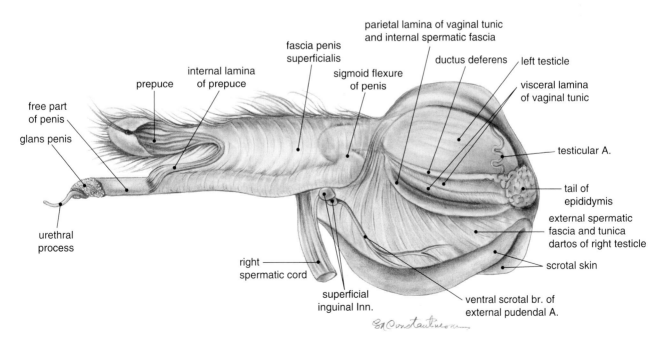

Figure 2.52. The penis and the left testicle—left lateral aspect—of the buck.

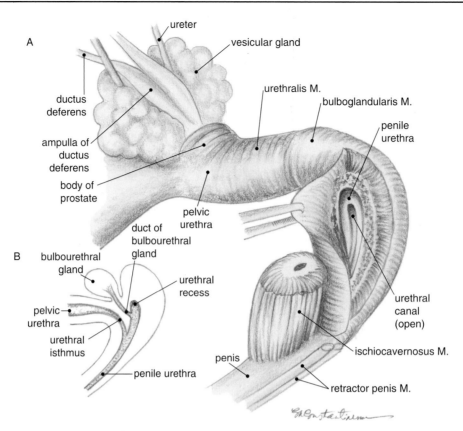

Figure 2.53. The urethral recess in the bull (redrawn from Garrett, 1987). **A.** Topography of urethral recess. **B.** Schematic representation of a median section.

exploration (see Figure 2.7). The hilus is distinct and located on the mesovarian border of the ovary. The uterine end is connected to the mesometrium by a short but strong proper ligament. The attachment of the mesosalpinx divides the mesovarium into a proximal and a distal mesovarium, the proximal one being by far the longest. The cranial border of the latter is marked by the suspensory ligament. The

distal mesovarium is thicker and provided with numerous muscular fibers. See Figure 2.55 to review these details and those that follow regarding the ovary and the uterine tube in ruminants.

In nulliparous and primiparous mature cows, the ovaries are found within the pelvic inlet. The more pregnancies the animal has had, the more cranially the ovaries are located; they drop within the abdominal cavity, pulled by the increasingly larger uterus.

The Uterine Tube

Flexuous, mobile, and from 20 cm to 28 cm long in the cow and 10 cm to 16 cm long in the small ruminants, the uterine tube is suspended by a short mesosalpinx. The tube surrounds and envelops the corresponding ovary, outlining a wide ovarian bursa whose opening is directed ventromedially. The infundibulum of the salpinx is provided with fimbriae, some of which are attached to the ovary (the ovarian fimbriae).

There is no precise delimitation between the isthmus and the apex of the uterine horn at the tubo-uterine junction. The tube is gradually continuous with the uterine horn.

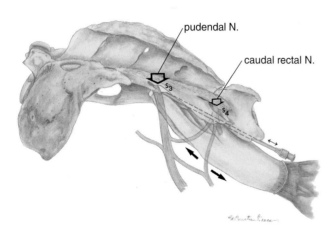

Figure 2.54. Landmarks for performing the subsacral anesthesia in the large ruminants (introduced by Popescu et al., 1958).

The Uterus

Ruminants have a typical uterus bicornis, with two horns, a body, and a cervix (see Figures 2.56, 2.57, 2.58,

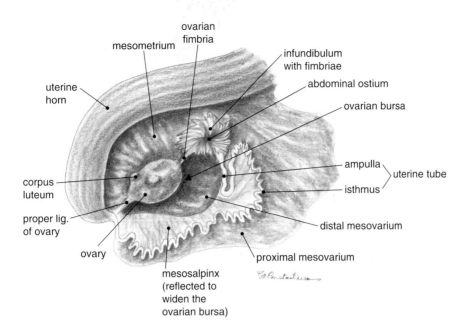

Figure 2.55. The ovary and uterine tube of the cow.

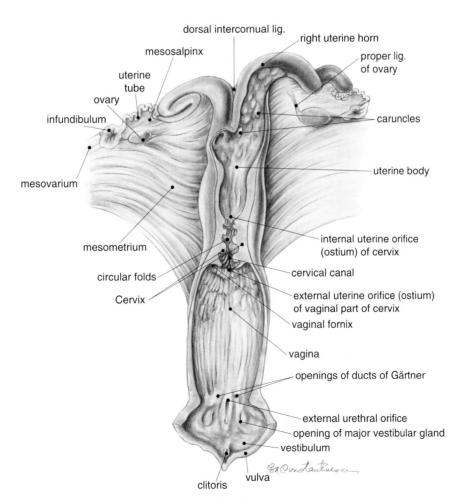

Figure 2.56. The uterus, vagina, and vestibulum of the cow—dorsal view.

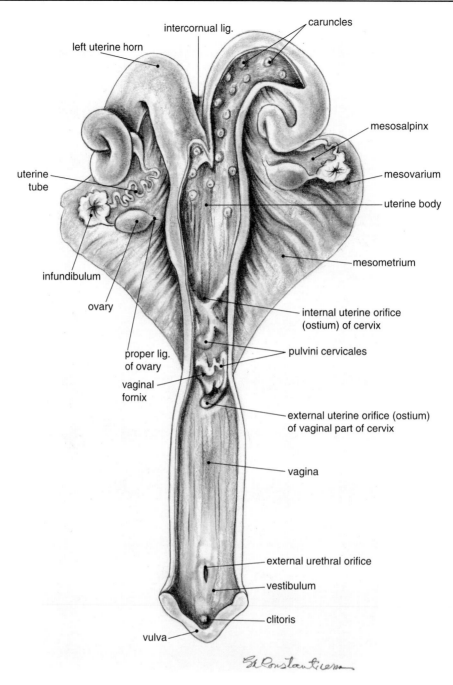

Figure 2.57. The genital tract of the ewe—dorsal view.

and 2.59 for this discussion). The uterine horns are from 35 cm to 45 cm long in the cow and from 12 cm to 15 cm long in the small ruminants; the horns diminish in size toward the apex. At their origin from the body of the uterus, the horns run side by side united by perimetrium (the visceral layer of the peritoneum that surrounds the uterus). Specific to the cow, at the point that they separate from each other, the horns are connected by two ligaments, the *dorsal* and the *ventral intercornual ligaments*. In small ruminants, one single intercornual ligament joins the two horns to one another. In the cow, these ligaments have a high clinical

importance, in that that for gestation diagnostics or the diagnosis of an abnormal condition of the ovaries by rectal palpation, the operator pulls the multiparous uterus back into the pelvic cavity, holding it from the intercornual ligaments. Cranially the horns separate from each other and start to shape themselves in a spiral motion, similar to the shape of the ram's horns, first curving ventrally, then caudally, and finally dorsally. The apices (singular, apex) of the uterine horns are "S" shaped. The free border of the horns is very convex, while the mesometrial border serves for the attachment of the mesometrium. The uterine horns are

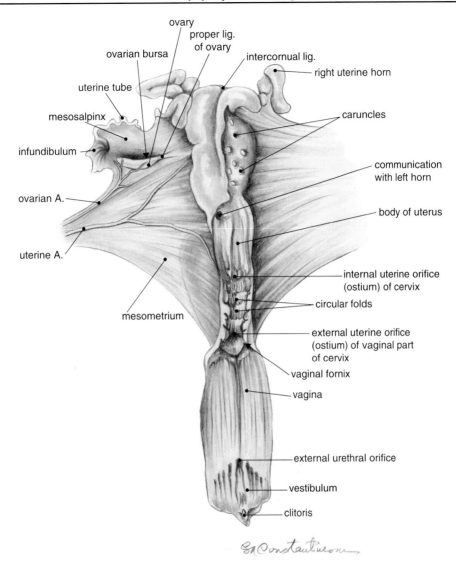

ovary
proper lig.
of ovary
ovarian bursa
intercornual lig.
uterine tube
right uterine horn
mesosalpinx
caruncles
infundibulum
communication
with left horn
ovarian A.
body of uterus
uterine A.
internal uterine orifice
(ostium) of cervix
mesometrium
circular folds
external uterine orifice
(ostium) of vaginal part
of cervix
vaginal fornix
vagina
external urethral orifice
vestibulum
clitoris

Figure 2.58. The genital tract of the female goat—dorsal aspect.

separated inside of the uterus by the uterine velum, similar to the configuration in the carnivores and the sow.

The body of the uterus, apparently long, is in reality only between 3 cm and 4 cm long in the cow and between 2 cm and 3 cm long in small ruminants. This body is suspended by a very large mesometrium, from which the round ligament of the uterus originates. Inside, the two horns open separately.

The endometrium (the mucosa) of each uterine horn and of the body has four prominent longitudinal folds separated by transverse grooves, which divide the mucosa in tens of segments. Two accessory folds are noticed, and as a result, each segment of the folds isolates itself and develops into an independent *caruncle*. There are from 80 to 120 caruncles in the cow, and more in the ewe and the goat, disposed on four rows. The caruncles are pediculated in all ruminants, but in the cow the surface is rounded, in the ewe, concave like a cup, and in the goat, flat, sometimes concave

(see Figures 2.60, 2.61, and 2.62). During pregnancy the caruncles get bigger, up to as large as a midsize potato in the cow. Their surface has a spongy aspect because of the numerous and deep crypts in which the villi of the *cotyledons* of the *placenta* implant (from this description, the placenta is of a cotyledonary type). Each caruncle and the corresponding cotyledon make a *placentome*.

The cervix is the third, last, and most caudal segment of the uterus. The cervix attains 10 cm in length in the cow and 4 cm in length in small ruminants. It is rigid in comparison to the rest of the uterus and the vagina; therefore, it is easy to identify it via the rectum. The cervical canal is irregular. The external uterine ostium (the communication between the uterus, the cervix, and the vagina) protrudes into the vagina and is surrounded by the vaginal fornix. In the cow, four circular folds of the endometrium and portions of the inner circular muscle layer interdigitate with each other in a very firm relationship, so that between

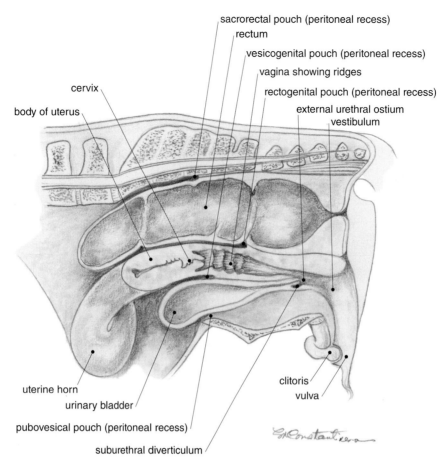

Figure 2.59. Sagittal section through the pelvic cavity in the cow (modified and redrawn in pencil from R. Barone, Laboratoire d'Anatomie École Nationale Vétérinaire, Lyon, 1978).

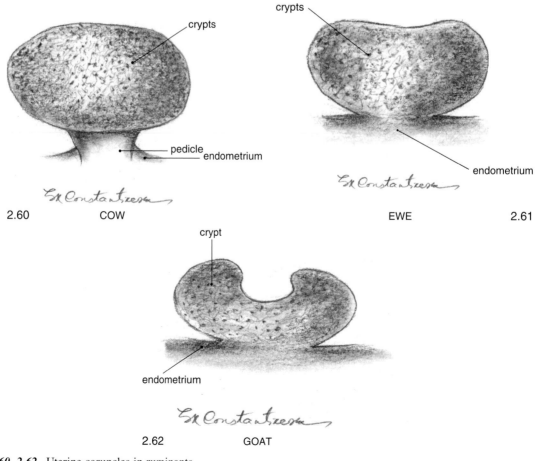

Figure 2.60–2.62. Uterine caruncles in ruminants.

two estrus periods the canal is practically impenetrable. In the small ruminants, the quantity of muscle fibers within the circular folds of the endometrium of the cervix is higher than in the cow. The protrusion of the cervix into the vagina (much more visible in the cow than in the small ruminants) consists of the last circular fold of the endometrium. The circular folds of the endometrium are crossed by longitudinal folds, which gives the appearance of an open flower.

In the cow, during the first 24 to 36 hours of estrus, the external uterine ostium allows the tip of the pipette for artificial insemination to enter for a couple of centimeters, and then it closes again. After birth, the cervical canal allows an operator to introduce a hand (for manual extraction of a retained placenta or for introducing medication) only for 36 to 48 hours. Also, artificial insemination nowadays is performed by guiding the pipette with one hand introduced within the rectum and palpating the firm cervix.

The broad ligaments are wide and divergent cranially. They are thick, strong, triangularly shaped, and consist of numerous smooth muscle fibers. The peritoneum covers the uterus as perimetrium; it continues to the rectum dorsally and the urinary bladder ventrally. Therefore, two peritoneal pouches are outlined: the *recto-genital* and the *vesico-genital pouch*, respectively. The recto-genital pouch is more caudally located, at the level of the first quarter of the vagina, while the vesico-genital pouch reaches only the origin of the vagina.

Between the perimetrium and the endometrium, a smooth muscle called the myometrium is found. The myometrium has two layers: a superficial, longitudinal layer visible under the perimetrium, and a deep, circular layer, which is thicker in the cervical region. At the base, the two uterine horns are connected to each other by oblique or transverse muscle fibers.

The Vagina

In the cow, the vagina measures 30 cm and is very expandable laterally. Its cranio-ventral inclination shows an uneven depth of the fornix, which is deeper dorsally (about 3 cm) than ventrally (about 1 cm). Vaginal annular ridges, thicker and more prominent toward the cervix and separated by grooves, are visible as part of the mucosa. The most cranial ridge is the closest to the vaginal portion of the cervix and surrounds it, looking apparently like a double cervix. A reduced hymen may be observed in some individuals, just cranial to the external urethral ostium. In small ruminants the vagina is only 10 cm long. Here and in the following subsection, refer again to Figures 2.56, 2.57, 2.58, and 2.59.

The Vestibule

In the cow, the vestibule is from 8 cm to 10 cm long and is caudo-ventrally oriented, hanging over the ischial arch. Therefore, exploration of the vestibule is easier than of the

vagina. On the floor, at the border between the vestibule and the vagina, the urethra opens by the external urethral ostium. The *suburethral diverticulum* (present only in the sow and ruminants) opens in the external urethral orifice. This is a blind sac, 2 cm deep, located behind the urethral orifice. To avoid this sac during the catheterization of the urinary bladder, one must introduce a finger into the diverticulum and pass the catheter over the finger into the urethra. The numerous *minor vestibular glands* open on the floor and lateral walls of the vestibule. Two symmetrical *Gärtner's ducts* usually are located on both sides of the urethral ostium, and in continuation caudally, the two *major vestibular glands* are shown. No major or minor vestibular glands are present in the goat; they are occasionally present in the ewe.

The Vulva and the Clitoris

The labiae of the vulva are thicker in the cow than in the small ruminants, and they are rounded. The ventral commissure is pointed and provided with fine hairs.

The 10 cm- to 12 cm-long clitoris in the cow—2 cm to 2.5 cm long in the small ruminants—is flexuous, practically has no glans, and is located in a very shallow fossa. The free part of the clitoris is slightly projected on the floor of the vulva, and the prepuce is less evident (see the vulva of the cow, ewe, and goat in Figures 2.63, 2.64, and 2.65).

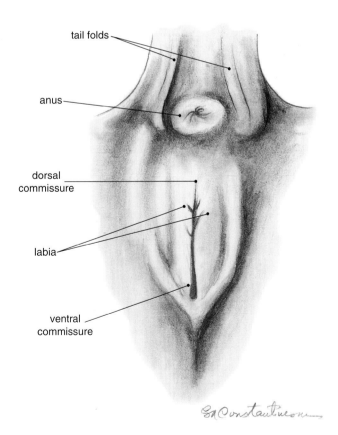

Figure 2.63. The vulva of the cow.

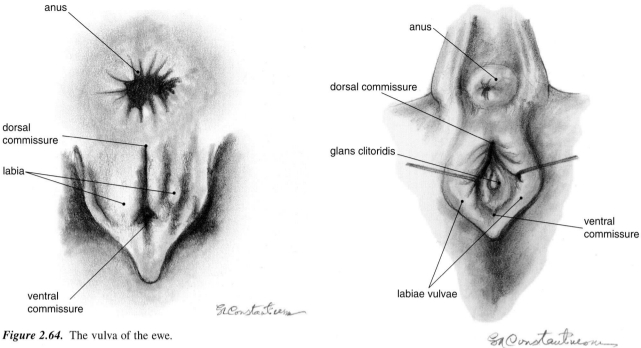

Figure 2.64. The vulva of the ewe.

Figure 2.65. The vulva of the goat.

The Female Urethra

There is no additional information regarding the female urethra (see Figure 2.59) other than the presence of the urethral diverticulum. As far as the blood supply is concerned, the uterine artery can be palpated in the cow by rectal exploration and compressed gently against the ilium bone. In a pregnant cow, if a fremitus is felt, the pregnancy is beyond the third month.

Part 2.6
The Genital Apparatus in the Horse

Male Genitalia

The male genitalia in the horse are presented in four subsections, following the same pattern as was chosen for the general description. Therefore, the first subsection covers the testicle, epididymis, ductus deferens, spermatic cord, and the tunics. The second subsection covers the accessory genital glands, the third subsection the penis, and the last subsection the male urethra.

The Testicle, Epidydimis, Ductus Deferens, Spermatic Cord, and the Tunics

Ovoidal shaped and measuring from 9 cm to 11 cm in length, 6 cm to 7 cm in height, and 5 cm to 6 cm in width, each testicle in the horse can weigh between 100 g and 300 g. The long axis is horizontal only in this species, with the head in the cranial position, and the tail caudal. The mediastinum testis is poorly developed and is closer to the head of the testicle. The proximal and distal mesorchium are separated by the attachment of the mesepididymis (refer to Figures 2.66 through 2.69 for this discussion).

The epididymis is located on the dorsal border of the testicle. The head of the epididymis doesn't exceed the head of the testicle, whereas the tail of the epididymis is very detached. The epididymal canal, which can be as long as 85 m, is the longest in the domestic species. The testicular bursa, the proper ligament of the testicle, the ligament of the tail of the epididymis, and the scrotal ligament are all well defined.

The ductus deferens is from 60 cm to 70 cm long, and the ampulla ranges from 15 cm to 25 cm long, with a diameter of from 2 cm to 2.5 cm. The ampullae, the seminal vesicles, and the two ureters are all together, connected by the genital fold. In the center of the fold, the rudimentary uterus masculinus is usually present in the horse.

The spermatic cord is short (from 12 cm to 13 cm) but voluminous. Vertically oriented in the proximal mesorchium, numerous smooth muscle fibers can be seen with the naked eye through transparency, formerly called internal cremaster muscle.

The cremaster muscle is strong and covers the craniolateral aspect of the thick internal spermatic fascia. The rest of the tunics are similar to those of the other species.

The Accessory Genital Glands

The seminal vesicles correspond to the vesicular glands of the ruminants and the pig (see the accessory genital glands in Figure 2.69). The surface of the seminal vesicles is even and smooth, and they look like 15 cm-long and 4 cm to 5 cm-wide small bladders. For a short distance at the end, the excretory duct of each vesicle joins the ipsilateral ampulla of the ductus deferens, a common duct which is the ejaculatory duct. The apices of the glands either exceed a

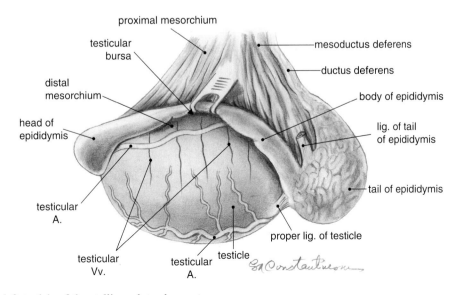

Figure 2.66. The left testicle of the stallion—lateral aspect.

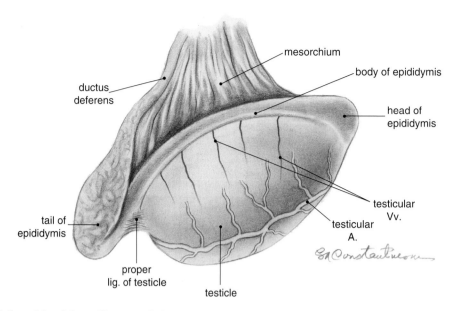

Figure 2.67. The left testicle of the stallion—medial aspect.

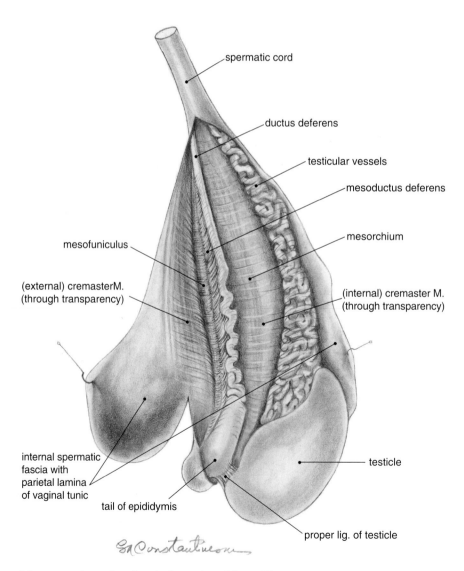

Figure 2.68. The testicle, spermatic cord, and testicular tunics of the stallion.

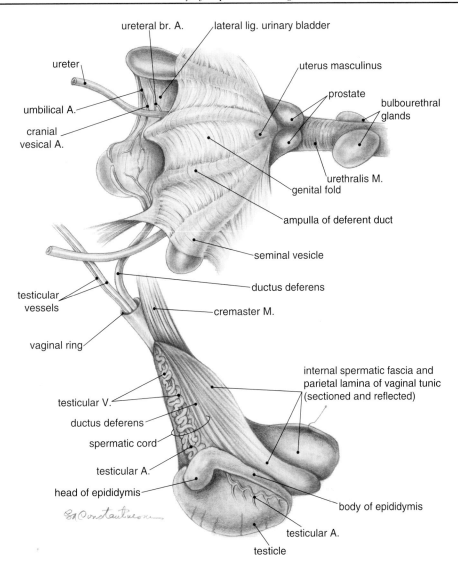

Figure 2.69. The genital apparatus, except the penis, of the stallion.

little the cranial border of the genital fold, or they are totally inside of the genital fold.

The prostate, located retroperitoneally, shows only the compact part, with two lobes connected by a thick isthmus. Each lobe is from 6 cm to 10 cm long and from 3 cm to 5 cm wide.

The bulbourethral glands are ovoidal shaped, from 4 cm to 6 cm long, and from 2 cm to 3 cm wide. The lobes are located on the dorsal aspect of the urethral isthmus (the urethra at the pelvic outlet) in a divergent position caudo-cranially. Covered by the bulboglandularis muscle, each gland opens within the urethra by way of six to eight excretory ducts. The prostate glands are difficult to feel via the rectum.

The Penis

The penis of the horse belongs to the musculocavernous type, with plenty of cavernous spaces and less trabeculae

(see figures 2.70 and 2.71 for this discussion). In a resting position, the penis measures from 50 cm to 60 cm, with 20 cm being held within the prepuce. In erection, the penis can be as long as 80 cm to 90 cm and from 5 cm to 6 cm in diameter.

The root of the penis is well represented by the two strong crura and the bulbus penis. The crura are overlapped by the ischiocavernosus muscles, which, in comparison to those of the bull, are less thick.

Distal to the junction of the crura, the body of the penis is attached to the pelvic symphysis by fibrous laminae from the aponeuroses of the gracilis muscles, collectively called the *suspensory ligament of the penis*. The body is flattened laterally at its origin, while in the free part the penis becomes cylindrical. Specific to the horse, there is a groove on the dorsal aspect of the penis. On the ventral surface, the urethral groove is sculptured to protect the urethra surrounded by the corpus spongiosum penis.

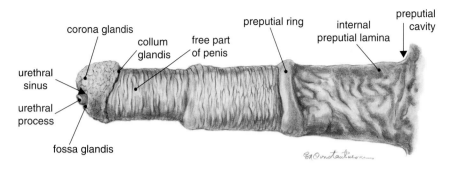

Figure 2.70. The penis of the horse.

The glans penis that contains the corpus spongiosum glandis is voluminous, and the corona glandis can reach the diameter of from 13 cm to 16 cm during erection. The corpus spongiosum glandis is a soft erectile tissue covered by a thin layer of skin, the continuation of the internal lamina of the prepuce. In the horse, the glans penis is a complex and unique structure. The circumference of the glans is called the *corona glandis*. The neck *(collum glandis)* separates the glans from the free part of the penis. Specific to the horse, the urethral process with the external urethral orifice exceeds the glans by 2 cm and is surrounded by the *fossa glandis*. Also in the horse only, the fossa glandis is provided with a dorsal bilobed diverticulum called the *urethral sinus*. An incomplete median ventral septum called the *septum of the glans* connects the urethral process to the glans. The glans covers the corpus cavernosum penis by a

10 cm-long dorsal process, which diminishes in size toward the caudal end.

The prepuce is unique in the horse. The external lamina continues with the internal lamina at the level at which the preputial orifice is outlined, as in any other species; but the internal lamina makes an additional fold called the *preputial fold*. This fold separates the internal lamina from the free part of the penis including the glans penis, and continues with the fine skin on the surface of the free part of the penis. The preputial fold has an external layer and an internal layer. The transition between the two layers outlines the preputial ring, which appears as a thick ring on the surface of the penis protruded from the prepuce. The preputial cavity is the space between the internal lamina of the prepuce and the free part of the penis, in which the preputial fold is lying in the resting position of the penis

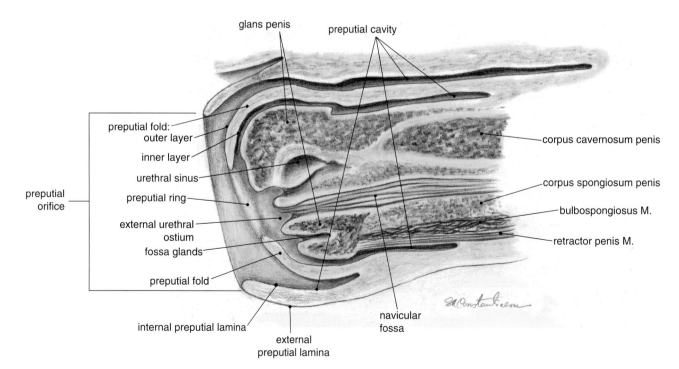

Figure 2.71. Median section through the free part of the penis and of the prepuce in the horse.

inside of the prepuce. There are no preputial muscles in the horse.

The muscles of the penis are similar to those of the other species. The retractor penis muscle is very long and ends at the proximity of the glans penis.

Blood Supply for the Penis

The blood supply of the horse penis is species specific. The penis is supplied by three symmetrical arteries: the external pudendal, the obturator, and the internal pudendal.

The external pudendal artery ends by the superficial caudal epigastric artery that supplies the prepuce, the cranial artery of the penis, and the ventral scrotal branch. The external pudendal artery also anastomoses with the middle artery of the penis (from the obturator artery) and contributes to the dorsal artery of the penis. The terminal branch of the internal pudendal artery is the artery of the penis. This artery branches into the artery of the bulbus penis, the deep artery of the penis and the dorsal artery of the penis. The latter is reinforced by the middle artery of the penis.

The veins are in general satellite to the arteries. On the dorsal aspect of the penis, the veins build up a dorsal venous plexus. In the horse only, there is a connection between the dorsal venous plexus of the penis and the deep femoral vein, called the accessory pudendal vein. The latter perforates the origin of the gracilis muscle on its way to reach the deep femoral vein (see Figure 2.72).

The Male Urethra

In the horse, the whole urethra is from 60 cm to 70 cm long, but the pelvic urethra measures only between 10 cm and 12 cm. The preprostatic and prostatic parts, as well as the urethral isthmus (from the pelvic urethra), have no specific features. The penile urethra surrounded by the corpus spongiosum penis and the urethral process were described with the penis. The bulbus penis in the horse is divided by a median septum. Also in the horse, and only in this species, there is a slight dilation of the urethra near its distal end; this dilation is called the *navicular fossa of the urethra.*

Female Genitalia

The female genitalia in the horse are discussed in seven subsections, starting with the ovaries and ending with the female urethra.

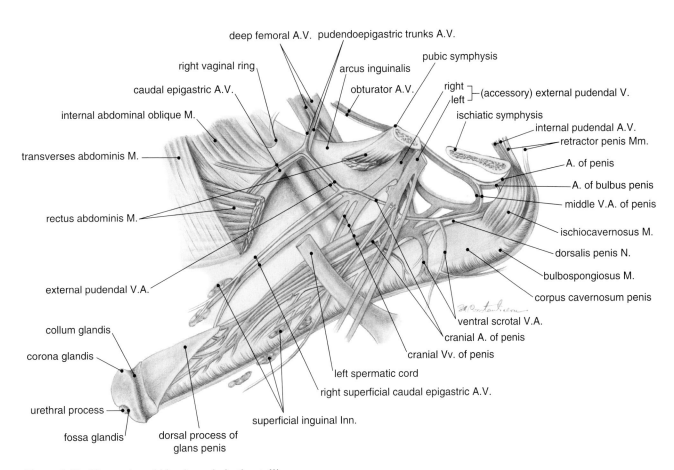

Figure 2.72. The penis and blood supply in the stallion.

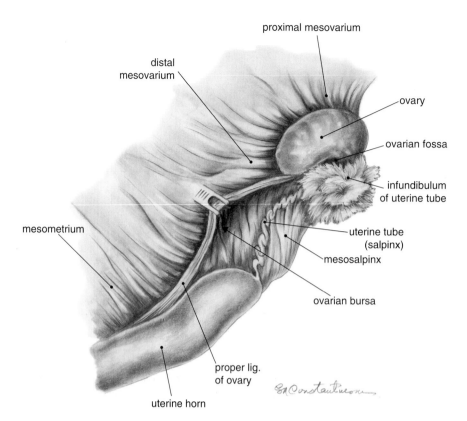

Figure 2.73. The ovary and uterine tube of the mare—medial aspect.

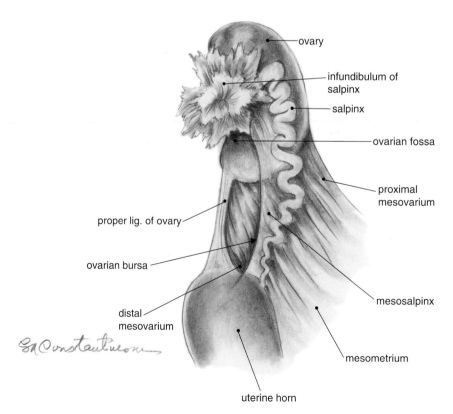

Figure 2.74. The ovary and uterine tube of the mare—ventral aspect.

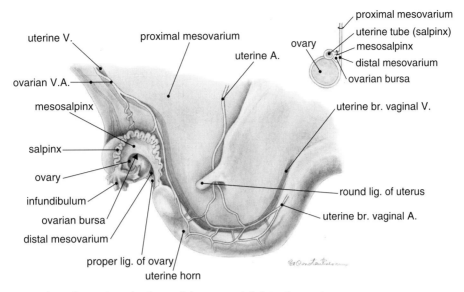

uterine V.
proximal mesovarium
uterine A.
ovary
proximal mesovarium
uterine tube (salpinx)
mesosalpinx
distal mesovarium
ovarian bursa
ovarian V.A.
mesosalpinx
salpinx
ovary
infundibulum
ovarian bursa
distal mesovarium
proper lig. of ovary
uterine horn
uterine br. vaginal V.
round lig. of uterus
uterine br. vaginal A.

Figure 2.75. The ovary, uterine tube, and uterine horn of the mare—left lateral aspect.

The Ovary

The ovary of the mare is totally different from the ovary of the other species (see Figures 2.73, 2.74, and 2.75 for this discussion). The cortex (the parenchymatous zone), which contains the follicles, is central, and the medulla (the vascular zone) is peripheral (see Figure 2.8). Bean-shaped and relatively large (from 5 cm to 8 cm long, 2 cm to 4 cm in diameter), and with an average weight of 60 g each, the ovaries are surrounded by peritoneum. The exception, specific to the mare, is one *ovarian fossa* for each ovary; these fossa are sculpted on the free borders of the ovaries. The free borders are ventrocranially oriented. Some clinicians call the ovarian fossa the ovulation fossa. The ovaries are connected to the corresponding uterine horns by strong and short proper ligaments of the ovaries. The mesovarium is typically divided into a proximal and a distal mesovarium by the attachment of the mesosalpinx.

The ovaries are located from 5 cm to 15 cm caudal to the kidneys, at the level of the 4th and 5th lumbar vertebrae, and 4 cm to 5 cm away from the apices of the uterine horns. For the benefit of the rectal exploration, the right ovary comes in contact with the base of the cecum, sometimes to the duodenum, while the left ovary is surrounded by loops of jejunum or descending colon. The ovarian bursa will be described with the uterine tube.

The Uterine Tube

Very flexuous and between 20 cm and 30 cm long, each uterine tube is connected to the mesovarium by a short mesosalpinx. The fimbriae of the uterine tube surrounding the infundibulum and the abdominal opening are abundant. The ovarian fimbriae are also present. In the mare only, the tube opens into the uterine horn in the center of a small *papilla*, provided with a small *sphincter*. The shallow

ovarian bursa is outlined between the mesosalpinx, the distal mesovarium, the ovary, and the proper ligament of the ovary.

The Uterus

In contrast to the other species, the uterus of the mare has a relatively short but large body, from 14 cm to 25 cm long. Each uterine horn is from 12 cm to 20 cm long, and the cervix is from 5 cm to 8 cm long. In the mare, the cranial end of the body is called the *uterine fundus* because the uterine body is not divided by the uterine velum, as in the other species. The two horns are projected cranially in a divergent position and are slightly curved ventrally. The endometrium of both the body and the horns has longitudinal folds. The cervix is centered by a straight cervical canal, which opens on the very prominent and plicated vaginal portion of the cervix. The endometrium of the cervical canal has many longitudinal folds. Figure 2.76 shows the genital tract of the Mare.

The vaginal portion of the uterine cervix is anchored to the walls of the vagina by vertical folds called *frenula* (singular, *frenulum*). In diestrus and estrus, only the dorsal frenulum can be identified. During pregnancy, a dorsal frenulum and a ventral frenulum anchor the vaginal portion of the cervix to the vaginal fornix (see Figures 2.77 through 2.82 for this discussion).

The horns and the cranial part of the uterus are located within the abdominal cavity, while the rest of the body and the whole cervix are located within the pelvic cavity.

The broad ligament is long and strong, and contains numerous smooth muscle fibers. The round ligament of the uterus originates from the broad ligament close to the apex of each uterine horn. The round ligament is enclosed in a lateral fold of the broad ligament, extends up to the deep

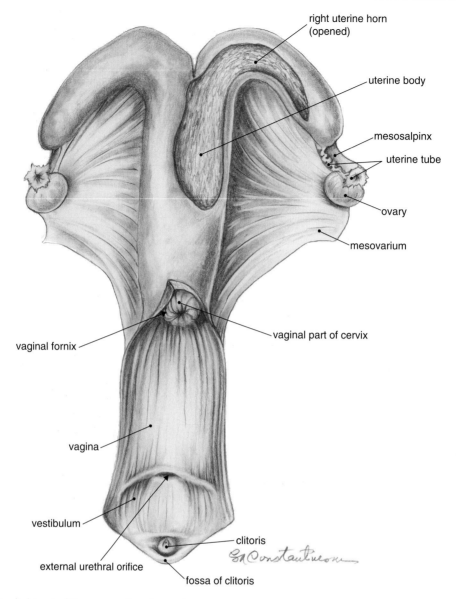

right uterine horn (opened)

uterine body

mesosalpinx

uterine tube

ovary

mesovarium

vaginal part of cervix

vaginal fornix

vagina

vestibulum

clitoris

external urethral orifice

fossa of clitoris

Figure 2.76. The genital tract of the mare—dorsal aspect.

inguinal ring, and looks like an appendix with a rounded end.

The Vagina

In the mare, the vagina (see Figure 2.76) is as long as 20 cm to 25 cm. The fornix is deep because of the extended protrusion of the vaginal portion of the cervix within the vagina. The mucosa has fine longitudinal folds. The hymen is well developed in almost all individuals, has different shapes, and is located just cranial to the external urethral ostium.

The Vestibule

The vestibule and the vulva hangs over the ischial arch. The external urethral ostium is located from 10 cm to 12 cm cranial to the ventral commissure of the vulva. Only the minor vestibular glands are present. The vestibular bulbs are very well developed (5 cm to 6 cm high and 3 cm wide) (see Figure 2.83).

The Vulva and the Clitoris

The labiae of the vulva are usually pigmented, and they contain many sweat and sebaceous glands. The dorsal commissure of the labia is pointed, while the ventral commissure is rounded.

The clitoris is very developed and from 7 cm to 9 cm long. The glans is voluminous, located within the fossa of the clitoris and attached to the prepuce by the frenulum of

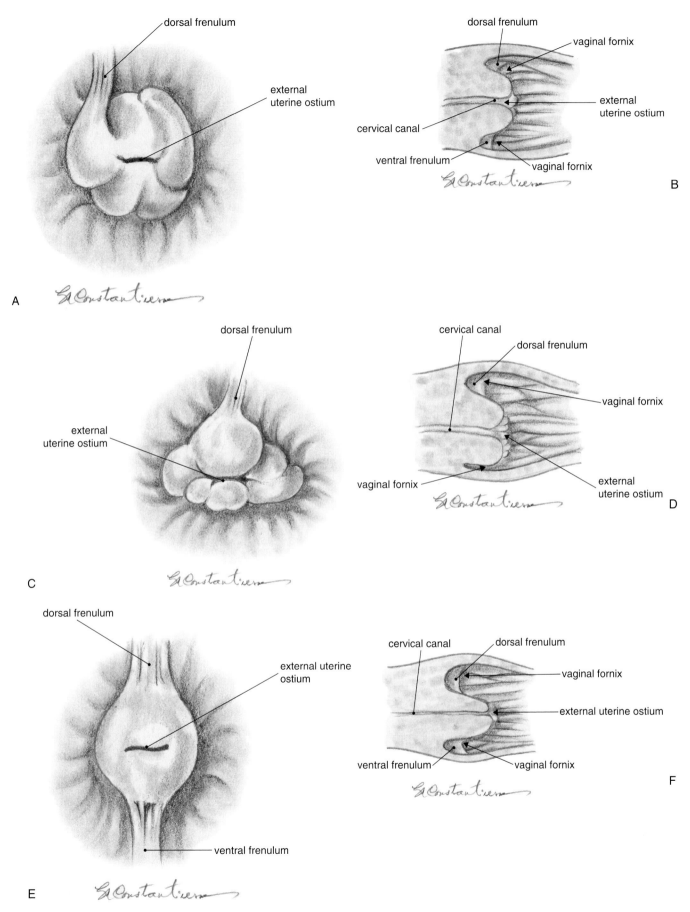

Figure 2.77–2.82. The vaginal part of the cervix in the mare during diestrus, estrus, and pregnancy. *Diestrus:* **A**. The cervix—caudal view. **B**. The vaginal portion of the cervix—median section. *Estrus:* **C**. The cervix—caudal view. **D**. The vaginal portion of the cervix—median section. *Pregnancy:* **E**. The cervix—caudal view. **F**. The vaginal portion of the cervix—median section.

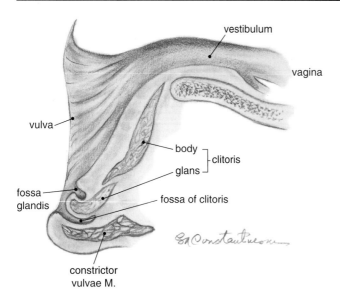

Figure 2.83. The vestibule of the mare—median section.

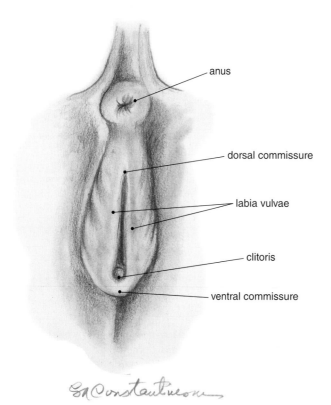

Figure 2.84. The vulva of the mare.

the clitoris. Lateral and ventral recesses can be identified around the glans. If the prepuce is pulled up, one median and two lateral additional sinuses can be identified (see Figures 2.84, 2.85, and 2.86).

Note

The size and weight of different parts of genital systems were adapted from Barone and Nickel, Schummer, Seiferle (op. cit.).

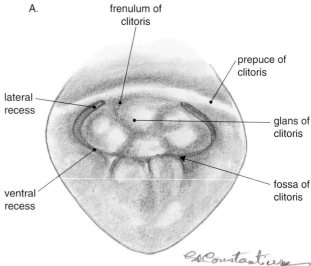

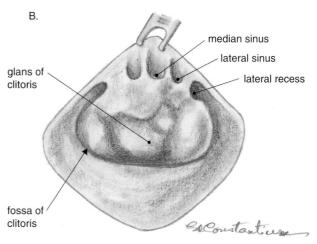

Figure 2.85–2.86. The clitoris of the mare. **A.** The clitoris in situ. **B.** The prepuce reflected.

Bibliography

Ashdown, Raymond R., and Stanley H. Done. 1996. *Color Atlas of Veterinary Anatomy, vol. I–II.* St. Louis: Mosby-Wolfe.

Barone, Robert. 1978. *Anatomie Comparée des Mammifères Domestiques, tome troisième, fascicule II, Appareil Uro-génital,* Lyon, France: Laboratoire d'Anatomie École Nationale Vétérinaire.

Budras, Klaus-Dieter, Wolfgang O. Sack, and Sabine Röck. 1994. *Anatomy of the Horse. An Illustrated Text,* 2nd ed. St. Louis: Mosby-Wolfe.

Budras, Klaus-Dieter, and Robert E. Habel. 2003. *Bovine Anatomy. An Illustrated Text,* 1st ed. Hannover: Schlütersche.

Budras, Klaus-Dieter, et al. 2002. *Anatomy of the Dog. An Illustrated Text,* 4th ed. Hannover: Schlütersche.

Constantinescu, Dan M., and Gheorghe M. Constantinescu. 2000. "Ethologia feto-maternală in timpul parturiției la vacă, cu argumente neurofiziologice pentru folosirea adecvată a technicilor obstetricale." *Analele Institutului de Cercetare şi Producţie pentru Creşterea Bovinelor,* 17:201–214.

Constantinescu, Gheorghe M. 2004. *Teaching Clinical Anatomy of Genital Organs in the Large Animals.* The XXVth Congress of the European Association of Veterinary Anatomists, Oslo, Norway.

Constantinescu, Gheorghe M. 2002. *Clinical Anatomy for Small Animal Practitioners.* Ames, IA: Iowa State University Press.

Constantinescu, Gheorghe M. 2001. *Guide to Regional Ruminant Anatomy Based on the Dissection of the Goat.* Ames, IA: Iowa State University Press.

Constantinescu, Gheorghe M. 1991. *Clinical Dissection Guide for Large Animals.* St. Louis: Mosby-Year Book.

Constantinescu, Gheorghe M., Brian L. Frappier, and Garry E. Brimer. 1996. *Reconsideration and Comparative View of the Internal Cremaster M. in Stallion, Bull, Goat, Boar, and Dog. Anatomia Histologia Embryologia,* 25:218.

Constantinescu Gheorghe M., and Dinu Theodorescu. 1977. *Aspecte practice privind topografia şi ramurile pre-si post-ganglionare ale plexului pelviperineal la vacă.* Symposium, Timişoara, Romania.

Constantinescu, Gheorghe M., Dinu Theodorescu, and Oliviu Fuciu. 1977. *L'anatomie clinique du plexus pelvi-périnéal chez la vache et le mouton. Zbl.für Vet. Med. C, G:367.*

Constantinescu, Gheorghe M., and Ileana A. Constantinescu. 2004. *Clinical Dissection Guide for Large Animals, Horse, and Large Ruminants,* 2nd ed. Ames, IA: Iowa State Press.

Constantinescu, Gheorghe M., Iustin Cosoroabă, and Dan M. Constantinescu. 1969. *Micul bazin la vacă.* Symposium, Timişoara, Romania.

Constantinescu, Gheorghe M., Iustin Cosoroabă, Liviu Rebreanu, Radu Palicica, and Grigore Fărcaş. 1970. *Contribuţii la studiul vascularizaţiei şi inervaţiei aparatului genital la scrofiţe între 0 şi 30 de zile.* Symposium, Timişoara, Romania.

deLahunta, Alexander, and Robert E. Habel. 1986. *Applied Veterinary Anatomy,* Philadelphia: Saunders.

Done, Stanley H., et al. 2000. *Color Atlas of Veterinary Anatomy, vol.3, The Dog and Cat.* St. Louis: Mosby.

Dyce, Keith M., Wolfgang O. Sack, and Cornelius J. G. Wensing. 2002. *Textbook of Veterinary Anatomy,* 3rd ed. Philadelphia: Saunders.

Ellenberger, Wilhelm, and Herman Baum. 1943. *Handbuch der vergleichenden Anatomie der Haustiere,* 18. Aufl., Berlin: Springer.

Evans, Howard. 1993. *Miller's Anatomy of the Dog,* 3rd ed., p. 527. Philadelphia: Saunders.

Getty, Robert. 1975. *Sisson and Grossman's The Anatomy of the Domestic Animals, vol.* 2, 5th ed. Philadelphia: Saunders.

Gheţie, Vasile, and Gheorghe M. Constantinescu. 1960. *Die morpho-physiologischen Grundlagen der Sexualreflexe beim Stier. Zuchthygiene* 4:285–291.

Gheţie, Vasile, Eugeniu Paştea, and Ilie T. Riga. 1955. *Anatomia Topografică a Calului,* Bucureşti: Editura Agro-Silvică de Stat.

Habel, Robert E. 1989. *Guide to the Dissection of Domestic Ruminants,* 4th ed. Ithaca, N.Y.: Robert E. Habel.

König, Horst E. 1992. *Anatomie der Katze,* Stuttgart: Fischer.

König, Horst E., and Hans-Georg Liebich. 2004. *Veterinary Anatomy of Domestic Mammals. Textbook and Colour Atlas.* Stuttgart: Schattauer.

Nickel, Richard, August Schummer, and Eugen Seiferle. 1979–1981. *The Anatomy of the Domestic Animals, vol. II* 2nd ed., *vol. III.* Berlin—Hamburg: Parey.

Nomina Anatomica Veterinaria. 5th edition. 2005. World Association of Veterinary Anatomists. Available on Website.

Palicica, Radu, Gheorghe M. Constantinescu, Tiberiu Ajtony, and Corneliu Radu. 1979. *Variaţii ale vascularizaţiei arteriale şi venoase ale aparatului genital la scroaf*ă. 2nd Symposium of Anatomy, Cluj-Napoca, Romania.

Popescu, Petre, Virgil Paraipan, and Valeriu Nicolescu. 1958. "Anestezia subsacrală la taur şi cal. In *Animal Anaesthesia, vol. 1,* edited by Melchior Westhues and Rudolf Fritsch. 1964, pp. 179–180. Edinburgh and London: Oliver and Boyd.

Radu, Corneliu, Gheorghe M. Constantinescu, Carmen Trandafir, and Radu Palicica. 1980. *Vascularizaţia aparatului genital femel la oaie.* Symposium Timişoara, Romania.

Rebreanu, Liviu, Gheorghe M. Constantinescu, Iustin Cosoroabă, Radu Palicica, and Grigore Fărcaş. 1970. *Cercetări de splanchnologie cantitativă la purcei între 0 şi 30 de zile: Aparatul genital mascul.* Symposium, Timişoara, Romania.

Rebreanu, Liviu, Radu Palicica, Iustin Cosoroabă, Gheorghe M. Constantinescu, and Grigore Fărcaş. 1972. "Splanchnolgia cantitativă la purcel: Aparatul genital femel." *Lucrări ştiinţifice ale Institutului Agronomic Timişoara seria Medicină Veterinar*ă 13:51–59.

Sack, Wolfgang O. 1991. *Rooney's Guide to the Dissection of the Horse,* 6th ed. Ithaca, N.Y.: Veterinary Textbooks.

Schaller, Oskar. 1992. *Illustrated Veterinary Anatomical Nomenclature.* Stuttgart: Enke.

Youngquist, Robert S., and W. R. Threlfall. 2007. *Current Therapy in Large Animal Theriogenology, Second Edition.* Saunders Elsevier.

Chapter 3

Histology, Cellular and Molecular Biology of Reproductive Organs

Heide Schatten, chapter editor

Part 3.1
Introduction to Histology, Cellular and Molecular Biology

Heide Schatten

Histology refers to the microscopic study of biological material and is employed to analyze cells and tissues that compose the various organs. In recent years, histology has increasingly included the study of tissue functions on cellular and molecular levels. Numerous staining techniques are available to investigate the mechanisms that underlie the variety of different functions that are carried out by cell organelles, cellular structures, macromolecular complexes, and other cellular components. In this concept, tissues, cells, and molecular pathways are visualized and analyzed by various microscopy methods, including the classic eosin-hematoxylin staining, and molecular tracers and probes that use fluorescence and immunofluorescence microscopy, electron microscopy, immunoelectron microscopy, autoradiography, in situ hybridization, and others.

Cellular and molecular aspects, staining methods, the histology of tissues that comprise the male and female reproductive systems, and fertilization will be presented in this section and those that follow in this chapter.

The Cell, Cellular Organelles, and Their Functions

Multicellular organisms are composed of cells that contain typical substructures as pictured in the first diagram. Figure 3.1 represents a basic overview of a cell in which the specific cellular components are shown.

The cellular organelles and cellular structures that are seen here are described as follows:

Cell membranes determine structural and biochemical boundaries of a cell and of cell organelles; cell membranes consist of lipids and proteins. The phospholipid bilayer is the basic membrane structure in which proteins are embedded. Most membranes consist of about 50 percent lipid and 50 percent protein, which represents a fluid mosaic model

in which both proteins and lipids are able to diffuse in lateral movements. Although the lipid bilayer is the fundamental structure, various peripheral and integral membrane proteins are responsible for the variations in membrane composition and play a significant role in transport and signal transduction.

In transmission electron microscopy, membranes are typically stained like railroad tracks, in which the outer lipophilic areas of the membrane stain heavily with osmium tetroxide, leaving the enclosed lipophobic area pale (for detailed information, see selected reading of books by Hayatt, 2000; Kessel and Smith, 1974; Banks, 1993; Kierszenbaum, 2002; and references within). More recently, fluorescence and immunofluorescence microscopy have been used to identify membranes and specific membrane components (for detailed information, see selected reading of books by Javois, 1999; Lacey, 1999; Alberts et al., 2002; Pollard and Earnshaw, 2002; Lodish et al., 2003; and references within).

The endoplasmic reticulum (ER) is characterized by a network of membranous tubes that traverse the entire cell. Rough ER (rER) is stubbed with ribosomes that are involved in protein synthesis. Smooth ER (sER) lacks ribosomes and is involved in detoxification processes.

The **Golgi apparatus** consists of stacks of membranous cisternae that are distributed throughout the cell. The main function of the Golgi complex is to modify and package proteins with specific functions to add oligosaccharides to proteins and lipids. The Golgi apparatus plays a major role in secretion. Vesicles derived from the Golgi complex serve as secretory and transport vesicles to shuttle components to the plasma membrane. Increased Golgi activity is seen in cells with abundant secretion.

The cell nucleus is the largest cellular organelle; it is distinguished from most other cellular organelles by a

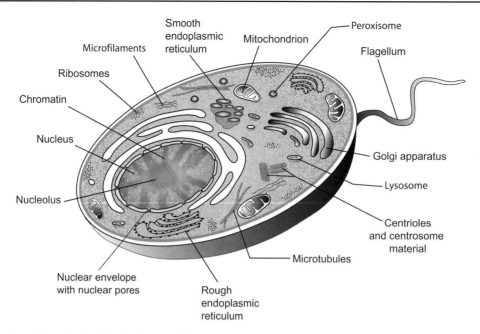

Figure 3.1. Overview of a typical cell and cell organelles.

double membrane organized around nuclear material that consists primarily of highly decondensed *chromatin*, one or several *nucleoli*, and *nuclear matrix* components. The inner nuclear membrane is associated with nuclear lamins, which are related to intermediate filaments (described below), while the outer nuclear membrane is continuous with endoplasmic reticulum. Nuclear pores are one prominent feature of the nuclear envelope. These tripartite structures embedded in the nuclear envelope allow transport of macromolecules in and out of the nucleus. Molecules smaller than 40 kD to 60 kD can diffuse through the nuclear pore complex freely. *Chromatin* consists primarily of very small particulate structures (nucleosomes that consist of histone octamer cores) organized on a double-stranded DNA string. Highly decondensed chromatin (called euchromatin; approximately 10 percent chromatin) is transcriptionally active and is the site for nonribosomal RNAs (mRNAs and tRNAs). Dense chromatin (called heterochromatin; about 90 percent chromatin) is transcriptionally inactive. Basic proteins (histones) and nonhistone chromosomal proteins are associated with chromatin.

Highly condensed chromatin is organized into chromosomes that are densely stained during meiosis and mitosis. The *nucleolus* is involved in ribosome and other ribonucleoprotein synthesis. The nucleolus is organized into three different zones, described as the granular region (pars granulosa), the fibrillar region, and the dense fibrillar region (pars fibrosa). Within the nucleus are nuclear matrix components, which are proteins thought to play a role in DNA transcription and replication.

Mitochondria are organelles of about 0.2 μm by 18 μm in size (approximately 1,000 to 10,000 per somatic cell) enveloped by a double membrane. Mature MII stage oocytes contain 90,000 to 350,000 mitochondria that arise during oogenesis from as few as 10 mitochondria in primary oocytes (reviewed in Schatten et al., 2005). The outer membrane of mitochondria is smooth and unfolded, while the inner membrane is highly complex and folded into cristae that project into the mitochondrial matrix. Mitochondria with tubular cristae are typically seen in steroid-producing cells such as the corpus luteum in the ovary and Leydig cells in the testis.

Mitochondria are often called the "powerhouses" of a cell. The inner mitochondrial membrane contains the enzymes for oxidative phosphorylation that play a role in the production of chemical energy in the form of ATP. Mitochondrial enzymes are also involved in programmed cell death (apoptosis, described below). Mitochondria contain DNA that shares similarities with bacterial DNA. Mitochondrial DNA is inherited maternally (strictly from the oocyte; paternal mitochondria are destroyed after fertilization) and is highly conserved. Proteins involved in mitochondrial structure and functions are encoded by both mitochondrial and nuclear DNA. Mitochondrial DNA is used in paternity tests and forensic applications.

In light microscopy, mitochondria can be visualized after staining with Janus Green B. More recently, Mito-Tracker staining is used to fluorescently label mitochondria and view them with fluorescence microscopy (as shown in Part 5 of this chapter, "Overview of Fertilization"; and in Katayama et al., 2006; Sun et al., 2001).

Lysosomes are membrane-bounded organelles with approximately 40 types of hydrolytic enzymes that function in an acidic environment (with a pH of about 5) and play a role in the degradation of proteins, nucleic acids, oligosaccharides, and phospholipids.

Peroxisomes are membrane-bounded vesicles that contain approximately 50 different enzymes that play a role in the synthesis of lipids, bile acids, and phospholipids. They also play a role in detoxification.

Ribosomes are 15×25 nm particles that are composed of a large and small subunit. They are the main cellular components for protein synthesis. Ribosomes can be seen freely dispersed in the cytoplasm, grouped into polysomes, or bound to endoplasmic reticulum (rER).

Glycogen particles are cell inclusions that are the major storage form of carbohydrate. They can be found as single particles or as multiple particles that form rosettes. Glycogen can be detected by light microscopy after staining with periodic acid-Schiff (PAS) reaction or Best's Carmine stain.

Lipids are cell inclusions that are stored in a variety of cell types, particularly in steroid-producing cells. Lipids are abundantly present in pig oocytes.

Glycocalyx is an extracellular domain of the plasma membrane that protects the cell surface and facilitates cell-to-cell interactions.

Annulate Lamellae are stacks of membrane cisternae that are characteristic of germ cells. Although their function is not entirely clear, it is thought that annulate lamellae provide stored membrane material needed in rapidly dividing germ cells.

The cytoskeleton is of particular importance in cell biology and modern histology because it plays multiple roles in numerous biological processes. The cytoskeleton is a complex, three-dimensional network of protein fibers that carries out numerous functions and is involved in cell motility, structural support, and changes in cell shape, signal transduction, phagocytosis, meiosis and mitosis, cell division, and many other processes.

The three major components of the cytoskeleton are microtubules (25 nm in diameter), intermediate filaments (10 nm in diameter) and microfilaments (7 nm in diameter); they are tube-like microstructures composed of their subunits, tubulin, actin, and intermediate filament monomers

and dimers, respectively. Numerous cytoskeleton-associated proteins are involved in carrying out specific cytoskeletal functions, including anchoring to the cell surface, interacting with each other, and severing preformed filaments.

All three cytoskeletal components play crucial roles in cell cycle progression. Microtubules and microfilaments are essential components for mitosis and meiosis, while intermediate filaments predominantly serve structural and signaling functions. Intermediate filaments are seen organized around the nucleus and in cellular junctions. A modified form of intermediate filaments is found underneath the nuclear envelope and composes the nuclear lamins.

Other critically important components of the cytoskeleton include centrosomes (for recent reviews, see Sun and Schatten, 2006a,b). Centrosomes are centers that nucleate, anchor, and organize microtubules. They are composed of numerous centrosomal proteins that typically surround a pair of centrioles, microtubule-based structures that resemble the structure of cilia (described in the next section); but centrosomes are composed of nine outer microtubule triplets and no central microtubules. Centrosomes undergo cell cycle-specific reorganization (reviewed in Sun and Schatten, 2006a,b).

While some centrosome proteins such as gamma-tubulin are permanently associated with centrosome structure, others are transiently associated with centrosome structure to perform cell cycle-specific centrosome functions. Transient centrosome proteins can be of nuclear or cytoplasmic origin (reviewed in Sun and Schatten, 2006a,b). The contribution of centrosomal proteins by egg and sperm cells has recently been reviewed by Manandhar et al. (2005). The following diagram (Figure 3.2) shows a typical organization of microfilaments, intermediate filaments, and microtubules within somatic cells.

The Cell Cycle

Although most somatic cells reside in a relatively quiescent state, renewal of cells takes place daily and follows specific and well-regulated events that are summarized as the cell

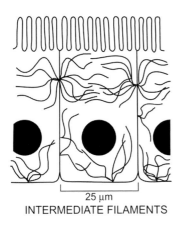
25 μm
INTERMEDIATE FILAMENTS

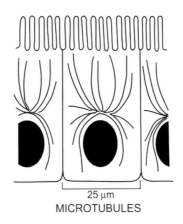
25 μm
MICROTUBULES

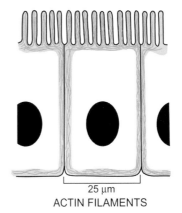
25 μm
ACTIN FILAMENTS

Figure 3.2. Cytoskeletal organization in epithelial cells.

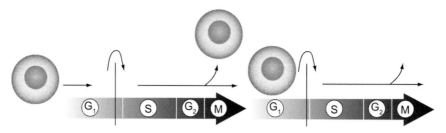

Figure 3.3. Phases of a typical cell cycle.

cycle. A typical cell cycle takes approximately 24 hours in mammalian cells. Two major phases are distinguished in a typical cell cycle; these phases are termed interphase and mitosis.

The interphase cycle is grouped into three phases characterized by specific events that are centered on DNA replication, the S (DNA synthesis) phase. The phase prior to DNA synthesis is called G1 (gap 1), and the phase following DNA synthesis is called G2 (gap 2). G1 contains one set of DNA (2n = diploid) and G2 contains two sets of DNA (4n). G1 and G2 are phases for cell growth to double

cell mass, prepare for DNA synthesis (G1), and provide check mechanisms (G2) before cells are allowed to enter into mitosis. Mitosis is the shortest phase of the cell cycle (see Figures 3.3 and 3.4).

Mitosis is grouped into four phases characterized by specific events that refer to the organization of microtubules by centrosomes into the mitotic apparatus, chromosome condensation, positioning, and reorganization into the reconstituted daughter cell nucleus. The main phases of mitosis are prophase, metaphase, anaphase, and telophase (see Figures 3.3, 3.4, and 3.5).

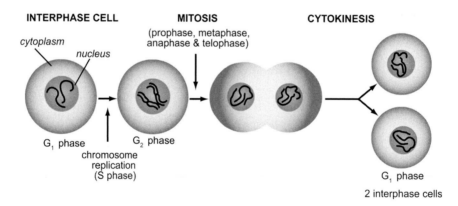

Figure 3.4. Interphase cells from G1 to cell division.

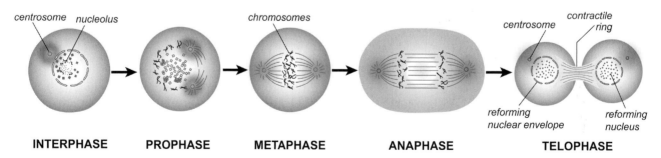

Figure 3.5. A cell undergoing mitosis and cell division. The nuclear envelope breaks down during prophase, chromatin condenses into chromosomes, and centrosomes move to the opposite poles. In metaphase, condensed chromosomes are organized at the metaphase plate and centrosomes are organized at the two mitotic poles. During anaphase, chromosomes move toward the two mitotic poles. Telophase describes the reformation of nuclei followed by cell division.

- Prophase is characterized by nuclear envelope breakdown, the beginning of chromosome condensation, centrosome splitting, and microtubule formation into the mitotic apparatus.
- Metaphase is characterized by maximally condensed chromosomes that are aligned at the central (metaphase) plate while microtubules are organized into the metaphase spindle by centrosomes that are positioned at the two opposite poles of the cell.
- Anaphase is characterized by chromosome separation to the opposite poles toward centrosomes while the spindle becomes reorganized into an anaphase spindle.
- Telophase is the last phase of mitosis, during which chromosomes decondense and become reorganized into daughter nuclei.

These highly dynamic mitotic events are followed by cell division, which results in two daughter cells with newly formed interphase nuclei. Cells that do not commit to DNA synthesis remain in a resting stage that is also called G0 and can be maintained for various lengths of time, often years.

Numerous cell-cycle control proteins and cell-cycle check points serve as assurances and regulators for accurate cell-cycle control. A Cdk2/cyclin B complex is one of the major triggers for cells to enter mitosis. Somatic cells have diploid sets of chromosomes; germ cells (male and female) have a haploid number of chromosomes. To achieve haploidy, diploid precursor cells undergo a process termed meiosis during which the number of chromosomes is reduced to haploidy (1n) (for review, see Yanagamachi, 1994). Diploidy is restored after fertilization when sperm and egg unite.

Apoptosis

Apoptosis (programmed cell death) is a programmed elimination of cells that are either damaged, affected by disease, or destined for destruction during embryo development. Precise genetic and molecular mechanisms are initiated to eliminate specific cells by coordinated signal transduction events. Cytochrome C released from mitochondria is one of the major triggers for programmed cell death.

Transmission electron microscopy has been used as a reliable technique to determine the morphological characteristics associated with apoptosis, which include local condensation and degradation of chromatin, destruction of the cytoskeleton by caspases, clustering of nuclear pores, and sequestration of chromatin into membrane-bound apoptotic bodies that are phagocytosed by macrophages. No inflammation is associated with apoptosis; this is different from necrosis, in which cell injury results in random cell destruction accompanied by inflammation.

Stem Cells

Stem cells are multipotent, undifferentiated cell populations that have properties of self-renewal, proliferation, and differentiation. Stem cells have been identified in numerous tissues where they are responsible for renewing diseased cells. It is thought that stem cells are also present in reproductive tissues.

Epithelial Tissue

The *epithelium* is a functional layer of cells that covers and lines organ surfaces and secretory glands. It is attached to the underlying connective tissue by the basement membrane. Three major categories of epithelia are distinguished based on the number of cell layers and shapes of cells.

- *Simple epithelia* are composed of one layer of cells and can be subdivided into simple squamous, simple cuboidal, and simple columnar, which refer to the height and width of cells. The term *endothelium* is used for the lining of blood and lymphatic vessels. The term *mesothelium* is used to describe the lining of all body cavities.
- *Stratified epithelia* consist of two or more cell layers. The shape of cells in the outer layer is used to describe the subdivisions into *stratified squamous*, *stratified cuboidal*, and *stratified columnar*.
- *Pseudostratified epithelia* are composed of basal and columnar cells that are layered onto the basal lamina. Pseudostratified columnar epithelium with stereocilia is visible in the epididymis of the male reproductive system. The basic epithelial classifications are presented in Figure 3.6.

This conventional classification of epithelial cells describes the basic morphology, but there are functional differences within epithelia of different organs. The epithelium is functionally highly significant because it serves important roles that include absorption and secretion, and it is a dynamic barrier for water and gas exchange. The ultrastructure of a typical epithelial cell reflects the functions as seen in surface modifications, number of cell organelles, and other characteristics. Tissue polarity refers to the domains of cells that are exposed to different microenvironments that influence tissue and organ functions. The *apical* domain of epithelial cells refers to the side that faces the lumen or external environment; the *lateral* domain interacts with surrounding cells through adhesion molecules and junctional complexes; the *basal* domain interacts with the underlying connective tissue and is typically associated with the basal lamina.

The polarity of epithelial cells is functionally highly important because functions between the internal and external environment vary, and different functions are required for different tissue organizations. Three major external epithelial cell surface modifications (*cilia, microvilli, stereocilia*) are known to serve varied cell functions in different tissue.

- Cilia are motile surface extensions composed primarily of microtubules that allow bending and cilia motility. Cilia are 0.2 µm in diameter and between 5 µm and 15 µm in length. In reproductive systems, ciliated

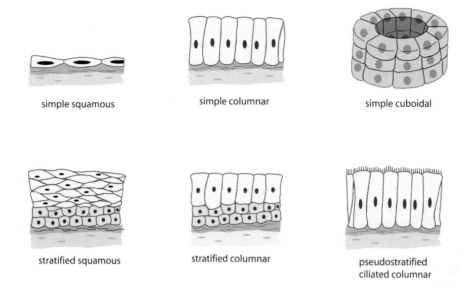

simple squamous

simple columnar

simple cuboidal

stratified squamous

stratified columnar

pseudostratified
ciliated columnar

Figure 3.6. Typical epithelial cell organizations.

epithelial cells are primarily found in the oviduct to allow transport of the fertilized egg to the uterine cavity. Other mechanisms may also play a role in this motility. A modified form of cilia is found in the sperm tail, where a set of nine doublet outer microtubules and two single central microtubules are the primary cytoskeletal components that allow sperm tail motility. Flagella can be a few hundred micrometers in length. A cross section of a cilium is shown in Figure 3.7.
- Microvilli are finger-like cell surface projections primarily composed of microfilaments. Microvilli are

approximately 0.1 μm in diameter and have various lengths. Microvilli abundantly line the intestine and are seen on the surface of cells. In the reproductive system, microvilli are seen at the luminal surface of the epididymis epithelium and on the surface of oocytes and embryos. Oocytes are densely stubbed with microvilli except for a small area that overlies the meiotic spindle.
- Stereocilia have the same substructure as microvilli, but not as cilia (as the name might suggest), and they do not contain microtubules. The major components of stereo-

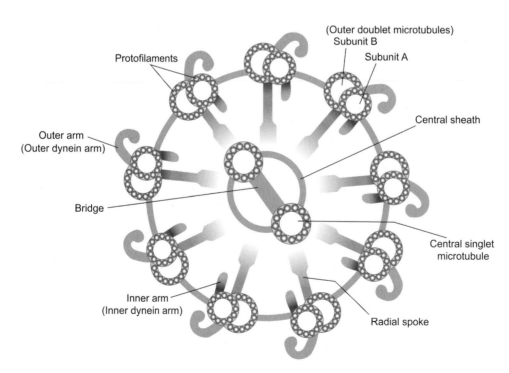

Figure 3.7. Cross-section through a cilium or flagellum.

cilia are microfilaments. Stereocilia are typical of the epithelial lining of the epididymis. They play a role in sperm maturation.

Several cell-adhesion molecules for inter-epithelial cell contact and cell junctions are associated with epithelial cell assemblies. Cell-adhesion molecules include Ca^{++}-dependent molecules such as cadherins and selectins, and Ca^{++}-independent molecules such as the immunoglobulin superfamily and integrins. Cell junctions provide stronger stability between cells and allow the movement of solutes, ions, and water. They are symmetrical structures between two cells; they can be divided into three major classes:

1. occluding junctions or tight junctions
2. anchoring junctions
3. gap or communicating junctions

These junctions can be well discerned on an ultrastructural level using transmission electron microscopy. Freeze-fracturing is a most useful technique to visualize occluding junctions. Dysfunctional cell junctions are associated with various diseases.

The *basement membrane* is the supporting sheet for most epithelia and is composed of laminin and fibronectin, two distinct proteins of the extracellular matrix associated with collagens, proteoglycans, and other proteins. The basement membrane is well recognizable with electron microscopy and can be visualized clearly in light microscopy with periodic acid-Schiff (PAS) stain. Immunocytochemical localization of antigens is commonly used to identify components in cells and tissue.

Epithelial Glands

Epithelial glands are generally classified into simple and compound glands. Simple epithelial glands are characterized by having their secretory area connected to the surface by an unbranched duct. They are subclassified into simple tubular glands, simple coiled tubular glands, simple tubular branched glands, and simple acinar or alveolar glands. Compound glands are characterized by branching ducts that contain secretary products.

Compound glands are classified into compound tubuloacinar glands, compound tubular glands, and compound alveolar glands. Most glands develop as epithelial outgrowth into the underlying connective tissue. Exocrine glands remain connected to the surface, while endocrine glands do not have an excretory duct. Examples of compound glands in the reproductive system are found in the prostate.

Cytology Methods

Many classic cytology methods are used for routine analysis (for detailed information, see Banks, 1993), including the classic eosin-hematoxylin staining. Immunofluorescence and fluorescence microscopy have become more frequently used techniques in recent years and are employed to analyze specific molecules with powerful and specific immunological and molecular probes. In this concept, specific fluorescent molecular markers are employed that either directly label the structure of interest, or they allow detection of the specific reactions, and, therefore, detection of the specific antigen, by using an antigen-antibody reaction followed by a fluorescently tagged second antibody staining (for detailed information, see Javois, 1999).

Examples of the most commonly used fluorescent labels are MitoTracker to label mitochondria, DAPI or Hoechst to label DNA, the anti-tubulin antibody to label microtubules, the anti-actin antibody to label microfilaments, and numerous others. The basic techniques have been extended to analyze live cells. Various modifications of fluorescence microscopy approaches include fluorescence recovery after photobleaching (FRAP) to study dynamic processes and fluorescence energy transfer (FRET) to study relationships between neighboring molecules within cells, among many others. Instrumentation that is used for analysis includes standard epifluorescence, confocal, or multiphoton microscopy.

The most commonly used classic stains include the periodic-acid-Schiff (PAS) reaction, which provides magenta staining to identify 1,2-glycol or 1,2-aminoalcohol groups that are found in glycogen, mucus, and glycoproteins. PAS is used preferentially to recognize the basement membrane that consists of laminin and fibronectin. Eosin stains many basic proteins. *Toluidine blue* is used to identify DNA and RNA, while the *Feulgen reaction* is specific for the localization of DNA. *Autoradiography* relies on radioactive labeling of a precursor, which is used to analyze synthesis of specific processes, such as DNA synthesis. This analysis uses radioactive thymidine labeling as the precursor.

Scanning and transmission electron microscopy are employed for *ultrastructural analysis* (Goldstein et al., 2003; Kierszenbaum, 2002). Both methods require fixation with strong protein crosslinkers such as glutaraldehyde. Scanning electron microscopy allows analysis of surface structures including internal structures that have been isolated or obtained by fracturing. Transmission electron microscopy allows analysis of thin-sectioned biological material that is stained with heavy metals, a process that typically is achieved by postfixation with osmium tetroxide and staining with uranyl acetate. Immunoelectron microscopy mainly employs antigen-antibody reactions. This is followed by labeling with secondary antibodies that are tagged with electron-dense gold particles of various sizes that typically range from 1nm to 20nm (this labeling is generally referred to as "immunogold labeling").

Acknowledgments

The author gratefully acknowledges Don Connor's help with the illustrations.

Bibliography

Alberts, B., Johnson, A., Lewis, J., Raff, M., Roberts, K., and Walter, P. (2002). *Molecular Biology of the Cell 4th edition.* New York and London: Garland Publishing Inc.

Banks, William, J. (1993). *Applied Veterinary Histology, 3rd edition.* St. Louis, London, Philadelphia, Sydney, Toronto: Mosby.

Goldstein, J., Newbury, D., Joy, D., Lyman, C., Echlin, P., Lifshin, E., Sawyer, L., and Michael, J. (2003). *Scanning Electron Microscopy and X-Ray Microanalysis.* New York, Boston, Dordrecht, London, Moscow: Kluwer Academic/Plenum Publishers.

Hayat, M.A. (2000). *Principles and Techniques of Electron Microscopy: Biological Applications, 4th edition.* Cambridge, UK: Cambridge University Press.

Javois, L.C. (1999). *Immunocytochemical Methods and Protocols.* Totowa, NJ: Humana Press.

Katayama, M., Zhong, Z.-S., Lai, L., Sutovsky, P., Prather, R.S., and Schatten, H. (2006). Mitochondrial distribution and microtubule organization in fertilized and cloned porcine embryos: Implications for developmental potential. *Dev. Biol.,* 299:206-220.

Kessel, R.G., and Smith, C.Y. (1974). *Scanning Electron Microscopy in Biology. A Students' Atlas on Biological Organization.* (With 22 Figures and 132 Plates). New York, Heidelberg, Berlin: Springer Verlag.

Kierszenbaum, A.L. (2002). *Histology and Cell Biology. An Introduction to Pathology.* St. Louis, London, Philadelphia, Sydney, Toronto: Mosby.

Lacey, A.J. (1999). *Light Microscopy in Biology. A Practical Approach.* Oxford, New York, Melbourne: Oxford University Press.

Lodish, H., Berk, A., Matsudaira, P., Kaiser, C.A., Krieger, M., Scott, M.P., Zipursky, S.L., and Darnell, J. (2003). *Molecular Cell Biology 5th edition.* New York: Freeman and Company.

Manandhar, G., Schatten, H., and Sutovsky, P. (2005). Centrosome reduction during gametogenesis and its significance. *Biol. Repro.,* 72:2–13.

Schatten, H., Prather, R.S., and Sun, Q.-Y. (2005). The significance of mitochondria for embryo development in cloned farm animals. *Mitochondrion* 5:303–321.

Sun, Q.-Y., and Schatten, H. (2006a). Centrosome inheritance after fertilization and nuclear transfer in mammals. In: Sutovsky, P. (ed). *Somatic Cell Nuclear Transfer,* New York: Springer.

Sun, Q.-Y., and Schatten, H. (2006b). Multiple roles of NuMA in vertebrate cells: Review of an intriguing multifunctional protein. *Frontiers in Bioscience* 11:1137-1146.

Sun, Q.-Y., Wu, G.M., Lai, L., Park, K.W., Day, B., Prather, R.S., and Schatten, H. (2001). Translocation of active mitochondria during pig oocyte maturation, fertilization, and early embryo development *in vitro.* Reproduction 122:155–163.

Pollard, T.D., and Earnshaw, W.C. (2002). *Cell Biology.* Philadelphia: Saunders.

Yanagimachi, R. (1994). Mammalian fertilization. In: Knobil, E., Neill, J.D. (eds). *The Physiology of Reproduction, 2nd edition, Vol. 1.* New York: Raven Press, pp 189–317.

Whitaker, M. (2006). Calcium at fertilization and in early development. *Physoiol. Rev* 86:25–88.

Part 3.2
Overview of Male Reproductive Organs

Cheryl S. Rosenfeld

The following overview of the male reproductive organs focuses on (1) the *testes*, which produce sperm and synthesize and secrete androgens; (2) the *epididymis, ductus (vas) deferens, ejaculatory duct*, and part of the *male urethra*, which are essential for transport of spermatozoa; (3) accessory glands, the *ampulla of the ductus deferens*, the *seminal vesicle (vesicular gland)*, the *prostate gland*, and the *bulbourethral (Cowper's) glands*, whose secretions provide nutrients to the ejaculated spermatozoa; and (4) the *penis*, the erectile tissue that forms the copulatory organ. The male reproductive system also includes the *prepuce*, which is typical skin that surrounds the penis, and the *scrotum*, which is the skin that encases the testes. The two main functions of the male reproductive system are production and transport of spermatozoa, and synthesis of testosterone and other hormones (for review of these systems, see Eurell and Frappier, 2006).

The Testes

The testes are comprised of two main areas: the connective tissue and vascular layers that associate and penetrate into the testes, and the parenchyma region that contains the convoluted seminiferous and straight tubules, which produce and transport the spermatozoa, respectively.

Connective Tissue and Vascular Layers Associated with the Testes

The *tunica vaginalis*, which includes the parietal and visceral lamina layers, surrounds each of the testes. The visceral lamina includes the mesothelial cells and underlying basement membrane. This layer blends insensibly into the *tunica albuginea* (see Figures 3.8 and 3.9), which is composed of dense, irregular connective tissue (DICCT) that also surrounds the epididymis (for review, see Eurell and Frappier, 2006). Branches of the testicular artery and pampiniform plexus (testicular vein) penetrate into this connective tissue layer.

These vascular areas are termed the *tunica vasculosa*, and they may be superficial or deep within the parenchyma of the testis (see Figures 3.9 and 3.10). Radiating from the tunica albuginea are thin connective tissue strands, called *septula*, that connect the tunica albuginea with the *mediastinum*, a connective tissue layer in the center of the testis. The septula divide the testis into lobules. The *rete testis* is located within the mediastinum region (see Figure 3.11).

Parenchyma of the Testis

The parenchyma of the testis is made up of various tubules, lobules, or ductules. The main tubules in this region are the

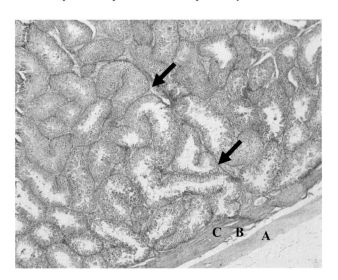

Figure 3.8. Low magnification of testis. **A.** Parietal lamina of vaginal tunic; **B.** visceral lamina of vaginal tunic; **C.** tunica albuginea. The **arrows** point at the septulum. (Also see color plate)

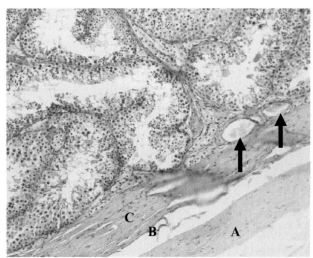

Figure 3.9. Low magnification of testis. **A.** Parietal lamina of vaginal tunic; **B.** Visceral lamina of vaginal tunic; **C.** Tunica albuginea. The **arrows** point at tunica vasculosa. (Also see color plate)

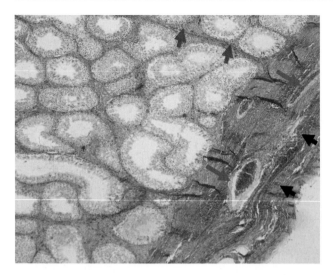

Figure 3.10. Testis. **Black arrows**, T. albuginea; **dark gray arrows**, T. vasculosa; and **light gray arrows**, septulum. (Also see color plate)

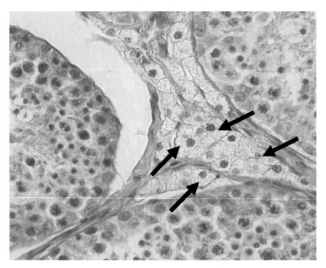

Figure 3.12. Convoluted seminiferous tubules and interstitium of the testis. The **arrows** point at Leydig cells, which appear very vacuolated. (Also see color plate)

convoluted seminiferous tubules (lobules), which produce the spermatozoa (see Figure 3.12). The spermatozoa are released from the seminiferous tubules into the *straight tubules*. These tubules are most prominent in the stallion, and the initial portion of these tubules are lined by Sertoli (Sustentacular) cells that, with their long filamentous morphology, act as a valve to prevent back-up of the sperm. The rest of the straight tubules are lined by simple cuboidal epithelium. From the straight tubules, the sperm then enters into the rete testis, which is located in the mediastinum region, and these channels secrete fluid to bathe the spermatozoa. The subsequent tubules are the efferent ductules, which in most species are outside the testis, but in other species, such as the boar, bull, goat and dog, are located within the testis.

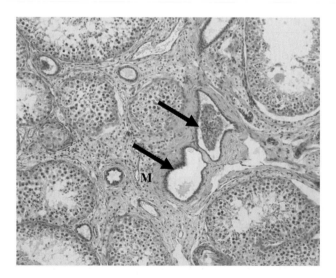

Figure 3.11. Low magnification of testis. **M.**, mediastinum. The **arrows** point at rete testis in mediastinum. (Also see color plate)

Convoluted Seminiferous Tubules
Convoluted seminiferous tubules are comprised of stratified spermatogenic epithelium with two main cell-types: *Sertoli (Sustentacular)* and *spermatogenic* cells (see Figures 3.13 and 3.14) (for review see Brehm and Steger, 2005). The *peri-tubular* or *myoid* cells with long elliptical nuclei surround the spermatogenic epithelium with its underlying basement membrane. While these cells are not true muscle cells, they possess numerous actin filaments. Thus, their contraction is thought to aid in releasing the sperm from the spermatogenic epithelium.

Spermatogenesis
The process of germ cell development from *spermatogonia* to *spermatozoa* is termed *spermatogenesis*, and this progression occurs within the *convoluted seminiferous tubules* (for further information see Franca et al., 2005; Liu, 2005). Spermatogenesis is further divided into three phases: *spermatocytogenesis*, *meiosis*, and *spermiogenesis*.

Spermatocytogenesis
The end product of spermatocytogenesis is the primary spermatocyte cell. The primordial germ cells give rise to *type A spermatogonia*, which are diploid. These cells remain close to the basement membrane and will continue to divide (see Figure 3.14). Type A spermatogonia are extremely resistant to toxic insult and if need be, can repopulate the germ cells within the seminiferous tubules. Some type A spermatogonia eventually differentiate into diploid *type B spermatogonia*, which further differentiate into diploid *primary spermatocytes* (see Figure 3.14).

Meiosis
Meiosis is the process by which the diploid primary spermatocytes eventually give rise to haploid round spermatids. The primary spematocytes (2N) undergo DNA duplication, and thus they are considered 4N in terms of DNA content.

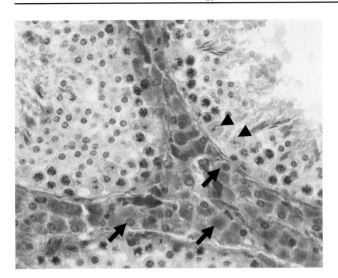

Figure 3.13. Testis. **Arrows**, Leydig (interstitial) cells; and **arrowheads**, Sertoli cells. (Also see color plate)

However, most individuals use N to refer to chromosomes rather than DNA. These cells will enter the first round of meiosis and one primary spermatocyte will give rise to *two secondary spermatocytes* (1N in terms of chromosomes and 2N for DNA content). These cells almost immediately initiate meiosis II, and thus they are transient and difficult to see in most histological sections of the testes. Two secondary spermatocytes will yield four *round spermatids* in the process of meiosis II (see Figures 3.14 and 3.15) (1N chromosomal content, 1N DNA content). The round spermatids are the end product of meiosis.

Spermiogenesis

The final stage of spermatogenesis is called *spermiogenesis*, and this process includes the development of the haploid *round spermatids* into haploid *elongated spermatozoa* that

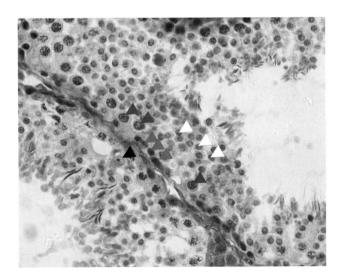

Figure 3.14. Testis. **Black arrowheads**, Sertoli cell; **light gray arrowheads**, spermatogonia; **dark grey arrowheads**, primary spermatocytes; and **white arrowheads**, spermatids. (Also see color plate)

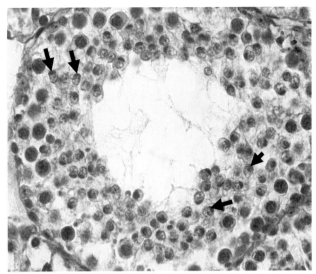

Figure 3.15. Testis. **Arrows** point at acrosomal cap surrounding the nucleus of the round spermatids. (Also see color plate)

are ready to be released from the convoluted seminiferous tubules (see Figures 3.14, 3.15, and 3.16). Four main events occur as part of this stage: *acrosome formation, condensation of the chromatin, flagellar formation,* and *the excess cytoplasm is shed as the residual body.*

The *acrosome* is a glycoprotein cap of digestive enzymes overlying the nucleus that is thought to aid the sperm in pentration through the corona radiata and zona pellucida surrounding the oocyte. Rough endoplasmic reticulum (RER) and the Golgi body are essential for the synthesis of this region. Initially the acrosome starts out as a granule, but as the cell develops further, the acrosome will expand to cover the nucleus.

The chromatin must undergo condensation to permit the spermatozoa to travel rapidly within the male and female reproductive tracts. The large spherical nucleus of the round spermatid becomes streamlined, but not pyknotic.

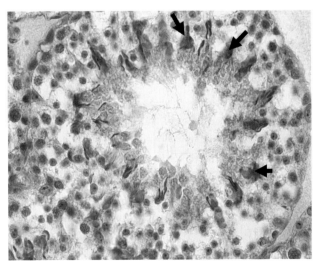

Figure 3.16. Testis. **Arrows** point at acrosomal cap surrounding the nucleus of the elongated spermatids. (Also see color plate)

The sperm must develop a *flagellum* for it to become motile within the male and female reproductive tracts. This structure will develop from one of the centrioles, and thus it is composed of microtubules in the classic 9 + 2 arrangement. The mitochondria orient alongside the flagella to generate ATP needed for flagellar movement. Finally, the round spermatids must shed their excess cytoplasm, as the *residual body*. The Sertoli cells then phagocytose the residual body.

Sertoli (Sustentacular) Cells

As their name implies, these cells support or nurse the germ cells. Innumerate functions have been attributed to the *Sertoli cells* (see Figures 3.13 and 3.14) (for review see Mruk and Cheng, 2004; Skinner and Griswold, 2004). We will examine just a few of these cells' functions, but first we will consider their morphology to understand some of their functions.

Morphology of the Sertoli Cells

The Sertoli cells are located within the convoluted seminiferous tubules, and the cytoplasmic boundaries of the Sertoli Cells cannot be discerned when the germ cells are present. However, these cells extend the entire length of the seminiferous epithelium. In most histological sections, the Sertoli cells are identified by their oval nucleus located near the basement membrane and they are oriented perpendicular to the seminiferous tubules. These cells also have a prominent nucleolus, but depending upon the plane of section, this structure is not evident in all Sertoli cells.

Functions of the Sertoli Cells

The general functions of the Sertoli cells are to support, protect, and nourish the developing germ cells. The Sertoli cells will also phagocytose the residual body formed during spermiogenesis and any dead germ cells.

These cells produce *androgen binding protein (ABP)* and *inhibin* in response to *Follicle Stimulating Hormone (FSH)*. ABP concentrates *testosterone* produced by the *Leydig cells*, and this concentration of testosterone and other androgens within the seminiferous epithelium is needed for normal spermatogenesis. Similar to females, inhibin from the Sertoli cells negatively inhibits FSH secretion in males.

Pre-pubertal Sertoli cells are capable of synthesizing *estrogen*. However, as they mature, they lose the ability to produce estrogen. In dogs and humans, neoplastic (cancerous) Sertoli cells can revert to producing estrogen. This synthesis of estrogen by Sertoli cell tumors can lead to a condition termed *gynecomastia* (enlarged mammary glands) that may produce milk and overall feminization of males.

In utero, the developing Sertoli cells produce *anti-Mullerian hormone (AMH)* or *Mullerian inhibiting substance (MIS)* that induces the regression of most of the *Mullerian (paramesonephric) duct*. However, even normal males have vestigial Mullerian duct tissue such as the uterus masculinis. Another important function of the Sertoli cells is to form the *blood-seminiferous tubular (testis) barrier* that is composed of the occluding junctions of the Sertoli cells. This barrier divides the convoluted seminiferous tubules into the *basal* and *adluminal compartments*. The function of this barrier is to protect germ cells that were not present at the time of immune maturation against attack by the immune system. Spermatogonia are the only germ cells present during immune maturation, and thus, these cells reside in the basal compartment. All of the other germ cells, including the primary spermatocytes, reside in the adluminal compartment. The primary spermatocytes are capable of moving past the tight junction and afterwards the tight junctions are re-established.

Interstitial (Leydig) Cells

The Leydig cells are located in the interstitium of the testis, between the convoluted seminiferous tubules. Leydig cells may appear either foamy (due to accumulation of many lipid droplets) or acidophilic (due to accumulation of numerous tubular cristate mitochondria) (see Figures 3.11 and 3.13). Boars and stallions have the greatest number of Leydig cells compared to other domestic animal species. In response to *interstitial cell stimulating hormone (ICSH)*, or as it is called in females, *luteinizing hormone (LH)*, these cells produce *testosterone* and some *estrogen* in adult animals. (For additional information on the Leydig cells see Payne, 1996).

Testicular Clinical Problems

We will consider just some of the pathological changes that can occur within the testis. Some of these, such as cryptorchidism and Sertoli cell tumors, may be linked together.

Testicular Tumors

There are three main types of testicular tumors: *Seminoma, Sertoli cell tumor,* and *Leydig (interstitial) cell tumor* (for review see McEntee, 2002). Most of these tumors are benign, but some of these can lead to other clinical sequelae.

Seminoma

This tumor is derived from germ cells, and of the three testicular tumors, is the most likely to become malignant. Just like normal germ cells, the neoplastic germ cells are located within the seminiferous tubules and they have high mitotic activity.

Sertoli Cell Tumor

Many Sertoli cell tumors produce large amounts of estrogen that can induce feminization, including enlarged mammary glands, and may cause urinary incontinence. This tumor is commonly seen in cryptorchid testes and is recognized by long filamentous cells that are within neoplastic convoluted seminiferous tubules devoid of germ cells.

Leydig (Interstitial) Cell Tumor

Leydig cell tumors are located in the interstitium. They are not known to produce any additional hormones, which induce secondary clinical problems.

Cryptorchidism

Normal spermatogenesis requires that the testes descend into the scrotum, which serves to provide the lower temperature necessary for germ cell development (for review see Wensing, 1988). Cryptorchidism occurs when the testes do not descend properly (for more information see Romagnoli, 1991).

Cryptorchid testes may be located as far cranial as the kidney or somewhere in the inguinal canal. The higher temperature exposure results in a lack of spermatogenesis in these testes. However, cryptorchid testes still have functional Sertoli and Leydig cells. One test to determine if an animal may have a retained testicle is to give him either GnRH or LH and then measure the serum testosterone concentrations. Cryptorchid animals have normal to elevated serum testosterone concentrations. Some have postulated that treatment of these animals with GnRH or LH may induce descent of the testes into the scrotum, but evidence to support this hypothesis is lacking. As mentioned above, Sertoli cell tumors are routinely observed in cryptorchid testes.

Epididymis

The *epididymis* connects the testis to the ductus (vas) deferens. Most individuals divide the epididymis into *efferent ductules* and *ductus epididymidis*.

Efferent Ductules

After traversing the rete testis, the sperm enters into the *efferent ductules*, which are composed of simple columnar epithelium with true motile cilia (kinocilia). The efferent ductules and initial portion of the ductus epididymidis absorb most of the rete testis fluid and the ciliated cells of the efferent ductules propel the sperm into the ductus epididymidis.

Ductus Epididymidis

The *ductus epididymidis* is divided into three regions: *initial segment* and *caput* (head), *corpus* (body), and *cauda* (tail). This organ stores and aids in the maturation of the spermatozoa. The spermatozoa is incapable of fertilization when it enters the epididymis. By the time they reach the cauda epididymis, the sperm are fully mature. All three regions of the ductus epidymidis are comprised of pseudo-stratified columnar epithelium with non-motile stereocilia (long microvilli), but the epithelial height decreases from the initial segment to the cauda region (see Figures 3.17 and 3.18).

Ductus Deferens

The *ductus deferens* is within the spermatic cord and is the continuation of the cauda epidymidis (see Figures 3.19, 3.20, and 3.21). This organ transports the sperm via peri-

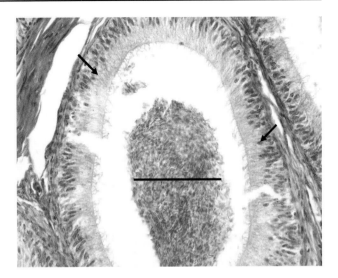

Figure 3.17. Cauda epididymis. **Arrows**, collections of spermatozoa in the ductus epididymis; **horizontal bar**, one epididymal tubule or ductule. (Also see color plate)

staltic action into the pelvic urethra. The *colliculis seminalis* is an eminence where the ductus deferens opens into the pelvic urethra. The ductus deferens is a typical tubular organ with pseudostratified columnar epithelium with or without stereocilia and a thick but ill-defined tunica muscularis that courses in all directions.

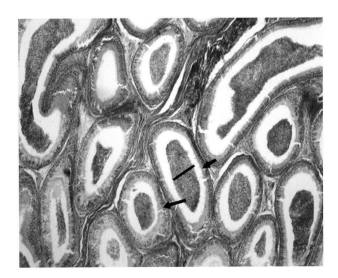

Figure 3.18. Cauda epididymis. Higher magnification of one epididymal tubule reveals that it is lined by a pseudostratified columnar epithelium. Within this epithelium, there are four main types of cells—basal, principal, narrow, and apical. Collections of spermatozoa are present in the center of the tubule. The spermatozoa that are stored in the cauda epididymis are fully mature and capable of fertilizing an ovum. The arrows point at the pseudostratified columnar epithelial lining of the epididymis. The horizontal bar is across the collection of spermatozoa in one epididymal tubule. (Also see color plate)

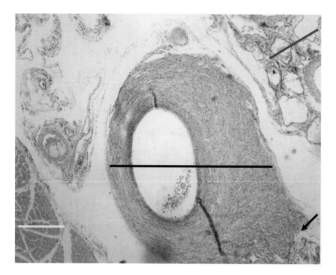

Figure 3.19. Spermatic cord. The four main structures that comprise the spermatic cord are visible. These include the ductus deferens, testicular artery, pamipiniform plexus and nerves. The visceral lamina of the vaginal tunic that surrounds the ductus deferens is called the mesoductus deferens, and that surrounds the arteries, nerves, and veins is called the mesorchium. **White horizontal bar**, cremaster muscle; **black horizontal bar**, ductus deferens; **dark gray bar**, pampiniform plexus, nerves, and testicular artery in this area; **black arrow**, mesoductus deferens. (Also see color plate)

Accessory Genital Glands

These organs produce the fluid of the ejaculate that nourishes, protects, and buffers the spermatozoa. As indicated in Table 3.1, these glands are not present in all species. The

Table 3.1. Summary of the accessory sex gland in the various species.

	Dog	Cat	Boar	Ruminants
Prostate	+	+	+	+
Bulbourethral gland	–	+	+	+
Seminal vesicles	–	–	+	+
Ampulla of ductus deferens	+	–	–	+

seminal vesicles (vesicular glands) are absent in the dog and tom cat, and dogs do not have a bulbourethral gland. Both the tom cat and boar lack an ampulla of the ductus deferens. All species have a prostate that can be predominantly as a body (in the case of the dog) or disseminate portion (as in the case of the boar).

Prostate

All domestic animal species have a *prostate*, but the dog has the most prominent prostatic body surrounding the urethra (see Figures 3.22, 3.23, and 3.24). In other species, such as the boar, the prostatic tissue is disseminated within the lamina propria-submucosa of the pelvic urethra. Simple cuboidal strikingly acidophilic epithelium characterizes the prostatic glands whether it is in the body or disseminate portion. These glands produce an alkaline product to neutralize the acidity of the semen, and the prostatic secretions are the bulk of the initial ejaculate.

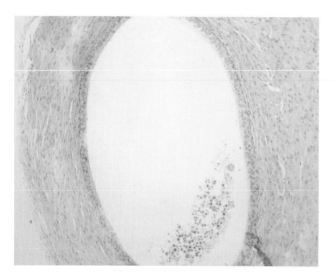

Figure 3.20. Ductus deferens in spermatic cord. The ductus deferens is lined by a pseudostratified columnar epithelium with long microvilli closest to the epididymis. The epithelium will decrease in height and in most cases the long microvilli will be lost. The smooth muscle surrounding the ductus deferens is irregularly arranged. The ductus deferens serves as a conduit to transport the spermatozoa. (Also see color plate)

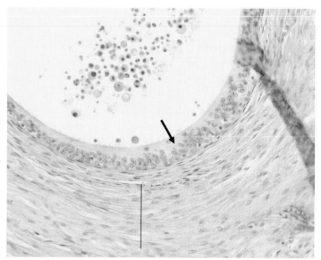

Figure 3.21. Higher magnification of ductus deferens in spermatic cord. **Black arrow**, pseudostratified columnar epithelium with long microvilli; **vertical bar**, tunica muscularis. (Also see color plate)

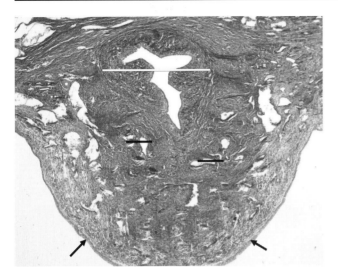

Figure 3.22. Canine prostate and prostatic urethra. The colliculus seminalis, where the ductus deferens empties into the urethra, is present. It is represented by multiple cross sections of the ductus deferens on each side. They are not to be confused with the uterus masculinis, which is a remnant of the paramesonephric duct. **Long white horizontal bar**, uterus masculinis; **short black horizontal bars**, cross sections of ductus deferens; **arrows**, epithelial lining of urethra. (Also see color plate)

Vesicular Glands (Seminal Vesicles)

This organ is made up of a fibrous to smooth muscle capsule surrounding large irregular alveolar glands with pseudo-stratified columnar epithelium (see Figures 3.25 and 3.26). In ruminants and boars, *basal cells* may be seen in this epithelial layer, and these cells may accumulate large lipid droplets, particularly in ruminants. The vesicular gland secretion is rich in fructose to nourish the spermatozoa.

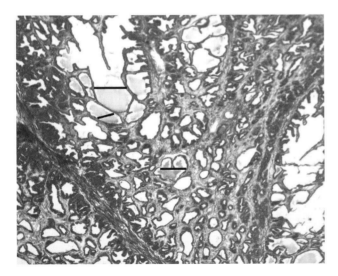

Figure 3.23. Higher magnification of prostate glands. **Horizontal bars**, tubuloalveolar prostatic glands of the dog. (Also see color plate)

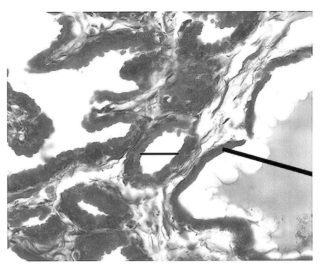

Figure 3.24. Canine prostate. The prostatic glands are lined by simple cuboidal to low columnar epithelium with apical blebs. The alkaline product buffers the spermatozoa. **Horizontal bars**, tubuloalveolar acidophilic staining prostatic glands that have apical blebs. (Also see color plate)

Ampulla of Ductus Deferens

The ampulla of ductus deferens is an enlargement of the terminal part of the ductus deferens, whose glands contain large irregular alveoli, but unlike the vesicular gland, lacks a capsule. This organ is best appreciated under low magnification. In the dog, the ampulla is grossly identified by a slight increase in the diameter of the ductus deferens. Similar to the ductus deferens, the ampulla contains a lamina propria-submucosa and

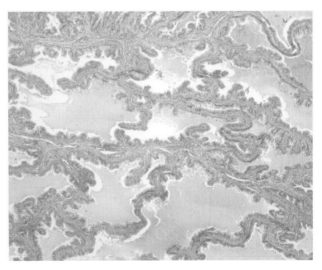

Figure 3.25. Vesicular glands of the boar. The vesicular glands are composed of irregularly shaped alveoli that are lined by a simple columnar to pseudostratified columnar epithelium. The fructose from these glands provides energy for the spermatozoa. Carnivores do not have vesicular glands. In ruminants and some boars, basal cells are present in the glandular epithelium, and in the case of ruminants, these cells may contain lipid droplets. (Also see color plate)

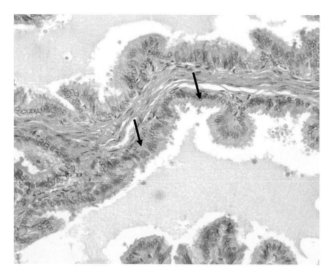

Figure 3.26. Higher magnification of the vesicular glands of the boar. The **arrows** point at simple columnar–pseudostratified columnar epithelium that lines the vesicular glands. (Also see color plate)

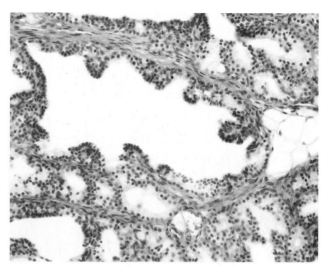

Figure 3.28. Feline bulbourethral gland. These glands are simple columnar tubuloalveolar glands. The nuclei of the cells is towards the base, and the cytoplasm stains pale to basophilic. (Also see color plate)

tunica muscularis arranged in ill-defined layers. As with the vesicular glands, the ampulla of the ductus deferens produces high concentrations of fructose for energy.

Bulbourethral (Cowper's) Gland

In the species that have a *bulbourethral gland*, this organ is located at the junction of the pelvic urethra and the penile urethra. The glands are arranged in tubules or alveoi or tubuloalveolar with simple columnar epithelium containing lipid droplets that push the nuclei towards the base (see Figures 3.27 and 3.28). The mucus secretion from these

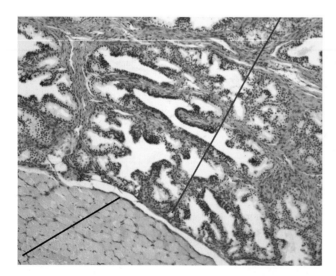

Figure 3.27. Feline bulbourethral glands and bulboglandularis muscle. The bulbourethral glands secrete a mucus product that coats the urethra prior to ejaculation. **Dark gray bar**, bulburethral gland in the cat; **black bar**, bulboglandularis muscle. (Also see color plate)

glands lubricates the urethra prior to ejaculation. In most histological sections, either the bulboglandularis or bulbospongiosis muscle may be seen in proximity to the bulbourethral gland.

External Genitalia

The external genitalia include the penis and scrotum. The penis is the male copulatory organ and contains the spongy or penile urethra. Thus, the penis is essential for transfer of the spermatozoa into the female reproductive tract. The scrotum encases the testes and helps provide the proper temperature for spermatozoa development.

Penis

The penis is composed of three parts: *root*, *body*, and *glans*. The glans region is the most variable in the domestic animals.

Root

The right and left crura attaches the root of the penis to the ischial tuberosities. The root comprises the two crura and the bulbus penis.

Body

The body consists of the *corpus cavernosa penis*, which is a continuation of the *crura of the penis*, and the penile urethra surrounded by the *corpus spongiosum* penis (see Figures 3.29 to 3.35). Both the corpora cavernosa and corpus spongiosum are considered erectile tissues and, depending on the species, may contain abundant elastic fibers and vascular sinuses. The paired

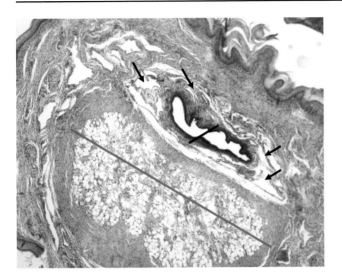

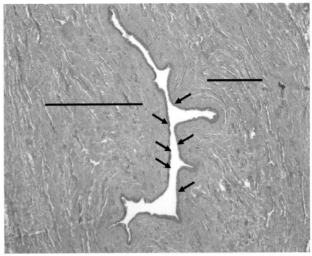

Figure 3.29. Feline penile urethra. Corpus spongiosum surrounds the penile urethra. Ventral to the urethra, corpus cavernosum that has been infiltrated with adipose tissue is present. Both the corpus spongiosum and corpus cavernosum are erectile tissue. **Black arrows**, corpus spongiosum; **long gray bar**, penile urethra; **short black bar**, corpus cavernosum. (Also see color plate)

Figure 3.31. Canine penis—pars longa glandis. This picture shows the penile urethra surrounded by corpus spongiosum. **Arrows**, urethral lining; **horizontal bars**, corpus spongiosum. (Also see color plate)

smooth muscle retractor penis muscles are below the corpus spongiosum. Similar to the testes and epididymis, the penis has a surrounding *tunica albuginea*.

Glans Penis

In the dog the glans consists of the *bulbus glandis* and *pars longa glandis*. Some species, such as the dog, tom cat, raccoon, otter, and walrus, have an *os penis* (a bony structure) in this region (see Figure 3.36), while others may have another area of erectile tissue called the corpus spongiosum glandis. In tom cats, the caudal end of the os penis can

collect calculi and thereby obstruct urination. This condition is called *feline urological syndrome (FUS)* and the calculi must be flushed out with a catheter or removed surgically by performing urethrotomy.

Unique Penile Anatomical Structures of the Tom Cat

The glans penis is conical and undivided in the tom cat. In the non-erect state, the urethra is dorsal to the os penis (see Figure 3.30); whereas it is in the reverse location in all other species. The intact tom cat has cornified spines on the glans penis that presumably induce ovulation in the queen. These structures regress in neutered cats.

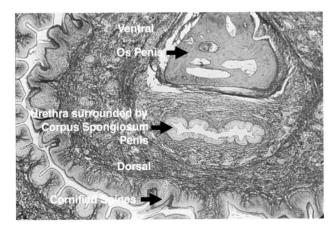

Figure 3.30. Feline penis. Unlike the other species, the cat penis is directed caudoventrally in the non-erect state so the urethra is dorsal to the os penis. Cats also have cornified spines that presumably induce ovulation in queens. These spines regress in neutered tom cats. (Also see color plate)

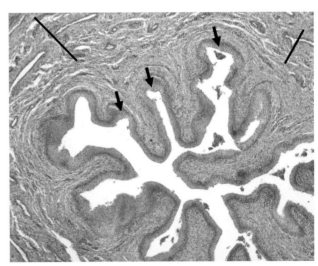

Figure 3.32. Equine penis. This pictures shows the penile urethra surrounded by corpus spongiosum. **Arrows**, urethral lining; **bars**, corpus spongiosum. (Also see color plate)

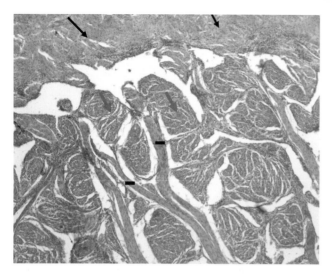

Figure 3.33. Equine penis. This picture shows the corpus cavernosum surrounded by the tunica albuginea. Helicine arteries supply blood to the corpus cavernosum. These arteries have epitheloid smooth muscle cells. When the cells are relaxed, the blood flows into the erectile tissue and the penis becomes erect. Contraction of these muscle fibers results in relaxation of the penis. **Black arrows**, tunica albuginea; **gray arrows**, corpus cavernosum; **horizontal bars**, trabeculae from the tunica albuginea that radiates into the corpus cavernosum. (Also see color plate)

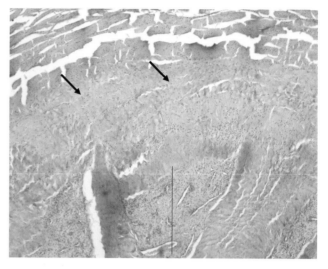

Figure 3.35. Bovine penis. This species has a fibrous type of penis with more fibrous connective tissue and less erectile tissue than the stallion. **Arrows**, tunica albuginea; **thin vertical bar**, corpus cavernosum. (Also see color plate)

Male Urethra

The pelvic urethra extends from the *neck of the urinary bladder* to the *bulb of the penis* (see Figure 3.37). The penile urethra is surrounded by the corpus spongiosum and eventually opens up into the *external urethral ostium*. The male urethra is a typical tubular organ with transitional to stratified squamous epithelium. The distal end of the penis may include portions that are stratified cuboidal to stratified columnar.

Scrotum

The scrotal skin is typical skin with an overlying epidermis and underlying *tunica dartos*, or subcutaneous layer, that contains smooth muscle which forms the scrotal septum.

For anatomical details see Chapter 2.

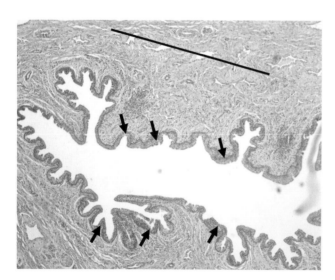

Figure 3.34. Bovine penis. This figure demonstrates the penile urethra surrounded by corpus spongiosum. **Arrows**, urethral lining; **bar**, corpus spongiosum. (Also see color plate)

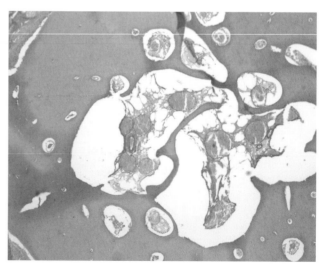

Figure 3.36. Canine penis—pars longa glandis. This figure shows the os penis in the pars longa glandis. Not pictured here is the corpus spongiosum glandis, which is erectile tissue that is the configuration of the corpus spongiosum penis. (Also see color plate)

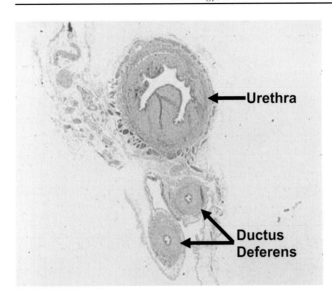

Figure 3.37. Pre-prostatic urethra of the cat and ductus deferens. The cat has a long pre-prostatic urethra, and thus it can be seen with the paired ductus deferens. (Also see color plate)

Acknowledgments

Photomicrographs were taken by Cheryl S. Rosenfeld from the University of Missouri, College of Veterinary Medicine Student Histology Slide Sets.

Bibliography

Brehm, R., and Steger, K. (2005). Regulation of Sertoli cell and germ cell differentation. *Adv Anat Embryol Cell Biol* 181:1–93.

Eurell J., and Frappier, B. (2006). *Dellman's Textbook of Veterinary Histology.* Ames: Blackwell Publishing Professional, 6th edition.

Franca, L.R., Avelar, G.F., and Almeida, F.F. (2005). Spermatogenesis and sperm transit through the epididymis in mammals with emphasis on pigs. *Theriogenology* 63:300–18.

Liu, Y.X. (2005). Control of spermatogenesis in primate and prospect of male contraception. *Arch Androl* 51:77–92.

McEntee, M.C. (2002) Reproductive oncology. *Clin Tech Small Anim Pract* 17:133–49.

Mruk, D.D., and Cheng, C.Y. (2004). Sertoli-Sertoli and Sertoligerm cell interactions and their significance in germ cell movement in the seminiferous epithelium during spermatogenesis. *Endocr Rev* 25:747–806.

Payne, A. (1996) *Leydig Cell.* St. Louis: Cache River Press.

Romagnoli, S.E. (1991)Canine cryptorchidism. *Vet Clin North Am Small Anim Pract.* 21:533–44.

Skinner, M.K., and Griswold, M.D. (editors). (2004). *Sertoli Cell Biology, Volume 1.* New York: Academic Press.

Wensing, C.J. (1988). The embryology of testicular descent. *Hormone Research.* 30:144–52.

Part 3.3
Comparative Histology and Subcellular Structure of Mammalian Spermatogenesis and Spermatozoa

Gaurishankar Manandhar and Peter Sutovsky

The purpose of spermatogenesis is to provide a continuous output of spermatozoa throughout the reproductive lifespan of an individual. This requires commensurate renewal of spermatogenic stem cells in the testes as well as certain stringency of sperm quality control aimed at avoiding fertilization of ova with the spermatozoa carrying nuclear or mitochondrial genomic defects. This process, which is flexible enough to permit evolutionary adaptation, assures the perpetuation of the species while lowering the likelihood of defective genome transmission that could lead to embryo loss or birth defects.

The goal of this section is to familiarize scientists and professional students who possess basic knowledge of the reproductive biology with details of the molecular composition of sperm organelles and their functions, emphasizing new findings yet to be incorporated in text books. It is illustrated by light and electron micrographs that compare spermatogenesis in laboratory rodents, large farm animals, ruminant and non-ruminant ungulates, and humans.

General Structure of Mammalian Spermatozoa

Mammalian spermatozoa are elongated motile cells specialized to deliver haploid male genomes to oocytes. A spermatozoon comprises a head and tail (see Figure 3.38). The head contains a nucleus with a highly compact, hypercondensed chromatin encapsulated by a perinuclear theca and acrosome that help the spermatozoon to penetrate the oocyte vestments and initiate an embryonic cell cycle after fertilization. The tail can be divided into a connecting piece, mid-piece, principle piece, and end-piece. The connecting piece encompasses the centrosome that plays an important role in bringing male and female gamete nuclei together in the zygotes and in organizing the bipolar cleavage spindle. The mid-piece harbors a mitochondrial sheath that is necessary to generate energy for the sperm motility. The tail propels the spermatozoa forward through the uterus and oviduct until meeting and penetrating the oocyte.

The length of human and common domestic animal spermatozoa is about 50 μm, while rodent spermatozoa measure 150 μm to 250 μm. Homey opossum (*Tarsipens rostratus*) has the longest spermatozoa (350 μm) among mammals. The spermatozoa of most mammalian species have compressed, spatulate heads (see Figure 3.39). Rodent spermatozoa have sickle-shaped, falciform heads. The marsupial spermatozoa become paired during epididymal maturation by adhering to the ventral side of the sperm head and remain paired until binding the zona pellucida (Moore and Taggart, 1995).

The Sperm Head

The head is the anterior-most part of spermatozoa, comprising the nucleus, perinuclear theca, acrosome, and plasma membrane. Its main function is to penetrate into the oocyte, deliver the haploid genome, and initiate embryonic development after fertilization.

Sperm Nucleus

The central core of the sperm head is the nucleus that encloses a haploid set of paternal chromosomes (see Figure 3.40). The chromatin of sperm head is 6 to 10 times more compact than the metaphase chromosomes of a somatic cell and is synthetically and transcriptionally inactive. Histochemical staining as well as electron microscopy shows that sperm chromatin is homogeneous in nature. However, primate sperm nuclei display vacuoles that are remarkably prominent in human spermatozoa (Zamboni et al., 1971). The nuclear vacuoles are irregular in outline, lack a limiting membrane, and probably formed as a result of incomplete chromatin condensation. Some nuclear vacuoles contain remnants of spermatid cytoplasm. The presence of vacuoles in the nuclei is regarded as a defect in most mammalian species (Barth and Oko, 1989). A nuclear diadem/crater defect caused by invagination of perinuclear cytoplasm and microtubules in the nucleus is occasionally observed in infertile ruminant males (Larsen and Chenoweth, 1990) and presumably fertile mice (Manandhar and Schatten, 1999).

The enormous compaction of sperm chromatin is due to replacement of the DNA-protecting proteins, histones, by protamines during the post-meiotic phase of sperm development. Protamines are arginine- and cysteine-rich (about 70 percent arginine and 15 percent cystein in protamine 1), basic, low molecular weight proteins (Brewer et al., 2002) that are capable of forming stable disulphide bonds (S-S) between their thiol groups.

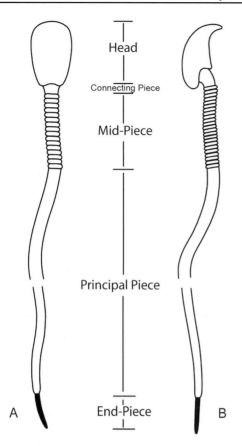

Figure 3.38. Schematic diagrams showing the internal structure of **A.** demembranated ungulate/primate and **B.** rodent spermatozoa.

Mammals have two protamine genes that encode for protamine 1 and protamine 2. Due to the presence of extensive, stable cross-linking by S-S bonds, the sperm chromatin is protected from damage by the external physical or chemical disruptive agents. However, transcriptional inactivation and initial condensation of chromatin seem to occur prior to the appearance of protamines during spermiogenesis. Protamine synthesis occurs after the complete repression of gene transcription in the post-meiotic period. Testis-specific transition proteins TP1 and TP2 (Meistrich et al., 2003) replace histones until they themselves are replaced by protamines.

Besides protamines, the sperm head chromatin also contains some testis-specific histones (Churikov et al., 2004). After fertilization, the disulphide bonds of protamines are reduced by the glutathione of oocyte cytoplasm causing relaxation of the chromatin folds, swelling of the nuclei, and replacement of the protamines by histones (Perreault et al., 1984). The sperm heads can be decondensed *in vitro* by treating them with reducing agents such as dithiothreitol (DTT) that breaks down the disulphide bonds.

Similar to somatic cell nuclei, the sperm head nuclei are also enveloped by a bilayered nuclear envelope. However, the sperm nuclear envelope lacks nuclear pore complexes

and perinuclear cisternae, both of which are lost during spermatid elongation (Sutovsky et al., 1999). Hence, the two layers of the nuclear envelope are closely adhered to each other and the underlying chromatin.

At the base of the sperm head, the nuclear envelope forms a redundant fold that hangs distally, separated from the chromatin. Some residual nuclear pore complexes are conserved in this region. A segment of nuclear membrane on the posterior surface that links capitulum and the connecting piece is called the *implantation fossa*. It is lined by a basal plate. The surface and intramembranous space of the implantation fossa possess dense particles that seem to provide attachment sites for the fine filaments extended from the capitulum and basal plate of the sperm tail.

The sperm nuclei contain one haploid set of chromosomes. The X and Y chromosomes become segregated after meiosis, resulting in 50 percent of the gametes receiving X chromosomes and the other 50 percent, Y chromosomes. There is no detectable morphological or biochemical difference between the X- or Y-bearing spermatozoa except for slightly smaller DNA content in the latter due to the lack of one arm in the Y chromosome. Both types of spermatozoa are equally capable of fertilization.

Human Y spermatozoa can be identified by fixing and staining with quinacrin dye which reveals the Y chromosomes as bright fluorescent spots under a UV microscope;

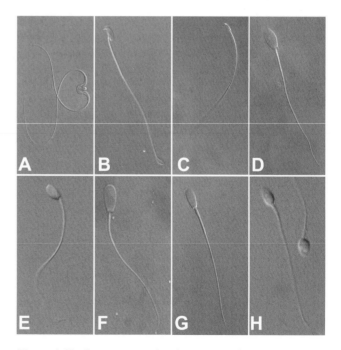

Figure 3.39. Spermatozoa of various mammalian species as visualized by differential interference contrast micrococopy. **A.** Common opossum (*Didelphis virginiana*); **B.** domestic mouse (*Mus musculus*); **C.** rat (*Rattus norvegicus*); **D.** rabbit (*Oryctolagus cuniculus*); **E.** stallion (*Equs caballus*); **F.** boar (*Sus scrofa*); **G.** bull (*Bos taurus*); and **H.** man (*Homo sapiens*).

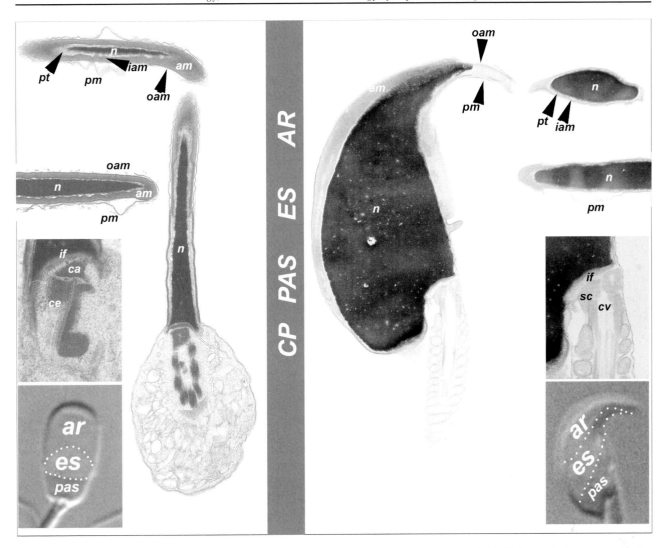

Figure 3.40. Transmission electron micrographs of porcine (left) and murine (right) sperm heads highlighting the inner acrosomal membrane (***iam***), outer acrosomal membrane (***oam***), acrosomal matrix (***am***), perinuclear theca (***pt***), nucleus (***n***), implantation fossa (***if***), and a basal plate (***bp***) as they pertain to the acrosomal region (***ar***), equatorial segment (***es***), and postacrosomal sheath (***pas***). Transmission electron micrograph insets show the fine structure of a connecting piece (***CP***) that comprises implantation fossa (***if***), capitulum (***ca***), striated columns (***sc***), and proximal centriole (***ce***), which is reduced to an empty centriolar vault (***cv***) in mouse spermatozoa.

however, the fixed and stained spermatozoa cannot be used for fertilization. With the advent of a high speed flow cytometry-based cell sorter and fluorescent DNA dyes that can label live spermatozoa, it has been possible to separate X and Y spermatozoa (Garner, 2006). The X chromosomes contain about 4 percent more DNA and therefore stain more brightly. The flow cytometer apparatus can detect the difference and separate X from Y spermatozoa at the rate of 10^6/h with 95 to 100 percent accuracy. The sorted spermatozoa have been used successfully for artificial insemination (Johnson et al., 2005), *in vitro* fertilization, and intracytoplasmic sperm injection (Abeydeera et al., 1998; Hollinshead et al., 2004). Sorted spermatozoa are commercially available and have been successfully used in animal breeding.

Perinuclear Theca

The mammalian sperm nuclei are surrounded by a compact cytoskeletal structure, the perinucelar theca (PT) (Oko, 1995; Sutovsky et al., 2003) from all sides except the base. Topographically, the PT can be divided into three regions: *subacrosomal layer*, *equatorial segment*, and *post-acrosomal sheath* (see Figure 3.40). The subacrosomal layer is the anterior portion of PT underlying the sac-like acrosome.

In rodents, the proximal part of the subacrosomal PT is hooked ventrally, forming a structure called the *perforatorium*. The inner acrosomal membrane (IAM) overlying the subacrosomal PT is exposed after acrosome reaction, possibly playing roles in binding and penetrating through the zona pellucida. The equatorial segment of PT that lies beneath the equatorial acrosome is not lost after acrosomal exocytosis. A small leaf of the equatorial PT curves upward between the acrosome and plasma membrane. It probably interacts with the equatorial plasma membrane, protecting from vesiculation during acrosome reaction and rendering it fusible with the oocyte plasma membrane (Toshimori et al., 1992).

The post-acrosomal sheath is a cup-like involucre extending below the acrosome sandwiched between the plasma membrane and the nuclear membrane. This segment of PT is not exposed after acrosome reaction or during zona penetration (Manandhar and Toshimori, 2003) but becomes the first sperm organelle to come in contact with the oocyte cytoplasm after sperm-oocyte plasma membrane fusion. Its content rapidly disperses in the oocyte after fusion (Sutovsky et al., 1997, 2003), and some proteins subsequently migrate to the polar regions of the meiotic/midzone spindle (Manandhar and Toshimori, 2003). Experimental evidence indicates that the post-acrosomal PT activates oocytes to initiate an embryonic cell cycle (Perry et al., 1999a).

Besides the specific roles played by the different segments, the PT as a whole is thought to be important for providing shape, mechanical rigidity, protection to the nucleus, adherence of acrosomes on the sperm nuclear surface, and possibly even storage of mRNAs and proteins for immediate use in the zygotes (Sutovsky et al., 2003). PT and the inner acrosomal membrane might play important roles in evolution by adhering to foreign DNA and inserting it into the oocytes after fertilization, hence introducing new genes into the population (Perry et al., 1999b).

Acrosome

An *acrosome* is a cap-like vesicle lying between the plasma membrane and the perinuclear theca on the frontal and lateral aspects of the nucleus. It is a membrane-bound organelle formed by the fusion of Golgi vesicles during spermiogenesis. Structurally and functionally it can be divided into two regions: (1) the anterior bulbous region that is exocytosed when spermatozoa pass through the cumulus cells or interact with the zona pellucida, and (2) a narrow pocket-like equatorial or posterior acrosome that is retained after acrosomal exocytosis and incorporated into an oocyte after fertilization (Manandhar and Toshimori, 2001).

Acrosomes are filled with hydrolytic enzymes (Tulsiani et al., 1998). The two most prominent enzymes are *hyaluronidase* and *acrosin*. Hyaluronidase (Myles and Primakoff, 1997) hydrolyses hyaluronic acid of the extracellular matrix that binds the cumulus cells around the oocytes. Spermatozoa penetrate the cumulus oophorus by releasing hyaluronidase, breaking down hyaluronic acid, and dispersing the cumulus cells. Addition of anti-hyaluronidase antibody in the culture medium can prevent *in vitro* fertilization without affecting the sperm motility (Zaneveld, 1982; Yanagimachi, 1994).

Acrosin (Honda et al., 2002) is a trypsin-like proteolytic enzyme mostly occurring as an inactive (zymogen) form

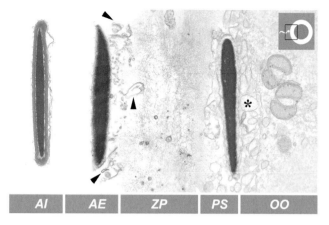

Figure 3.41. Fate of sperm acrosome during penetration through oocyte vestments in pigs. Spermatozoa have intact acrosomes prior to sperm-oocyte binding (**AI**). It undergoes exocytosis (acrosome reaction) when the sperm binds the zona pellucida of oocyte (**AE**). Acrosome exocytosis is visible as an extensive vesiculation of the outer acrosomal membrane on the zona pellucida (**ZP**) surface. The zona-penetrated spermatozoa found in the perivitelline space (**PS**) are without acrosomes. **Asterisk** indicates cross-section of one of the numerous oocyte microvilli which help in sperm-oocyte plasma membrane fusion.

(proacrosin) in the intact acrosomal matrix. Earlier experiments suggested that acrosin might be involved in zona dissolution and penetration of spermatozoa. According to this viewpoint, spermatozoa undergo acrosomal exocytosis when they bind to the zona pellucida (Florman and Storey, 1982; Gerton, 2002) (see Figure 3.41).

The acrosomal matrix and its resident proteolytic enzymes are released on the ZP surface, opening a fertilization slit. Acrosin inhibitors and anti-acrosin antibodies prevent fertilization by inhibiting acrosome reaction, sperm binding, and penetration through the zona pellucida (Liu and Baker, 1993; Fraser, 1982; Valdivia et al., 1999). Paradoxically, spermatozoa of acrosin knock-out mice can still penetrate zona pellucida and fertilize (Baba et al., 1994).

According to an alternative hypothesis, spermatozoa penetrate the zona pellucida by mechanical shearing force but not by enzymatic digestion (Bedford, 1998). Thus, the mechanism of sperm penetration of mammalian zona pellucida is still not fully understood (Olds-Clarke, 2003).

In addition to hyaluronidase and acrosin, the sperm acrosome contains several other glycolytic and proteolytic enzymes such as aryl sulphatase A, neuraminidase, collagenase, esterase, glycosidase, acid-alkaline phosphatages, cathepsins, 26 S proteasome, etc. It is possible that some of these proteases remain associated with the inner acrosomal membrane after acrosomal exocytosis, thus securing the proteolytic activity on the leading edge of the sperm head throughout the process of zona penetration (Sutovsky et al., 2004).

Sperm Tail and Flagellum

The sperm tail is the entire slender organelle extending behind the head. The functions of the tail are to propel spermatozoa forward by a whiplash-like movement and to generate energy for the movement. On the basis of external morphology, the tail can be further divided into four regions: the connecting piece, mid-piece, principal piece, and end-piece. Internally, the tail has complex structural components, described as follows:

Connecting Piece

The "neck" region of mammalian spermatozoa is a complex and specialized structure that joins the head and tail together (see Figures 3.40 and 3.42). The interface between the head

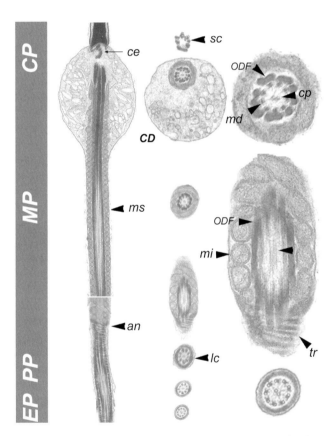

Figure 3.42. Ultrastructure of boar sperm tail. The proximal end of the sperm tail comprises a connecting piece (*CP*) that is composed of striated columns (*sc*). Residual centrioles (*ce*) are enclosed inside the vault of striated columns. The tail is made up of a central core of mirotubular axoneme surrounded by nine strands of outer dense fibers (*ODF*). In the mid-piece (*MP*), the axoneme-ODF cylinder is encircled by a mitochondrial sheath (*ms*). The testicular spermatozoa usually have cytoplasmic droplets (*CD*) in the mid-piece region. The principal piece (*PP*) of sperm tail is separated from the mid-piece by an annulus (*an*). The axoneme-ODF cylinder of the principal piece is surrounded by a fibrous sheath consisting of a twin longitudinal columns (*lc*) interconnected by a series of transversal ribs (*tr*). The outer dense fibers are absent in the end piece (*EP*) of the sperm tail.

and tail is analogous to a ball-and-socket joint; the concave surface of the head is referred to as the *basal plate* and the convex surface of the tail as the *capitulum*. Both are electron-dense structures interconnected with fine filaments. Head and tail are separated when these filaments are severed. The capitulum extends caudally as nine striated columns that continue distally as the nine outer dense fibers (ODF) of the sperm tail. The striated appearance of the columns is due to the presence of dense segments alternating with narrow light bands. The striated columns are rapidly disassembled after the spermatozoa are incorporated into the ooplasm, possibly mediated by the reducing activity of oocyte glutathione (Sutovsky et al., 1996).

Sperm Centrosome

The space enclosed by the striated columns is occupied by the *centrosomal apparatus* (Manandhar et al., 2005). The centrosome is the major microtubule organizing center (MTOC) of mammalian cells, composed of two centrioles and a loose pericentriolar material. Centrioles are the structural core of centrosomes comprising nine microtubular triplets symmetrically displaced in a pinwheel-like arrangement. In a centrosome, two centrioles are positioned together in an orthogonal orientation. The pericentriolar centrosomal proteins emanate microtubules by anchoring and stabilizing their minus-ends and radiating the plus-ends. The spermatozoan centrosomes are reduced and inactive.

Spermatozoa of most mammalian species possess intact proximal centrioles, devoid of MTOCs but enclosed within dense pericentriolar vaults. The distal centrioles are partially or almost completely degenerated (Manandhar et al., 2000, 2005). Their microtubules extend posteriorly as the microtubule doublets of the tail axoneme. In mice and rats, both distal and proximal centrioles are completely degenerated (Manandhar et al., 1998; Wooley and Fawcett, 1973).

The residual centrosomal apparatus is inactive in spermatozoa, but plays an important role during fertilization by organizing microtubular structures. Soon after sperm-egg fusion, the sperm centrioles recruit centrosomal proteins from the oocyte cytoplasm, reconstruct functional zygotic centrosomes, and organize the sperm aster (Schatten, 1994). The female pronuclei move along the sperm aster microtubules to appose closely with the male pronuclei (Payne et al., 2003). During zygotic interphase, the centrosomes duplicate and form two poles of the bipolar spindles (Paweletz et al., 1987a; 1987b).

Axoneme

The entire elongated structure behind the connecting piece/ "neck" region is the sperm tail or flagellum. It can be divided into a mid-piece, a principle piece, and an end-piece (see Figure 3.42). The core structure of the tail is an axoneme surrounded by outer dense fibers and a fibrous sheath. An *axoneme* is a cylindrical structure consisting of a pair of central microtubules surrounded by nine microtubule doublets displaced circumferentially in a radial-symmetrical manner (9 + 2 arrangement).

Each of the nine peripheral doublets is composed of two subfibers, B and A (the annotations correspond to clockwise arrangement). The A-subfiber of each doublet projects one dynein arm toward the B-subfiber of the adjacent doublet and one dynein arm toward the central doublet (see Figure 3.42). By hydrolyzing ATP, the dyneins undergo conformational change and stretch toward the minus end of the B-subfiber. This activity causes the adjacent doublets to slide past one another. Due to the synchronous and coordinated sliding movement of the doublets, a bending wave is propagated down the tail, resulting in sperm motility.

Outer Dense Fibers

The *outer dense fibers (ODF)* and *fibrous sheath (FS)* are the non-contractile cytoskeletal structures of sperm tails. The ODF are confined to the mid-piece and principal piece, whereas the FS is found only in the principal piece of the tail. Though non-contractile, they provide elastic recoil necessary for tail motility.

The sperm tail has nine ODF fibers, one opposite each microtubule doublet. Two diagonally opposite ODFs at the 3 and 8 positions are attached to the longitudinal strands of FS that lie outside the ODF. In the lower part of the tail, these two ODF strands are replaced by the inward growth of FS, linking directly to the corresponding microtubule doublets. The molecular composition of ODF comprises unique proteins—odf1, odf2, odf3, heat-shock proteins (hspB10), keratin-like proteins (SAK3), cystein-rich proteins (tpx-1), and some other accessory proteins (Fouquet and Kan, 1994; Oko, 1998). The specific function of these proteins in spermatozoa is not known; but odf2, the most abundant ODF protein, associates with the centrosomes in a microtubule-dependant manner in various types of somatic cells (Hoyer-Fender et al., 2003).

Fibrous Sheath

The FS is composed of two longitudinal columns connected by an array of circumferential, transversally oriented ribs (Eddy et al., 2003). Compositionally, FS mainly comprises two classes of proteins: those involved in signal transduction and those involved in glycolysis. More than 40 percent of FS proteins are A-kinase anchoring protein 4 (AKAP4) (Eddy et al., 1991). Other signaling proteins of FS are AKAP3, tAKAP80, and rapporin (Eddy et al., 2003). These molecules sequester protein kinase-A to the flagellum, and possibly play roles in signaling reactions leading to sperm maturation, acquisition of progressive motility, capacitation, and hyperactivation during sperm transport in the oviduct (Turner et al., 1999).

The glycolytic proteins found in the FS are *glyceraldehyde-3-phosphate dehydrogenases* (Miki et al., 2004) and *hexokinase type 1s* (Fernandez-Novell et al., 2004) that are possibly active in glycolysis, producing energy for tail motility. The structural scaffold of FS includes unique myosin- and keratin-like proteins (Eddy et al., 1991).

Mitochondrial Sheath

The mid-piece has a larger diameter due to the presence of mitochondria lined up end-to-end forming a helix around the central core of the mid-piece axoneme-ODF complex. Human spermatozoa have 15 gyres of mitochondrial helix while rodent spermatozoa may have more than 30 gyres. The sperm mitochondria are physiologically active and can aerobically oxidize various substrates to synthesize ATP (Aitken, 2000). After fertilization they enter oocytes but are soon degraded, averting inheritance of potentially mutated paternal mitochondrial DNA to the progeny (Cummins, 2000).

It has been shown that mitochondria of spermatozoa are tagged with proteolytic marker ubiquitin and possibly broken down by the proteasomal machinery of the oocyte cytoplasm (Sutovsky et al., 1999). Hence, the mammalian embryos receive mitochondria and mitochondrial genes only through maternal contribution.

Cytoplasmic Droplet

When spermatozoa are released free into the seminiferous tubule lumen they shed most of the unused cytoplasm as residual bodies that are phagocytosed by the Sertoli cells (deKretser and Kerr, 1994). Small remnants of cytoplasm left behind in the neck region of the mature, free spermatozoa are called the *cytoplasmic droplets (CD)*.

The size of sperm CD is variable in different animal spermatozoa. Ultrastructural analysis of the sperm CD (see Figure 3.42) reveals various types of membranes, lipid droplets, Golgi-derived saccules and vesicles, and diverse cytoplasmic structures (Oko et al., 1993). Biochemically, the CD is composed of lipids, lipoproteins, RNAs, and numerous hydrolytic enzymes (Cooper and Yeung, 2003).

CDs are not known to perform any definite function during spermatogenesis or fertilization. They migrate from the distal to proximal region of the mid-piece and finally are sloughed off as the spermatozoa travel through the epididymis (Kaplan et al., 1984). The spermatozoa that fail to get rid of CDs show impaired motility and are unable to fertilize. High retention of sperm CDs is most commonly seen in boar ejaculates (Fischer, 2003).

Sperm Plasma Membrane

Live spermatozoa are covered with intact and continuous plasma membrane. The sperm plasma membrane deserves special attention because of its important role in sperm functions, particularly capacitation, acrosome reaction, and fusion with the egg plasma membrane. It undergoes dynamic changes and remodeling concomitant with the maturation process.

While passing through the epididymis, the sperm plasma membrane adsorbs various secretory proteins that have been shown to be important for rendering it fusogenic

(Cuasnicu et al., 2001). By this process, the epididymal spermatozoa acquire fertilizing capability.

Acrosin inhibitors (acrostatin) present in the epididymal fluid and seminal plasma are absorbed by the plasma membrane overlying the acrosome, possibly preventing premature capacitation/acrosomal exocytosis (Guraya, 1987). The immature spermatozoa taken out directly from the epididymis cannot fertilize oocytes. They attain fertilizing capability while traveling through the uterus and oviduct, a phenomenon referred to as *capacitation* (Chang, 1951; Yanagimachi, 1994).

The underlying event of capacitation appears to be changes in the plasma membrane fluidity caused by the loss of cholesterol and redistribution of phospholipids. The epididymal and ejaculated spermatozoa can be capacitated *in vitro* if they are cultured for several hours in the presence of serum albumin and bicarbonate ions or specific capacitation-promoting culture conditions (Jaiswal and Eisenbach, 2002). Several integral proteins of the plasma membrane are modified and rearranged after capacitation or acrosome reaction. For example, fertilin (antigen recognized by the antibody PH30) is uniformly distributed in the epididymal spermatozoa.

After capacitation, fertilin is proteolytically cleaved and redistributed to the post-acrosomal region (Evans 2002; Myles and Primakoff 1997). *Basigin*, a protein initially occurring on the principal piece of the sperm tail, moves to the mid-piece during epididymal transit and finally to the head after capacitation (Saxena et al., 2002). *Equatorin*, originally residing in the equatorial acrosome, is released and redistributed on the equatorial plasma membrane after acrosomal exocytosis (Manandhar and Toshimori, 2001).

The acrosin inhibitors adsorbed by the acrosomes and plasma membranes are removed during sperm migration in the female genital tract, an event that parallels capacitation (Guraya, 1987). The lipid rafts of plasma membrane of the sperm head region diffuse freely, but their movement to the tail region is restricted by the junction formed by the annulus at the mid-piece/principal piece joint.

Spermatogenesis

The spermatozoa develop from progenitor somatic cells (spermatogonia) in the testis and then undergo functional maturity in the epididymis. The entire process of spermatozoa development is called the *spermatogenesis*. The testicular phase of spermatogenesis consists of diploid and haploid phases.

Diploid Phase

The developing testis is invaded by the epiblast-derived male *primordial germ cells (PGCs)* at an early stage of embryonic development, following the migration of the PGCs from the allantois to the genital ridge (Clark and Eddy, 1975). The diploid testicular germ cells, spermatogonia, remain quiescent until the peri-pubertal stage of

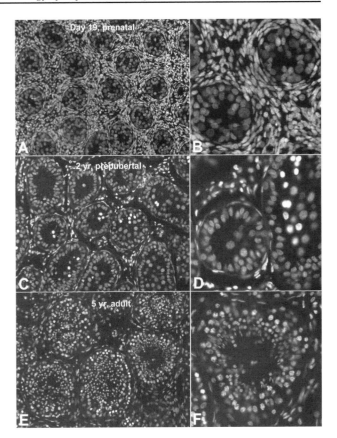

Figure 3.43. Germ cells in prenatal and postnatal rhesus monkey (*Macaca mulatto*) testes. Low (**A, C, E**) and corresponding high magnification images (**B, D, F**) of testicular tissue sections stained with blue fluorescent DNA stain DAPI. A high proportion of stromal cells and few spermatogonia are seen in the prenatal seminiferous tubules. Spermatogonial proliferation at or shortly before the onset of puberty causes dilation of the seminiferous tubules and a proportional reduction in the volume of testicular stroma. Diploid and haploid stage spermatogenic cells are visible in the fully differentiated seminiferous tubules of adult testis.

postnatal development (see Figure 3.43). They are activated at puberty and stimulated to proliferate by mitosis. Spermatogonia are found in the outer circumference of the seminiferous tubules, adjacent to the inner face of the basement membrane (see Figures 3.44–47).

From the reservoir of self regenerating stem cells, a group of type A-spermatogonia emerges that are destined to develop into spermatozoa (Clermont, 1969; Clermont and Antar, 1973; Foquet and Dadoune, 1986). Spermatogenesis begins from this stage. The type A-spermatogonia undergo a limited number of mitoses to produce a clone of cells that are linked together with cytoplasmic bridges, formed due to incomplete cytokinesis. The cytoplasmic bridges are retained until the spermatozoa are fully developed. After the final mitosis, the type A spermatogonia differentiate into type B-spermatogonia characterized by a unique morphology. All type B-spermatogonia

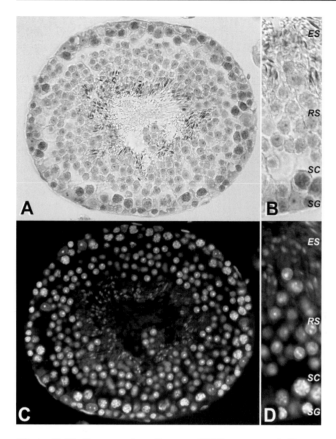

Figure 3.44. Cross-section of a stage II-III mouse seminiferous tubule, double stained with hematoxylin-eosin, DAPI, observed under a transmitted light microscope (**A, B**) and an epifluorescence microscope (**C, D**). The figures demonstrate a varied resolution of the cellular structures by the two histochemical techniques commonly used for staging of seminiferous epithelium. SG, spermatogonia; SC, pachytene spermatocytes; RS, round spermatids; and ES, late elongating spermatids.

undergo mitosis and finally enter meiosis as primary spermatocytes.

The seminiferous tubules have two compartments. The Basal Compartment located immediately beneath the basement membrane is bathed by blood from the peripheral endings of the testicular blood vessels. Hence, the blood serum components, paracrine secretions of the stromal Leydig cells and the endocrine secretions of the pituitary-gonadal axis, directly affect the cells of the basal compartment. The spermatogonia are located in these compartments. The Sertoli cells form tight junctions (blood-testis barrier) on the lateral membranes, restricting diffusion of the blood components from the basal compartment toward the lumen of the seminiferous tubule.

The region of the seminiferous tubules from the blood-testis barrier inward is called the Adluminal Compartment. The primary spermatocytes migrate into the adluminal compartment by crossing the blood-testis barrier. Spermatogenic cells in the adluminal compartment are not

directly affected by the blood or lymphatic fluid. Consequently, the adluminal compartment is an immunologically privileged site.

Though many proteins of the sperm plasma membrane are immunogenic, the spermatozoa develop normally without being attacked by the immune system. Once the spermatocytes cross the blood-testis barrier, their development is less prone to the systemic hormonal or physiological imbalances, a mechanism that secures reproductive fecundity under unfavorable conditions. A notable exception is the testicular pathology targeting Sertoli cells, which has a profound effect on both the basal and adluminal compartments (Figure 3.48).

After entering meiosis, the primary spermatocytes again become quiescent at the *pachytene stage* for some time, and then undergo meiosis I division, producing two secondary spermatocytes. Immediately each secondary spermatocyte undergoes meiosis II division, giving rise to two haploid spermatids. Due to random chromosome segregation and crossing-over, every spermatid is genetically unique, expressing unique haploid gene products. Nevertheless, the group of spermatids (clones) derived from one type A spermatogonium develops synchronously to maturity by

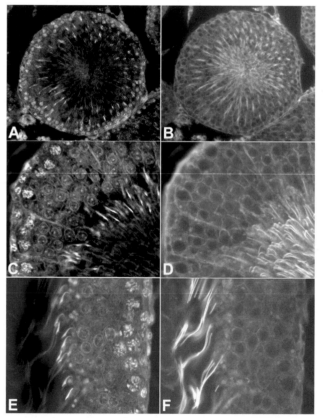

Figure 3.45. Seminiferous tubule sections double-stained with DAPI revealing the nuclei (**A, C, E**); anti-tubulin antibody revealing the microtubule cytoskeleton of spermatogenic cells (**B, D, F**) and axonemes of the elongating spermatids.

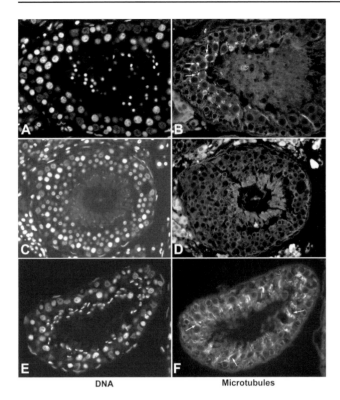

DNA   Microtubules

Figure 3.46. Spermatogenesis in a common opossum (*Didelphis virginiana*) as visualized by DNA labeling with DAPI (**A, C, E**) and microtubule labeling with anti-tubulin antibody (**B, D, F**) in testicular tissue sections. Note the bundling of microtubules in the cytoplasmic bridges (**arrows, B**) and Sertoli cells projecting their cytoplasmic extensions from the basal to the adluminal compartment (**arrows, F**).

exchanging their gametic gene products through the cytoplasmic bridges. Selection of the most vigorous spermatozoan for fertilization takes place during their journey through the uterus and oviduct to meet the oocyte.

Haploid Phase—Spermiogenesis

The testicular phase of sperm development after meiosis is called the *haploid phase* of spermatogenesis. During this phase, the immature sperm cells, or spermatids, develop in the crypts of Sertoli cells in the seminiferous tubules until they are fully formed and released into the lumen. The haploid spermatids develop various organelles, finally transforming themselves into spermatozoa.

Spermatid Elongation and Biogenesis of Sperm Accessory Structures

The early spermatids have round shapes, isodiametric nuclei, and somatic cell-like subcellular organization. They undergo complex morphogenesis, producing elongated and motile spermatozoa, the process referred to as the *spermiogenesis*. The duration of testicular spermiogenesis varies among individual mammals. The most prominent morphological changes are the compaction of nuclei, formation

of acrosomes, and biogenesis of the sperm tail (see Figure 3.49).

Acrosome formation begins at the earliest stage of spermiogenesis. The Golgi cisternae pinch off proacrosomal vesicles containing dense granules. These vesicles fuse and the granules coalesce and adhere on the nuclear surface. Additional vesicles are docked to the proacrosome that becomes anchored to the nascent subacrosomal perinuclear theca and gradually spreads on the nuclear surface, developing into a cap-like acrosome.

The *perinuclear theca (PT)* is formed in the early stage spermatids. Some PT gene transcripts are synthesized even before the meiotic division. The PT proteins first associate peripherally on the acrosomal vesicles, then becomes localized between the acrosome and nucleus at the subacrosomal region (Oko and Maravei, 1995; Oko, 1995). Later the PT extends caudally around the elongating spermatid nuclei.

Biogenesis of the sperm tail is also initiated at the early stage by the distal centriole (see Figure 3.49). In the beginning, the centrioles are randomly localized in the spermatid cytoplasm. The microtubule triplets of the distal centriole

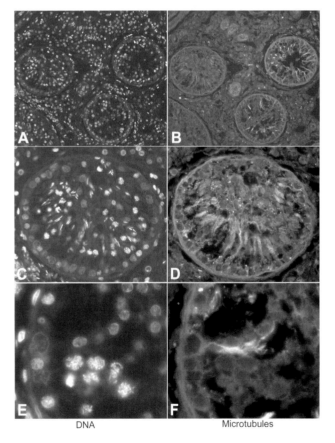

DNA   Microtubules

Figure 3.47. Double staining of DNA (**A, C, E**) and microtubules (**B, D, F**) of bull mediastinum. Compared to testicular parenchyma, a higher proportion of stromal cells are seen in the mediastinum where the ends of the seminiferous tubules converge into rete testis.

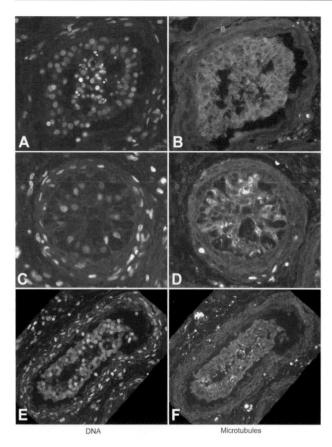

DNA   Microtubules

Figure 3.48. Testicular pathology in human chemotherapy patients, as shown by DNA (**A, C, E**) and tubulin (**B, D, F**) immunofluorescent labeling. Note the absence of germ cells and sloughing of Sertoli cells into the lumen of seminiferous tubules.

eventually extend posteriorly as axoneme doublets that meander through the intercellular spaces. The centriolar pair along with the nascent axoneme implants on the nuclear surface opposite the acrosome. The proximal centriole rotates tangentially to the nuclear surface while the distal centriole lies perpendicularly. At the site of implantation, the nuclear envelope becomes modified into an implantation fossa with a thick basal plate. Development of the outer dense fibers begins in the mid-piece region and progresses distally (Oko and Clermont, 1989). Initially they are attached to the wall of axonemal microtubules, but later separate from those. The fibrous sheath, however, is assembled first in the lower part of the principal piece, and then progresses upward up to the region of the annulus (Oko and Clermont, 1989).

The isodiametric nuclei of the round spermatids undergo a remarkable metamorphosis during spermatid elongation, resulting in highly compact, dorsiventrally flat, and uniquely shaped sperm heads characteristic of the particular animal species. Changes in nuclear shape take place concomitantly with chromatin condensation and development of perinuclear theca and Sertoli cell cytoskeletons. Histones of the spermatid chromatin are replaced by transition proteins that are finally replaced by protamines.

The sperm *nuclear envelope (NE)* is devoid of the nuclear pore complexes except in the redundant NE-folds of the posterior edges (Sutovsky et al., 1999). The nuclei move upward; the plasma membrane is closely applied over the anterior part of the nucleus where the acrosome spreads. The Sertoli cells develop actin-based junctional complexes at the interface with the spermatids. These unique structures, also referred to as *ectoplasmic special-*

Figure 3.49. Ultrastructure of developing spermatids. (**A**) A step 2 rhesus spermatid. The cell has freely localized Golgi apparatus (GA), proacrosomal vesicle (PV), and centriolar pair (**arrowhead**), not associated with the nucleus. The distal centriole has generated microtubular axoneme (**arrow**) that extends into the *intercellular* space. (**B**) A step 3 rhesus spermatid. The pro-acrosomal vesicle with a single pro-acrosomal granule has docked (**asterisk**) to the nascent subacrosomal perinuclear theca layer (**arrowheads**) on the anterior surface of nucleus. (**C**) A step 6 rhesus spermatid. The acrosomal cap has spread on the nuclear surface subtending an angle of 120°. Note a prominent Golgi apparatus (GA) adjacent to the nascent acrosomal cap (**asterisk**). (**D**) A step 10 rhesus spermatid. The membranous folds below the posterior edges of the acrosome have emanated manchette microtubules (**arrows**). Note that the sperm tail has attached to the implantation fossa of the sperm nucleus (**arrowheads**) and annuli (an) have begun to form. (**E**) Magnified view of a portion of sperm head as indicated by the boxed region in (D) showing nuclear membrane (NM), subacrosomal layer (SAL) of the perinuclear theca, and actin bundles (AB) of the Sertoli cells ectoplasmic specializations. (**F**) Centriolar complex of a step 10 mouse spermatid. The distal centriole appears dark due to accumulation of a thick pericentriolar vault and formation of striated columns. The proximal centriole extends a short adjunct (AJ) enveloped with a fibrous material that emanates microtubular aster. The nuclear membrane at the docking site has been remarkably thickened forming an implantation fossa (**arrowheads**). (**G**) Neck region of a mouse epididymal (fully mature) spermatozoon. The proximal and distal centriolar vaults (PCV, DCV) appear empty due to complete degeneration of centriolar microtubules. Mitochondria encircle the axoneme-ODF cylinder forming a sheath. (**H**) Cross section of the proximal centriole of a step 14 rhesus monkey spermatid, showing the typical pinwheel-like arrangement of nine microtubule triplets. (**I**) Cross-section of the neck region of a rhesus mature spermatozoon, approximately at the plane indicated by the line "**I**" in the figure (G). The centriolar microtubules are absent, but nine ODF are quite distinct. The central doublet of axoneme extends upward occupying the center of the cylinder. (**J**) Cross section of the mid-piece region of rhesus mature spermatozoon showing typical axoneme-ODF cylinder. (**K**) Cross section of the end-piece of a rhesus spermatozoan sperm tail. The two longitudinal columns (**asterisks**) and the horizontal ribs of fibrous sheath are well defined. Note the radial spoke-like dynein arms extending from the peripheral microtubules toward the central doublet.

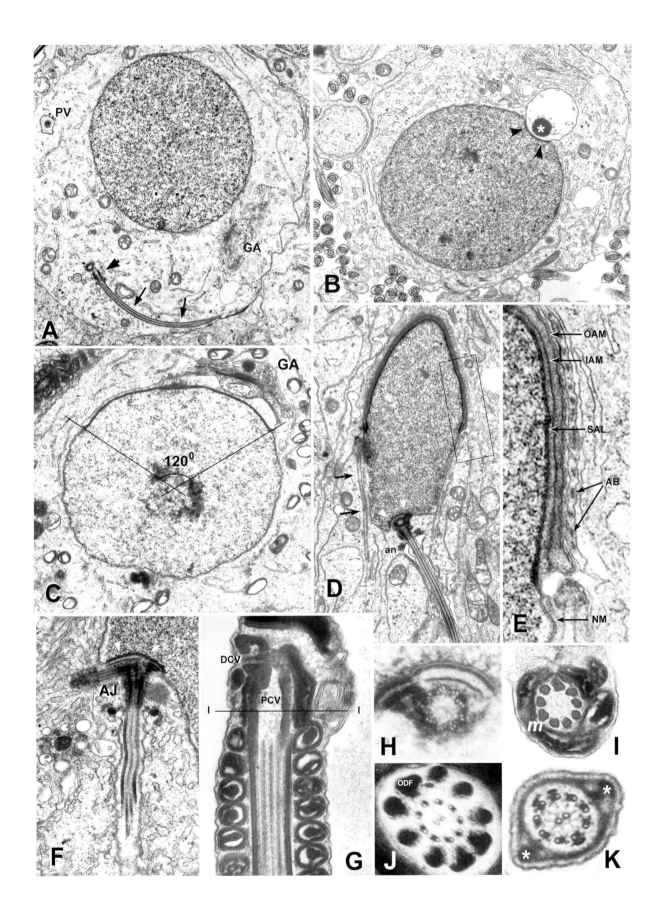

ization (Russell et al., 1988; Vogl et al., 1991), help maintain the proper orientation of spermatids and nuclear morphogenesis.

During the elongation stage, a narrow membranous fold encircling the nucleus below the posterior edge of the acrosome emanates a veil-like collection of microtubules, the *manchette*. It probably plays a role in nuclear shaping and transporting unused cytoplasmic materials to the residual bodies for disposal (Kierszenbaum, 2002). The proximal centrioles transiently produce short adjuncts that are surrounded by flocculent fibrous material nucleating microtubular asters (Manandhar et al., 1998, 2000). The annulus descends during the late stages of spermiogenesis. The evacuated proximal region of the axoneme-ODF cylinder is encircled by a mitochondrial helix. This part of the tail becomes the mid-piece.

Spermatids develop in the crypts of Sertoli cells in the adluminal compartment until fully differentiated. Morphologically mature spermatozoa are released as individual cells into the lumen of the seminiferous tubule, a process called *spermiation*. Before release, excess cytoplasm of the elongated spermatids is pinched off as residual bodies that are phagocytosed by the Sertoli cells. In mammalian species with poor semen quality, residual bodies often contaminate the ejaculated semen. Testicular spermatozoa are immotile; they are transported into the epididymis by the pressure of luminal fluid secreted by the Sertoli cells and by the motile force of the ciliated cells of efferent ducts.

Steps of Spermiogenesis

Spermiogenesis is a long and strictly regulated process that can be divided into smaller steps characterized by distinct morphogenetic features, particularly the shape of acrosome and nucleus and the degree of chromatin condensation. Several comprehensive reviews and book chapters have described the morphological features of this intricate process (Barth and Oko, 1989; deKretser and Kerr, 1994; Hess and Moore, 1993; Russell et al., 1990). Mouse spermiogenesis comprises 16 steps of morphogenesis as described below (see Figure 3.50):

Step 1. Newly formed spermatid nuclei display a finely granular texture and a dense heterochromatin in the center. Some late-stage dividing meiotic II cells are seen at the vicinity of step 1 spermatids. The spermatids do not yet have acrosomes, but a prominent Golgi apparatus localizes randomly in the cytoplasm or at the juxtanuclear position.

Step 2. Proacrosomal granules are seen between the Golgi apparatus and nuclei, but they are unattached to the nuclear envelope.

Step 3. Proacrosomal granules fuse, forming a single round acrosomal vesicle that attaches to the nuclear envelope with the help of a newly deposited nascent subacrosomal layer of perinuclear theca (see Figure 3.49, section B).

Step 4. The acrosomal vesicle begins to flatten out and spread on the nucleus. Step 4 continues until the margins of the acrosome make a 40° wedge with respect to the nuclear center.

Step 5. The acrosomal vesicle spreads until its margins stretch up to 95° from the center of the nucleus.

Step 6. The acrosomal margins extend up to 120° (see Figure 3.49, section C).

Step 7. The acrosomal margins extend to an angle of 120° to 150°. The centrioles subtending axonemes dock to the nucleus at the site opposite the acrosome.

Step 8. The nuclei elongate slightly, becoming pear-shaped. The nucleus migrates upward and the acrosomal region contacts the inner face of the spermatid plasma membrane.

Step 9. Nuclear shaping begins as it elongates and flattens laterally. The dorsal side curves, but the ventral side remains flat. The apical hook begins to take shape. The acrosome extends mostly on the dorsal surface and the curved tip of the nucleus. The caudal surface is narrow and flat. A microtubule-based manchette (see Color Figures 1 and 2) is formed.

Step 10. The nuclei flatten and elongate further. The acrosome reaches almost to the caudal end of the dorsal nuclear surface. The angle between the ventral and caudal surfaces becomes sharp due to development of implantation fossa. Proximal centriolar adjunct and adjunct-asters are formed (see Figure 3.49, section F).

Step 11. Nuclei appear compact due to chromatin condensation. The angle between the dorsal and caudal surfaces also makes a sharp turn.

Step 12. The nuclei have the longest size and compact chromatin. Dividing-stage meiotic cells are seen in the surroundings.

Step 13. The spermatid heads shorten further.

Step 14. The heads become shorter and broader.

Step 15. The mitochondria begin to align around the proximal axoneme-ODF cylinder.

Step 16. The mitochondrial sheath formation is complete. The apical hook of the sperm head is distinct. Structurally mature spermatozoa are released from the seminiferous epithelium into the lumens of seminiferous tubules. The loose spermatozoa from the seminiferous tubule's lumens are collected in the rete testis and transported via efferent duct to the initial segment of the epididymis. The sperm biogenesis continues in the epididymis. Structurally and functionally mature spermatozoa are finally stored in the cauda epididymis, the cavernous distal compartment.

Cycle of the Seminiferous Epithelium

As described above, a group of spermatids originated by common lineage from a spermatogonium develop synchronously. Hence, the seminiferous tubules in cross sections display groups of spermatogenic cells in specific stages of spermatogenesis (see Figures 3.44 to 3.47). At a given time

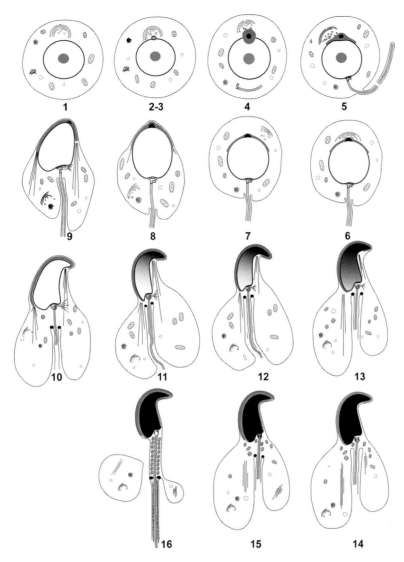

Figure 3.50. Schematic diagrams elucidating steps 1 through 16 of mouse spermiogenesis. The haploid germ cells produced immediately after meiosis II are the step 1 spermatids. They have isodiametric nuclei with distinct heterochromatin, randomly localized Golgi apparatus, and centriolar complex. As the spermatids develop, the Golgi apparatus moves to the anterior surface of the nucleus where the acrosome stretches as a cap-like structure. The centriolar apparatus along with the axoneme docks on the posterior side of the nucleus in step-5 spermatids. From step-6 onward the nuclear heterochromatin disappears. In step-8, the nuclei move upward, resulting in its acrosomal side becoming closely apposed with the plasma membrane. The nuclei assume the characteristic pear-shape. In the step-9 spermatids, the membrane folds below the posterior edges of the acrosome emanate manchette microtubules. The proximal centrioles also extend adjuncts radiating microtubule aster. Anterior hook and falciform shape of nuclei are evident in step-10 spermatids. Formation of annulus and striated columns are also notable. From step-11 onward, the nuclei become progressively narrower and elongated. The chromatin condensation apparently progress from the proximal to the distal direction in the nuclei. Nuclear chromatins are homogeneously compact in step-14 to step-16 spermatids. The annuli begin to descend in step 15 and step-16 spermatids, and the space around the axoneme-ODF cylinder evacuated by the annuli is encircled by the mitochondrial sheath. After step-16 spermiogenesis, the testicular spermatozoa are released into the seminiferous tubule lumen, pinching off and leaving behind the residual cytoplasm in the Sertoli cell crypts.

and location in the seminiferous tubule, a group of type-A spermatogonia enters spermatogenesis. After a definite interval, a new group of type-A spermatogonia enters spermatogenesis. By this time the previous spermatogenic cells would advance to a higher stage of development. Thus, spermatogenesis is initiated and propagated at a definite periodicity, mimicking a spiral cycle called the *spermatogenic cycle* or *cycle of seminiferous epithelium* (see Figure 3.51).

The duration of the spermatogenic cycle, i.e. the pitch of the spiral cycle and the progress of spermatogenesis during this period, are always constant in a given species, but vary

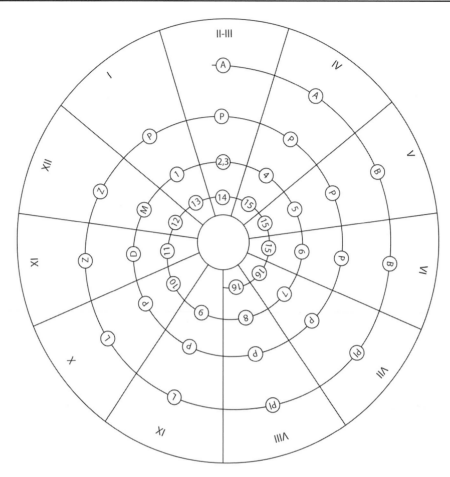

Figure 3.51. Schematic interpretation of the cycle of seminiferous epithelium modeled after mouse spermatogenesis. Roman numerals represent stages I through XII of spermatogenesis. Arabic numerals represent steps 1 through 16 of spermiogenesis.

in different species (Table 3.2). For example, in mice the spermatogenic cycle of the seminiferous epithelium is 8.6 days long and complete spermatogenesis comprises 4.5 cycles. Thus, mature spermatozoa are shed from the given segment of seminiferous epithelium every 8.6 days; however, a complete testicular spermatogenesis, from spermatogonium stage to spermiation, requires 39 days. During one spermatogenic cycle in mice, the germ cells undergo 12 stages of spermatogenesis, which are by consensus assigned roman numerals I to XII.

A constant periodicity applies not only to the overall cycle, but also to each stage of spermatogenesis. Therefore, each spermatogenic stage coexists with three or four preceding or following stages of the corresponding cycles. Because there are 12 spermatogenic stages in one mouse spermatogenic cycle, there would be 12 different combinations of germ cells (14 in the rat) designated as the stages of seminiferous epithelium.

The seminiferous tubule of each stage consists of the germ cells belonging to various cycles in concentric layers, progressing from the basement membrane to the lumen. For example, the mouse stage II seminiferous tubule shows concentric layers of type B spermatogonial cells, pachytene spermatocytes, step 5 spermatids, and step 15 spermatids sequentially from the basement to the lumen. Thus, the cycle of seminiferous epithelium can be defined as the successive, synchronous evolution of one stage of spermatogenesis to the next.

Table 3.2. Kinetics of spermatogenesis in selected mammalian species.

Animals	Duration of spermatogenesis (Days)	Duration of cycle (days)	No. of stages of semf tubules	No. of steps of spermiogenesis
Man	64	16	6	8–9
Monkey	?	10	12	?
Dog	49	13.6	8	12
Bull	54	13.5	8	?
Ram	49	10.4	8	?
Boar	34	8.6	8	?
Rat	48	12	14	19
Mouse	39	8.6	12	16

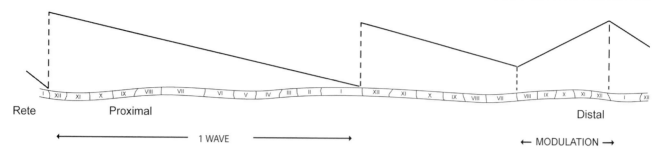

Figure 3.52. A schematic interpretation of the wave of seminiferous epithelium, incorporating the concept of wave modulation.

Some common characteristics can be used to simplify the staging of seminiferous epithelium. For example, round spermatids are found in stages I to VII. Dividing primary and secondary spermatocytes with meiotic spindles and condensed chromosomes occur in stage XII tubules (stage XIV in rat) (Hess and Moore, 1993).

In contrast to other mammals, spermatogenesis in humans appears to be synchronized in small areas (Clermont, 1963; Schulze and Rehder, 1984). When examined in transverse sections, the organized germ cell association belonging to one stage is confined to a segment of the tubule as a wedge; the adjacent sectors are occupied by the preceding or following developmental stages. The demarcation lines between the adjacent stages are not quite distinct. A cross section of tubules usually shows three stages of spermatogenesis. Some regions of the tubules may lack one or even two generations of spermatogenic cells. This anomaly is more frequent in individuals showing lower sperm count. The human spermatogenic cycle comprises six stages of cellular associations (Clermont, 1963).

Spermatogenic Wave

As described above, groups of germ cells progress through successive stages of development with defined periodicity at any location of seminiferous tubules. Spermatogenesis is a highly organized developmental process in time as well as space. The seminiferous tubules thus exhibit orderly progression of spermatogenic stages along the length. Distally from the rete testis, segments of tubule exhibit sequentially earlier spermatogenetic stages until reaching stage I, followed by a new sequence of orderly descending spermatogenic stages. In other words, spermatogenetic stages progress in a wave-like pattern along the length of the tubule, a phenomenon referred to as the spermatogenic wave. Hence, the wave of the seminiferous epithelium can be defined as the arrangement of successive stages of the cycle along the length of the seminiferous tubule.

The sequence of spermatogenic wave may be reversed (ascending order) in some segments of a seminiferous tubule. Such segments are called the *modulations* (see Figure 3.52). The modulated wave eventually returns to the normal, descending order. Because the spermatogenic waves progress in descending order distally from both ends

of the seminiferous tubule, they meet at a common stage somewhere in the middle of the seminiferous tubule. The average spermatogenic wave length, i.e. the length of seminiferous tubule segment comprising all 12 stages, in mice is 2.6 cm.

Conclusion

Spermatogenesis is an intricate process by which haploid, individualized spermatozoa with unique accessory structures and fertilizing capability are produced from immotile, diploid, somatic-cell-like spermatogonia. The spermatogenic stem cells undergo proliferation with two distinct end points: self renewal by mitosis and transformation into spermatocytes. Each spermatocyte divides by two cycles of meiotic division, giving rise to four haploid spermatids that undergo spermiogenesis, forming highly elongated and free-swimming spermatozoa.

Spermatogenesis is made possible by the unique architecture of seminiferous epithelium in which the diploid phase of spermatogenesis occurs in the nutrient-rich basal compartment and the haploid cells, expressing unique, male germ cell-specific surface receptors, develop in the adluminal compartments, protected from the body's immune system by the blood-testis barrier.

By building on the existing knowledge of mammalian spermatogenesis, it will become possible to produce normal spermatozoa *in vitro* to treat infertility caused by trauma, cancer, toxic exposure, congenital condition, etc. On the other hand, seminiferous epithelium can be an important target for reversible male contraceptive drugs that will alter the blood-testis barrier, halt spermatogenesis/spermiogenesis, or prevent spermiation.

Acknowledgments

We thank Dr. Richard Oko for critical reading of the manuscript, and Kathryn Craighead for proofreading and editing. The support of our lab mates Kathleen Baska, Dawn Feng, Nicole Leitman, Kyle Lovercamp, Miriam Sutovsky, and Youg-Joo Yi, and our many external and internal collaborators, is greatly appreciated. Our research on mammalian spermatogenesis is currently supported by USDA-NRI award #2002-02069 and by funding from the Pfizer

Foundation and Food for the 21st Century Program of the University of Missouri-Columbia.

Bibliography

Abeydeera, L.R., Johnson, L.A., Welch, G.R., Wang, W.H., Boquest, A.C., Cantley, T.C., Rieke, A., and Day, B.N. (1998). Birth of piglets preselected for gender following in-vitro fertilization of in-vitro matured pig oocytes by X and Y chromosome bearing spermatozoa sorted by high speed flow cytometry. *Theriogenology* 50(7):981–988.

Aitken, J.R. (2000). Possible redox regulation of sperm motility activation. *J Androl* 21(4):491–496.

Baba, T., Azuma, S., Kashiwabara, S., and Toyoda, Y. (1994). Sperm from mice carrying a targeted mutation of the acrosin gene can penetrate the oocyte zona pellucida and effect fertilization. *J Biol Chem* 69(50):31845–31849.

Barth, A.D., and Oko, R.J. (1989). *Abnormal morphology of bovine spermatozoa*. Ames: Iowa State University Press.

Bedford, J.M. (1998). Mammalian fertilization misread? Sperm penetration of the eutherian zona pellucida is unlikely to be a lytic event. *Biol Reprod* 59(6):1275–1287.

Brewer L., Corzett, M., and Balhorn, R. (2002). Condensation of DNA by nuclear basic nuclear proteins. *J Biol Chem* 277(41): 38895–388900.

Churikov, D., Zalenskaya, I.A., and Zalensky, A.O. (2004). Male germline-specific histones in mouse and man. *Cytogenet Genome Res* 105(2–4):203–214.

Clark, J.M., and Eddy, E.M. (1975). Fine structural observations on the origin and associations of primordial germ cells of the mouse. *Dev Biol* 47(1):136–155.

Clermont, Y. (1963). The cycle of the seminiferous epithelium in man. *Am J Anat* 112:35–51.

Clermont, Y., and Antar, M. (1973). Duration of the cycle of the seminiferous epithelium and the spermatogonial renewal in the monkey *Macaca arctoides*. *Am J Anat* 136(2):153–165.

Cooper, T.G., and Yeung, C.H. (2003). Acquisition of volume regulatory response of sperm upon maturation in the epididymis and the role of the cytoplasmic droplet. *Microsc Res Tech* 61(1):28–38.

Cuasnicu, P.S., Ellerman, D.A., Cohen, D.J., Busso, D., Morgenfeld, M.M., and Da Ros, V.G. (2001). Molecular mechanisms involved in mammalian gamete fusion. *Arch Med Res* 32(6):614–618.

Cummins, J. (2000). Fertilization and elimination of the paternal mitochondrial genome. *Hum Reprod* 15 Suppl 2:92–101.

deKretser, D.M., and Kerr, J.B. (1994). The cytology of testis. In: Knobil, E., and Neill, J.D. (eds) *The Physiology of Reproduction*, Ames: Raven Press, New York, pp 1177–1290.

Eddy, E.M., O'Brien, D.A., Fenderson, B.A., and Welch, J.E. (1991). Intermediate filament—like proteins in the fibrous sheath of the mouse sperm flagellum. *Ann N Y Acad Sci* 637:224–239.

Eddy, E.M., Toshimori, K., and O'Brien, D.A. (2003). Fibrous sheath of mammalian spermatozoa. *Microsc Res Tech* 61(1): 103–115.

Evans, J.P. (2002). The molecular basis of sperm-oocyte membrane interactions during mammalian fertilization. *Hum Reprod Update* 8(4):297–311.

Fernandez-Novell, J.M., Ballester, J., Medrano, A., Otaegui, P.J., Rigau, T., Guinovart, J.J., and Rodriguez-Gil, J.E. (2004). The presence of a high-Km hexokinase activity in dog, but not in boar, sperm. *FEBS Lett* 570(1–3):211–216.

Fischer, K. (2003). Proteins of the 15-lipoxygenase and ubiquitin-proteasome pathways colocalize in the boar sperm cytoplasmic droplet. Master of Science Thesis, Graduate School, University of Missouri-Columbia, Columbia, MO.

Florman, H.M., and Storey, B.T. (1982). Mouse gamete interactions: the zona pellucida is the site of the acrosome reaction leading to fertilization in-vitro. *Dev Biol* 91(1):121–130.

Fouquet, J.P., and Dadoune, J.P. (1986). Renewal of spermatogonia in the monkey (*Macaca fascicularis*). *Biol Reprod* 35(1):199–207.

Fouquet, J.P., and Kann, M.L. (1994). The cytoskeleton of mammalian spermatozoa. *Biol Cell* 81(2):89–93.

Fraser, L.R. (1982). p-Aminobenzamidine, an acrosin inhibitor, inhibits mouse sperm penetration of the zona pellucida but not the acrosome reaction. *J Reprod Fertil* 65(1):185–94.

Garner, D.L. (2006). Flow cytometric sexing of mammalian sperm. *Theriogenology* 65(5):943–957.

Gerton, J.L. (2002). Function of the sperm acrosome. In: Hardy, D. (ed), *Fertilization*, Ames: Academic Press, San Diego, pp 265–302.

Guraya, S.S. (1987). *Biology of Spermatogenesis and Spermatozoa in Mammals*. Ames: Springer-Verlag, Berlin.

Hollinshead, F.K., Evans, G., Evans, K.M., Catt, S.L., Maxwell, W.M., and O'Brien, J.K. (2004). Birth of lambs of a predetermined sex after in-vitro production of embryos using frozen-thawed sex-sorted and re-frozen-thawed ram spermatozoa. *Reproduction* 127(5):557–568.

Honda, A., Siruntawineti, J., and Baba, T. (2002). Role of acrosomal matrix proteases in sperm-zona pellucida interactions. *Hum Reprod Update* 8(5):405–412.

Hess, R.A., and Moore, G.L. (1993). Histological Methods for the Evaluation of the Testis. In Chapin, R.E., and Heindel, J.J. (eds), *Methods in Reproductive Toxicology*, Ames: Academic Press, San Diego, pp 52–85.

Hoyer-Fender, S., Neesen, J., Szpirer, J., and Szpirer, C. (2003). Genomic organisation and chromosomal assignment of ODF2 (outer dense fiber 2), encoding the main component of sperm tail outer dense fibers and a centrosomal scaffold protein. *Cytogenet Genome Res* 103(1–2):122–127.

Jaiswal, B.S., and Eisenbach, M. (2002). Capacitation. In Hardy, D. (ed), *Fertilization*, San Diego: Academic Press, pp 57–118.

Johnson, L.A., Rath, D., Vazquez, J.M., Maxwell, W.M., and Dobrinsky, J.R. (2005). Preselection of sex of offspring in swine for production: current status of the process and its application. *Theriogenology* 63(2):615–624.

Kaplan, M., Russell, L.D., Peterson, R.N., and Martan, J. (1984). Boar sperm cytoplasmic droplets: their ultrastructure, their numbers in the epididymis and at ejaculation and their removal during isolation of sperm plasma membranes. *Tissue Cell* 16:455–468.

Kierszenbaum, A.L. (2002). Intramanchette transport (IMT): managing the making of the spermatid head, centrosome, and tail. *Mol Reprod Dev* 63(1):1–4.

Larsen, R.E., and Chenoweth, P.J. (1990). Diadem/crater defects in spermatozoa from two related angus bulls. *Mol Reprod Dev* 25(1):87–96.

Liu, D.Y., and Baker, H.W. (1993). Inhibition of acrosin activity with a trypsin inhibitor blocks human sperm penetration of the zona pellucida. *Biol Reprod* 48(2):340–348.

Manandhar, G., Simerly, C., and Schatten, G. (2000). Centrosome reduction during mammalian spermiogenesis. *Curr Top Dev Biol* 49:343–363.

Manandhar, G., and Toshimori, K. (2003). Fate of postacrosomal perinuclear theca recognized by monoclonal antibody MN13 after sperm head microinjection and its role in oocyte activation in mice. *Biol Reprod* 68(2):655–663.

Manandhar, G., Schatten, H., and Sutovsky, P. (2005). Centrosome reduction during gametogenesis and its significance. *Biol Reprod* 72(1):2–13.

Manandhar, G., and Toshimori, K. (2001). Exposure of sperm head equatorin after acrosome reaction and its fate after fertilization in mice. *Biol Reprod* 65(5):1425–1436.

Manandhar, G., Sutovsky, P., Joshi, H., Stearns, T., and Schatten, G. (1998). Centrosome reduction during mouse spermiogenesis. *Dev Biol* 203:424–434.

Manandhar, G., and Schatten, G. (1999). Formation of synchytial spermatids and their development in mice. 32nd Annual Meeting of the Society for the Study of Reproduction, Pullman, WA.

Meistrich, M.L., Mohapatra, B., Shirley, C.R., and Zhao, M. (2003). Roles of transition nuclear proteins in spermiogenesis. *Chromosoma* 111(8):483–488.

Miki, K., Qu, W., Goulding, E.H., Willis, W.D., Bunch, D.O., Strader, L.F., Perreault, S.D., Eddy, E.M., and O'Brien, D.A. (2004). Glyceraldehyde 3-phosphate dehydrogenase-S, a sperm-specific glycolytic enzyme, is required for sperm motility and male fertility. *Proc Natl Acad Sci USA* 101(47):16501–16506.

Myles, D.G., and Primakoff, P. (1997). Why did the sperm cross the cumulus? To get to the oocyte. Functions of the sperm surface proteins PH-20 and fertilin in arriving at, and fusing with, the egg. *Biol Reprod* 56(2):320–327.

Oko, R., and Clermont, Y. (1989). Light microscopic immuno-cytochemical study of fibrous sheath and outer dense fiber formation in the rat spermatid. *Anat Rec* 225(1):46–55.

Oko, R. (1995). Developmental expression and possible role of perinuclear theca proteins in mammalian spermatozoa. *Reprod Fertil Dev* 7(4):777–797.

Oko, R. (1998). Occurrence and formation of cytoskeletal proteins in mammalian spermatozoa. *Andrologia* 30(4–5):193–206.

Oko, R., Hermo, L., Chan, P.T, Fazel, A., and Bergeron, J.J. (1993). The cytoplasmic droplet of rat epididymal spermatozoa contains saccular elements with Golgi characteristics. *J Cell Biol* 123(4):809–821.

Olds-Clarke, P. (2003). Unresolved issues in mammalian fertilization. *Int Rev Cytol* 232:129–84.

Paweletz, N., Mazia, D., and Finze, E.M. (1987a). Fine structural studies of the bipolarization of the mitotic apparatus in the fertilized sea urchin egg. I. The structure and behavior of centrosomes before fusion of the pronuclei. *Eur J Cell Biol* 44:195–204.

Paweletz, N., Mazia, D., and Finze, E.M. (1987b). Fine structural studies of the bipolarization of the mitotic apparatus in the fertilized sea urchin egg. II. Bipolarization before the first mitosis. *Eur J Cell Biol* 44:205–213.

Payne, C., Rawe, V., Ramalho-Santos, J., Simerly, C., and Schatten, G. (2003). Preferentially localized dynein and peri-nuclear dynactin associate with nuclear pore complex proteins to mediate genomic union during mammalian fertilization. *J Cell Sci* 116:4727–4738.

Perreault, S.D., Wolf, R.A., and Zirkin, B.R. (1984). The role of disulfide bond reduction during mammalian sperm nuclear decondensation in-vivo. *Dev Biol* 101:160–167.

Perry, A.C., Wakayama, T., and Yanagimachi, R. (1999a). A novel trans-complementation assay suggests full mammalian oocyte activation is coordinately initiated by multiple, submembrane sperm components. *Biol Reprod* 60(3):747–755.

Perry, A.C., Wakayama, T., Kishikawa, H., Kasai, T., Okabe, M., Toyoda, Y., and Yanagimachi, R. (1999b). Mammalian transgenesis by intracytoplasmic sperm injection. *Science* 284(5417):1180–1183.

Russell, L.D., Goh, J.C., Rashed, R.M., and Vogl, A.W. (1988). The consequences of actin disruption at Sertoli ectoplasmic specialization sites facing spermatids after in-vivo exposure of rat testis to cytochalasin D. *Biol Reprod* 39(1):105–18.

Russell, L.D., Ettlin, R., Hikim, A.P.S., and Clegg, E.D. (1990). *Histological Pathological Evaluation of the Testis.* Clearwater, FL: Cache River Press.

Saxena, D.K., Oh-Oka, T., Kadomatsu, K., Muramatsu, T., and Toshimori, K. (2002). Behaviour of a sperm surface trans-membrane glycoprotein basigin during epididymal maturation and its role in fertilization in mice. *Reproduction* 123: 435–444.

Schatten, G. (1994). The centrosome and its mode of inheritance: the reduction of the centrosome during gametogenesis and its restoration during fertilization. *Dev Biol* 165(2):299–335.

Schulze, W., and Rehder, U. (1984). Organization and orphogen-esis of the human seminiferous epithelium. *Cell Tissue Res* 237(3):395–407.

Sutovsky, P., Navara, C., and Schatten, G. (1996). The fate of the sperm mitochondria and the incorporation, conversion and disassembly of the sperm tail structures during bovine fertil-ization in-vitro. *Biol. Reprod* 55:1195–1205.

Sutovsky, P., Oko, R., Hewitson, L., and Schatten, G. (1997). The removal of the sperm perinuclear theca and its association with the bovine oocyte surface during fertilization. *Dev Biol* 188(1):75–84.

Sutovsky, P., Ramalho-Santos, J., Moreno, R., Oko, R., Hewitson, L., and Schatten, G. (1999). On-stage selection of single round spermatids using a vital, mitochondrion-specific fluorescent probe MitoTracker(TM) and high resolution differential interference contrast microscopy. *Hum Reprod* 14(9):2301–2312.

Sutovsky, P., Manandhar, G., Wu, A., and Oko, R. (2003). Interactions of sperm perinuclear theca with the oocyte: implications for oocyte activation, anti-polyspermy defense, and assisted reproduction. *Microsc Res Tech* 61(4):362–378.

Sutovsky, P., Manandhar, G., McCauley, T.C., Caamano, J.N., Sutovsky, M., Thompson, W.E., and Day, B.N.(2004). Proteasomal interference prevents zona pellucida penetration and fertilization in mammals. *Biol Reprod* 71(5):1625–37.

Toshimori, K., Tanii, I., Araki, S., and Oura, C. (1992). Characterization of the antigen recognized by a monoclonal antibody MN9: unique transport pathway to the equatorial segment of sperm head during spermiogenesis. *Cell Tissue Res* 270(3): 459–468.

Tulsiani, D.R., Abou-Haila, A., Loeser, C.R., and Pereira, B.M. (1998). The biological and functional significance of the sperm acrosome and acrosomal enzymes in mammalian fertilization. *Exp Cell Res* 240(2):151–164.

Turner, R.M., Eriksson, R.L., Gerton, G.L., and Moss, S.B. (1999). Relationship between sperm motility and the processing and tyrosine phosphorylation of two human sperm fibrous sheath proteins, pro-hAKAP82 and hAKAP82. *Mol Hum Reprod* 5(9):816–824.

Valdivia, M., Sillerico, T., De Ioannes, A., and Barros, C. (1999). Proteolytic activity of rabbit perivitelline spermatozoa. *Zygote* 7(2):143–9.

Vogl, A.W., Pfeiffer, D.C., and Redenbach, D.M. (1991). Ectoplasmic ("junctional") specializations in mammalian Sertoli cells: influence on spermatogenic cells. *Ann N Y Acad Sci* 637: 175–202.

Wooley, D.M., and Fawcett, D.W. (1973). The degeneration and disappearance of the centrioles during the development of the rat spermatozoa. *Anat Rec* 177:289–203.

Yanagimachi, R. (1994). Mammalian fertilization. In: Knobil, E., and Neill, J.D. (eds), *The Physiology of Reproduction*, 2nd ed., Ames: Raven Press, New York, pp 189–317.

Zamboni, L., Zemjanis, R., and Stefanini, M. (1971). The fine structure of monkey and human spermatozoa. *Anat Rec* 169(2): 129–53.

Zaneveld, L.J. 1982. *Research Frontier in Fertility Regulation, Vol III*, Gerland, G.I. (ed) Ames: Northwestern University, Chicago, pp 1–15.

Part 3.4
Overview of Female Reproductive Organs

Cheryl S. Rosenfeld and Heide Schatten

The anatomy and developmental anatomy of the female reproductive organs have been described in detail in Chapters 1 and 2, respectively. Please see these chapters and chapter 5 on reproductive physiology for complete descriptions. In this chapter we show representative histological images of the paired ovaries, the ducts (oviduct, uterus, and vagina) that are derived from the Paramesonephric or Müllerian duct, and the external genitalia (labia majora, labia minora, and clitoris)(for review on these systems see Hafez and Hafez, 2000; Eurell and Frappier, 2006).

Ovary

The four main functions of the ovaries are production of female gametes (ova), secretion of steroid hormones (estrogen and progesterone), regulation of postnatal growth, and secondary sexual characteristics.

Primordial Germ Cells and Oogonia

Primordial germ cells (PGC) first appear in the yolk sac endoderm at around 17 days post-coitus (dpc) in the dog and 19 dpc in cattle. These cells then migrate from the dorsal mesentery of the hindgut to the gonadal ridge, which at this time is undifferentiated and has the potential to become an ovary or testes (Motta et al., 1997; Bendel-Stenzel et al., 1998; Pereda et al., 2006). In females, the primordial germ cells will give rise to *oogonia* that undergo extensive mitosis during prenatal development. After birth, the oogonia presumably undergo mitotic arrest, but some reports indicate that these cells retain limited mitotic potential after birth. In general, though, females have little to no ability to replenish their germ cells after birth; whereas, males have lifetime replenishment of their germ cells. Oogonia eventually differentiate into primary oocytes.

Primary and Secondary Oocytes

At birth, most females have approximately 1 million primary oocytes, but only several hundred of these will ovulate. The fate of most oocytes is to undergo degeneration or atresia. All of the oocytes contained within ovarian follicles are primary oocytes. Those oocytes that are ovulated will enter the first round of meiosis and give rise to a secondary oocyte and first polar body. The secondary oocyte will complete the second round of meiosis and a haploid ovum and secondary polar body result from this last round of division.

Ovarian Morphology

The ovary is divided into a cortex and medulla. In most species the cortex contains the ovarian follicles and corpora lutea (CL), but in equid species, these structures are instead located in the medullary region. In all other species, the medulla solely contains blood and lymph vessels and nerves.

Ovarian Cortex

The ovarian cortex is covered by a superficial simple squamous to cuboidal epithelium that is also referred to as *germinal epithelium* because it used to be thought that these cells gave rise to the germ cells (see Figures 3.53, 3.54, and 3.55). However, it is now recognized that these cells do not produce germs cells but are instead similar to mesothelial cells. Deep to these epithelial cells is a dense irregular connective tissue called *tunica albuginea* that blends into the *ovarian stroma* of loose connective tissue that contains the ovarian follicles in most species (see Figure 3.53).

Ovarian Medulla

The ovarian medulla contains blood and lymph vessels and nerves. Connective tissue with some smooth muscle is also present in this region, as well as the rete ovarii, which are blind ending tubules. In equid species, ovarian follicles are located within the ovarian medulla.

Ovarian Follicular Development

The primary oocyte and its surrounding epithelial cells are considered an ovarian follicle at all stages of development. Ovarian follicular development is divided into four recognizable stages: primordial, primary, secondary, and tertiary (vesicular, pre-ovulatory or Graafian) follicles.

Primordial Follicle

The primordial follicle is classified by the primary oocyte surrounded by a single layer of simple squamous follicular epithelial cells (see Figure 3.53). Along with the primary follicles, they are located below the tunica albuginea in the superficial cortex region and are generally at a resting phase.

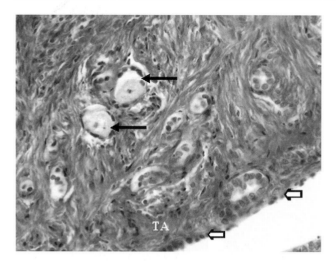

Figure 3.53. Low magnification of canine ovarian cortex region. **Block arrows** point at the lining superficial or germinal epithelium, which are mesothelial cells. **Arrows** point at primordial follicles with simple squamous epithelial cells surrounding a primary oocyte. **TA**, tunica albuginea, it is the connective tissue below the superficial epithelium and blends into the ovarian stroma. (Also see color plate)

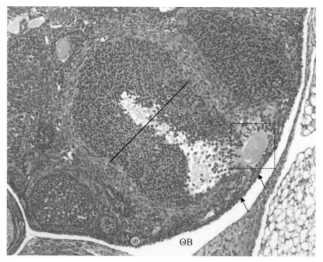

Figure 3.55. Mouse ovary with tertiary (Graafian) follicle undergoing ovulation (**bar**). **Boxed area**, primary oocyte, corona radiata, and cumulus oophoros that are in the process of ovulation. **Arrows** point at the superficial or germinal epithelium that surrounds the ovary. **OB**, ovarian bursa, which is the region that the primary oocyte will be released into after ovulation. (Also see color plate)

Primary Follicle

The primary follicle includes the primary oocyte and an encasing single layer of cuboidal follicular epithelial cells (see Figure 3.54). Clusters of primordial and primary follicles are called an *egg nest* and are commonly seen in species that ovulate more than one oocyte at a time.

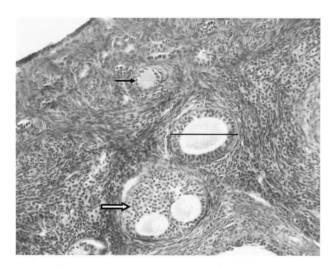

Figure 3.54. Low magnification of canine ovarian cortex region. The **black arrow** points at a primary follicle with simple cuboidal epithelium surrounding a primary oocyte. The **bar** spans a secondary follicle with stratified follicular epithelium around the primary oocyte. The **block arrow** points at a polyovulatory follicle, which is atypical. If this follicle ovulates, two primary oocytes will be released. (Also see color plate)

Secondary Follicle

At this stage of development, the primary oocyte is surrounded by stratified follicular epithelial (granulosa) cells and inner and outer theca (interstitial) cells are developing beyond the basement membrane of the follicle (see Figure 3.54). The oocyte and surrounding granulosa cells have produced a well-defined zona pellucida (glycoprotein coat) that encases the primary oocyte.

Tertiary (Vesicular, Pre-Ovulatory, or Graafian) Follicle

The main feature that characterizes the tertiary follicle is the development of a *follicular antrum* or fluid, which is also called *liquor folliculi*, within the follicular epithelium (see Figures 3.55 to 3.58). By this stage, the surrounding interstitial cells are well-differentiated into a *theca interna* and *theca externa* layers. The follicular epithelial cells (granulosa cells) are classified according to their location within the ovarian follicle. Those epithelial cells that surround the primary oocyte and are just beyond the zona pellucida are called *corona radiata cells* (see Figure 3.58), and those that protrude from the main follicular epithelial wall are termed *cumulus oophoros cells* (see Figure 3.58). The corona radiata and cumulus oophoros cells will eventually be ovulated along with primary oocyte (see Figures 3.53 and 3.59). The follicular epithelial cells that form the wall of the follicle are called stratum or mural granulosa cells, and rest on a basement membrane (see Figure 3.58).

At the tertiary follicle stage, the theca interna cells will produce *androgens* that are converted by the granulosa cells to *estrogens*. The tertiary follicle may also be referred to as

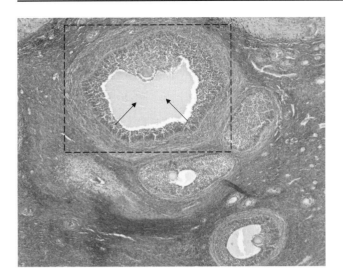

Figure 3.56. Low magnification of pig ovary. **Boxed area**, one tertiary or vesicular ovarian follicle that is comprised of stratum granulosum and theca cells. Within the stratum granulosum is a follicular antrum or liquor folliculi (**arrows**). (Also see color plate)

a *vesicular, pre-ovulatory,* or *Graafian follicle,* but the last two terms are only applicable to tertiary follicles that are fully mature and ready to undergo ovulation. Species variability exists in the size of mature tertiary follicles; it is approximately 2 mm in the cat and dog, 10 mm in small ruminants, 10 to 20 mm in cows, and 50 to 70 mm in the mare.

Atretic Follicles

Most follicles do not culminate in ovulation but instead undergo degeneration or *atresia. Atretic follicles* are char-

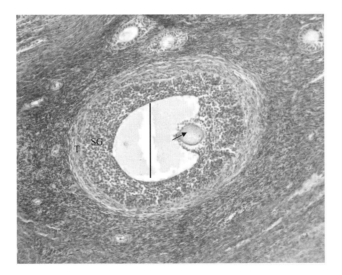

Figure 3.57. Higher magnification of ovarian section from Figure 3.56. One tertiary follicle is featured. The **arrow** points to the primary oocyte and the **bar** spans the follicular antrum. **SG**, stratum granulosum; and **T**, thecal layers. (Also see color plate)

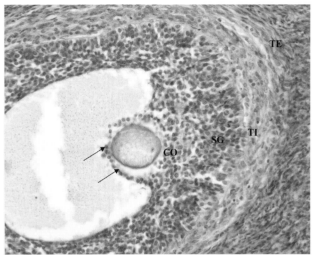

Figure 3.58. Further magnification of tertiary follicle from Figure 3.57. The **arrows** point to the corona radiata cells that are just beyond the zona pellucida surrounding the primary oocyte. **CO**, cumulus oophoros cells that project from the stratum granulosum (**SG**). **TI**, theca interna, and **TE**, theca externa. (Also see color plate)

acterized by having several pyknotic granulosa cells and chromatolytic cells and the formation of a thick glassy membrane surrounding the follicle (see Figure 3.60). The dead cells of these follicles are phagocytosed by macrophages.

Species Differences in Follicular Development and Associated Cells

In equid species, ovarian follicles are located in the medullary region and are ovulated into the *ovulation fossa* that borders the cortical tissue rather than an ovarian bursa. Dogs and cats have *interstitial endocrine cells*

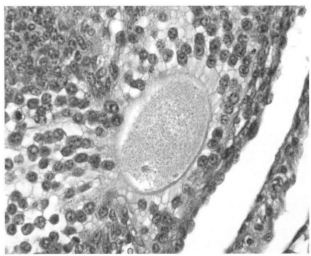

Figure 3.59. Higher magnification of primary oocyte that is being extruded from the tertiary follicle in Figure 3.55. (Also see color plate)

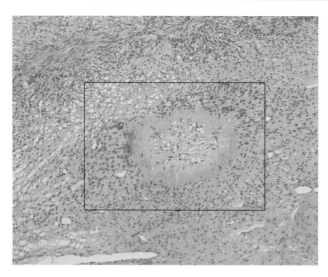

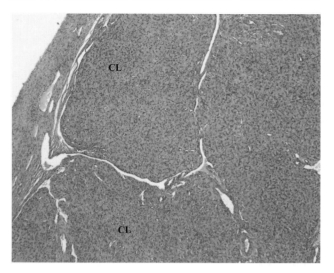

Figure 3.60. Atretic follicle within the ovary (**boxed region**). This follicle is characterized by hyalinization (thickening) of the basement membrane and many pyknotic and necrotic granulosa cells. No oocyte is present in this atretic follicle. (Also see color plate)

Figure 3.61. Sheep ovary with many corpora lutea (**CL**). After ovulation the granulosa and theca cells undergo luteinization and begin to secrete progesterone. (Also see color plate)

that originate from theca interna and granulosa cells of atretic follicles, and these cells produce various steroid hormones.

Ovulation and Fertilization

Pulsatile secretion of *luteinizing hormone (LH)* from the *pars distalis* region of the anterior pituitary gland induces an increase in prostaglandins and various collagenases that enzymatically degrade the follicular wall. Thus, the LH pulse culminates in ovulation of the tertiary follicle. The cumulus oophoros, corona radiata, and primary oocyte are released from the follicle into the *ovarian bursa* and peritoneal cavity, and finally transcend into the ampulla of the oviduct to await fertilization. During this time, the primary oocyte completes the first round of meiosis. A *corpora hemorrhagicum* (characterized by hemorrhage into this area) forms after the follicular wall collapses. The remaining granulosa and theca cells undergo luteinization and fill in this open area to form a corpora lutea.

Cats, llamas and other species are induced ovulators and thus, the act of copulation is necessary to trigger ovulation. Most other domestic animal species ovulate spontaneously. The second meiotic division is completed at the time of fertilization. More information on fertilization is provided in Chapter 5.

Corpora Lutea

Luteinized granulosa and theca cells form the luteal cells of the corpora lutea (CL). In some species, the CL is comprised of recognizable *small and large luteal cells* that are thought to originate from the theca or granulosa cells, respectively (see Figures 3.61 and 3.62). However, not all

scientists agree with this hypothesis. The process of luteinization is characterized by an increase in cell size and number and in some species the formation of a yellow pigment (lutein). The luteal cells produce progesterone in high concentrations that in most species is required to support a pregnancy.

Progesterone inhibits LH secretion, and thus high concentrations of this steroid hormone inhibit ovulation. Many blood vessels are present in the CL to transport progesterone to its target sites and to nourish the luteal cells. In most species, if the animal does not become pregnant, the uterus will produce prostaglandin $F_{2\alpha}$ ($PGF_{2\alpha}$) that destroys the

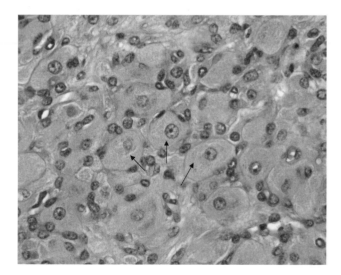

Figure 3.62. Higher magnification of sheep CL from Figure 3.61 revealing the large (**arrows**) and small luteal cells that comprise the CL. Each CL contains numerous blood vessels to nourish the luteal cells and transport the secreted progesterone to their target sites. (Also see color plate)

CL (induces luteolysis). A corpus albicans develops after luteolysis. The destruction of the CL results in a precipitous drop of progesterone and thereby permits further ovarian follicular development, LH surge, and ensuing ovulation to occur again.

Estrous Cycle

The estrous cycle is defined by recurring periods of physiological and behavioral changes with each reproductive cycle. Estrus or heat is the period of sexual receptivity, and in Latin, it means "mad desire." Four to five phases compose a single estrous cycle. These are *proestrus, estrus, metestrus* (not present in all species), *diestrus, and anestrus.*

Initiation of the Estrous Cycle
The estrous cycle is regulated by several extrinsic or environmental factors and intrinsic factors. The combination of the extrinsic or intrinsic factors governs when female animals enter into the estrus or heat period of the cycle.

Environmental Factors
Several environmental factors can influence when an animal enters estrus. These factors include hours of daylight (*photoperiod*), temperature, and food supply. In the ewe and mare, hours of daylight dictate when the animal will come into heat. Daylight affects *melatonin* production by the *pineal gland,* which in turn affects gonadotropin releasing hormone (GnRH) and gonadrotropins that regulate the estrous cycle. Mares come into estrus during long day length/decreased melatonin concentrations. In contrast, short day length/increased melatonin concentrations induce ewes to come into heat. In lower vertebrates, temperature exerts an important role in regulation of sexual function, but in mammals, seasonal temperature variations do not exert as much control of the estrous cycle. However, excessive heat or cold conditions or starvation can negatively impact the estrous cycle and post-fertilization embryonic development. Temperature might affect photoperiod control of the estrous cycle.

Intrinsic Factors
Age and genetics are the two main intrinsic factors that influence when an animal comes into heat. The initiation of estrus (puberty) varies across species with some coming into heat at a relatively early age and others having delayed puberty. In contrast to the male, the female can only reproduce for a finite time because of limited numbers of oocytes and other endocrine disturbances that manifest with age. Aged females have delayed return to estrus, decreased ovulation and fertilization rates, and less ability of the uterus to support the developing conceptus.

Hormonal Regulation of the Estrous Cycle
GnRH (factor) from the hypothalamus induces the anterior pituitary (adenohypophysis) to produce and release follicle stimulating hormone (FSH). FSH promotes ovarian follicular development and stimulates the granulosa cells to convert androgens from the theca cells into estrogens.

Estrogen exerts pleiotropic effects in several organs. In the uterus, estrogen stimulates the growth and branching of the endometrial glands and accumulation of fluid in the uterine stroma (uterine edema). Estrogen stimulates the cervix to produce the mucous plug and increases the thickness of the vaginal epithelium. Peak estrogen levels occur at the time when the female is receptive to the male (estrus or heat). Finally, in response to estrogen, the anterior pituitary gland releases the ovulatory surge of luteinizing hormone (LH), which culminates in rupture of the follicle.

Proestrus and Estrus
These two portions of the cycle are considered the follicular phase of the cycle; it is during these times that the ovarian follicle to be ovulated develops into the tertiary follicle. Proestrus is the phase of the estrous cycle characterized by follicular growth, rising estrogen concentrations, and endometrial development. Estrus is characterized by peak estrogen concentrations and more importantly the period when the female is receptive to being mounted by the male. Ovulation occurs at the end of estrus and at this time, estrogen concentrations decline in most species.

Metestrus and Diestrus
Metestrus and diestrus are the luteal phase of the cycle. Initial CL development and progesterone secretion occurs during metestrus. During diestrus, the CL produces voluminous concentrations of progesterone. In most species, if pregnancy does not occur the CL undergoes luteolysis in response to $PGF_{2\alpha}$ from the uterus, and progesterone concentrations decline, which permits the gonadrotropin concentrations to increase and trigger the next estrus period. After luteolysis, the CL is replaced by a corpus albicans. In contrast to other species, dogs have a prolonged diestrus phase regardless if they are pregnant.

Anestrus
Anestrus is the period of ovarian inactivity. Depending on the species this can be prolonged or it may be short with a small gap between estrous cycles.

Species Differences in the Estrous Cycle
Dogs are monestrous with generally one estrous cycle per year. The cow and sow are polyestrous and can come into estrus at any point during the year. The mare, ewe, doe, and queen are seasonally polyestrous with the time of year influencing when they will come into heat.

Oviduct (Uterine or Fallopian Tube)

The oviduct is divided into the infundibulium (which has fimbriae), ampulla, and isthmus regions. After the oocytes

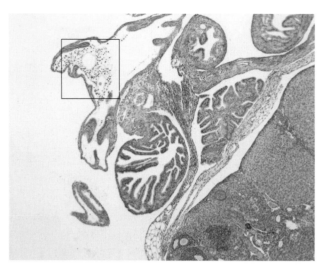

Figure 3.63. Mouse ovary and oviduct after ovulation. The ampulla of the oviduct contains the newly released ova and surrounding cumulus cells (**boxed region**). Fertilization will take place in this area. (Also see color plate)

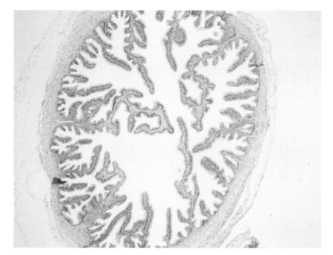

Figure 3.65. Low magnification of bovine oviduct that reveals the many foldings of the tunica mucosa and the relatively thin wall appearance to this tubular organ. The connective tissue beyond the tunica serosa is termed mesosalpinx. (Also see color plate)

are ovulated into the ovarian bursa, they then traverse from the infundibulum to the ampulla to await fertilization (see Figures 3.63 and 3.64). If the ova are fertilized, then the resulting embryos will undergo cleavage and move into the isthmus region and eventually into the uterus. The wall thickness of the oviduct increases from the infundibulium to the isthmus region, but the infundibulum and ampulla region are more tortuous than the isthmus region. The oviduct is a classic tubular organ with a tunica mucosa, submucosa, and muscularis layers (see Figure 3.65).

The mucosa-submucosa includes primary, secondary, and tertiary folds or plicae, and this region contains simple columnar to pseudostratified epithelial cells that include

ciliated (kinocilia) and non-ciliated secretory cells with microvilli, also called peg cells (see Figure 3.66). The secreted oviductal glycoproteins are thought to aid in embryonic development, sperm capacitation, and hyperactivation, but pre-implantational embryos can develop in the culture dish without these glycoproteins. Thus, the significance of these secretory products *in vivo* is uncertain. Ovarian steroid hormones regulate the secretion of these glycoproteins. Smooth muscle comprises the tunica muscularis region, and this layer is predominantly made up of smooth muscle fibers arranged in a circular format.

The fimbriae of the infundibulum are unattached except for at the upper pole of the ovary, and this anatomical

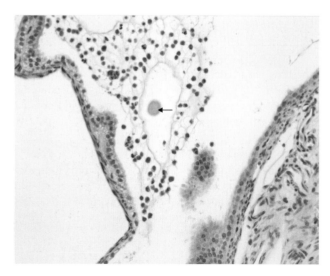

Figure 3.64. Higher magnification of mouse oviduct from Figure 3.63. The **arrow** points to an ovulated ovum within the ampulla of the oviduct. (Also see color plate)

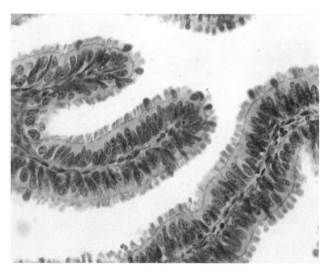

Figure 3.66. Higher magnification of the oviduct reveals the ciliated and non-ciliated cells that line the folded tunica mucosa. (Also see color plate)

arrangement helps to secure the ovulated oocyte. The oocyte or fertilized zygote is transported by the ciliary activity of the ciliated cells and by the peristaltic contraction of the muscular wall. Ovarian steroid hormones regulate the ciliary beat such that ciliary activity is greatest at ovulation. Muscular contraction of the uterus and oviduct transport the spermatozoa to the ampullary region.

Uterus (Uterine Horn)

The uterus is a typical tubular organ with two uterine horns, a body, and a cervix, but the layers of the uterus are defined differently than other tubular organs. The uterine layers are the endometrium (tunica mucosa), myometrium (tunica muscularis), and perimetrium (tunica serosa) (see Figures 3.67 to 74). The endometrium is comprised of simple columnar endometrial epithelial cells, connective tissue stroma, and simple coiled to branched tubular endometrial glands. Estrogen stimulates the development of these glands, and progesterone governs the secretion of the endometrial glands. The myometrium consists of smooth muscle arranged in an inner circular and outer longitudinal layer, and during pregnancy these smooth muscle cells can increase in number (undergo hyperplasia) (see Figure 3.68). The collection of blood vessels between the two muscle layers is termed *stratum vasculare* (see Figure 3.68). The perimetrium is made up of the connective tissue beyond the myometrium and mesothelial cell lining.

The developing embryo implants within the uterus. Depending on the species this implantation may be relatively superficial with the fetal epithelium directly abutting the uterine epithelium or rather invasive with the fetal epithelium eroding the uterine epithelium and connective

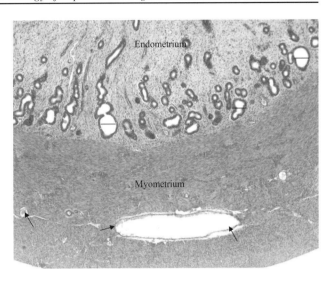

Figure 3.68. Canine uterus. This section depicts the endometrium with connective tissue stroma and endometrial glands and the myometrium that is comprised of inner circular and outer longitudinal smooth muscle layers. The stratum vasculare (**arrows**), which are collections of blood vessels, resides between the two muscular layers. (Also see color plate)

tissue and directly contacting the uterine blood vessels. The uterus nourishes the developing conceptus either through uterine secretions (histiotrophe) or from nutrients within the uterine blood vessels (hemotrophe). When the conceptus is ready to be born, the smooth muscle of the myometrium contracts to result in expulsion of the implanted conceptus and ensuing parturition (birth). At the end of a non-fertile estrous cycle, the uterus produces $PGF_{2\alpha}$ to induce luteolysis and the beginning of a new estrous cycle.

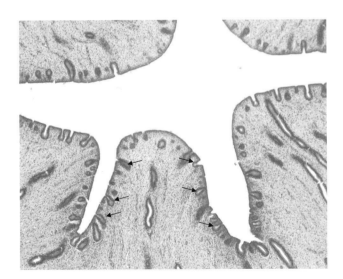

Figure 3.67. Low magnification of canine uterus revealing the endometrium made up of the endometrial lining cells, connective tissue stroma, and endometrial glands. The canine uterus has short endometrial glands that project downward from the endometrial lining (**arrows**). (Also see color plate)

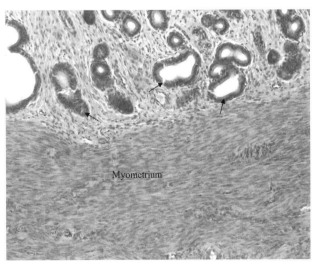

Figure 3.69. Higher magnification of canine uterus from Figure 3.68. The **arrows** point at endometrial glands. The myometrium is below the endometrial region. (Also see color plate)

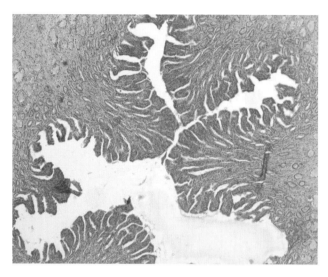

Figure 3.70. Low magnification of pregnant cat uterus. Estrogen stimulates proliferation of the endometrial glands, and progesterone stimulates these glands to secrete histiotrophe to nourish the developing conceptus. Numerous endometrial glands are evident in this section. (Also see color plate)

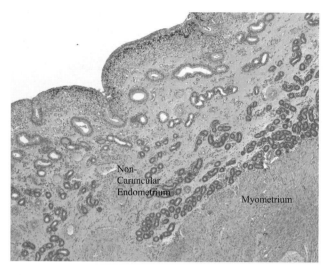

Figure 3.72. Low magnification of sheep uterus in the non-caruncular endometrial region. The non-caruncular region is characterized by the presence of endometrial gland. The myometrium is below the endometrium. (Also see color plate)

Certain species differences exist in the uterus. The canid uterus has endometrial crypts that are small endometrial glands projecting downward from the endometrial lining (see Figure 3.67). Ruminant animals have a caruncular and non-caruncular uterine region (see Figures 3.72 to 3.74). The caruncular region is where the conceptus implants and the fetal placenta (cotyledon) combines with the maternal caruncle to form a placentome. This region is characterized histologically by the lack of endometrial glands below the endometrial lining (see Figure 3.74). In contrast, the non-caruncular region of the ruminant uterus contains endometrial glands (see Figures 3.72 and 3.73). In sheep, particularly

black-faced ones, ectopic melanocytes may be located within the endometrial stroma, and these cells impart multifocal black areas within the uterus (see Figures 3.72 and 3.73). However, the function of these cells in this region is unknown.

Cervix

The cervix acts a sphincter-like fibrous organ, and the main function of this organ is to produce a mucus secretion (mucous plug) that is thought to aid in movement of the

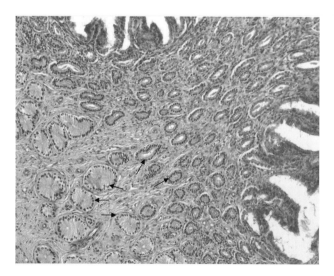

Figure 3.71. Higher magnification of pregnant cat uterus from Figure 3.70. The **arrows** point to a few of the abundant endometrial glands. (Also see color plate)

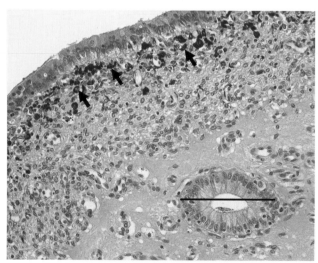

Figure 3.73. Higher magnification of ovine uterus from Figure 3.72. Below the endometrial lining cells are several ectopic melanocytes (**arrows**). These cells are routinely seen in sheep uteri, particularly sections from black-faced sheep. The **bar** spans one endometrial gland that characterizes the non-caruncular region. (Also see color plate)

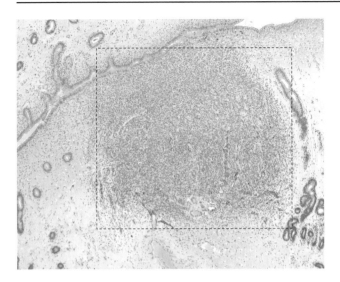

Figure 3.74. Ovine uterus—caruncular region. No endometrial glands are present in the caruncular region. Instead, in this region, the connective tissue stroma proliferates below the endometrial lining cells (**boxed area**). (Also see color plate)

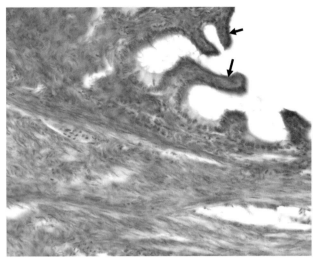

Figure 3.76. Higher magnification of bovine cervix from Figure 3.75. The **arrows** point at the secondary folds that branch from the primary folds. The epithelial cells that line these folds produce a mucous secretion that forms the "mucous plug." (Also see color plate)

sperm within the female reproductive tract. This secretion is stimulated by estrogen and is produced by the simple columnar epithelial lining cells, which include mucous-producing and ciliated cells (see Figures 3.75 and 3.76). The tunica mucosa of the cervix is organized into primary and secondary folds to increase the surface area of this organ. An inner circular and outer longitudinal layer with smooth muscle and elastic fibers compose the tunica muscularis, and the cervix has a typical tunica serosa.

Vagina-Vetstibule

These organs include a tunica mucosa-submucosa, tunica muscularis, and tunica serosa (cranial end)/adventitia

(caudal end). The tunica mucosa-submucosa is made up of non-kerartinized stratified squamous epithelium with abundant loose to dense irregular connective tissue below this epithelial lining (see Figure 3.77). Estrogen secreted during proestrus and estrus increases the thickness of this epithelial lining and in canids and rodents, analysis of vaginal smears can aid in determining which phase of the estrous cycle the animal is in at a given time. Lymphatic nodules are commonly seen in the caudal end of the vagina. Smooth muscle arranged in a thick inner circular and thin outer longitudinal layer comprise the tunica muscularis.

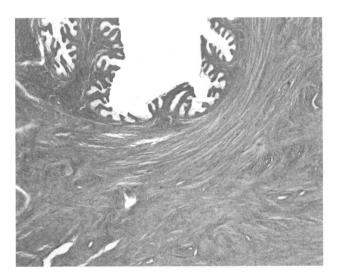

Figure 3.75. Bovine cervix. The tunica mucosa of the cervix has many primary, secondary, and tertiary folds. (Also see color plate)

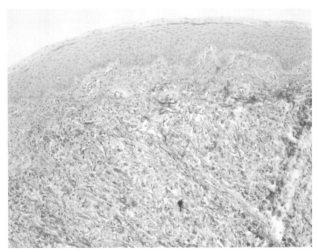

Figure 3.77. Low magnification of canine vagina. The tunica mucosa is comprised of non-keratinized stratified squamous epithelium. Deep to the epithelial lining is loose to dense irregular connective tissue that is devoid of glands in contrast to other tubular organs. (Also see color plate)

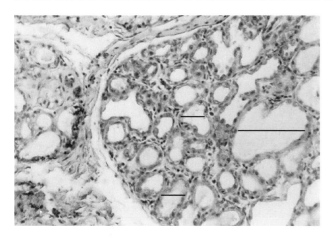

Figure 3.78. Active bovine mammary gland that consists of many lobules containing alveolar glands (**bars**). (Also see color plate)

External Genitalia (Labia Majora, Labia Minora, and Clitoris)

The labia majora and labia minora are modified skin structures. The labia majora contains hair follicles and glands, and smooth muscle fibers. The labia minora contains blood vessels, elastic fibers, and apocrine sweat and sebaceous glands. The clitoris consists of vascular tissue (corpora cavernosa) surrounded by fibrous collagen, and sensory nerves.

Mammary Gland and Teat

Mammary glands are modified sweat glands that have evolved to provide nourishment to post-natal animals. The mammary gland secretion (milk) is made up various proteins and lipids, and can contain whole cells. The exact percentage of lipids and proteins in the milk depends on the

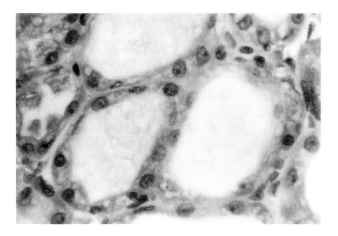

Figure 3.79. Higher magnification of mammary gland alveoli from Figure 3.78. The mammary gland secretion (milk) includes a mixture of proteins (secreted via merocrine mode) and lipids (produced via apocrine secretion). Within the lumen of the alveoli some sloughed epithelial and inflammatory cells may be observed. (Also see color plate)

animal species. For instance, seals have the most amount of lipids within their milk.

The mammary glands are alveolar in appearance with simple cuboidal to columnar epithelium (see Figures 3.78 and 3.79). The lipid portion is produced via apocrine secretion, and the protein portion is released via merocrine secretion. Various inflammatory cells may be seen within the lumen of the glands. A certain amount of these cells is considered normal, but if the number of cells exceeds a certain limit in dairy species, the milk is considered mastitic and must be rejected.

Similar to sweat glands, myoepithelial cells surround each of the glands, and their contraction results in expulsion of the milk into the intralobular followed by the interlobular ducts, which fuse to form the lactiferous ducts. These ducts then drain into the lactiferous sinus and the milk is then expelled from the teat, which is comprised of an extremely thick keratinized stratified squamous epithelium. In dogs, the myoepithelial cells may de-differentiate and form a tumor called a mixed mammary gland tumor that consists of cartilage and bone. Most mammary tumors in dogs are benign, but in cats approximately 80 percent are malignant.

Development and Hormonal Regulation of the Mammary Gland

The mammary gland develops from invagination of the surface ectoderm into the underlying mesoderm. Puberty triggers an increase in this growth with estrogen stimulating branching of the duct system and fat accumulation within the organ. During pregnancy, estrogen, progesterone, and prolactin stimulate the growth of the alveoli. Prolactin from the anterior pituitary gland further promotes lactation or secretion of the milk. Oxytocin released from the poster pituitary gland stimulates contraction of the myoepithelial cells around the alveoli to induce the milk ejection reflex.

Involution

After lactation, the alveolar cells degenerate with only a few small alveoli remaining. Most of the organ is occupied at this time with the ducts and abundant fat and connective tissue.

Acknowledgments

Photomicrographs were taken by Cheryl S. Rosenfeld from the University of Missouri, College of Veterinary Medicine Student Histology Slide Sets, or from mouse sections obtained from Dr. Dennis B. Lubahn's mouse colony (Figures 3.55, 3.59, 3.63, and 3.64).

Bibliography

Bendel-Stenzel, M., Anderson, R., Heasman, J., and Wylie, C. (1998). The origin and migration of primordial germ cells in the mouse. *Semin Cell Dev Biol* 9:393–400.

Eurell, J., and Frappier, B. (2006). *Dellman's Textbook of Veterinary Histology 6th ed.* Ames: Blackwell Publishing Professional.

Hafez, E.S.E., and Hafez, B. (2000) *Reproduction in Farm Animals 7th ed.* Philadelphia: Lippincott Williams and Wilkins.

Motta, P.M., Nottola, S.A., and Makabe, S. (1997). Natural history of the female germ cell from its origin to full maturation through prenatal ovarian development. *Eur J Obstet Gynecol Reprod Biol* 75:5–10.

Pereda, J., Zorn, T., and Soto-Suazo, M. (2006). Migration of human and mouse primordial germ cells and colonization of the developing ovary: an ultrastructural and cytochemical study. *Microsc Res Tech* 69:386–395.

Part 3.5
Overview of Fertilization

Heide Schatten

Fertilization initiates the formation of a new individual. For fertilization to occur, the oocyte must have enlarged, undergone meiosis, and matured in its ovarian follicle to the metaphase II stage. The follicle then releases the haploid metaphase II oocyte in the oviduct, where fertilization occurs with a haploid sperm cell, restoring the diploid chromosome set of the developing embryo. After fertilization, the zygote is translocated to the uterus, which takes four to seven days depending on the species. The first diagram (Figure 3.80) provides an overview of fertilization and subsequent developmental stages to blastocyst formation as observed in the sow.

Fertilization involves a cascade of events that begins with the fusion and union of a sperm and egg cell and concludes when chromosomal diploidy is restored. On molecular levels, the fertilization process is complex and is well detailed in a recent review (Whitaker, 2006). For fertilization to occur sperm must have been matured in the epididymis and capacitated in the female reproductive tract. The egg must have matured into a Graafian follicle.

Binding and Fusion of Spermatozoa and Oocyte Plasma Membrane

Capacitation involves changes induced by oviductal fluid and includes modifications of the sperm surface (redistribution and removal of membrane proteins), metabolism, and motility. It is associated with a rise in intracellular calcium ions, pH, and cAMP, and with hyperpolarization of the sperm plasmalemma. Sperm motility is increased in a process that takes place in the oviduct and results in hyperactivation, which is associated with high-amplitude flagellar bending that allows penetration of viscous fluids, as is encountered in the oviduct. It is thought that specific oviductal signals may influence hyperactivity, because it is seen more frequently during the time of ovulation.

The acrosome is a species-specific, membrane-bounded organelle containing numerous hydrolytic enzymes. During fertilization, specific glycoproteins in the oocyte are responsible for sperm recognition and acrosome reaction. The acrosome reaction is triggered by specific binding in the oocyte's zona pellucida and is absolutely necessary for successful fertilization. The zona pellucida consists of three sulfated glycoproteins called ZP1, ZP2, and ZP3. The plasma membrane of the sperm overlying the acrosome binds to ZP3 in the oocyte's zona pellucida, which induces the acrosome reaction. ZP2 acts as a secondary sperm receptor. Sperm then is able to penetrate the zona pellucida (for detailed review, please see Yanagimachi, 1994).

Fertilization is species-specific and only eggs from the same species trigger the acrosome reaction in sperm. Only acrosome-reacted sperm can penetrate the zona pellucida and fuse with the oocyte. Aside from ZP3 there are other agents that can induce the acrosome reaction, including progesterone, prostaglandins, calcium ionophore, diacylglycerol, and others. Once one sperm has entered the oocyte the zona pellucida hardens, which prevents further sperm from entering and provides a block to polyspermy.

Oocyte Activation

Gamete interaction triggers a cascade of signaling events within the egg, collectively referred to as egg activation (see Figure 3.81A). Maximal activation competence is achieved when the oocyte has reached the MII stage, after germinal vesicle (GV) breakdown and after cortical granule migration to their subcortical region at the oocyte's surface. Ca^{2+} influx from the external environment results in Ca^{2+} release from internal stores such as endoplasmic reticulum and cortical granules.

Cortical granules show great diversity; they contain carbohydrates and proteins, and they may also have protease, glycosidase, or peroxidase activity. Increase in Ca^{2+} causes cortical granule exocytosis which leads to morphological and biochemical changes of the oocyte surface. The cascade of egg activation includes release of Ca^{2+} from the endoplasmic reticulum and cortical granules, cortical granule exocytosis and membrane reorganization, recruitment and translation of maternal mRNAs, cytoskeletal activity and reorganizations, and resumption of meiosis. Transient increase in $[Ca^{2+}]_i$ is one of the first indicators of oocyte activation and is necessary for cytoskeletal activity (discussed below) that facilitates numerous processes during the early and late activation events.

Multiple cytosolic Ca^{2+} pulses or oscillations are seen in most mammalian species, which ultimately results in release of oocytes from meiotic arrest (reviewed by Stricker, 1999). Ca^{2+}–dependent early events of activation include cortical reactions that are triggered by protein kinase C (PKC) which is activated by the first rise in Ca^{2+} while the later events of activation triggered by Ca^{2+} include resumption of

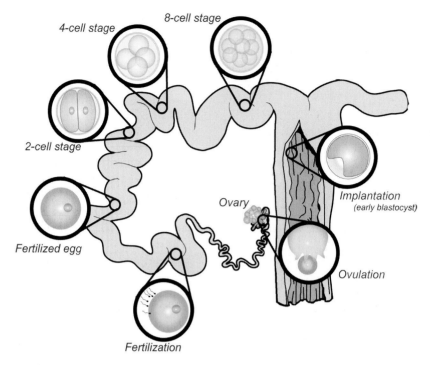

Figure 3.80. Stages of fertilization and development to the preimplantation blastocyst in the sow.

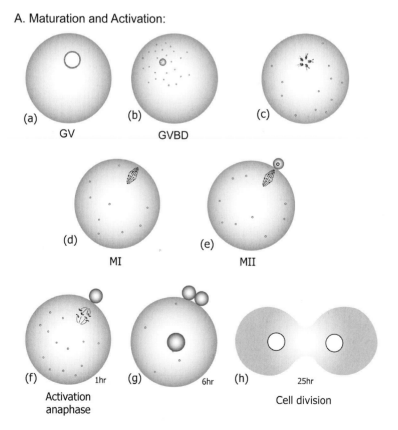

Figure 3.81A. Stages of oocyte maturation and activation.

meiosis requiring higher amounts of Ca^{2+}. Ca^{2+} is required from external sources to replenish Ca^{2+} pools and maintain Ca^{2+} oscillations. The increase in $[Ca^{2+}]_i$ is accomplished by inositol 1,4,5-triphosphate ($InsP_3$)-mediated release of calcium from intracellular stores (reviewed by Whitaker, 2006, and references within).

Egg activation by sperm or artificially induced egg activation results in meiotic maturation. This involves activation and inactivation of maturation-promoting factor (MPF), which is a serine/threonine protein kinase composed of a catalytic subunit ($p34^{cdc2}$) and a regulatory subunit (cyclin B). GV-intact oocytes have low MPF activity which transiently increases after completion of MI. It is most elevated during MII (Choi et al., 1991). Chromosomal condensation is induced by MPF activation. It is thought that the arrest of MII oocytes is maintained by a cytostatic factor (CSF or p39mos) that is responsible for the maintenance of MPF. MPF becomes inactivated as intracellular Ca^{2+} rises as a result of gamete fusion, which causes destruction of MPF's cyclin B component.

Another protein kinase that is critically important for the oocyte's signaling pathways is the mitogen-activated protein kinase (MAPK) (reviewed by Sun et al., 1999; Fan and Sun, 2004). MAPK increases following activation of MPF. It remains elevated from MI to MII and in the MII-arrested oocyte. After fertilization, MAPK is temporally correlated with the formation of pronuclear envelopes of male and female pronuclei.

Development of Male Pronucleus

The sperm undergoes significant changes after entering the oocyte. The sperm's pore-less nuclear envelope rapidly disintegrates and is replaced by a pronuclear double membrane that now contains nuclear pores. The sperm's nuclear lamins disassemble and become replaced by a new set of lamins. Factors within the oocyte cytoplasm are involved in decondensation of the sperm's tightly packed DNA by modifying the disulphide-stabilized protamines that are characteristic for sperm chromatin. The sperm protamines are replaced by oocyte histones and sperm chromatin is packaged into nucleosomal chromatin which is similar to histones of somatic cell nuclei. Swelling of the nucleus takes place (Poccia and Collas, 1997). The formation of a new envelope typically occurs when the activated oocyte's MII spindle undergoes telophase, which correlates with the absence of MAP kinase (Moos et al., 1996) and MPF (Usui et al., 1997) in the oocyte.

Cytoskeletal Dynamics, Cytoplasmic and Pronuclear Movements

Cytoskeletal dynamics and cytoskeletal reorganizations play significant roles during fertilization (see Figure 3.81B)

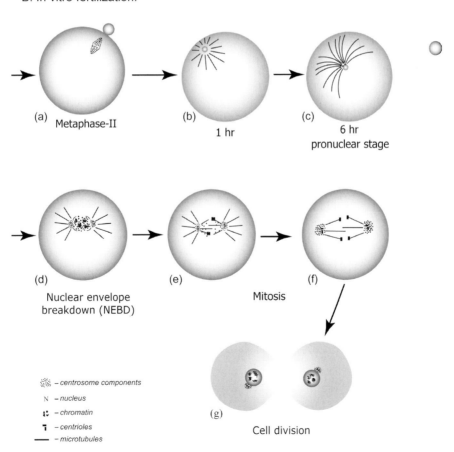

B. In vitro fertilization:

(a) Metaphase-II

(b) 1 hr

(c) 6 hr pronuclear stage

(d) Nuclear envelope breakdown (NEBD)

(e) Mitosis

(f)

— centrosome components
N — nucleus
— chromatin
— centrioles
— microtubules

(g) Cell division

Figure 3.81B. Stages of *in vitro* fertilization. Modified from Liu et al., 2006; and Sun and Schatten, 2006a.

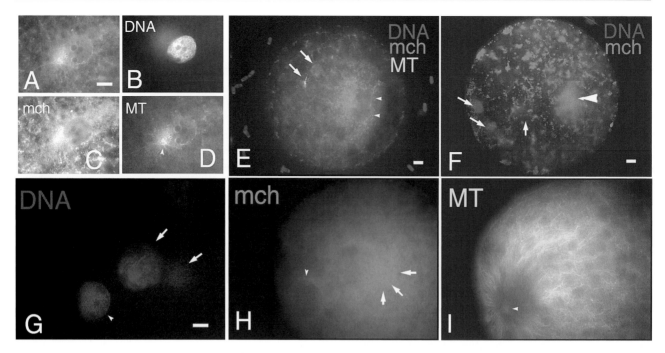

Figure 3.82. Distribution of mitochondria (**mch**) and microtubules (**MT**) in fertilized oocytes. (**A–D**), the enlarged sperm head is surrounded by mch which aggregate (**C**) at the sperm aster (**arrowhead** in (**D**)). (**E**), at 10 h after insemination, three pronuclei are formed due to polyspermy which often occurs during porcine IVF. No mch aggregation is seen around the female pronucleus (**arrow**) judged from the close association of the second polar body (**arrow**) extruded by cytokinetic MTs (green signal). On the other hand, mch aggregate around two male pronuclei (**arrowheads**). Cluster formation of mch is observed at the cortex. (**F**), the female pronucleus is closely localized to the two polar bodies (**arrows**) and displays a rare association of mch, whereas the male pronucleus displays a diffuse pattern of mch association (**arrowhead**). (**G–I**), a continuous ring of mch (**arrowhead** in **H**) is formed at the rim of male pronuclei (**arrowhead** in **G**) surrounded by well-developed MTs from the sperm aster (**arrowhead** in **I**). Mch are not observed around female pronuclei (**arrow** in **G**) but are associated with the second polar body (**arrow** in **G** and **H**). Bar, 10 μm. Reprinted with permission from Katayama et al., 2006. (Also see color plate)

and throughout embryo development. The activated oocyte undergoes surface reorganizations in which microfilaments play a major role (reviewed by Sun and Schatten, 2006c). In most fertilized eggs short microvilli elevate into longer microvilli. This is the result of increases in intracellular calcium followed by actin polymerization into microfilaments that provide the structural components within microvilli. Membranes of the exocytosed cortical granules contribute to plasma membrane reorganization and microvillar elongation.

Shortly after sperm incorporation a microtubule-based sperm aster is formed that originates from centrosomal material at the sperm nucleus (recently reviewed in Sun and Schatten, 2006a,b) and is responsible for the union of female and male pronuclei. Functional centrosomes are formed by combining oocyte and sperm centrosomal proteins (reviewed by Manandhar et al., 2005; Sun and Schatten, 2006a,b). As the microtubular rays of the sperm aster elongate and reach the female pronucleus both pronuclei move to the center of the oocyte, forming a large radial microtubule-based aster that fills the cytoplasm and connects to the oocyte's surface. The sperm aster and radial aster serve as the major transport system for translocation of macromolecular com-

plexes, mitochondria, vesicles, endoplasmic reticulum (ER), pigment granules, and other cellular components that are crucial for embryo development (reviewed in Schatten et al., 2005; mitochondrial translocations described in Katayama et al., 2006).

Abnormal microtubule formation can lead to developmental failures. The assembly of microtubules and microfilaments is vital for pronuclear formation and all subsequent cell divisions. The diploid nucleus undergoes cell cycles that will result in first and subsequent cell divisions. Asymmetric microtubule-based mitotic formations are associated with asymmetric cell divisions during embryo differentiation. Figure 3.82 depicts microtubule organization and mitochondria translocations in fertilized porcine oocytes (from Katayama et al., 2006).

Figures 3.81A and 3.81B summarize the events of oocyte maturation, activation, and fertilization (modified from Liu et al., 2006 and Sun and Schatten, 2006a).

Acknowledgments

The author gratefully acknowledges Don Connor's help with the illustrations.

Bibliography

Choi, T., Aoki, F., Mori, M., Yamashita, M., Nagahama, Y., and Kohmoto, K. (1991). Activation of p34^{cdc2} protein kinase activity in meiotic and mitotic cell cycles in mouse oocytes and embryos. *Development* 113:789–795.

Fan, H.-Y., and Sun, Q.-Y. (2004). Involvement of mitogen-activated protein kinase cascade during oocyte maturation and fertilization in mammals. *Biol. Reprod.* 70:535–547.

Katayama, M., Zhong, Z.-S., Lai, L., Sutovsky, P., Prather, R.S., and Schatten, H. (2006). Mitochondrial distribution and microtubule organization in fertilized and cloned porcine embryos: Implications for developmental potential. *Dev. Biol.* 299:206–220.

Liu, Z.H., Schatten, H., Hao, Y.H., Lai, L., Wax, D., Samuel, M., Zhong, Z.-S., Sun, Q.-Y., and Prather, R.S. (2006). The nuclear mitotic apparatus (NuMA) protein is contributed by the donor cell nucleus in cloned porcine embryos. *Frontiers in Bioscience* 11:1945–1957.

Manandhar, G., Schatten, H., and Sutovsky, P. (2005). Centrosome reduction during gametogenesis and its significance. *Biol. Repro.* 72:2–13.

Moos, J., Xu, Z., Schultz, R.M., and Kopf, G.S. (1996). Regulation of nuclear envelope assembly/disassembly by MAP kinase. *Dev. Biol.* 175:358–361.

Poccia, D., and Collas, P. (1997). Nuclear envelope dynamics during male pronuclear development. *Dev. Growth Differ.* 39:541–550.

Schatten, H., Prather, R.S., and Sun, Q.-Y. (2005). The significance of mitochondria for embryo development in cloned farm animals. *Mitochondrion* 5:303–321.

Stricker, S.A. (1999). Comparative biology of calcium signaling during fertilization and egg activation in animals. *Dev. Biol.* 211:157–176.

Sun, Q.Y., Breitbart, H., and Schatten, H. (1999). The role of MAPK cascade in mammalian germ cells. *Reproduction, Fertility and Development* 11:443–450.

Sun, Q.-Y., and Schatten, H. (2006a). Centrosome inheritance after fertilization and nuclear transfer in mammals. In: Sutovsky, P. (ed). *Somatic Cell Nuclear Transfer*, New York: Springer, in press.

Sun, Q.-Y., and Schatten, H. (2006b). Multiple roles of NuMA in vertebrate cells: review of an intriguing multifunctional protein. *Frontiers in Bioscience* 11:1137–1146.

Sun, Q.-Y., and Schatten, H. (2006c). Regulation of dynamic events by microfilaments during oocyte maturation and fertilization. *Reproduction* 131:193–205.

Usui, N., Ogura, A., Kimura, Y., and Yanagimachi, R. (1997). Sperm nuclear envelope: breakdown of intrinsic envelope and de *novo* formation in hamster oocytes or eggs. *Zygote* 5:35–46.

Whitaker, M. (2006). Calcium at fertilization and in early development. *Physiol. Rev* 86:25–88.

Yanagimachi, R. (1994). Mammalian fertilization. In: Knobil, E., and Neill, J.D. (eds). *The physiology of reproduction, 2nd ed., Vol. 1,* New York: Raven Press, pp. 189–317.

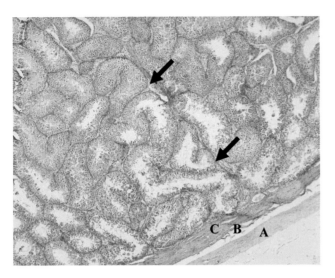

Figure 3.8. Low magnification of testis. **A.** Parietal lamina of vaginal tunic; **B.** visceral lamina of vaginal tunic; **C.** tunica albuginea. The **arrows** point at the septulum.

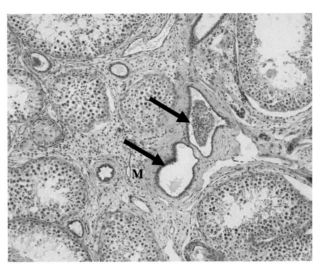

Figure 3.11. Low magnification of testis. **M.**, mediastinum. The **arrows** point at rete testis in mediastinum.

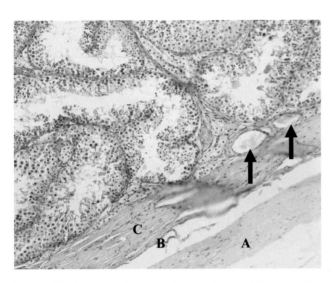

Figure 3.9. Low magnification of testis. **A.** Parietal lamina of vaginal tunic; **B.** Visceral lamina of vaginal tunic; **C.** Tunica albuginea. The **arrows** point at tunica vasculosa.

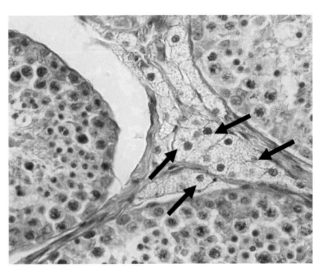

Figure 3.12. Convoluted seminiferous tubules and interstitium of the testis. The **arrows** point at Leydig cells, which appear very vacuolated.

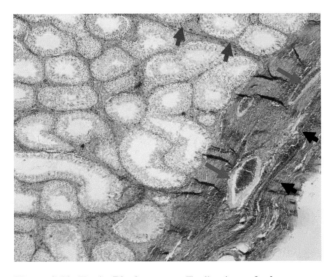

Figure 3.10. Testis. **Black arrows**, T. albuginea; **dark gray arrows**, T. vasculosa; and **light gray arrows**, septulum.

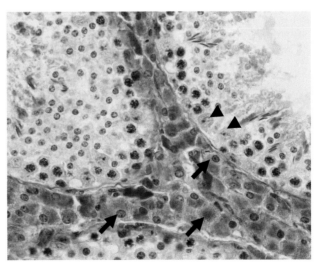

Figure 3.13. Testis. **Arrows**, Leydig (interstitial) cells; and **arrowheads**, Sertoli cells.

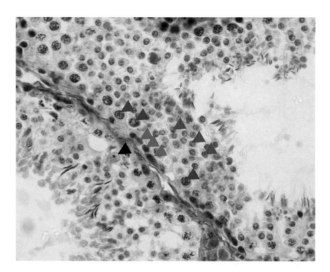

Figure 3.14. Testis. **Black arrowheads**, Sertoli cell; **light gray arrowheads**, spermatogonia; **dark grey arrowheads**, primary spermatocytes; and **white arrowheads**, spermatids.

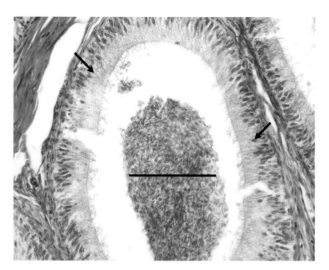

Figure 3.17. Cauda epididymis. **Arrows**, collections of spermatozoa in the ductus epididymis; **horizontal bar**, one epididymal tubule or ductule.

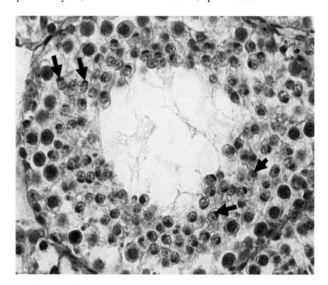

Figure 3.15. Testis. **Arrows** point at acrosomal cap surrounding the nucleus of the round spermatids.

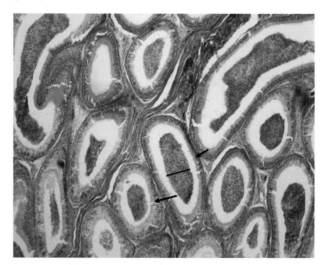

Figure 3.18. Cauda epididymis. The **arrows** point at the pseudostratified columnar epithelial lining of the epididymis. The **horizontal bar** is across the collection of spermatozoa in one epididymal tubule.

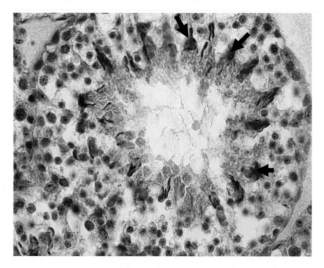

Figure 3.16. Testis. **Arrows** point at acrosomal cap surrounding the nucleus of the elongated spermatids.

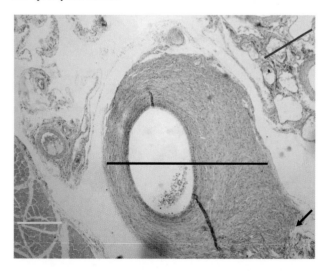

Figure 3.19. Spermatic cord. **White horizontal bar**, cremaster muscle; **black horizontal bar**, ductus deferens; **dark gray bar**, pampiniform plexus, nerves, and testicular artery in this area; **black arrow**, mesoductus deferens.

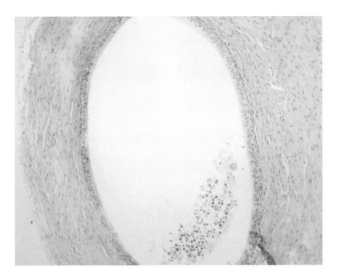

Figure 3.20. Ductus deferens in spermatic cord. The ductus deferens is lined by a pseudostratified columnar epithelium with long microvilli closest to the epididymis.

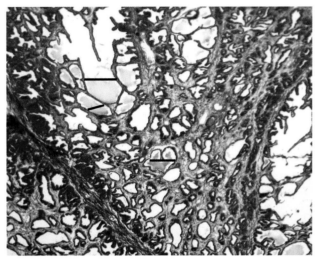

Figure 3.23. Higher magnification of prostate glands. **Horizontal bars**, tubuloalveolar prostatic glands of the dog.

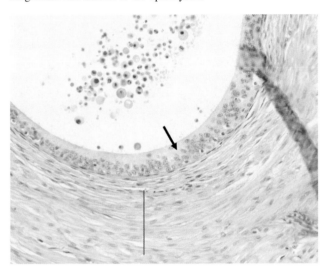

Figure 3.21. Higher magnification of ductus deferens in spermatic cord. **Black arrow**, pseudostratified columnar epithelium with long microvilli; **vertical bar**, tunica muscularis.

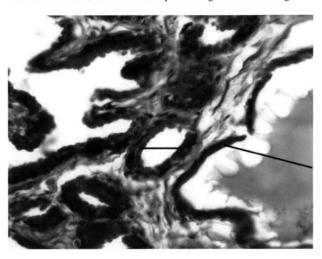

Figure 3.24. Canine prostate. The prostatic glands are lined by simple cuboidal to low columnar epithelium with apical blebs. **Horizontal bars**, tubuloalveolar acidophilic staining prostatic glands that have apical blebs.

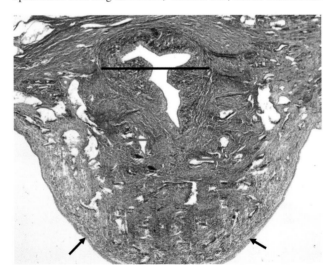

Figure 3.22. Canine prostate and prostatic urethra. **Long white horizontal bar**, uterus masculinis; **short black horizontal bars**, cross sections of ductus deferens; **arrows**, epithelial lining of urethra.

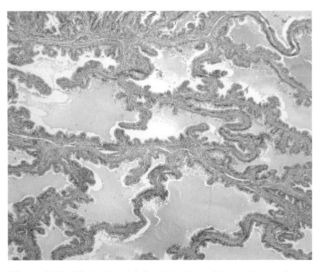

Figure 3.25. Vesicular glands of the boar. The vesicular glands are composed of irregularly shaped alveoli that are lined by a simple columnar to pseudostratified columnar epithelium.

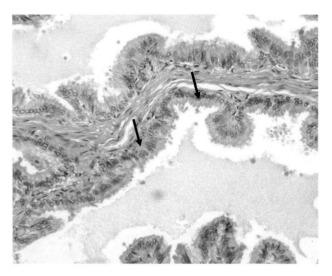

Figure 3.26. Higher magnification of the vesicular glands of the boar. The **arrows** point at simple columnar–pseudostratified columnar epithelium that lines the vesicular glands.

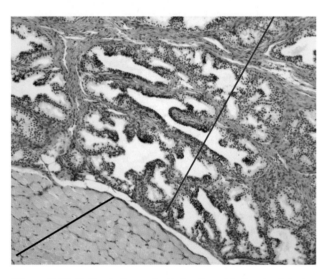

Figure 3.27. Feline bulbourethral glands and bulboglandularis muscle. **Dark gray bar**, bulburethral gland in the cat; **black bar**, bulboglandularis muscle.

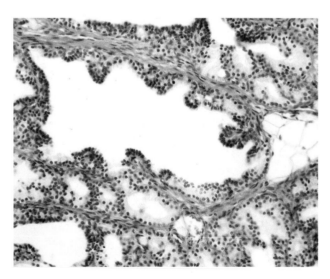

Figure 3.28. Feline bulbourethral gland. These glands are simple columnar tubuloalveolar glands. The nuclei of the cells is towards the base, and the cytoplasm stains pale to basophilic.

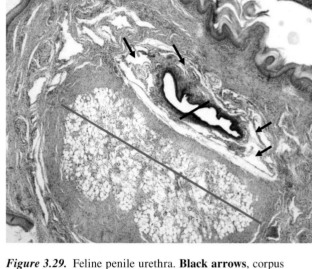

Figure 3.29. Feline penile urethra. **Black arrows**, corpus spongiosum; **long gray bar**, penile urethra; **short black bar**, corpus cavernosum.

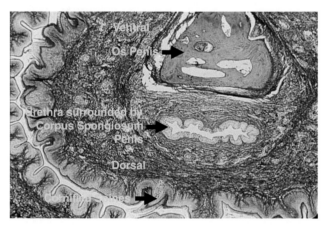

Figure 3.30. Feline penis. Unlike the other species, the cat penis is directed caudoventrally in the non-erect state so the urethra is dorsal to the os penis.

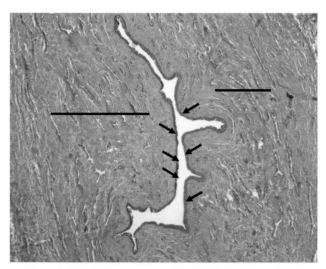

Figure 3.31. Canine penis—pars longa glandis. This picture shows the penile urethra surrounded by corpus spongiosum. **Arrows**, urethral lining; **horizontal bars**, corpus spongiosum.

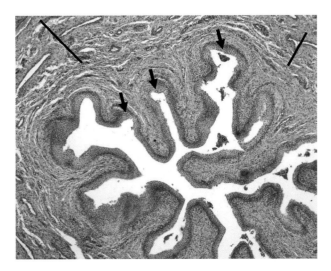

Figure 3.32. Equine penis. This pictures shows the penile urethra surrounded by corpus spongiosum. **Arrows**, urethral lining; **bars**, corpus spongiosum.

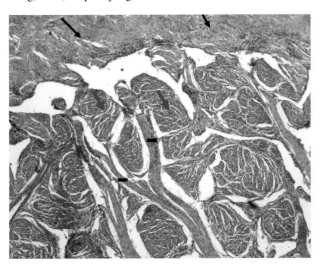

Figure 3.33. Equine penis. **Black arrows**, tunica albuginea; **gray arrows**, corpus cavernosum; **horizontal bars**, trabeculae from the tunica albuginea that radiates into the corpus cavernosum.

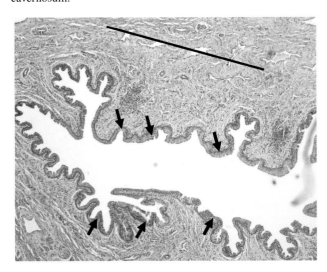

Figure 3.34. Bovine penis. This figure demonstrates the penile urethra surrounded by corpus spongiosum. **Arrows**, urethral lining; **bar**, corpus spongiosum.

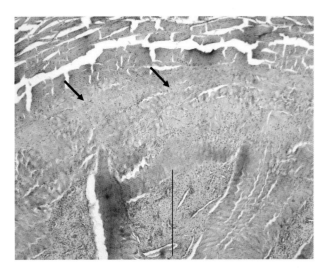

Figure 3.35. Bovine penis. This species has a fibrous type of penis with more fibrous connective tissue and less erectile tissue than the stallion. **Arrows**, tunica albuginea; **thin vertical bar**, corpus cavernosum.

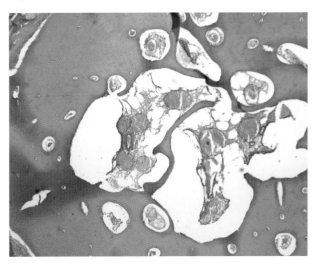

Figure 3.36. Canine penis—pars longa glandis. This figure shows the os penis in the pars longa glandis. Not pictured here is the corpus spongiosum glandis.

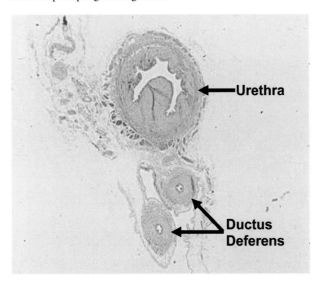

Figure 3.37. Pre-prostatic urethra of the cat and ductus deferens. The cat has a long pre-prostatic urethra, and thus it can be seen with the paired ductus deferens.

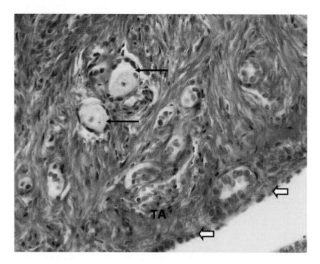

Figure 3.53. Low magnification of canine ovarian cortex region. **Block arrows**, lining superficial or germinal epithelium, which are mesothelial cells. **Arrows**, primordial follicles. **TA**, tunica albuginea.

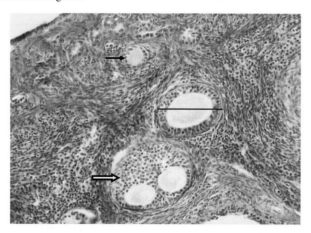

Figure 3.54. Low magnification of canine ovarian cortex region. The **black arrow** points at a primary follicle with simple cuboidal epithelium surrounding a primary oocyte. The **bar** spans a secondary follicle with stratified follicular epithelium around the primary oocyte. The **block arrow** points at a polyovulatory follicle, which is atypical. If this follicle ovulates, two primary oocytes will be released.

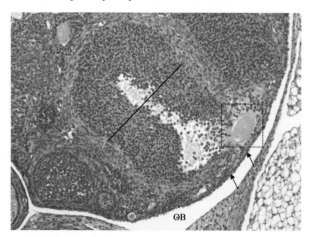

Figure 3.55. Mouse ovary with tertiary (Graafian) follicle undergoing ovulation (**bar**). **Boxed area**, primary oocyte, corona radiata, and cumulus oophoros that are in the process of ovulation. **Arrows** point at the superficial or germinal epithelium that surrounds the ovary. **OB**, ovarian bursa.

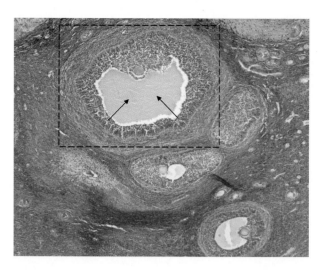

Figure 3.56. Low magnification of pig ovary. **Boxed area**, one tertiary or vesicular ovarian follicle that is comprised of stratum granulosum and theca cells. Within the stratum granulosum is a follicular antrum or liquor folliculi (**arrows**).

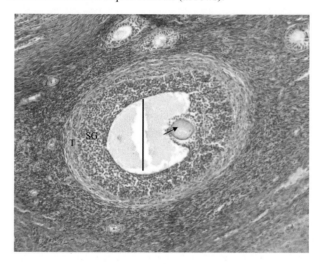

Figure 3.57. Higher magnification of ovarian section from Figure 3.56. One tertiary follicle is featured. The **arrow** points to the primary oocyte and the **bar** spans the follicular antrum. **SG**, stratum granulosum; and **T**, thecal layers.

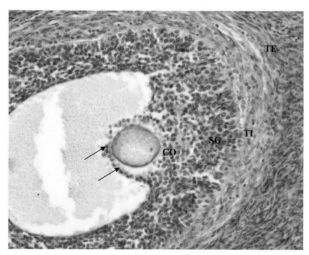

Figure 3.58. Further magnification of tertiary follicle from Figure 3.57. The **arrows** point to the corona radiata cells. **CO**, cumulus oophoros cells that project from the stratum granulosum (**SG**). **TI**, theca interna, and **TE**, theca externa.

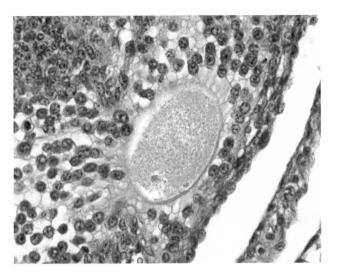

Figure 3.59. Higher magnification of primary oocyte that is being extruded from the tertiary follicle in Figure 3.55.

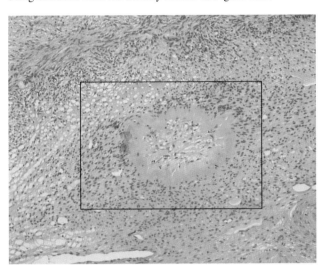

Figure 3.60. Atretic follicle within the ovary (**boxed region**). This follicle is characterized by hyalinization (thickening) of the basement membrane and many pyknotic and necrotic granulosa cells. No oocyte is present in this atretic follicle.

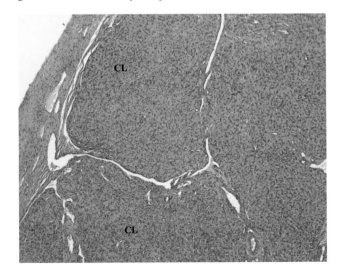

Figure 3.61. Sheep ovary with many corpora lutea (**CL**). After ovulation the granulosa and theca cells undergo luteinization and begin to secrete progesterone.

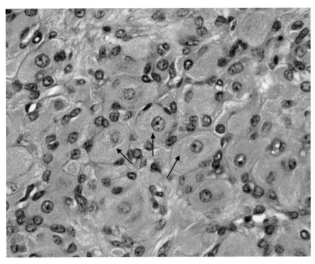

Figure 3.62. Higher magnification of sheep CL from Figure 3.61 revealing the large (**arrows**) and small luteal cells that comprise the CL.

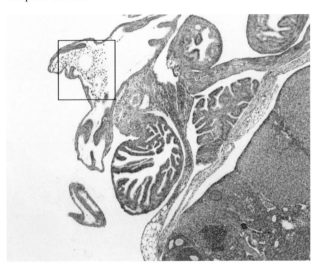

Figure 3.63. Mouse ovary and oviduct after ovulation. The ampulla of the oviduct contains the newly released ova and surrounding cumulus cells (**boxed region**). Fertilization will take place in this area.

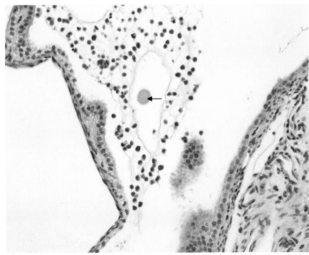

Figure 3.64. Higher magnification of mouse oviduct from Figure 3.63. The **arrow** points to an ovulated ovum within the ampulla of the oviduct.

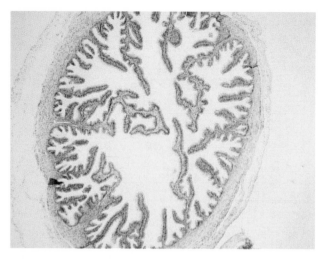

Figure 3.65. Low magnification of bovine oviduct that reveals the many foldings of the tunica mucosa and the relatively thin wall appearance to this tubular organ.

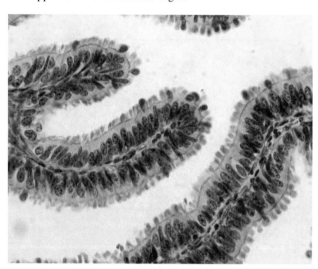

Figure 3.66. Higher magnification of the oviduct reveals the ciliated and non-ciliated cells that line the folded tunica mucosa.

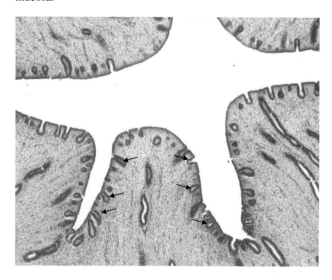

Figure 3.67. Low magnification of canine uterus revealing the endometrium made up of the endometrial lining cells, connective tissue stroma, and endometrial glands. The canine uterus has short endometrial glands that project downward from the endometrial lining (**arrows**).

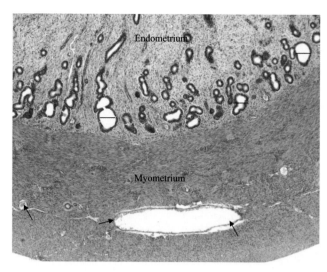

Figure 3.68. Canine uterus. The stratum vasculare (**arrows**), which are collections of blood vessels, resides between the two muscular layers.

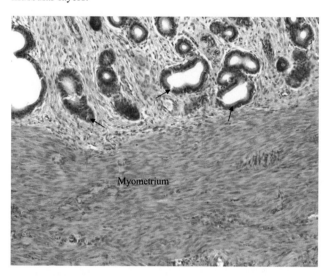

Figure 3.69. Higher magnification of canine uterus from Figure 3.68. The **arrows** point at endometrial glands. The myometrium is below the endometrial region.

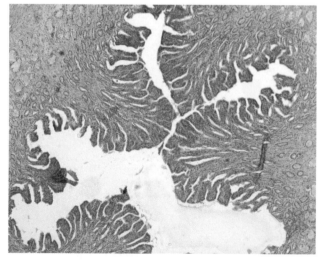

Figure 3.70. Low magnification of pregnant cat uterus. Numerous endometrial glands are evident in this section.

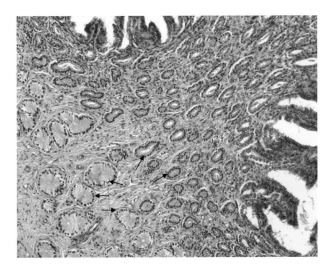

Figure 3.71. Higher magnification of pregnant cat uterus from Figure 3.70. The **arrows** point to a few of the abundant endometrial glands.

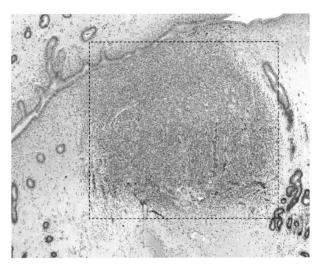

Figure 3.74. Ovine uterus—caruncular region. The connective tissue stroma proliferates below the endometrial lining cells (**boxed area**).

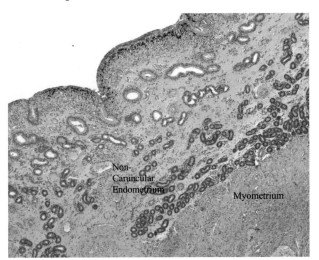

Figure 3.72. Low magnification of sheep uterus in the non-caruncular endometrial region. The non-caruncular region is characterized by the presence of endometrial gland.

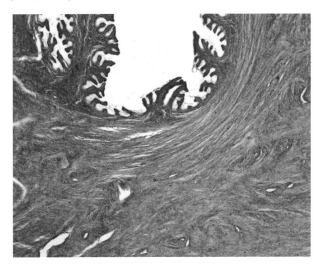

Figure 3.75. Bovine cervix. The tunica mucosa of the cervix has many primary, secondary, and tertiary folds.

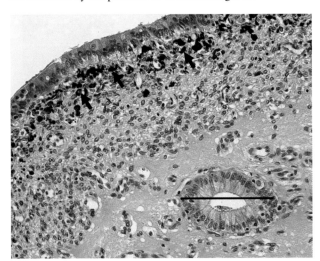

Figure 3.73. Higher magnification of ovine uterus from Figure 3.72. Below the endometrial lining cells are several ectopic melanocytes (**arrows**). These cells are routinely seen in sheep uteri. The **bar** spans one endometrial gland that characterizes the non-caruncular region.

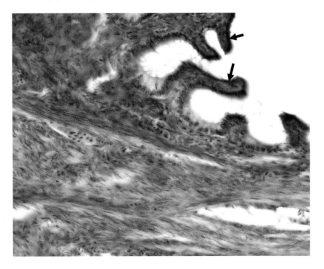

Figure 3.76. Higher magnification of bovine cervix from Figure 3.75. The **arrows** point at the secondary folds that branch from the primary folds.

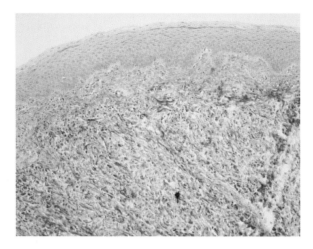

Figure 3.77. Low magnification of canine vagina. The tunica mucosa is comprised of non-keratinised stratified squamous epithelium.

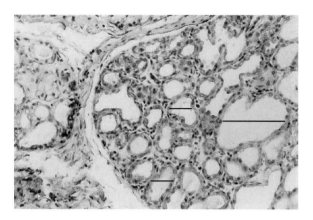

Figure 3.78. Active bovine mammary gland that consists of many lobules containing alveolar glands (**bars**).

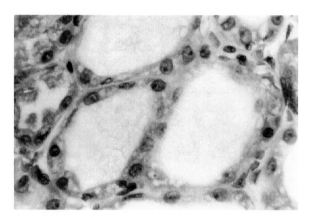

Figure 3.79. Higher magnification of mammary gland alveoli from Figure 3.78.

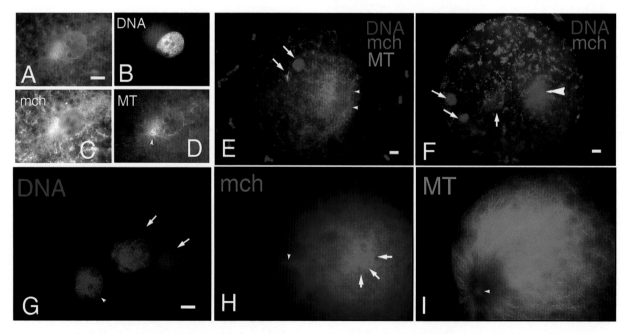

Figure 3.82. Distribution of mitochondria (**mch**) and microtubules (**MT**) in fertilized oocytes. (**A–D**), the enlarged sperm head is surrounded by mch which aggregate (**C**) at the sperm aster (**arrowhead** in (**D**)). (**E**), at 10 h after insemination, three pronuclei are formed due to polyspermy which often occurs during porcine IVF. No mch aggregation is seen around the female pronucleus (**arrow**) judged from the close association of the second polar body (**arrow**) extruded by cytokinetic MTs (green signal). On the other hand, mch aggregate around two male pronuclei (**arrowheads**). Cluster formation of mch is observed at the cortex. (**F**), the female pronucleus is closely localized to the two polar bodies (**arrows**) and displays a rare association of mch, whereas the male pronucleus displays a diffuse pattern of mch association (**arrowhead**). (**G–I**), a continuous ring of mch (**arrowhead** in **H**) is formed at the rim of male pronuclei (**arrowhead** in **G**) surrounded by well-developed MTs from the sperm aster (**arrowhead** in **I**). Mch are not observed around female pronuclei (**arrow** in **G**) but are associated with the second polar body (**arrow** in **G** and **H**). Bar, 10 μm. Reprinted with permission from Katayama et al., 2006.

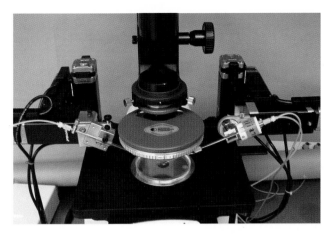

Figure 5.1. Micromanipulation system used for pronuclear microinjection and somatic cell nuclear transfer.

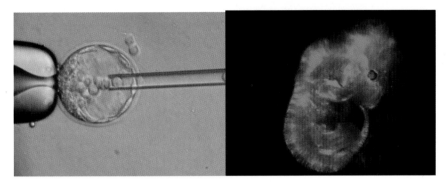

Figure 5.3. Embryonic stem cell micro-injection into mouse blastocyst (left) and resulting chimeric mouse after embryo transfer (right).

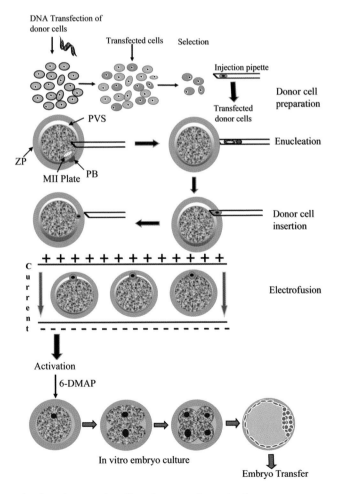

Figure 5.5. Transgenic animal production via somatic cell nuclear transfer technology.

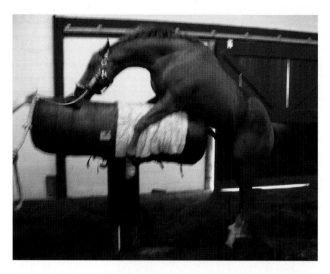

Figure 7.3. A stallion mounting a phantom dummy for semen collection.

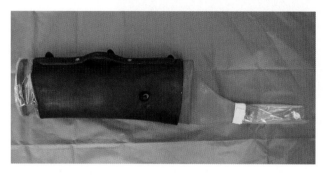

Figure 7.4. A Missouri artificial vagina for stallion semen collection.

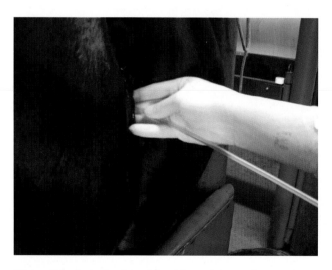

Figure 7.5. A sterile sleeved hand is used to part the mare's labia and introduce the insemination pipette.

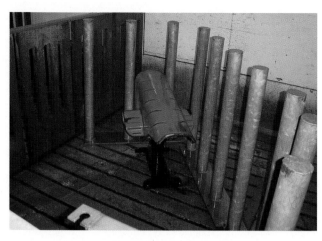

Figure 7.7. A typical boar semen collection pen and phantom mount. Note the spacing of vertical posts to allow the technician easy access and escape from the pen, while yet keeping the boar within the pen.

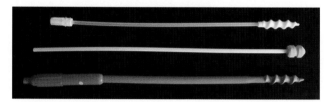

Figure 7.8. Swine artificial insemination pipettes. **(A):** single-use, disposable spiral tip pipette; **(B):** single-use, disposable foam-tip pipette; and **(C):** re-usable Melrose catheter.

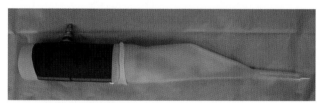

Figure 7.9. A complete ram/buck artificial vagina.

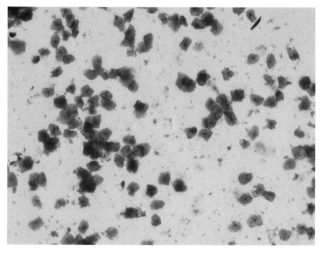

Figure 7.12. Vaginal cytology in a bitch. Sample shows predominantly keratinized epithelial cells, indicative of an estrus bitch.

Chapter 4

Comparative Reproductive Physiology of Domestic Animals

Eric M. Walters

Introduction

Reproduction is an exciting area of investigation because associated events reoccur on a scheduled and predictable time frame. Reproduction relies heavily on the basic well-being of the animal; it is one of the first systems in the body to shut down under periods of stress and imbalance in homeostasis, and during infection. Basic knowledge of reproduction is critical to successfully manipulating the reproductive system in many assisted reproductive technologies.

Many of the assisted reproductive technologies discussed in this book require the investigator to manipulate some aspect of reproduction, whether it's superovulation, embryo transfer into a suitable recipient, or transvaginal oocyte aspiration. Many of these assisted reproductive technologies are similar across species, yet appropriate techniques to manipulate different stages of the reproductive cycle differ. This chapter is intended to give a comparative overview of physiology of reproduction in several domestic animal species, starting with the endocrine system that controls the different stages of reproduction to the male and female physiology of reproduction, and ending with parturition and lactation.

Endocrine Glands

The endocrine glands are those glands whose secretion, called *hormones*, empties into the blood stream. All of the hormones that have involvement in the reproductive system will be discussed further in this chapter.

Hypothalamus

The diencephalon is the region of the brain just above the brainstem which includes the thalamus, hypothalamus with the hypophysis, epithalamus including the pineal gland, metathalamus, and subthalamus. The hypothalamus is located at the basal part of the diencephalon ventral to the thalamus. The hypothalamus is stimulated by higher brain centers to work in an inhibitory and stimulatory manner (by releasing several hormone-specific releasing factors) to control the pituitary gland. In terms of reproduction, the major hypothalamic hormone is the gonadotropin releasing hormone (GnRH); however there are other hormones released by the hypothalamus that have effects on the reproductive system. For example, the hypothalamus releases thyrotropin-releasing hormone (TRH). TRH in cattle and ewes stimulates the release of prolactin. In cattle it also stimulates growth hormone.

Hypophysis

The hypophysis (pituitary gland) has been referred to as the master endocrine gland because it controls the major endocrine glands (adrenal, thyroid, and gonads) as well as the mammary gland, uterus, and others. In addition, if the pituitary gland is removed or nonfunctional, there is a loss of function in the gonads and adrenal and thyroid glands.

The main parts of the pituitary gland are the anterior lobe (andenohypophysis) and the posterior lobe (neurohypophysis) that secrete different hormones. Hormones that are released by the anterior lobe of the pituitary gland include luteinizing hormone (LH), follicle stimulating hormone (FSH), thyroid stimulating hormone (TSH), adrenal cortical stimulating hormone (ACTH), corticotropin, growth hormone, somatotropin, and prolactin. The posterior lobe releases oxytocin and vasopressin. All of the pituitary hormones in combination with the target organ products work in a positive and negative feedback loop to the hypothalamus, pituitary, and higher brain centers to regulate production and secretion of the hormone.

Adrenal and Thyroid Glands

Hormones from other glands directly or indirectly affect the reproductive system. The adrenal and thyroid glands produce several hormones that affect some aspect of the reproductive process. The thyroid gland contains several thyroid follicles which are the functional unit of the gland. The follicles within the thyroid gland are not identical and contain a single layer of cuboidal epithelium. The thyroid gland has many functions that are independent of reproduction, including Ca^{2+} homeostasis.

Thyroid stimulating hormone (TSH) production and secretion is from the anterior pituitary gland, stimulating the thyroid gland to begin synthesis of thyroid hormones (T_3 and T_4). Thyroxine (T_4) is typically found in larger amounts than triiodothyronin (T_3). The mode of action for the thyroid hormones is analogous to that of the steroid hormones. It is believed that T_3 is the physiologically active thyroid hormone, regulating many cellular events, and T_4 is believed to be involved in the negative feedback loop on the hypothalamus.

Some of the functions of the thyroid hormones' effects on the reproductive system are: (1) required for early embryonic differentiation of the nervous system, (2) required for pituitary production of prolactin and growth hormone, (3) induction of enzyme synthesis such as the α-lactalbumin (critical for milk production), and (4) induction of cellular proteins such as prolactin.

The adrenal gland is composed of chromaffin and steroidogenic tissue. Similar to the thyroid gland, the adrenal gland has many functions that are independent of the reproductive system but also has an effect on the reproductive system. The adrenal gland is another source of steroid hormones that are synthesized from cholesterol.

Steroid production in the adrenal gland is similar to gondal steroid production in that cholesterol is converted through several enzymatic pathways to produce the steroid of interest. Adrenal steroids can be categorized into three types: glucocorticoids (cortisol), mineralocorticoids (aldosterone), and androgens. The steroids produced by the adrenal gland require the double bond between positions 4 and 5 and the keto group at position 3 of the A ring for biological activity.

Glucocorticoids production by the adrenal gland is regulated by pituitary adrenal cortisol-stimulating hormone (ACTH). In addition, cortisol is involved in the feedback loop of the pituitary (release of ACTH), hypothalamus (block release of CRH), and high brain centers. The mode of action is believed to involve *de novo* synthesis of cellular proteins and most often enzymes. Glucocorticoids also inhibit prostaglandin synthesis, potentially by inhibiting phospholipase A_2 activity.

One of the major effects of the glucocorticoids on reproduction is during stress response. As the animal is stressed the levels of glucocorticoids increase and reproduction is suppressed. The glucocorticoids and other hormones inhibit the release of GnRH at the hypothalamic level. With the inhibition of GnRH, the levels of LH and FSH decrease, which ultimately decreases the gondal activity.

Aldosterone is a mineralocorticoid which mediates its action by the induction of protein synthesis within the target tissue. Aldosterone levels begin to increase and are maintained during pregnancy. Aldosterone is also involved in the homeostasis of the pregnant mother in terms of blood pressure and other cellular events.

Endocrinology

As the female progresses through these different stages of the estrous cycle, hormone concentrations undergo cyclical changes to induce the necessary responses in the ovary, uterus, and brain. Similar events occur in the male as spermatozoa are being produced. Reproduction is regulated by a series of hormones that both originate in and alter the physiology of the reproductive and nervous systems. These two systems work together to initiate and coordinate the reproductive system on a predictable time frame.

Hormones affect metabolism, synthetic activity, and secretory activity of the target tissue. Dramatic physiological responses can be caused by small quantities (nanograms to picograms) of hormones. The half-life of hormones is defined as the amount of time required to remove half of the hormone from the blood supply or from the body. Some hormones have short half-lives so they can cause the necessary response only and not trigger unwanted responses. Others have longer half-lives that maintain a sustained activity.

Hormones are classified by their origin, primary mode of action, and biochemical structure. Hypothalamic hormones are produced by neurons of the hypothalamus, whose primary role is to cause the release of hormones from the hypophysis. GnRH is the primary hypothalamic hormone of the reproductive system (see Figure 4.1). It is a decapeptide with a molecular weight of 1.1 kDa.

GnRH targets the adenohypophysis and neurohypophysis of the pituitary gland which cause release of pituitary hormones from both lobes. The primary anterior pituitary hormones affecting reproduction are FSH, LH, and prolactin, whereas oxytocin is from the posterior pituitary gland.

Gonadal hormones originate from the gonads and have target tissues that range from the hypothalamus and pituitary gland to other tissues of the reproductive tract. The development of secondary sex characteristics (in other words, "femaleness" or "maleness") is initiated by gonadal hormones such as estrogen or testosterone. In the female several gonadal hormones are produced by the ovary: estrogen, progesterone, inhibin, limited testosterone, oxytocin, and relaxin. In the male, the testis produces: testosterone, other androgens, inhibin, and limited estrogen.

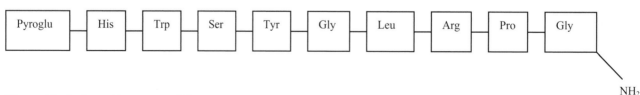

Figure 4.1. Amino acid sequence of GnRH.

Other reproductive hormones are produced by the uterus as well as the placenta, which maintains of pregnancy and the animal's cyclicity. Prostaglandin $F_{2\alpha}$ is a uterine hormone that helps govern cyclicity in the animal. Placental hormones include progesterone, estrogen, equine chorionic gonadotropin (eCG), and human chorionic gonadotropin (hCG).

In addition to being classified by their source, hormones are also classified by mode of action. For example, there are those hormones that are synthesized by neurons and others that are synthesized by the gonads. Neurohormones such as oxytocin are synthesized by neurons and released into the bloodstream and can cause a response in tissues that have receptors for them. Releasing hormones such as GnRH are also classified as neurohormones because they are also synthesized by neurons and cause the release of other hormones.

Gonadotropins have an affinity for the gonad of either the male or female. Gonadotroph cells within the anterior pituitary gland synthesize and release hormones such as LH and FSH. In the male of some species, FSH is believed to be a "key regulator" of spermatogenesis; in the female it promotes the development of the antral follicle(s) to the dominant/ovulatory follicle(s).

The gonadotropins also stimulate the production of steroids (estrogen, progesterone, and testosterone) within the gonads. These steroids stimulate the reproductive tract. They also feed back to regulate the production of gonadotropins (LH and FSH) and regulate reproductive behavior and secondary sex characteristics. In the ovary, LH causes ovulation of the dominant follicle(s) and formation of the corpus luteum; however, in the male LH promotes the production of testosterone.

FSH has a similar action but different effects on the gonads. In the female, FSH begins to recruit the follicles prior to ovulation and in the male it affects spermatogenesis. Pregnancy hormones are at their highest level during pregnancy and help to maintain pregnancy (progesterone in some species) and develop the mammary gland (placental lactogen).

Another mode of action is the luteolysis which leads to the regression of the corpus luteum. Prostaglandin $F_{2\alpha}$ ($PGF_{2\alpha}$) is the major luteolytic hormone of the reproductive system which is secreted by the uterus. $PGF_{2\alpha}$ causes regression of the CL at defined points in time in the reproductive cycle.

Finally, hormones can be classified by their biochemical structure: peptides, glycoproteins, steroids, and prostaglandins. Glycoproteins contain a carbohydrate group (to protect the hormone from degradation) and are typically small polypeptides. The number of carbohydrates on the surface of the glycoprotein determines the half-life of the protein. Glycoproteins have an alpha and beta subunit that are linked by hydrogen bonds with carbohydrate groups covalently linked on the alpha and beta subunit. In the case of LH and FSH, the alpha subunit is identical, but function and receptor specificity are determined by the beta subunit. Inhibin is another glycoprotein hormone that contains an alpha and beta subunit, but with inhibin there are two beta subunits with similar activity. Not all proteins have an alpha and beta subunit. Prolactin is an example of a single polypeptide chain protein.

Steroid hormones are among the predominant biochemically active hormones in the reproductive system. They have a cyclopentanoperhydrophenanthrene nucleus and are composed of four rings designated A, B, C, and D, with a molecular weight of 300. Steroid hormones are synthesized from cholesterol through a series of enzymatic conversions resulting in steroids with minor but biologically significant differences.

Cholesterol enters into the mitochondria and then is converted to pregnenolone, which is released into the cytoplasm of the cell where there are further conversions to produce androgens and further conversions to estrogen (see Figure 4.2). There are three sources of cholesterol for steroidogenesis: *de novo* synthesis, intracellular stores, and blood lipoprotein (LDL) cholesterol.

All steroidogenic cells have the capacity to produce cholesterol from *de novo* synthesis, but gondal tissue converts acetyl-CoA to cholesterol. However, with this process there is a rate-limiting step which is the cytoplasmic hydroxymethyl glutaryl (HMG)-CoA reductase. In the ovary, placenta, and adrenal glands there is evidence that the primary source of cholesterol for steroidogenesis is from the LDLs. This is less evident in the male. Steroid hormone production is highly regulated by controlling the enzyme levels and localizing the enzymes. An additional rate-limiting step in steroidogenesis is the production of steroidogenic acute regulatory protein (StAR). StAR delivers cholesterol from the outer to inner membranes of the mitochondria. Despite the fact that steroidogenesis is highly regulated, steroid hormones have a pronounced effect on the reproductive system in the male and female because they act as sexual promoters. Estrogen, progesterone, androgens, and testosterone are steroid hormones that have effects on the reproductive tract.

Prostaglandins were first thought to be produced by the prostate gland because they were initially discovered in seminal plasma. Prostaglandins are lipids composed of 20-carbon unsaturated hydroxyl fatty acids. There are several prostaglandins and metabolites but only two are of primary importance for reproduction, $PGF_{2\alpha}$ and prostaglandin E_2. The discovery that prostaglandins cause luteolysis of the corpus luteum has laid the foundation for the use of prostaglandins as a tool for manipulating the reproductive cycle.

The mode of action for hormones can be classified by the type of hormones (e.g. protein vs. steroid). Protein hormones use the hormone receptor binding on the cell surface to initiate a primary response. Protein hormones diffuse from the blood into the interstitial compartment, then bind to the specific hormone receptor at the target tissue. This

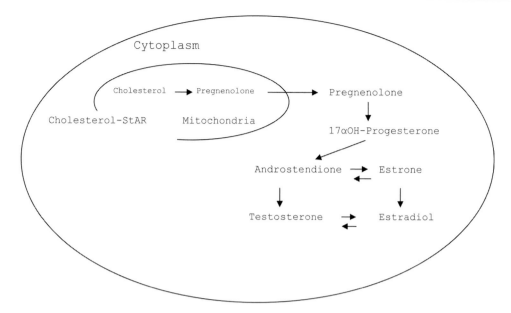

Figure 4.2. Steroid biosynthesis pathway.

hormone binding is believed to be specific by the geometry of the protein and the receptor. Only certain configurations of the protein "fit/bind" the receptor, or in other words there are only two adjacent pieces that will combine into one piece.

Once the protein hormone has bound to the receptor, in the cytoplasm of the cell there is activation of the G-protein pathway which then activates adenylate cyclase. Adenylate cyclase causes the conversion of ATP to cyclic AMP (cAMP; second messenger) which then triggers downstream events. cAMP has been termed a "second messenger" because it must be present for the activation of protein kinases. Several different protein kinases within the cytoplasm of the cell trigger different events to occur, such as conversion of substrates to product or synthesis of a new product. Depending on which protein kinase is activated, the subsequent events that occur downstream and the end result (e.g. flagellum movement or production of estradiol) will differ.

Steroid hormones have a similar but different mode of action compared to the glycoproteins. Steroid hormones are transported through the blood supply as protein hormones are, but steroid hormones are not water-soluble. Therefore, steroid hormones must form a complex with water-soluble steroid-specific carrier proteins or plasma proteins. These carrier proteins help transport the steroid in the bloodstream and to the cell membrane.

Once the complex has reached the cell membrane, the steroid hormone diffuses into the cytoplasm of the cell as a result of the lipid solubility of the steroid hormones. In the cell, the steroid hormone diffuses through the cytoplasm into the nucleus. Upon entering the nucleus the steroid hormone binds to its specific receptor just as the protein hormones. DNA-directed messenger RNA synthesis or transcription is initiated by the binding of the steroid to the receptor (see Figure 4.3). The freshly synthesized mRNA leaves the nucleus and then directs synthesis of proteins, thus causing the end result to occur.

Male Physiology

The male reproductive system has often been referred to as a "manufacturing plant," largely because of the continuous production of fertile spermatozoa. As with manufacturing any product, whether it is spermatozoa or anything else, there are many factors that impend or enhance production and delivery. For anatomical details see Chapter 2, "Anatomy of Reproductive Organs" and for histological details see Chapter 3 Part 2, "Overview of Male Reproductive Organs." If we continue to think about the male reproductive system as a manufacturing plant, then all the basic components have to be functional to reach full productivity. In terms of production, sperm output per day for both testis ranges from less than 1 to 25 billion, or 35,000 to 290,000 spermatozoa per second depending on species.

There are several basic components to the male reproductive system, such as the spermatic cord (for details see Chapter 2, "Anatomy of Reproductive Organs"), which are critical to the daily production of sperm. One of the major functions of the spermatic cord involves heat exchange via the pampiniform plexus. In general, in most mammals the testes must be 4°C to 6°C cooler than body temperature of that mammal for proper spermatogenesis. The pampiniform plexus is a vascular system consisting of an intertwined artery and veins. This system forms a countercurrent heat exchanger in which heat is transferred from the warm blood coming from the body to the cooler blood returning from the testes. Disruption of this heat exchanger severely compromises spermatogenesis.

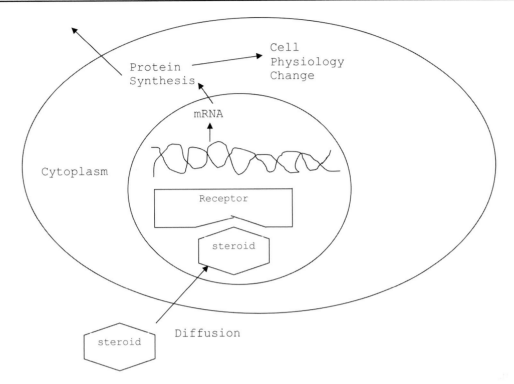

Figure 4.3. Mode of action for a steroid hormone.

The cremaster muscle has two important functions in the male reproductive system. It contributes to the support system of the testis as a part of the internal abdominal oblique muscle. It also helps regulate scrotal temperature by contraction and relaxation.

The scrotum is the most superficial testicular tunic, which is involved in temperature regulation and protects and supports the testis. For details, see Chapter 2, "Anatomy of Reproductive Organs" and Chapter 3 Part 2, "Overview of Male Reproductive Organs." Because the scrotum is involved in temperature regulation, it has a large number of sweat glands and thermosensitive nerves. The thermosensitive nerves help control the amount of scrotal sweating as well as the respiration of the animal. In species that have pendulous scrotum such as the ruminants, the scrotum via the tunica dartos raises and lower the scrotum in response to changes in temperature. As the temperature decreases, the scrotum is pulled closer to the body to maintain the proper scrotal temperature and the opposite occurs as the temperature rises.

The testes are the main site for production of spermatozoa in the male. Sperm production is based on the length and number of tubules present in the testis which in turn is based on the size of the testis. In farm animals, the boar has the largest testis, thus making it the best in terms of sperm production per gm of testis. Sperm production relies heavily of the machinery of the testes, which include the seminiferous tubules, Leydig (interstitial endocrine) cells, Sertoli (sustentacular) cells, germinal or spermatogenic cells, and rete testis.

A seminiferous tubule consists of tubulus seminiferous contortus (the majority of spermatogenesis occurs in this region) and tubulus seminiferous rectus (straight section). The seminiferous tubules join in the rete testis, which is protected within the mediastinum testis, and transport sperm to the epididymis via the efferent ductulus for final maturation prior to ejaculation. For details, see Chapter 3 Part 2, "Overview of Male Reproductive Organs."

Spermatogenesis occurs within the tubulus contortus. Of the components in the tubules, two cell types are critical for spermatogenesis to occur properly: Sertoli cell, which is considered to be the nurse cell of the spermatozoa during spermatogenesis, and Leydig cell, which produces the testosterone needed for spermatogenesis.

Accessory Sex Glands

In most mammals, the accessory sex gland secretions make up the majority of the seminal plasma during ejaculation. The species differences are mainly anatomical in terms of the accessory glands for the production of seminal plasma during ejaculation. In the bull and stallion, the accessory sex glands can be manipulated via the rectum to stimulate ejaculation for collecting semen for a fertility check (breeding soundness exam). In the pig, the bulbourethral (Cowper's) glands are large and are the source of the gelatinous material found in boar semen. For anatomical details, see Chapter 2, "Anatomy of Reproductive Organs."

Spermatogenesis

Spermatogenesis is a complex chronological series of events which involves divisions and differentiation and takes several weeks to produce partial mature sperm cells. The process starts with a self-renewing stem cell population that undergoes mitosis to maintain the stem cell population and produces primary spermatocytes that will then undergo meiosis to produce the haploid spermatid. The haploid spermatid is then differentiated into spermatozoa that are transported to the lumen of the seminiferous tubules. Spermatogenesis can be divided into four phases: (1) spermatocytogenesis (mitosis), (2) meiosis, (3) spermiogenesis, and (4) spermiation (release of the sperm into the lumen). For specific structural details, see Chapter 3, "Histology, Cellular and Molecular Biology of Reproductive Organs."

Endocrine Control of Spermatogenesis

Initiation of spermatogenesis is due largely to the amount of hormones, in particular testosterone and follicle-stimulating hormone (FSH). The Leydig cells are stimulated by luteinizing hormone (LH) to produce testosterone, which maintains spermatogenesis in the adult animal. The testosterone that is produced by the Leydig cells diffuses into the adjacent Sertoli cells which is then released into the bloodstream to feed back to the hypothalamus and pituitary gland to prevent further secretions of LH and FSH.

FSH action is on the Sertoli cells within the testis. The FSH stimulates production of estradiol by converting testosterone and stimulating production of inhibin and androgen binding protein (ABP). FSH is required for the formation and maintenance of the tight junctions between the Sertoli cells.

Testosterone is required for spermatid maturation and maintenance of spermatogenesis. Testosterone has several functions in the male system: (1) maintenance of germ cells, (2) increase in seminiferous tubule fluid, (3) development of secondary sex characteristics, (4) sexual differentiation of the brain, and (5) increase in meiosis, vasomotion, and spermatid development. Although high levels of testosterone are required for proper spermatogenesis, some of the testosterone is converted to dihydrotestosterone as well as estradiol.

Estradiol levels in the male are relatively low compared to testosterone. However estrogen does have an important role (water re-absorption in the epididymis) in the male. Nevertheless, exposure to high levels of estrogenic compounds has a negative affect on spermatogenesis.

The Sertoli cells are also stimulated by FSH to produce ABP, except in the pig. The ABP forms a complex with androgens and is transported with the sperm to the epididymis. ABP also helps carry androgens (mainly testosterone) within the Sertoli cells, and transports androgens to the liver.

FSH and LH are both secreted by the anterior lobe of the pituitary gland under the control of GnRH as well as the negative feedback of testosterone and estradiol. In addition, inhibin is used in the negative feedback loop from the testis to the pituitary gland. Inhibin blocks the release of FSH but not LH. Furthermore, it is believed that prolactin may play a critical role in regulating LH receptors in Leydig cells.

Another important player is transferrin, which transports Fe to the germ cells in the testis. Transferrin is up-regulated by several factors such as FSH, testosterone, retinol, and retinoic acid. Sperm production can be determined by the amount of transferrin present; for example, when sperm counts are low so is transferrin.

There are species differences in the hormone(s) that are necessary to support spermatogenesis. For example, in the ram FSH is necessary and LH may also have a direct role. In addition, there is also a seasonal effect on spermatogenesis and the levels of hormones present. For example, the levels of FSH and LH in the horse are higher in the summer because sperm production is at it highest level.

Sperm Transport in the Male

Once the sperm is released to the lumen of the seminiferous tubules, it is transported from the rete testis to the epididymis for final maturation and storage until ejaculation. The epididymis consists of three sections: head or caput, body or corpus, and tail or cauda, and its function as a whole is stimulated by androgens.

The head is the region of the epididymis where maturation of the sperm occurs; the sperm is then transported to the body and the tail of the epididymis.. The sperm gain motility and fertilization capability in the epididymis without undergoing capacitation. There are decapacitation factors (proteins, glycolipids, and/or lipids) present in the epididymis to stabilize the sperm membrane. The tail of the epididymis is the storage location for the sperm prior to ejaculation.

Erection and Ejaculation

During mating the male mounts the female in estrus and deposits semen into the reproductive tract. Erection of the penis depends on the general aspects of sexual behavior and is controlled by the nervous system. With erection, the penis begins to elongate and it becomes more rigid. Stimulation of the sympathetic and parasympathetic nerves is caused by sensory input and psychic stimuli. The sympathetic nerves inhibit vasoconstriction and the parasympathetic nerves affect the dilation of blood vessels and enlargement of the corpus cavernosum. In addition, in all farm animals there is a relaxation of the penile retractor muscle.

Ejaculation involves muscle contractions of various parts of the male reproductive system that is mediated by the nervous system (parasympathetic nerves). Tonic and rhythmic muscle contractions of the epididymis, penis, accessory glands, and ductus deferens, and closure of the neck of the bladder, aid in the movement of sperm and seminal plasma and final expulsion of the semen through the penis.

Some species such as the boar and stallion have a very prolonged ejaculation compared to other species. In the stallion and the boar, the penis is primarily responsive to pressure, whereas ruminants are more responsive to temperature. In these species the semen can be divided into pre-sperm, sperm-rich fraction, and post-sperm (gel/plug fraction).

The site of ejaculation is also species-dependent. Ruminants deposit semen in the vagina, whereas the stallion deposits semen in the uterus. The pig deposits in two locations—the cervix and the body of the uterus—largely due to the retention of the penis during copulation.

Capacitation and Acrosome Reaction

Even though it is known that the sperm in the epididymis has the ability to fertilize an oocyte, it still has to undergo several changes to complete the process of fertilization. Freshly ejaculated sperm have to undergo further changes to be able to fertilize the oocyte and these changes usually occur in the female reproductive tract. The changes consist of process that has been called "capacitation." There are species differences in the time required for capacitation in the female tract; for example, boar sperm requires three to six hours.

Capacitation involves the alteration of the plasma membrane, such as the removal of decapacitation factors, removal of cholesterol, influx of calcium, an increase in intracellular pH, and an increase in protein tyrosine phosphorylation (not fully understood). Capacitation of the sperm can occur in either the utenine tube or uterus and appears to be under the control of estrogens. In contrast to estrogen's positive effect on capacitation, progesterone appears to have an inhibitory effect.

The majority of the changes that occur during capacitation involve the sperm head; however, no morphological changes occur. Capacitation is believed to allow the sperm to undergo the acrosome reaction. The lifespan of capacitated sperm is limited; as a result, precise timing between capacitation and the acrosome reaction is necessary for proper fertilization to occur.

The acrosome reaction is the progressive breakdown and fusion of the plasma membrane and the outer acrosomal membrane. This fusion allows release of the enzymes from the acrosome which causes the ultimate loss of the plasma-membrane-acrosome complex. Furthermore, there are changes in the equatorial region of the sperm that are essential for sperm-egg binding. In addition, this release of the enzymes from the acrosome is critical for the penetration of the cumulus cells and zona pellucida (ZP).

Female Physiology

For details on the female anatomy of the reproductive system see Chapter 2, "Anatomy of Reproductive Organs" and for histological details see Chapter 3 Part 4, "Overview of Female Reproductive Organs." The female is less productive than the male in terms of gamete production. She produces one to 15 follicles depending on species during the estrus cycle but undergoes predictable and dramatic series of changes. In addition, the female reproductive tract is responsible for the development of the offspring.

The ovary is the site of gamete production in the female. It has both an endocrine and exocrine function because it performs steroidogenesis and egg release, respectively. The ovary consists of the cortex which houses the oocytes arrested at prophase in most species, and the medulla.

Several different types of ovarian follicles can be found at a given time within the ovary cortex. These different types of follicles represent the different stages of follicular development (discussed in Folliculogenesis and Oogenesis). In the center of the ovary is the medulla housing the nerves, vasculature, and lymphatic systems. The primordial germ cells (those that give rise to the oocyte) have migrated to the genital ridge to form the ovary with surrounding cells.

As prenatal development continues the oogonia are produced by mitotic replication followed by meiotic division, giving rise to millions of oocytes arrested at prophase. At the time of birth, the number of oocytes has been significantly reduced by atresia. Additional oocytes are lost as the animal reaches puberty so there are only a few hundred oocytes left during the reproductive life span of the animal. In addition to producing the oocytes for fertilization, the ovary produces steroids, especially estrogen and progesterone, during different stages of the estrus cycle, and maintains pregnancy.

The uterine or fallopian tube (salpinx) is the site of fertilization. There are three sections of the uterine tube: infundibulum, ampulla, and isthmus. The primary function of the uterine tube is the transportation of the freshly ovulated oocyte and sperm to the site of fertilization, followed by the transport of the fertilized egg to the uterus. The infundibulum collects the freshly ovulated oocyte in some species. The infundibulum contains finger-like projections called fimbriae which increase the surface area of the infundibulum. Once the oocyte is ovulated and collected by the infundibulum, it is transported to the ampulla of the uterine tube. An undefined area where the ampulla continues with the isthmus (also conventionally called the ampullary-isthmic junction) is the site of fertilization. The isthmus of the uterine tube is smaller in diameter and transports the fertilized oocyte to the uterus for subsequent embryonic development. Limited embryonic development occurs in the isthmus of the uterine tube, depending on species (see Fertilization and Embryo development).

The point at which the uterine tube connects to the uterus is conventionally called the uterotubal junction; it is closed until three to five days post-ovulation. In some species, such as the cow, the uterotubal junction (UTJ) controls the movement of the embryo from the oviduct to the uterus by estradiol regulation. High concentrations of estradiol are believed to cause a blockage in the UTJ, which is reversed/opened when estradiol levels decrease, thus allowing the movement of the embryo into the uterus. In other species, there is no obvious blockage at the UTJ;

however pigs have a constriction at the UTJ which is believed to be the mechanism for blockage of polyspermy in the pig. This constriction acts as a major barrier for sperm transport and limits the number of sperm released into the ampulla region of the uterine tube.

The uterus is critical for the development of the fetus and maintenance of pregnancy. For anatomical details, see Chapter 2, "Anatomy of Reproductive Organs" and for histological details see Chapter 3 Part 4, "Overview of Female Reproductive Organs." The myometrium is the combination of longitudinal and the inner circular muscle fibers which also have several physiological functions. The most critical function of the myometrium is transport of the embryos, sperm, and the fetus by contraction. In response to estradiol, most species (with the exception of the mare) the myometrium has a high level of tone. Uterine tone is believed to be related to the function of the uterus; in other words, there is more tone as sperm is transported to the oviduct than when the progesterone level is high.

The innermost section of the uterus is the endometrium, which is composed of the mucosa and submucosa. The secretions of the uterus are provided by the mucosal epithelium, which is believed to enhance embryonic development and sperm survival in the uterus. The uterine glands also release their secretion into the lumen of the uterus which is under the control of both estrogen and progesterone (secretions change with the different days of the estrous cycle). Under the influence of estrogen, the uterine glands begin to coil and secrete into the uterus; however, is not at full secretory capacity until it is under the influence of progesterone. The uterine glands are believed to secrete substances that are essential for embryonic development in the uterus. The endometrium in domestic mammals does not slough; however, humans slough the endometrium and uterine glands on a monthly basis (i.e. each estrous cycle).

The uterus has several functions, including sperm transport, control of cyclicity by production of prostaglandin $F_{2\alpha}$, embryonic development of the pre-/post-implantation embryo, contribution to the development of the placenta, and expulsion of the fetus and placenta.

The cervix produces various amounts of mucus; for example, ruminants produce large amounts of mucus whereas in the sow and mare a much smaller amount is produced. The mucus lubricates the cervix for copulation, in the stallion and boar. An additional function of the cervical mucus is to protect the fetus from the outside environment. During pregnancy, the cervical mucus acts as a "glue" of the cervical folds so foreign material does not disrupt the pregnancy.

The vagina and the vestibulum are considered together as the copulatory organ of the reproductive tract. The major function of the vagina and the vestibulum in some species is the movement of sperm from the site of deposit to the site of fertilization.

The vulva is the external part of the female reproductive tract and its primary function is to protect the reproductive tract from the environment.

Folliculogenesis and Oogenesis

The process of follicular development occurs continuously throughout the estrous cycle. The follicles are developed in waves throughout the estrous cycle. There are two types of follicular waves: anovulatory wave and ovulatory wave. The only difference between these two or three waves (one to two anovulatory waves and one ovulatory wave) is the timing of the wave in the estrous cycle. In the ovulatory wave the levels of LH continue to increase and result in an LH surge, causing the ovulation of the oocyte. Folliculogenesis is the development of the follicles and then the recruitment, selection, dominance/ovulation, and atresia of an antral follicle(s) in the ovary. The number of follicles that develop and ovulate somewhat depends on the species. Some species are polytocous (litter-bearing; multiple ovulation), whereas others are monotocous (one offspring; single ovulation).

There are different types of ovarian follicles that represent the different stages of development and maturity at any time of the estrous cycle. There are four stages of follicles present in the ovary: primordial follicle, primary follicle, secondary follicle, and antral follicle. For specific details see Chapter 3, "Histology, Cellular and Molecular Biology of Reproductive Organs."

The smallest and most immature follicle is the primordial follicle. It is surrounded by only a single layer of flattened cells that are derived from the primordial germ cells that migrated to the genital ridges during prenatal development. The primordial follicle matures into the primary follicle, which is characterized by the changing of the cells that surround the oocyte. Whereas the cells are flattened in the primordial follicle, they have become cuboidal in the primary follicle.

The number of primordial and primary follicles present in the ovary is set at birth; in other words, primary follicles do not regenerate. The primary follicle either develops into a secondary follicle or degenerates. As the primary follicle develops into the secondary follicle layers of follicle cells are added, but without the development of a cavity (antrum). In addition to the additional layers of follicle cells, the oocyte obtains a translucent layer of glycoproteins called the zona pellucida (ZP). The ZP is made of three glycoproteins (zp1, zp2, zp3). Up to this point all the follicles have been microscopic.

The antral follicle, also known as the tertiary follicle, is characterized by the formation of a cavity (antrum) which is filled with fluid, called follicular fluid. Depending on the species, the antral follicle can be seen on the ovary with the naked eye and appears as a blister-like structure ranging in size from less than 1 mm to several centimeters. As the animal goes through the estrous cycle, the antral follicles are selected for further development and ovulation. The dominant follicle (ovulatory follicle) is also called the Graafian follicle.

The antral follicles are the pool of follicles that can be selected from during the follicular phase of the estrous cycle. As the antral follicle develops, the layers of follicular cells can be divided into distinct layers: theca externa, theca interna, and granulosal cell layer. The theca externa is composed primarily of loose connective tissue that surrounds and supports the antral follicle. Just beneath the theca externa is the theca interna, which provides the androgens needed and is influenced by LH.

A basement membrane separates the theca interna from the granulosal cell layer. This layer has the FSH receptors and produces several different materials needed for development. Estrogen, inhibin, and follicular fluid are the important factors that the granulosal cells produce. It is believed that the granulosal cells are the governing cells of oocyte maturation.

The follicular phase accounts for a small amount of the estrous cycle of the female (discussed in the next section). During this phase several antral follicles are lost to either atresia or ovulation. This phase is when the recruitment, selection, dominance of the antral follicles occurs. Antral follicles can be lost to atresia during each stage of the follicular phase. Recruitment of a small group of follicles (a cohort) occurs when the levels of FSH are high, LH is low, there is no inhibin, and estrogen is increasing. As recruitment ends, the antral follicles that have not undergone atresia are selected for further development and the dominant follicle(s) begin to emerge.

As development continues, the estrogen levels also continue to increase, and there is moderate FSH and LH and low inhibin. At the time of dominance, the follicles are pre-ovulatory and the levels of FSH are low, there is high LH and high inhibin, and the non-dominant follicles begin to undergo atresia.

Ovulation is the rupture of the dominant follicle(s) which releases the oocyte(s) from the follicle. Small blood vessels rupture at the time of ovulation, causing local hemorrhage. The combination of ruptured blood vessels and protrusion of tissue forms a structure known as the corpus hemorrhagicum. After this is formed, there is luteinization/differentiation of the theca interna and the granulosal cells into luteal cells. The collection of luteal cells forms the structure of the corpus luteum which produces the progesterone for maintenance of pregnancy. If there is no pregnancy, then the uterus will produce $PGF_{2\alpha}$ to regress the CL and the next estrous cycle begins. However, if a pregnancy occurs, then the CL will be maintained until parturition.

Simultaneously as the follicle undergoes folliculogenesis, the oocyte within the follicle changes as well. These events of maturation which occur throughout the lifespan of the female are known as oogenesis. Prenatally, the primordial germ cells undergo mitosis to ensure that there are enough primary oocytes at birth for future follicular development. As the oogonia performs its last mitotic activity to form the primary oocyte, it makes an important transition as the primary oocyte enters the first meiotic prophase where it is arrested until puberty.

The primary oocyte is arrested at prophase I of meiosis until it is stimulated by gonadotropins or it can remain arrested throughout the reproductive lifespan of the female.

As stated earlier, during the transition from the primary follicle to the secondary follicle the oocyte develops a translucent band of glycoproteins called the ZP. The ZP is an important developmental step because it is a protective coating for the developing embryo that has several functions. These include protecting the embryo from the outside environment by limiting diffusion, blocking polyspermy, and restricting the blastomeres of the embryo and thus promoting good cell-to-cell contact.

In the secondary oocyte, the zona begins to form junctional complexes with the neighboring follicular cells. Also known as gap junctions, these are critical for the cell-to-cell communication between the oocyte and granulosal cells. The gap junctions are believed to be critical for the growth of the oocyte within the follicle and they remain intact with the plasma membrane until the preovulatory LH surge.

The oocyte has reached its full cytoplasmic size once the follicle has begun forming the antrum. At the time of the ovulatory LH surge, several events occur with the oocyte such as the loss/breakdown of the gap junctions and the resumption of meiosis. Prior to ovulation the oocyte is still diploid (2N) during the resumption of meiosis. During the metaphase the oocyte extrudes the first polar body which contains half of the genetic material, thus forming a haploid (1N) oocyte arrested at metaphase II. The oocyte then remains arrested at metaphase II until fertilization or subsequent degeneration (see fertilization and embryonic development).

Estrous Cycle

After a female has reached puberty and enters into her productive life, she also enters a reproductive cyclicity ranging from four to 28 days depending on the species of interest. This reproductive cyclicity is termed "estrous cycle" and by definition lasts from one estrus to the subsequent estrus. The cycle is a series of scheduled events in which the female has repeated opportunities to become pregnant as she is receptive to the male. However, many factors affect the reproductive cyclicity, such as season, nutrition, lactation, and illness. With the exception of seasonality, many of these factors are influenced by management of the species. Later, we will discuss the species differences in seasonality (e.g. short-day breeders vs. long-day breeders).

The estrous cycle (see Figure 4.4) can be divided into luteal and follicular phases. The luteal phase (days one to 18, based on a 21-day cycle) is when there is lutenization of the follicle and subsequent regression of the CL if the female is not pregnant. The follicular phase (days 18 to 21) is when new follicles are recruited, developed, and ovulated.

The follicular phase can be divided into four sections: estrus, metestrus, diestrus, and proestrus. In each section there are defined events that must occur on time for the subsequent events to occur. Estrus (day 21; hours long) is the period when the female is sexually receptive to the

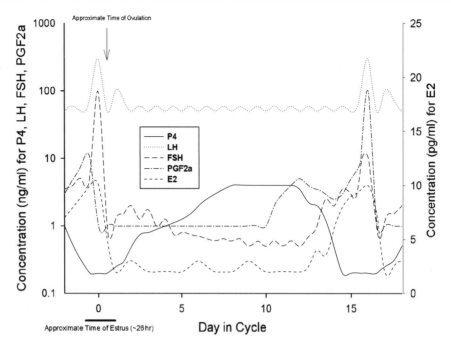

Figure 4.4. Diagram of the hormone levels during the estrous cycle of the ewe. Redrawn by Steve Mullen, University of Missouri-Columbia.

male, estradiol (E_2) is at its peak level, and ovulation occurs. Estrus also typically lasts hours compared to days of the other phases of the estrous cycle.

After estrus, the female enters into metestrus (days one to five based on a 21-day cycle) when estradiol levels are decreasing and progesterone (P_4) levels are increasing because the corpus luteum is forming on the ovary at the site of ovulation. Diestrus (days six to 18) is the period after metestrus when P_4 is at its peak level and E_2 is at its lowest level. In addition, maternal recognition of pregnancy occurs at this time as the embryo(s) begin signaling the female to maintain the pregnancy (discussed in detail in a later section) and not to begin cycling again. However, with no maternal recognition of pregnancy, the female enters proestrus (days 18 to 21). Proestrus is defined by a decrease in P_4 and an increase of E_2 as well as the formation of the next cohort of follicles that will ovulate during estrus.

Anestrus and Seasonality
Anestrus is a condition that may be caused by many factors that prevent reproductive cyclicity, including pregnancy, lactation, seasonality, stress caused by environmental or management factors, and pathological conditions. During this period, the ovary is in a semi-inactive state; in other words, there is no new recruitment of dominant/ovulatory follicles. While most of the factors that cause anestrus are abnormal conditions, seasonal anestrus in some species is normal.

Seasonality or seasonal anestrus is believed to have evolved to prevent mating at times when survival of the offspring would be low. Species that exhibit seasonality normally make a transition from anestrus to cyclicity on an

annual basis which is controlled by the photoperiod (e.g. long-day breeders and short-day breeders), a hormone called melatonin. The mare is an example of a long-day breeder; she begins to cycle as the day length increases in the spring. The ewe, a short-day breeder, is the opposite. She begins to cycle and her hormone levels increase as the day length shortens (see Table 4.1) . The hormone melatonin is released by the pineal gland (the epiphysis) during the night hours and is inhibited during the daylight hours. It affects the pulse generator of the pulsatile release of GnRH, LH, and FSH.

Estrus Behavior
Observing changes in the female's behavior is the main way to visually determine if the animal is coming into estrus. During the proestrus period the female's activity increases, she begins searching for the male, other animals begin to mount the female. At estrus the female will stand for

Table 4.1. Length of estrous cycle and estrus in various species.

Species	Estrous cycle length (Avg. days)	Estrus length
Cow	21	18 hours
Ewe	17	24–36 hours
Sow	21	24–60 hours
Mare	21	4–8 days

mounting by other animals. In some species, such as the pig, the ears will stand straight back. It will be difficult for any female species to move from one location to another. These behavioral changes are associated with the changing endocrine profile of the female. As the female becomes receptive to the male and her activity increases, E_2 also increases as P_4. Estradiol appears to be the driving force of the behavioral changes associated with the estrous cycle.

Fertilization and Embryo Development

The female becomes more receptive to mating by the male and begins to enter her productive life span as she begins her cyclicity. During the estrus stage of the estrous cycle, there is a peak of LH causing ovulation of the dominant follicle(s), which releases a Metaphase II (MII) oocyte into the oviduct. The freshly ovulated MII oocyte is cytoplasm surrounded by the plasma membrane, the zona pellucida, and the cumulus oophorus. For details see Chapter 3, "Histology, Cellular and Molecular Biology of Reproductive Organs."

The ZP has many functions but one of the most important is that it contains the receptors for binding the spermatozoa as well as protecting the oocyte from penetration of multiple spermatozoa. The cumulus oophorus is loosely packed cumulus cells that also protect the oocyte. The cumulus cells are lost after ovulation; however, timing is species-dependent. For example the pig, cow, and sheep lose their cumulus cells shortly after ovulation.

At the time of ovulation the oocyte is arrested at the metaphase stage of meiosis II for most species, with the exception of the dog. During meiosis II, the oocytes extrude the first polar body which contains half of the genetic material [e.g. from diploid (2N) to haploid (1N)] and does not resume meiosis until activation by the sperm. At sperm binding/penetration, the oocyte undergoes a series of changes that causes extrusion of the second polar body, activation of the oocyte, formation of the pronuclei, and preparation for subsequent embryonic development.

Prior to binding of the sperm to the oocyte, the oocyte must be transported to the site of fertilization, the ampulla-isthmus region. The oocytes are transported from the ovulation site to the fertilization site by the contractile movement of the uterine tube. Next, the cilia action and fluid movement (in some species) transport the oocyte through the ampulla. The cumulus cells either are transported with the oocytes as one unit or are removed during the movement of the oocytes through the oviduct.

The female is receptive to the male during estrus. Depending on the species, the semen is deposited into the vagina, cervix, or uterus and then transported to the site of fertilization (see the Erection and Ejaculation section earlier in this chapter for species differences). The mechanism of transport depends on species-specific factors such as volume of ejaculate, anatomy of the female tract, and site of deposit. Despite the mechanism for transport, in all species only a limited number of sperm reach the site of fertilization (see

Table 4.2. Characteristics of mating in various species.

Species	Site of semen deposit	Number of sperm at the ampulla-isthamus junction
Cow	Vagina	Few
Ewe	Vagina	650
Sow	Cervix and uterus	1,000
Mare	Vagina and vaginal portion of the cervix	Few

Table 4.2). As the sperm are transported to the site of fertilization, they gain the ability to fertilize, e.g. capacitation (previously discussed in the section on male physiology).

Fertilization occurs once the sperm and oocyte have reached the ampulla-isthmus junction of the uterine tube. Fertilization is defined as the penetration of the oocyte with one spermatozoa which leads to the normal development of the fertilized oocyte. Fertilization triggers several events that are required for subsequent embryonic development: block to polyspermy; resumption of meiosis II; and pronuclei formation, syngamy, and cleavage. The block to polyspermy is a series of events that occurs at fertilization and which prevents the oocyte from being fertilized by multiple sperm. Upon binding of the spermatozoa, the oocyte causes the cortical granules to undergo exocytosis, releasing their contents into the perivitelline space causing changes in the ZP. This change hardens the ZP which is caused by the enzymes of the cortical granules and ultimately blocks penetration of the oocyte by multiple spermatozoa.

Initially the sperm binds to ZP3 which has been exposed during capacitation and initiates the acrosome reaction. Then the inner acrosome membrane binds to ZP2. The motility of the sperm forces the sperm into the egg at an oblique angle. The penetration of the oocyte by the sperm triggers a series of events to allow the oocyte to undergo subsequent embryonic development and implantation.

Oocyte activation is critical for subsequent embryonic development. With sperm fusion, there is an increase in intracellular calcium (calcium oscillations) within the oocyte that repeats at different intervals (five to 60 minutes) depending on the species. Calcium oscillations are important to aid in the release of sperm factor, bind to the egg receptor, break down the maturation promoting factor, and activate sperm head decongestion.

The sperm head begins to decongest and form the male pronucleus (1N) and simultaneously the oocyte is activated to resume meiosis and begin the formation of the female pronucleus (1N). After the formation of both the male and female pronucleus, the zygote begins the event of syngamy (fusion of the male and female pronuclei) by the migration of the pronuclei to the middle of the oocyte and subsequent fusion.

The developing zygote becomes an embryo at the time of syngamy. An embryo is defined as a species in the early

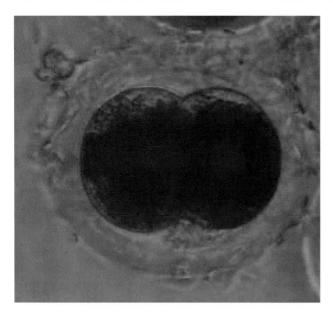

Figure 4.5. Photograph illustrating the developing embryo (two-cell stage embryo) in the pig. Notice the blackness of the pig embryo as it contains a high lipid content.

developmental stages (see Figure 4.5). At this point, there are no anatomical differences between species. The difference between a developing embryo of a cow, pig, and human can only be distinguished by a skilled embryologist at this stage of embryonic development. In general terms, embryonic development of many species is similar in patterns of divisions and embryonic stages; however, the differences in the embryos among the species are largely due to the length of embryonic development, transition from maternal to zygotic genome, and length of the gestation (development of the fetus in utero). In other words, the timing from fertilization to implantation and length of embryonic stage are different among species as gestation length increases or decreases.

After syngamy, the developing embryo undergoes a series of cleavage divisions that begin to reduce the size of the cytoplasm into smaller and smaller cellular units. The first division is a two-cell embryo, in which the blastomeres (cells of the embryo) are equal in size. The embryo then completes subsequent divisions to the four-, eight-, and 16-cell stages, and then fewer divisions to the morula and blastocyst stage. In the first few divisions the embryo relies heavily on the maternal stores of mRNA, proteins, etc. for the requirements to undergo the cleavage divisions.

The time at which the embryo relies on the maternal stores depends on species. For example, in the pig the transition called the "maternal to zygotic transition" occurs at the four cell-stage. This transition is when the embryo begins producing embryonic mRNA, proteins, etc. required for subsequent cleavage divisions. During this time the embryo is being transported to different locations in the reproductive tract (i.e. from the uterine tube to the

uterus). The species vary in their timing of transportation of the embryo to the uterus (see Table 4.3). Again, these changes are largely due to the length of gestation. In addition, in species such as the pig, the embryo can migrate from one uterine horn to another.

In the early stages of embryonic development, the blastomeres have the potential to develop into any cell type of the individual; this has been defined as "totipotent." Until the morula/compacted morula stage, all of the blastomeres in the embryo are totipotent; however, at this stage some of the blastomeres have been programmed to differentiate into the trophoblast cells (TE) of the blastocyst. The remaining cells remain totipotent as the inner cell mass cells (ICM). There are two populations of cells in the resulting blastocyst, TE, which gives rise to the extraembryonic membranes, and ICM, which gives rise to the developing fetus.

During development to the blastocyst stage, the embryo begins to form the blastocoele, which partitions the embryo into two distinct cell populations. The formation of the blastocoele is due to a large influx of fluid across the ZP. The blastocyst hatch from the ZP with the combination of growth and influx of fluid and enzymes produced by the trophoblast. For some species (pigs, ruminants) at this point in development more cellular changes have to occur prior to implantation.

In the sow, between embryonic days (E7 to E10), the embryo is still spherical and growing in cell numbers and diameter. However, at E10, the pig embryo begins to elongate into a filamentous embryo and begins to prepare for implantation. Similar events in embryonic development occur in ruminants but differ in timing, diameter, and cell numbers. The embryo undergoes tremendous growth during this period. For example, the embryo in the cow at day 15 is 1 mm to 2 mm in length and by days 18 to 19 the embryo is 10 cm to 20 cm in length.

During these morphological changes, the blastocyst also initiates differentiation of the ICM, forming three distinct layers: endoderm, mesoderm, and ectoderm. The endoderm layer forms first as an outgrowth of the ICM, and develops into the lining of the gut, glands, and bladder. Connective tissue, the vascular system, bones, muscles, and adrenal cortex are derived from the mesoderm layer. Finally, the

Table 4.3. Location and timing of preimplantation embryogenesis in various species.

Species	Oviducts (days)	Uterus (days)
Cow	Zygote—8-cell (0–3)	8-cell—blastocyst (3–11)
Ewe	Zygote—8-cell (0–2.5)	8-cell—blastocyst (2.5–8)
Sow	Zygote—4-cell (0–3)	4-cell—blastocyst (3–9)
Mare	Zygote—4-cell (0–2)	4-cell—blastocyst (2–8)

nervous system and covering of the body are derived from the ectoderm layer.

Another interesting embryonic difference between ruminants, the mare, and the sow is the migration of embryos prior to implantation. In ruminants, the embryos remain in the uterine horn on the side of ovulation. However, in the sow and the mare, the embryos migrate between uterine horns and the embryo may implant on the side of ovulation or on the contralateral side.

Pregnancy

The blastocyst is located in the uterus prior to implantation in all species. The uterus undergoes changes during embryonic development to prepare for implantation, independent of the presence of a viable (one that will implant) developing embryo. As the uterus prepares, the developing embryo begins to signal to the mother that the embryo(s) is (are) here and ready to implant; this event is called maternal recognition of pregnancy. The signal for maternal recognition of pregnancy and the timing for the signal to occur are species-dependent (see Table 4.4). If no viable embryo produces a signal during this period or if there is a problem with the developing embryo, the animal will cycle back and enter into the next estrous cycle. However, if the embryo is present and the signal for maternal recognition of pregnancy occurs during the critical period, then progesterone (P_4) levels will remain high. The embryo attaches to the uterus several days after it has signaled the mother that it is there and ready and the mother recognizes the signal.

Placenta and Implantation

The attachment of the developing embryo and the uterine endometrium is a transient relationship that provides an advantage to the developing conceptus by providing nutrients and protection during development. As the embryo develops it forms the placenta, which is a metabolic and endocrine organ between the developing conceptus and the uterine endometrium. It has a lifespan of the gestational length of the species. For more details, see Chapter 11, "Introduction to Comparative Placentation" and Chapter 12, "Comparative Placentation." The placenta is typically composed of a fetal component (chorion) and a maternal

Table 4.4. Maternal recognition of pregnancy for domestic animals.

Species	Signal for maternal recognition	Days of signal
Cow	Interferon tau	15–18
Ewe	Interferon tau	12–14
Sow	Estradiol/two embryos/horn	10–12
Mare	Proteins/embryo migration	12–14

component (uterine endometrium), which are the site of metabolic exchange. In addition to the metabolic function, the placenta acts as an endocrine organ by producing a variety of hormones which are critical for the maintenance of pregnancy.

Chorionic villi are finger-like projections on the surface of the chorion and serve as the functional unit of the fetal placenta. The distribution of the chorionic villi on the placenta, which gives each placenta a distinct anatomical appearance, serves as the method of classifying and separating the species. The classification of the placenta is: diffuse, cotyledonary, zonary, and discoidal.

Chorionic villi are uniformly distributed over the surface of the chorion in diffuse placentas. The sow has a diffuse attachment of the placenta to the uterine endometrium, which is a velvet-like surface with closely spaced chorionic villi.

Cows and small ruminants have cotyledonary placentas which have a large number of button-like structures called caruncles. These are convex in the cow, concave in the ewe, and flat or very deep in the goat. For more details on anatomical differences see Chapter 2, "Anatomy of Reproductive Organs." Briefly, the numbers of caruncles differ among species: in the cow there are approximately 80 to 120 caruncles distributed across the uterine mucosa, whereas small ruminants have more caruncles. The corresponding structure of the placenta to each caruncle is called cotyledon. It is trophoblastic in origin and consists of blood vessels and connective tissue. The interface between the fetal cotyledon and the maternal caruncle is called the placentome.

Zonary placentas have a band-like zone of the chorionic villi and are typically found in dogs and cats. Even within this zone there are regions with different functions. The prodominant region near the middle of the conceptus is the primary region of exchange. The second region is pigmented due to hematomas (the function of this region is not fully understood). The transparent region on the distal ends of the conceptus may be involved in the uptake of material directly from the uterine lumen.

The discoidal placenta is found in primates, including humans.

The placenta, in addition to serving as the metabolic and waste exchanger between the fetus and the mother, is a transient endocrine organ that produces a wide variety of hormones. These hormones can gain access to both the maternal and fetal blood supply. In some species, such as the ruminants, production of progesterone is taken over by another source such as the placenta at a different time in gestation. Furthermore, the CL could be removed at a specific time in the pregnancy and the other source could maintain the pregnancy. For example, in the ewe the CL is required for the first 55 days but after that the placenta produces enough P_4 to maintain the pregnancy. In the cow, the CL is required for 215 days of the 283 but from day 215 on the maternal adrenal produces enough P_4 to maintain the pregnancy to term. The mare is different than the other farm animals in that it maintains the original CL, but at

Table 4.5. Average gestational length of domestic animals.

Species	Gestational length
Cow	283 days
Sow	114 days
Ewe	148 days
Mare	338 days

day 40 the placenta begins to produce equine chorionic gonadotropin (eCG). The mare also has follicular waves that result in ovulation of follicles producing accessory CLs that produce P_4.

In some species (such as the sow), loss of the CL at any point will terminate the pregnancy. During the first quarter of gestation in the sow, each uterine horn must have at least two piglets (for a total of four) to produce enough estradiol to maintain the pregnancy. In addition to progesterone, the placenta mares and humans produces chorionic gonadotropin, which provides the stimulus for the CL maintenance during pregnancy. Furthermore, the placenta produces relaxin in mares, cats, and sows, but it is not found at any gestational age in cows. Relaxin prepares the birth canal by softening the connective tissue in the cervix and promotes elasticity of the pelvic ligaments. Placental lactogen, also called somatomammotropin, has been found in sheep and cows. It is believed to be similar to growth hormone; it promotes the growth of the fetus and stimulates the mammary gland.

Gestational Length

Gestational length varies among species—it varies by fetal sex in some species—and is largely due to the survival aspect (Table 4.5). For example, mice and rats have many predators that can affect their existence, so reproduction capacity and gestational length is critical. On the other hand, cows and pigs have fewer predators so reproduction capacity and gestational length is not as important. Many of the differences that have been seen thus far in the female reproductive system have been due to differences in the gestational length of the animals.

Parturition

Parturition, the act of giving birth, is a series of complex physiological events: (1) initiation of myometrial contractions by removal of the P_4 inhibition, (2) expulsion of the fetus, and (3) expulsion of the fetal membranes. The fetal pituitary-adrenal complex initiates the endocrine events by limitations of the uterus, making the fetus believe that it is under stress. In response, the fetal anterior pituitary lobe releases the adrenocorticotropic hormone which then stimulates the adrenal cortex to produce corticoids. The elevation of fetal corticoids causes a cascade of endocrine/biochemical events to initiate parturition.

As the levels of fetal corticoids increase the level of P_4 decreases as it is converted to E_2. The increase in E_2 begins to cause another series of events, such as the increase of myometrial contractions and secretions in the tract to provide lubrication for the fetus. $PGF_{2\alpha}$ is also produced, causing luteolysis of the CL and further decreasing the levels of P_4.

For those species in which relaxin is produced and is important in parturition, $PGF_{2\alpha}$ stimulates the production of relaxin, thus preparing the tract for parturition by softening the connective tissues and promoting elasticity of the pelvic ligaments. Myometrial contractions begin at this time and continue to increase in numbers and pressure.

At this point, stage II of parturition (expulsion of the fetus) begins. As myometrial contractions increase, the levels of E_2 also continue to increase, causing more changes in the cervix and vagina. In response to increased estradiol levels they begin to produce mucus which removes the cervical plug of pregnancy and moistens the cervical canal and vagina. In addition to estradiol, oxytocin—a glycoprotein that causes an increase in myometrial contractions and aids in milk let-down—is released from the posterior lobe of the pituitary gland. As myometrial contractions increase in frequency and duration, the fetus(es) is (are) expelled in a timely manner which can range from minutes to hours.

The final stage of parturition is the expulsion of the fetal membranes. This event typically follows quickly after the expulsion of the fetus. The release of the fetal membranes from the uterus is from a powerful vasoconstriction of the arteries, thus reducing the pressure and releasing the membranes.

Dystocia are difficulties that are encountered during parturition. There are several factors that influence the incidence of dystocia. The first is the size, typically excessive, of the fetus. Fetal size is controlled by the sires and dams, but the last half of gestation nutrition also influences fetal size.

The second factor is fetal position within the uterus. The normal birthing position of the fetus is front feet first, followed by the head. In cattle the fetus does not finalize its position until the end of the gestation, just prior to parturition. Of all the births in cattle, approximately 5 percent can be characterized by an abnormal position of the fetus, thus requiring assisted births or Caesarean section.

The third factor is multiple births in monotocous (one offspring) species such as the mare. Twins can cause problems when both present at the same time. One twin may be in an abnormal position, blocking both fetuses, and animal be fatigued by the birthing process. Another cause of trouble may be a deformed calus of the coxal bones. In mares, ultrasounds are performed to determine pregnancy but also to determine twin status. In the mare, if twins are present, one of the fetuses is aborted so that one foal has the best chance of survival.

Lactation

Lactation is the production of milk to nourish a newborn animal to an age of independence. The young are exposed to an extremely different environment following parturition than they were in utero. The new environment can be cold and dry, and one in which the newborns are exposed to different types of bacteria and viruses. The production of milk is a critical component to survival of the newborn because it is the only source for water, minerals, vitamins, and nutrients, and it is the initial source of antibodies (passive immunity).

The mammary gland is considered to be an accessory reproductive organ. The relationship between reproduction and lactation is critical because most of the development of the mammary gland (mammogenesis) occurs during pregnancy. Many of the hormones used during pregnancy are also critical for lactation. Initially during parturition, there is a release of prolactin and oxytocin, causing production of milk (colostrum, a nutrient-rich milk with high antibody levels for passive immunity). Despite the fact that these hormone levels are sufficient for initializing lactation, it is not enough for a sustained lactation period. However, these two hormones are used in a positive feedback loop to continue the production of milk during the lactation period.

Lactation can be divided into three sections: mammogenesis, lactogenesis, and galactopoiesis. Mammogenesis is the development of the mammary gland for lactation; this event occurs simultaneously with pregnancy. Hormones required for maintenance of the pregnancy also aid in the development of the mammary gland.

Lactogenesis is the synthesis and secretion of milk. It occurs slightly (hours) prior to parturition, and milk synthesis is one indication that parturition is beginning. The main hormonal regulation of lactogenesis is the level of P_4, which inhibits milk production. In addition, there is cytologic and enzymatic differentiation of the mammary gland for sustained milk production, and an increase in lactose production.

Galactopoiesis (enhancement or maintenance of lactation) subsequently begins and continues until the young is removed or no longer requires milk. The key regulator of galactopoiesis is the removal of the milk from the gland. There is a difference in lactation in farm animals. For example, the sow typically lactates for two to three weeks before the piglets are removed; however, the cow lactates for several months depending on management (early wean vs. normal wean).

Mammary glands vary by species in terms of the number of glands and their location. Mammals that are monotocous have mammary glands in the inguinal region, whereas mammals that are polytocous have paired mammary glands on both sides of the ventral midline. Even within the monotocous species there are differences in the gland's anatomy. One reason for the differences is the frequency of nursing in polytocous vs. monotocous mammals. The sow nurses her piglets on an hourly basis, whereas the cow nurses less frequently basis. This is largely due to the amount that each animal receives at each nurse, i.e., piglets receive less milk at a nursing than do calves.

Milk can be divided into several different components, including water, lactose, fat, protein, and minerals. Water is the largest component of milk is water. Lactose (composed of glucose and galactose) is the major carbohydrate and osmole (which draws the water into the gland) of milk. Fat is highly variable both between species and within species. Triglycerides are the largest lipid type, or energy source, found in milk. Milk proteins are unique to the milk; they have the composition that is appropriate for growth and development of the young. Minerals in the milk provide components for bone development. Some of the minerals form complexes with proteins such as the casein. Other components are vitamins, milk cells (white blood cells), and others.

References

Bahr, J. (1997). *AnSc 431 Advanced Endocrinology.* University of Illinois Reproductive Training Program. Champaign-Urbana. University of Illinois.

Cupps, P.T. (1991). *Reproduction in Domestic Animals 4th ed.* San Diego, CA.: Academic Press, Inc., 1–655.

Hadley, M.E. (1996). *Endocrinology. 4th ed.* Upper Saddle River, NJ.: Prentice Hall, Inc., 1–518.

Hafez, E.S.E (1993). *Reproduction in Farm Animals 6th ed.* Malvern, PA.: Lea and Febiger, 1–526.

Hurley, W. (1998). *AnSc 308 Lactation Biology.* University of Illinois Reproductive Training Program. Champaign-Urbana, University of Illinois.

Parrish, J.J. *AnSci 434 Reproductive Physiology.* University of Wisconsin-Madison. www.wisc.edu/ansci_repro/

Senger, P.L. (1999). *Pathway to Pregnancy and Parturition 1st revised ed.* Pullman, WA: Current Conceptions, Inc., 1–247.

Chapter 5

Transgenic Animals

Yuksel Agca and Anthony W.S. Chan

Introduction and Background

Gene delivery to the mammalian germplasm (i.e., gametes and embryos) is one of the most significant scientific achievements of the last several decades. Since its introduction, transgenesis has evolved in many ways and has been widely applied in many fields of biomedicine, agriculture, and basic research.

Transgenesis facilitates a better understanding of the function of a specific gene by either its overexpression or deletion from various model systems. The technology has allowed scientists to ask and answer many relevant questions in life sciences. The impact of transgenesis on biomedical and commercial pharmaceutical industrial research programs has also been overwhelming (Schnieke et al., 1997; Niemann et al., 2003).

However, despite all of the significant advancements, one of the most important tasks that remains is the search for the most efficient and reliable gene delivery system for creating transgenic animals from various mammalian species. The ability to produce transgenic animals in a wide spectrum of species would further broaden the application of transgenic technology for studying human health and disease and increasing animal production and biopharming for pharmaceutical development as well as gene therapy and disease resistance.

The introduction of a new gene (or genes) into an animal plays a key role in determining the relationship between genotype and phenotype. Although transgenic rodents have been valuable animal models for comparative biomedical research, the physiological similarities between humans and pigs and monkeys make these non-rodent species potentially superior models for human diseases (Lai et al., 2002; Wolf et al., 1999).

Currently, there are only a handful of transgenic livestock as compared to thousands of transgenic rodents. This is due to both technical and biological obstacles, which include low transgenic efficiency, longer generation interval, and high maintenance cost. Advancements in two particular areas of scientific research have enormously helped the development of novel methods of gene delivery in mammals and have accelerated the development of transgenic technology. The first is assisted reproductive tech-

nologies (ART). ART such as manipulation of oocyte/embryo development and ovulation, non-surgical artificial insemination (AI) and embryo transfer (ET), *in vitro* fertilization (IVF) and embryo culture, and intracytoplasmic sperm injection (ICSI) have revolutionized animal research and production. The second area is the development of molecular biological techniques, such as polymerase chain reaction, fluorescent in-situ hybridization, DNA microarray, and transgene reporters.

Transgenic Markers and Methods of Transgenic Animal Production

The ability to select embryos with a higher probability of being transgenic before their transfer into surrogate mothers would significantly reduce the number of non-transgenic animals born. In addition, easily detectable reporter genes would help test the efficiency of transgenic techniques, as well as compare the impact of different promoters on ubiquitous or tissue-specific expression of a particular transgene. Transgenic reporters such as β-galactosidase (Vernet et al., 1993), secreted placental alkaline phosphatase (Chan et al., 1995), firefly luciferase (Miranda et al., 1993), and green fluorescent protein (GFP) (Ikawa et al., 1999) have been developed over the last several decades. GFP appears to be an almost ideal transgenic marker, and its use has greatly accelerated the development of an efficient gene delivery system. GFP allows the selection of transgenic embryos soon after gene transfer or prior to embryo transfer (Takada et al., 1997; Chen et al., 2002).

Green Fluorescent Protein (GFP)

GFP was first introduced as an expression marker by Chalfie and colleagues in 1994. GFP is derived from the jellyfish *Aequorea* and was cloned in 1992 (Prasher et al., 1992). It is a single peptide composed of 238 amino acids which absorbs blue light and emits green light without the need of substrate or any pretreatment (Ikawa et al., 1999). GFP expression has been shown in a wide range of mammalian cells, embryos, and live animals (Takada et al., 1997).

The unique properties of GFP include its small size, ease of detection method, and non-species specific expression. It is nontoxic to the host and is resistant to high temperature, alkaline pH, detergents, chaotropic salts, organic solvents, and many proteases (Ikawa et al., 1999). A fusion protein of GFP or a peptide tagged with GFP can be used as a marker to follow *in vivo* gene expression and real-time protein localization (Wacker et al., 1997). Transgenic studies in mammals have significantly benefited from the use of GFP. The majority of transgenic studies have used GFP gene expression and translation as proof-of-principle to evaluate various transgenic methods and promoters and to better understand temporal and spatial expression patterns after using different gene transfer methods in various mammalian species.

Gene Delivery Methods

To date, the following major gene delivery methods have been successfully demonstrated: (1) pronuclear microinjection (Gordon et al., 1980), (2) embryonic stem cells (Doetschman, 2002), (3) viral infection (Jaenisch and Mintz, 1974; Chan et al., 1998), (4) sperm mediated gene delivery (Brackett et al., 1971; Lavitrano et al., 1989), and (5) somatic cell nuclear transfer (Schnieke et al., 1997; Cibelli et al., 1998a).

Each of these methods has its advantages and disadvantages, depending on the species of interest. It is important to perform studies investigating transgene stability and correlations between transgene inheritance and persistent transgene phenotypic expression in transgenic animals. The significance of transgenic animals to the development of human or animal disease models, cell-based therapeutic approaches, and bioreactors is evident. Therefore, the availability of a simple and reliable methodology to create transgenic animals with a specific genetic background in desired species is urgently needed. The following sections are intended to provide a general overview of gene delivery strategies using various approaches that may advance transgenic technology in large animals.

Pronuclear Microinjection (PI)

Pronuclear microinjection of linearized plasmid DNA into one-cell murine zygotes was first introduced in the 1980s (Gordon et al., 1980). Using this method, one of the pronuclei is injected with a DNA solution (4 to 10 ng/μl) using a micropipette attached to a micromanipulator with the aid of a microscope (see Figures 5.1 and 5.2). PI is the predomi-

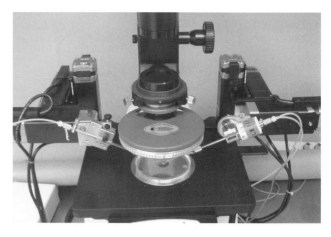

Figure 5.1. Micromanipulation system used for pronuclear microinjection and somatic cell nuclear transfer. (Also see color plate)

nant method currently used for creating transgenic rodents. PI has several advantages over other gene delivery systems and it is considered a safe and consistent method for gene transfer (Brem and Muller, 1994). There is no practical limit on the size of the DNA fragment being injected (Evans et al., 1994; Brem et al., 1996), and the efficiency of integration has no apparent correlation with DNA length (Brinster et al., 1985).

Despite the need for transgenic large domestic animals, the production of transgenic livestock by PI has been very inefficient. This is due, in part, to difficulties associated with visualizing the pronuclei in zygotes with high intracellular lipid content and the lack of synchronization of pronuclei in large domestic animal species. Waiting for the appropriate moment for visualization and injection of the pronucleus is time-consuming and labor-intensive. Due to the opacity of the cytoplasm, the eggs of most domestic animal species require the use of centrifugation for visualization of pronuclei (Hammer et al., 1985).

In addition, there is a very low gene integration efficiency associated with PI, especially in large domestic animals, which require the transfer of multiple injected embryos into a large number of recipients to obtain a few transgenic founders. For example, one transgenic animal can be expected after injection of approximately 40, 100,

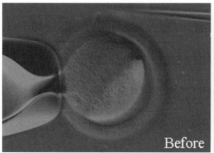
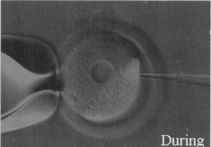
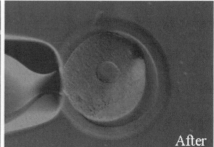

Figure 5.2. Pronuclear microinjection of plasmid DNA into cattle zygote.

110, 90, and 1,600 zygote in mice, pigs, sheep, goats, and cattle, respectively (Wall et al., 1997). The differences in efficiency point to fundamental differences between species. For example, the timing of the maternal-to-embryonic transition in transcription in mouse embryos occurs at the 2-cell stage (Bouniol et al., 1995) versus the 8-cell stage in cattle and pigs (Barnes et al., 1991). The S-phase (DNA replication) during the first embryonic cell cycle occurs between 11 and 18 hours post-insemination in mice (Hogan et al., 1986) and eight and 18 hours post-insemination in cattle (Eid et al., 1994; Gagne et al., 1995).

Because DNA insertion is most likely to occur during DNA replication (Coffin, 1990), delivery of a DNA fragment during or before S-phase should, theoretically, enhance gene transfer efficiency. Pronuclear microinjection has a higher chance of success when mouse zygotes are injected at 12 hours post-insemination, which is at the beginning of S-phase (Hogan et al., 1986). On the other hand, the optimal time for bovine PI is between 18 and 26 hours post-insemination, which is close to the end of DNA replication (Krisher et al., 1994).

PI usually results in multiple transgene copies at a single insertion site called the tandem repeat (Bishop and Smith, 1989). Although gene expression is not always related to the transgene copy number, multiple copies hinder the analysis of gene function (Davis and MacDonald, 1988). Approximately 20 percent to 30 percent of founder transgenic mice are mosaic despite PI being performed at the pronuclear stage (Wall and Seidel, 1992). An even higher rate of mosaicism is observed in transgenic livestock (Brem and Muller, 1994). In cattle, a high rate of mosaicism (more than 80 percent) in embryos suggests a similar outcome in transgenic founders (Kubisch et al., 1995).

Embryonic Stem (ES) Cells

The establishment of pluripotent cell lines from mouse embryos in 1981 has led to a new dimension in transgenic technology which enabled gene disruption (Evans and Kaufman, 1981). Embryonic stem (ES) cells are usually derived from inner cell mass cells (ICM) of a blastocyst stage embryo, which are undifferentiated and capable of differentiating into derivatives of the three germ layers (ectoderm, mesoderm, and endoderm) (Robertson, 1987). ES cells allow genetic manipulation and modification *in vitro* using conventional gene delivery methods that are used for tissue culture systems. When transgenic ES cells are injected into a host blastocyst, they proliferate and differentiate into all tissue types resulting in chimeric animals after transfer into foster mothers (see Figure 5.3). However, these chimeric animals need to be further tested for germline transmission because of the random distribution of ES cells. Since this technology was introduced, thousands of knockout mice have been produced to elucidate loss of gene function (Doetschman, 2002).

After the establishment of embryonic cell lines from mouse blastocysts, there has been a desire to create identical transgenic large animals using ES cells, embryonic cells, and primordial germ cells. Unfortunately, attempts made for the translation ES cell technology to other animals, even one of the widely used laboratory animals (rats), have largely failed (Iannaccone and Galat, 2002). In this regard, although a significant milestone was reached with the production of a calf after nuclear transfer of embryonic derived cell lines (Sims and First, 1994), little effort has been made to establish ES cells in large animals.

Pluripotency of pig primordial germ cells and the production of transgenic chimeric embryos have been demonstrated by Piedrahita et al. (1998). Problems with the use of ES cell technology are two-fold, especially in large animals. First, it has been difficult to establish stable ES cell lines that have the ability to maintain pluripotency under long term *in vitro* culture condition. Second, the long generation interval in large animals makes testing germline transmission of chimeric animals costly due to the maintenance of so many potential founders. These shortcomings, as well as the recent success with SCNT, have diminished the overall enthusiasm for the establishment of ES cells in large animals.

Viral Mediated Gene Transfer

Another approach for generating transgenic animals is infection of germ cells or preimplantation embryos using viral

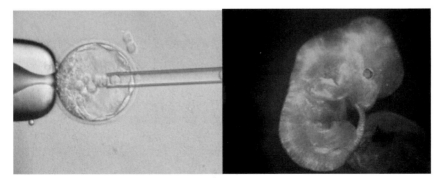

Figure 5.3. Embryonic stem cell micro-injection into mouse blastocyst (left) and resulting chimeric mouse after embryo transfer (right). (Also see color plate)

vectors (Chan et al., 1998; Hofmann et al., 2003). This is generally achieved by microinjection of viral vectors into the perivitelline space (PVS) of zygotes or metaphase II (MII) oocytes using a micromanipulator. There is no need to visualize the pronuclei, which is one of the limiting factors in transgenic livestock production via PI.

To date, retroviral and lentiviral vectors have been introduced and used to create transgenic animals. Transgenic mice were first produced by infecting preimplantation mouse embryos using competent retrovirus (Jaenisch and Mintz, 1974). However, retrovirus infection was not widely accepted for transgenic animal production until the development of Moloney murine leukemia virus (MoMLV) based replication-defective retroviral vector (Temin, 1989). The development of a pseudotyped retroviral vector has also broadened the applicable host range, as compared to that of the conventional retroviral vector (Burns et al., 1993).

Due to the species-specificity of retroviruses, most of the research has concentrated on mice and chickens (Mitrani et al., 1987; Sanes et al., 1986). Reports in other species were rarely seen until 1993, when Kim and colleagues demonstrated successful infection of bovine preimplantation embryos by replacing the endogenous MoMLV envelope glycoprotein with that of the gibbon ape leukemia virus (Kim et al., 1993).

One of the limitations of conventional retroviral rectors is the low titre ($1 \times 10^{5-6}$ colony forming units (cfu)/ml) (Kim et al., 1993). Recently, a pseudotyped vesicular stomatitis virus envelop glycoprotein VSVG- MoMLV-derived retroviral vector has been developed (Burns et al., 1993). This vector can be concentrated up to a high titer ($1 \times 10^{9-10}$ cfu/ml) and has a very broad host cell range. With the high titer of VSV-G pseudotype, virus-containing solutions can be injected into the PVS (see Figure 5.4).

In bovine oocytes, the volume of PVS is estimated to be between 200 and 300 picoliters. With a virus titer at $1 \times 10^{9-10}$ cfu/ml, an injection of 10 picoliters can deliver approximately 10 to 100 infectious viral particles into the PVS. Transgenic large animals, including cattle, pigs, and monkeys, have been successfully produced by the infection of mature oocytes using a VSVG pseudotyped retroviral vector with high efficiency (Chan et al., 1998; Cabot et al.,

2002; Chan et al., 2001). A retroviral vector carrying a hepatitis B surface antigen gene controlled by the viral LTR promoter, with a titer of 10^9 cfu/ml, was used to infect MII bovine oocytes, resulting in 100 percent transgenic calves. In addition to viral titer, the bovine studies suggest the critical role of the target cell (i.e., unfertilized vs. fertilized oocytes) in gene transfer efficiency. Using the same retroviral vector carrying enhanced GFP (EGFP), Cabot et al. (2001) transfected *in vitro* matured porcine MII oocytes and subsequently fertilized them to obtain embryos. They obtained two litters after embryo transfer. One pig from each litter was identified as transgenic and both expressed EGFP.

One of the significant drawbacks of retroviral vectors, which has significantly reduced their use in large animals, is the down regulation or silencing of the transgene by methylation after integration into the genome (Jahner et al., 1982). It has been suggested that methylation has evolved as a self-defense mechanism, suppressing mobile elements (Yoder et al., 1997). As an alternative, the recent use of a self-inactivating lentiviral vector system, which minimizes the interference on internal promoter control (Miyoshi et al., 1998), has bypassed the retrovirus-associated problem of transgene suppression. VSVG pseudotyped lentiviral vectors can infect non-dividing cells, whereas retroviral vectors can only infect mitotic cells. Recent studies have shown that unlike traditional oncoretroviral vectors, transgenes introduced by lentiviral vectors into oocyte, male germline cells, embryos, and ES cells provided stable gene expression (Pfeifer et al., 2002; Hamra et al., 2002; Lois et al., 2002; Hofmann et al., 2004).

Germline transmission as well as ubiquitous expression of EGFP has been demonstrated in transgenic mice and rats created by infection of one-cell embryos using a lentiviral vector (Lois et al., 2002). Hofmann et al. (2003) performed studies on swine with a lentiviral vector carrying a ubiquitously active phosphoglycerate kinase promoter to deliver GFP transgene. Of the 46 piglets born, 32 (70 percent) carried the transgene and 30 (94 percent) expressed GFP. The results were also confirmed by direct fluorescence imaging. GFP expression was present in all tissues, including germ cells.

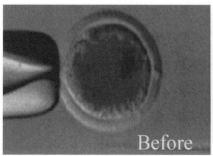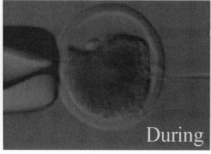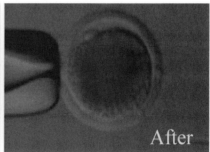

Figure 5.4. Perivitelline space microinjection of viral vector into cattle zygote.

transgenic sheep by NT requires fewer than half the animals needed for PI.

In cattle, Kato et al. (1998) produced eight genetically identical healthy calves by SCNT, using fully differentiated cumulus and oviductal cells from a single adult cow. This study was shortly followed up with the production of transgenic calves using SCNT by genetically modifying fetal fibroblasts cells with β-galactosidase-neomycin resistance fusion gene driven by a cytomegalovirus promoter (Cibelli et al., 1998a). Later, McCreath et al. (2000) targeted ovine α-1-procollagen (COL1A1) locus in fetal fibroblasts to place a therapeutic transgene and produced live sheep via SCNT.

In the context of tissue and organ transplantation, the presence of galactose α-1, 3-galactose residues on the surface of pig cells is a major barrier for successful xenotransplantation due to hyperacute rejection. Lai et al. (2002) successfully generated miniature swine with a null allele of the α-1, 3-galactosyl transferase locus (GGTA1) via SCNT using gene-targeted fibroblast cells. They obtained four live pigs in which one allele of the GGTA1 locus had been knocked out. To expedite the production of GGTA1 null pigs, Kolber-Simonds et al. (2004) later selected spontaneous null mutant cells from fibroblast cultures of heterozygous pigs to use in a second round of SCNT. Three healthy male piglets, which were hemizygous and homozygous for the gene-targeted allele, were produced in this study.

Behboodi et al. (2005) have recently produced transgenic goats via SCNT in an effort to develop a malaria vaccine. Two donor cell lines, transfected with a transgene expressing a modified version of the MSP-1(42) malaria antigen (glycosylated or non-glycosylated), were used to produce the vaccine. Two female kids were produced per cell line and a total of nine kids were produced after the cloned does were bred. The cloned does that were expressing the non-glycosylated antigen had normal milk yields with recombinant protein production.

Cibelli et al. (1998a) reported an interesting approach using SCNT to produce transgenic ES-like cells from fetal bovine fibroblasts. These cells, when reintroduced into preimplantation embryos, differentiated into three embryonic germ layers. Six out of seven (86 percent) of the calves born were chimeric for at least one tissue. These experiments elegantly showed that somatic cells can be genetically modified and then de-differentiated by nuclear transfer into ES-like cells, opening the possibility of using them in differentiation studies and human cell-based therapy.

The impact of SCNT cloning and transgenesis on life science and biomedical research, as well as on transgenic technology, has been immense (Schnieke et al., 1997; Cibelli et al., 1998a; Onishi et al., 2000; Polejaeva et al., 2000). This cloning technique has ushered basic, biomedical, and agricultural research into a new era (First, 1990; First and Prather, 1991; Fulka et al., 1998; Fan et al., 1999; Gurdon, 1999). We are now able to create a herd of identical animals that carries a unique genotype and, potentially,

an identical phenotype. Pharmaceutical, therapeutic and vaccine testing, as well as xenotransplantation, all benefit from this scientific advance (Dormont, 1990; Letvin, 1992; Kent and Lewis, 1998; Nathanson et al., 1999; Chan et al., 2000b; Lai et al., 2002).

The production of pharmaceutically valuable recombinant proteins (Schnieke et al., 1997; Cibelli et al., 1998a) and therapeutic cloning (Renard, 1998; Wolf et al., 1998; De Sousa et al., 1999; Gurdon, 1999; Kikyo and Wolffe, 2000; Kondo and Raff, 2000; McKay, 2000) are further applications of SCNT transgenic techniques. SCNT advances basic research efforts to understand the underlying molecular and cellular mechanisms of recipient oocyte reprogramming of the donor nucleus and the bases for gene function and differentiation (Latham, 2004).

Regardless of the animal species, the wider use of SCNT is limited by the major health problems, collectively referred to as large offspring syndrome (LOS), commonly observed in cloned animals. LOS is currently thought to be caused by failed reprogramming of the donor nucleus and suboptimal *in vitro* culture conditions (Farin et al., 2004). LOS is generally manifested by placental abnormalities, high birth weight, respiratory problems, and metabolic deficiencies in the newborns. Due to these potentially lethal clinical problems, intensive peri- and postnatal care is required for increased survival rates in cloned animals. Research efforts to better understand the mechanisms of nuclear reprogramming and to develop more efficient gene targeting and colony selection methodologies in somatic cells will likely increase transgenesis using SCNT.

Transgenesis in Large Domestic Animals

The significance of creating transgenic large animals was widely recognized after the delivery of a human growth hormone gene into a mouse zygote and subsequent dramatic growth in the resulting transgenic mice (Palmiter et al., 1982). In addition, many reports have urged the limitations of rodents as a sole animal model (Petters et al., 1997; Thomson and Marshall, 1998) and stressed the importance of producing alternative transgenic large animals. The desire for the large scale production of human recombinant proteins (α-1-antitrypsin, antithrombin, and monoclonal antibodies) in the milk by the pharmaceutical industry has been the driving force for the creation of transgenic large animals. In this regard, the mammary gland of livestock such as cattle and goats is well suited.

Creation of transgenic farm animals was first reported in 1985 (Hammer et al., 1985) using the PI method. There are numerous practical values in creating transgenic livestock, including improved milk production and composition, increased growth rate, diseases resistance, reproductive performance, and cell-and organ-based therapy (Niemann et al., 2003). The possibilities for diverse applications of this technology were soon recognized, especially with the establishment of "pharming," which became the major driving force for the application in large animals and today's transgenic research (Wall et al., 1997).

Pharming is the use of farm animals as bioreactors for production of gene products of interest, such as blood clotting factors (Clark, 1989) and antibodies (Edmunds et al., 1998) in milk (Clark et al., 1989), blood (Sharma et al., 1994), or urine (Wall et al., 1998). In addition, the need for appropriate animal models in biomedical studies (Petters et al., 1997) and organ donors for xenotransplantation (Cozzi and White, 1995; Lai et al., 2002; Kolber-Simonds et al., 2004), disease resistances (Muller and Brem, 1994), and genetic improvements in farm animals (Brem, 1994) intensified the interest in transgenic large animals. As a result, cattle, pigs, goats, sheep, and rhesus monkeys have received significant attention from the agricultural and biomedical community. However, low transgenic efficiency in these species led to the development of alternative means of transgenic production which are described above.

Transgenesis in Nonhuman Primates (NHP)

Nonhuman primates (NHP), the closest phylogenetic relatives to humans, have contributed significantly to the advancement of biomedicine. These species have played important roles in the development of vaccines against rubella and Hepatitis B, the improvement of human infertility problems, and the development of cures for elevations in blood cholesterol concentrations and diseases such as sickle cell anemia.

It is clear that NHP share many physiologic, neurologic, and genetic similarities with humans. NHP models are generally considered the best for understanding human physiology and diseases. In general, NHP are excellent models for healthy individuals, unless extrinsic stimuli such as psychological assault and chemicals are administered. These interventions generally lead to similar physiologic conditions found in human patients. In fear studies, animals are subjected to persistent insult with fear factors, such that their brain function can be monitored under various conditions. Limited cognitive and behavioral tests are available for rodents, and these are not always applicable to studying neurodegenerative diseases. Therefore, due to progressive neurodegeneration, deleterious alterations in behavior, and altered mental states associated with neurodegenerative diseases in humans, the NHP is the only animal model that provides accessibility to a wide range of testing methods and high resolution brain imaging techniques.

The creation of a transgenic NHP model with genetic alterations will further mimic patient conditions and will have a great impact on our understanding of human disease development, thereby paving the way for effective therapeutic approaches.

The major barrier for advancing NHP models for human diseases is the difficulty of implementing recently emerging genomic tools. To date, few reports have described the generation of transgenic monkeys (Chan et al., 2001;

Wolfgang et al., 2001). In fact, the development of successful transgenic NHP models for human genetic disorders requires many levels of validation. Unlike the generation of transgenic animals as bioreactors and beyond the introduction of disease-causing genes with high expression levels, the spatial expression of the transgene and its correlation with the pattern of disease onset are important determinants of whether an NHP model is a good representative of human patients. The manifestation of phenotype, such as behavioral imbalance, diminished cognitive function, and pathologic changes (i.e., selective loss of neurons) in neurodegenerative disorders, is an important clinical feature that should be observed in such animal models.

Nevertheless, the development of transgenic NHP models of human disease is a lengthy process which requires characterization at molecular, cellular, and clinical levels. Development of NHP models of human genetic disorders proceeds in four stages: (1) the development of a gene construct composed of the disease-causing genes with an effective regulatory unit, (2) the determination of gene expression pattern and phenotypic characteristics in tissue culture and small animal models, (3) the generation of transgenic NHP, and (4) the preservation and generation of a sufficient number of NHP with unique genetic composition and expected phenotype.

The first steps in creating an ideal NHP model of human genetic disease are to identify the mutant gene, characterize its biological function, and determine the possible adverse consequences of its inclusion in the NHP genome. In addition to the mutant gene, an effective regulatory unit that achieves sufficient expression is also a critical component. So far, due to the limitation of gene transfer technology in NHP, transgenic NHP models for human diseases are limited to those caused by dominant genetic defects.

Except for SCNT, all other gene transfer methods result in random integration of the transgene. Because of the presence of the endogenous homolog in the target cell genome, a recessive gene defect that requires mutation at both alleles cannot be achieved with the currently available gene transfer techniques. Therefore, it is necessary to develop transgenic NHP models for diseases caused by single dominant genetic disorders which would result from the gain-of-function of the mutant gene. Additionally, a single dominant genetic disorder has other advantages over complex genetic disorders. Complex diseases often involve multiple genetic defects, requiring long selection and breeding programs to establish animal colonies with stable genotypes and phenotypes for further study. Thus, an NHP model which has a relatively long generation interval may not be appropriate for complex genetic disorders.

The development of transgenic NHP models for human diseases attempts to mimic a patient's condition by introducing similar genetic defects into the genome of NHP. An effective regulatory unit should be carefully selected for controlling the expression of the mutant genes to ensure the success of the transgenic NHP model. Because of the high cost and ethical concerns in NHP research, strategic planning and effective evaluation systems should identify genetic and epigenetic factors and determine the likelihood of the gene construct, resulting in a successful transgenic NHP model.

An appropriate transgenic NHP model for human disease is not only determined by the efficient spatial expression of the mutant gene, but also by the development of phenotypes that lead to the clinical features observed in human patients. Indeed, the disease onset and progression, as well as the development of clinical signs caused by the genetic defect, often take a long period of time, involving accumulative effects of epigenetic and environmental factors. The challenges after the generation of well-characterized transgenic NHP models for human diseases are the preservation of these unique genotypes and the availability of these animal models to the biomedical community. One of the foreseeable tasks is the generation of a significant number of NHP models that have similar if not identical genetic composition and pathogenetic patterns to those found in the founder transgenic NHP.

Traditionally, a breeding scheme of crossing transgenic founder with non-transgenic animals has been followed by back-crossing in murine models. However, due to their long generation interval in NHP, traditional breeding protocols are not practical approaches for NHP transgenic models. Moreover, the natural breeding process will result in unpredictable transgene segregation patterns, especially if multiple integration events occur. Alternative strategies need to be developed to preserve the unique genotypes of valuable NHP animal models.

One of the challenges in developing transgenic NHP models is the limitation of gene transfer methods. Although great success and advancement have been achieved in the production of transgenic cloned rodents and large domestic animals, generation of a cloned monkey has been consistently unsuccessful (Chan et al., 2001). Cloning NHP using ES cells or somatic cells has, thus far, been unsuccessful (Wolf et al., 1999; Wolf et al., 2004; Simerly et al., 2004).

The only successful method in generating transgenic NHP, thus far, has been the infection NHP oocytes with retroviral vectors. Although the production of transgenic NHP models for human genetic diseases by cloning remains in the distant future for the time-being, efforts will continue to develop NHP cloning techniques because of the foreseeable, revolutionary impact of transgenic NHP models in comparative biomedical research. The production of identical animals carrying a unique genotype and, potentially, an identical phenotype, has great promise for pharmaceutical, therapeutic, and vaccine development, as well as the study of cell differentiation.

Conclusion

Tremendous progress has been made in gamete and embryo biotechnologies, molecular biological techniques, gene and cell cycle regulation, and gene delivery methodologies over the past three decades. These advancements have collectively provided a solid basis for future breakthroughs in transgenesis in a wide array of mammalian species. Species-specific and more efficient gene delivery systems (e.g., inducible and conditional viral vectors), together with the development of cloning techniques using nuclear transfer, will provide alternative transgenic approaches for species in which PI and ES cell technology has not been successful. Specific gene replacement, specific-site insertion of transgenes, tissue-specific expression of transgenes, artificial mammalian chromosomes, *in vitro* differentiation, and many other, newly developed research areas will benefit from successful transgenesis in animals. Our scientific knowledge has benefited greatly from transgenic rodent studies of gene function and genotypic interactions with various environmental cues. The future holds great promise for the translation of this research to the large scale production of transgenic animal species for xenotransplantation, biopharming, production of animal models for human diseases, and other biomedical and agricultural uses which can improve the quality of life for humans as well as animals.

Acknowledgement

We thank Dr. Tim Evans for his thoughtful comments and critical reading of the manuscript, and Mr. Howard Wilson for his assistance with the images.

References

Bachiller, D., Schellander, K., Peli, J., and Ruther, U. (1991). Liposome-mediated DNA uptake by sperm cells. *Mol. Reprod. Dev.* 30:194–200.

Barnes, F.L., and First, N.L. (1991). Embryonic transcription in in-vitro cultured bovine embryos. *Mol. Reprod. Dev.* 29: 117–123.

Behboodi, E., Ayres, S.L., Memili, E., O'Coin, M., Chen, L.H., Reggio, B.C., Landry, A.M., Gavin, W.G., Meade, H.M., Godke, R.A., and Echelard, Y. (2005). Health and reproductive profiles of malaria antigen-producing transgenic goats derived by somatic cell nuclear transfer. *Cloning Stem Cells.* 7:107–118.

Bishop, J.O., and Smith, P. (1989). Mechanism of chromosomal integration of microinjected DNA. *Mol. Biol. Med.* 6:283–298.

Bouniol, C., Nguyen, E., and Debey, P. (1995). Endogenous transcription occurs at the 1-cell stage in the mouse. *Exp. Cell Res.* 218:57–62.

Brackett, B.G., Baranska, W., Sawicki, W., and Koprowski, H. (1971). Uptake of heterologous genome by mammalian spermatozoa and its transfer to ova through fertilization. *Proc. Natl. Acad. Sci.* USA. 68:353–357.

Brem, G.M., and Muller, M. (1994). *Large transgenic mammals.* In: N. Maclean, ed., *Animals with Novel Genes.* Cambridge: Cambridge University Press, pp. 179–245.

Brem, G.M., Besenfelder, U., Aigner, B., Muller, M., Libel, I., Schutz, G., and Montoliu, L. (1996). YAC transgenesis in farm animals: rescue of albinism in rabbits. *Mol. Reprod. Dev.* 44:56–62.

Brinster, R.L., Chen, H.Y., Trumbauer, M.E., Yagle, M.K., and Palmiter, R.D. (1985). Factors affecting the efficiency of introducing foreign DNA into mice by microinjecting eggs. *Proc. Natl. Acad. Sci. USA.* 82:4438–4442.

Burns, J.C., Friedmann, T., Driever, W., Burrascano, M., and Yee, J.K. (1993). Vesicular stomatitis virus G glycoprotein pseudotyped retroviral vectors: Concentration to very high titer and efficient gene transfer into mammalian and nonmammalian cells. *Proc. Natl. Acad. Sci. USA.* 90:8033–8037.

Cabot, R.A., Kuhholzer, B., Chan, A.W., Lai, L., Park, K.W., Chong, K.Y., Schatten, G., Murphy, C.N., Abeydeera, L.R., Day, B.N., and Prather, R.S. (2001). Transgenic pigs produced using in vitro matured oocytes infected with a retroviral vector. *Anim Biotechnol.* 12:205–214.

Camaioni, A., Russo, M.A., Odorisio, T., Gandolfi, F., Fazio, V.M., and Siracusa, G. (1992). Uptake of exogenous DNA by mammalian spermatozoa: specific localization of DNA on sperm head. *J. Reprod. Fertil.* 96:203–212.

Campbell, K.H.S., McWhir, J., Ritchie, W.A., and Wilmut, I. (1996). Sheep cloned by nuclear transfer from a cultured cell line. *Nature.* 380:64–66.

Campbell, K.H., Alberio, R., Choi, I., Fisher, P., Kelly, R.D., Lee, J.H., and Maalouf, W. (2005). Cloning: eight years after Dolly. *Reprod Domest Anim.* 40:256–268.

Cappello, F., Stassi, G., Lazzereschi, D., Renzi, L., Di Stefano, C., Marfe, G., Giancotti, P., Wang, H.J., Stoppacciaro, A., Forni, M., Bacci, M.L., Turchi, V., Sinibaldi, P., Rossi, M., Bruzzone, P., Pretagostini, R., Della Casa, G., Cortesini, R., Frati, L., and Lavitrano, M. (2000). hDAF expression in hearts of transgenic pigs obtained by sperm-mediated gene transfer. *Transplant Proc.* 32:895–896.

Castro, F.O., Hernández, O., Uliver, C., Solano, R., Milanés, C., Aguilar, A., Pérez, A., de Armas, R., Herrera, L., and De la Fuente, J. (1990). Introduction of foreign DNA into the spermatozoa of farm animals. *Theriogenololgy.* 34:1099–1110.

Chalfie, M., Tu, Y., Euskirchen, G., Ward, W.W., and Prasher, D.C. (1994). Green fluorescent protein as a marker for gene expression. *Science.* 263:802–805.

Chan, A.W.S., Homan, E.J., Ballou, L.U., Burns, J.C., and Bremel, R.D. (1998). Transgenic cattle produced by reverse-transcribed gene transfer in oocytes. *Proc. Natl. Acad. Sci. USA.* 95:14028–14033.

Chan, A.W.S., Chong, K.Y., Martinovich, C., Simerly, C., and Schatten, G. (2001). Transgenic monkeys produced by retroviral gene transfer into mature oocytes. *Science.* 291:309–312.

Chan, A.W.S., Luetjens, C.M., Dominko, T., Ramalho-Santos, J., Simerly, C.R., Hewitson, L., and Schatten, G. (2000a). Foreign DNA transmission by intracytoplasmic sperm injection: Injection of sperm bound with exogenous DNA results in embryonic GFP expression and live rhesus births. *Mol. Hum. Reprod.* 6:26–33.

Chan, A.W.S., Dominko, T., Luetjens, C.M., Neuber, E., Martinovich, C., Hewitson, L., Simerly, C., and Schatten, G. (2000b). Clonal propagation of primate offspring by embryo splitting. *Science.* 287:317–319.

Chen, S.H., Vaught, T.D., Monahan, J.A., Boone, J., Emslie, E., Jobst, P.M., Lamborn, A.E., Schnieke, A., Robertson, L., Colman, A., Dai, Y., Polejaeva, I.A., and Ayares, D.L. (2002). Efficient production of transgenic cloned calves using preimplantation screening. *Biol. Reprod.* 67:1488–1492.

Cibelli, J.B., Stice, S.L., Golueke, P.J., Kane, J.J, Jerry, J., Blackwell, C., Ponce de Leon, F.A., and Robl, J.M. (1998a). Transgenic bovine chimeric offspring produced from somatic cell-derived stem-like cells. *Nat. Biotechnol.* 16:642–646.

Cibelli, J.B., Stice, S.L., Golueke, P.J., Kane, J.J, Jerry, J., Blackwell, C., Ponce de Leon, F.A., and Robl, J.M. (1998b). Cloned transgenic calves produced from nonquiescent fetal fibroblasts. *Science.* 280:1256–1258.

Clark, A.J., Bessoa, H., Bishop, J.O., Brown, P., Harris, S., Lathe, R., McClenaghen, M., Prowse, C., Simons, J.P., Whitelaw, C.B.A., and Wilmut, I. (1989). Expression of human antihemophilic factor IX in milk of transgenic sheep. *Biotechnolology.* 7:487–492.

Coffin, J.M. (1990). Molecular mechanism of nucleic acid integration. *J. Med. Virol.* 31:43–49.

Cozzi, W., and White, D.J.G. (1995). The generation of transgenic pigs as potential organ donors for human. *Nat. Med.* 1:964–966.

Davis, B.P., and MacDonald, R.J. (1988). Limited transcription of rat elastase I transgene repeats in transgenic mice. *Genes Dev.* 2:13–22.

De Sousa, P.A., Winger, Q., Hill, J.R., Jones, K., Watson, A.J., and Westhusin, M.E. (1999). Reprogramming of fibroblast nuclei after transfer into bovine oocytes. *Cloning.* 1:63–69.

Doetschman, T. (2002). Gene targeting in embryonic stem cells: history and methodology. In: C. Pinkert, ed. *Transgenic Animal Technology.* San Diego: Academic Press, pp. 113–141.

Dormont, D. (1990). Primates as a model for the study of lentiviruses and AIDS. *Pathol. Biol.* (Paris) 38:182–188.

Edmunds, T., Van Patten, S.M., Pollock, J., Hanson, E., Bernasconi, R., Higgins, E., Manavalan, P., Ziomek, C., Meade, H., McPherson, J.M., and Cole, E.S. (1998). Transgenically produced human antithrombin: structural and functional comparison to human plasma-derived antithrombin. *Blood.* 91:4561–4571.

Eid, L.N., Lorton, S.P., and Parrish, J.J. (1994). Paternal influence on S-phase in the first cell cycle of the bovine embryos. *Biol. Reprod.* 51:1232–1237.

Evans, M.J., Gilmour, D.T., and Colledge, W.H. (1994). Transgenic rodents. In: N. Maclean, ed. *Animal with Novel Genes.* Cambridge: Cambridge University Press, pp. 138–178.

Evans, M.J., and Kaufman, M.H. (1981). Establishment in culture of pluripotential cells from mouse embryos. *Nature.* 9:154–156.

Fan, J., Challah, M., and Watanabe, T. (1999). Transgenic rabbit models for biomedical research: current status, basic methods and future perspectives. *Pathol. Int.* 49:583–94.

Farin, C.E., Farin, P.W., and Piedrahita, J.A. (2004). Development of fetuses from in vitro-produced and cloned bovine embryos. *J. Anim. Sci.* 82 E-Suppl:E53–62.

First, N.L. (1990). New animal breeding techniques and their application. *J. Reprod. Fertil.* Suppl 41:3–14.

First, N.L., and Prather, R.S. (1991). Genomic potential in mammals. *Differentiation.* 48:1–8.

Francolini, M., Lavitrano, M., Lamia, C.L., French, D., Frati, L., Cotelli, F., and Spadafora, C. (1993). Evidence for nuclear internalization of exogenous DNA into mammalian sperm cells. *Mol. Reprod. Dev.* 34:133–139.

Fulka, J., First, N.L., Loi, P., and Moor, R.M. (1998). Cloning by somatic cell nuclear transfer. *Bioessays* 20:847–851.

Gagne, M.B., Pothier, F., and Sirard, M.A. (1995). Effect of microinjection time during postfertilization S-phase in bovine embryonic development. *Mol. Reprod. Dev.* 41:184–194.

Gandolfi, F., Lavitrano, M., Camaioni, A., Spadafora, C., Siracusa, G., and Lauria, A. (1989). The use of sperm-mediated gene transfer for the generation of transgenic pigs. *J. Reprod. Fertil.* Abstr 4:10.

Gordon, J.W., Scangos, G.A., Plotkin, D.J., Barbosa, J.A., and Ruddle, F.H. (1980). Genetic transformation of mouse embryos by microinjection of purified DNA. *Proc. Natl. Acad. Sci. USA.* 77:7380–7384.

Gurdon, J.B. (1999). Genetic reprogramming following nuclear transplantation in amphibia. *Semin. Cell. Dev. Biol.* 10:239–243.

Hammer, R.E., Pursel, V.G., Rexroad, C.E. Jr., Wall, R.J., Bolt, K.M., Ebert, R.D., Palmiter, R.D., and Brinster, R.L. (1985). Production of transgenic rabbits, sheep and pigs by microinjection. *Nature.* 315:680.

Hamra, F.K., Gatlin, J., Chapman, K.M., Grellhesl, D.M., Garcia, J.V., Hammer, R.E., and Garbers, D.L. (2002). Production of transgenic rats by lentiviral transduction of male germ-line stem cells. *Proc. Natl. Acad. Sci. USA.* 99:14931–14936.

Hofmann, A., Kessler, B., Ewerling, S., Weppert, M., Vogg, B., Ludwig, H., Stojkovic, M., Boelhauve, M., Brem, G., Wolf, E., and Pfeifer, A. (2003). Efficient transgenesis in farm animals by lentiviral vectors. *EMBO Rep.* 4:1054–1060.

Hofmann, A., Zakhartchenko, V., Weppert, M., Sebald, H., Wenigerkind, H., Brem, G., Wolf, E., and Pfeifer, A. (2004). Generation of transgenic cattle by lentiviral gene transfer into oocytes. *Biol Reprod.* 71:405–409.

Hogan, B., Costantini, F., and Lacy, E. (1986.) *Manipulating the Mouse Emrbyo.* Cold Spring Harbor, NY: Cold Spring Harbor Laboratory.

Huguet, E., and Esponda, P. (1998). Foreign DNA introduced into the vas deferens is gained by mammalian spermatozoa. *Mol. Reprod. Dev.* 51:42–52.

Iannaccone, P.M., and Galat, V. (2002). Production of Transgenic Rats. In: C. Pinkert, ed. *Transgenic Animal Technology.* San Diego: Academic Press, pp. 235–250.

Ikawa, M., Yamada, S., Nakanishi, T., and Okabe, M. (1999). Green fluorescent protein (GFP) as a vital marker in mammals. *Curr. Top. Dev. Biol.* 44:1–20.

Jaenisch, R. (1974). Infection of mouse blastocysts with SV 40 DNA: Normal development of infected embryos and persistence SV 40-specific DNA sequences in the adult animals. *Cold Spring Harbor Symp.* 39:375–380.

Jahner, D., Stuhlmann, H., Stewart, C.L., Harbers, K., Lohler, J., Simon, I., and Jaenisch, R. (1982). De novo methylation and expression of retroviral genomes during mouse embryogenesis. *Nature.* 12:623–628.

Kato, Y., Tani, T., Sotomaru, Y., Kurokawa, K., Kato, J.Y., Doguchi, H., Yasue, H., and Tsunoda, Y. (1998). Eight calves cloned from somatic cells of a single adult. *Science.* 282:2095–2098.

Kent, S.J., and Lewis, I.M. (1998). Genetically identical primate modelling systems for HIV vaccines. *Reprod. Fertil. Dev.* 10:651–657.

Kikyo, N., Wade, P.A., Guschin, D., Ge, H., and Wolffe, A.P. (2000). Active remodeling of somatic nuclei in egg cytoplasm by the nucleosomal ATPase ISWI. *Science.* 289:2360–2362.

Kim, J.H., Jung-Ha, H.S., Lee, H.T., and Chung, K.S. (1997). Development of a positive method for male stem cell-mediated gene transfer in mouse and pig. *Mol. Reprod. Dev.* 46:1–12.

Kim, T., Leifried-Rutledge, M.L., and First, N.L. (1993). Gene transfer in bovine blastocysts using replication-defective retroviral vectors packaged with Gibbon ape leukemia virus envelope. *Mol. Reprod. Dev.* 35:105–113.

Kolber-Simonds, D., Lai, L., Watt, S.R., Denaro, M., Arn, S., Augenstein, M.L., Betthauser, J., Carter, D.B., Greenstein, J.L., Hao, Y., Im, G.S., Liu, Z., Mell, G.D., Murphy, C.N., Park, K.W., Rieke, A., Ryan, D.J., Sachs, D.H., Forsberg, E.J., Prather, R.S., and Hawley, R.J. (2004). Production of alpha-1,3-galactosyltransferase null pigs by means of nuclear transfer with fibroblasts bearing loss of heterozygosity mutations. *Proc. Natl. Acad. Sci. USA.* 101:7335–7340.

Kondo, T., and Raff, M. (2000). Oligodendrocyte precursor cells reprogrammed to become multipotential CNS stem cells. *Science.* 289:1754–1757.

Krisher, R.L., Gibbons, J.R., Canseco, R.S., Johnson, J.L., Russell, C.G., Notter, D.R., Velander, W.H., and Gwazdauskas, F.C. (1994). Influence of time of gene microinjection on development and DNA detection frequency in bovine embryos. *Trans. Res.* 3:226–231.

Kubisch, H.M., Hernandez-Ledezma, J.J., Larson, M.A., Sikes, J.D., and Roberts, R.M. (1995). Expression of two transgenes in in-vitro matured and fertilized bovine zygotes after DNA microinjection. *J. Reprod. Fertil.* 104:133–139.

Lai, L., Kolber-Simonds, D., Park, K.W., Cheong, H.T., Greenstein, J.L., Im, G.S., Samuel, M., Bonk, A., Rieke, A., Day, B.N., Murphy, C.N., Carter, D.B., Hawley, R.J., and Prather, R.S. (2002). Production of alpha-1,3-galactosyltransferase knock-out pigs by nuclear transfer cloning. *Science.* 295:1089–1092.

Latham, K.E. (2004). Cloning: questions answered and unsolved. *Differentiation.* 72:11–22.

Lauria, A., and Gandolfi, F. (1993). Recent advances in sperm cell mediated gene transfer. *Mol. Reprod. Dev.* 36:255–257.

Lavitrano, M., Bacci, M.L., Forni, M., Lazzereschi, D., Di Stefano, C., Fioretti, D., Giancotti, P., Marfe, G., Pucci, L., Renzi, L.,

Wang, H., Stoppacciaro, A., Stassi, G., Sargiacomo, M., Sinibaldi, P., Turchi, V., Giovannoni, R., Della Casa, G., Seren, E., and Rossi, G. (2002). Efficient production by sperm-mediated gene transfer of human decay accelerating factor (hDAF) transgenic pigs for xenotransplantation. *Proc. Natl. Acad. Sci. USA.* 99:14230–14235.

Lavitrano, M., Camaioni, A., Frati, V.M., Dolci, S., Farace, M.G., and Spadafora, C. (1989). Sperm cells as vectors for introducing foreign DNA into eggs: genetic transformation of mice. *Cell.* 57:717–723.

Lavitrano, M., French, D., Zanim, M., Frati, L., and Spadafora, C. (1992). The interaction between exogenous DNA and sperm cells. *Mol. Reprod. Dev.* 31:161–169.

Letvin, N.L. (1992). Nonhuman primate models for HIV vaccine development. *Immunodefic. Rev.* 3(3), 247–260.

Lois, C., Hong, E.J., Pease, S., Brown, E.J., and Baltimore, D. (2002). Germline transmission and tissue-specific expression of transgenes delivered by lentiviral vectors. *Science.* 295:868–872.

Maione, B., Lavitrano, M., Spadafora, C., and Kiessling, A.A. (1998). Sperm-mediated gene transfer in mice. *Mol. Reprod. Dev.* 50:406–409.

McCreath, K.J., Howcroft, J., Campbell, K.H., Colman, A., Schnieke, A.E., and Kind, A.J. (2000). Production of gene-targeted sheep by nuclear transfer from cultured somatic cells. *Nature.* 405:1066–1069.

McKay, R. (2000). Mammalian deconstruction for stem cell reconstruction. *Nat. Med.* 6:747–748.

Meng, L., Ely, J., Stouffer, R.L., and Wolf, D.P. (1997). Rhesus monkeys produced by nuclear transfer. *Biol. Reprod.* 57:454–459.

Miller, D.G., Adam, M.A., and Miller, V. (1990). Gene transfer by retrovirus vectors occurs only in cells that are actively replicating at the time of infection. *Mol. Cell. Biol.* 10:4239–4242.

Miranda, M., Majumder, S., Wiekouski, M., and DePamphilis, M.L. (1993). Application of firefly luciferase to preimplantation development. *Methods Enzymol.* 225:412–433.

Mitrani, E., Coffin, J., Boedtker, H., and Doty, P. (1987). Rous sarcoma virus is integrated but not expressed in chicken early embryonic cells. *Proc. Natl. Acad. Sci. USA.* 84:2781–2784.

Miyoshi, H., Blomer, U., Takahashi, M., Gage, F.H., and Verma, I.M. (1998). Development of a self-inactivating lentivirus vector. *J. Virol.* 72:8150–8157.

Muller, M., and Brem, G. (1994). Transgenic strategies to increase disease resistance in livestock. *Reprod. Fertil. Dev.* 6: 605–613.

Nathanson, N., Hirsch, V.M., and Mathieson, B.J. (1999). The role of nonhuman primates in the development of an AIDS vaccine. *Aids* 13(Suppl A(2)):S113–120.

Niemann, H., Rath, D., and Wrenzycki, C. (2003). Advances in biotechnology: new tools in future pig production for agriculture and biomedicine. *Reprod Domest Anim.* 38:82–89.

Onishi, A., Iwamoto, M., Akita, T., Mikawa, S., Takeda, K., Awata, T., Hanada, H., and Perry, A.C.F. (2000). Pig cloning by microinjection of fetal fibroblast nuclei. *Science.* 289:1188–1190.

Palmiter, R.D., Brinster, R.L., Hammer, R.E., Trumbauer, M.E., Rosenfeld, M.G., Birnberg, N.C., and Evans, R.M. (1982). Dramatic growth of mice that develop from eggs microinjected with metallothionein-growth hormone fusion genes. *Nature.* 300:611–615.

Petters, R.M., Alexander, C.A., Wells, K.D., Collins, E.B., Sommer, J.R., Blanton, M.R., Rojas, G., Hao, Y., Flowers, W.L., Banin, E., Cideciyan, A.V., Jacobson, S.G., and Wong, F. (1997). Genetically engineered large animal model for studying cone photoreceptor survival and degeneration in retinitis pigmentosa. *Nat. Biotechnol.* 15:965–970.

Pfeifer, A., Ikawa, M., Dayn, Y., and Verma, I.M. (2002). Transgenesis by lentiviral vectors: lack of gene silencing in mammalian embryonic stem cells and preimplantation embryos. *Proc. Natl. Acad. Sci. USA.* 99:2140–2145.

Piedrahita, J.A., Moore, K., Oetama, B., Lee, C.K., Scales, N., Ramsoondar, J., Bazer, F.W., and Ott, T. (1998). Generation of transgenic porcine chimeras using primordial germ cell-derived colonies. *Biol. Reprod.* 58:1321–1329.

Polejaeva, I.A., Chen, S.H., Vaught, T.D., Page, R.L., Mullins, J., Ball, S., Dai, Y., Boone, J., Walker, S., Ayares, D.L., Colman, A., and Campbell, K.H.S. (2000). Cloned pigs produced by nuclear transfer from adult somatic cells. *Nature.* 407:86–90.

Prasher, D., Eckenrode, V., Ward, W., Prendergast, F., and Cormier, M. (1992). Primary structure of the Aequorea Victoria green-fluorescent protein. *Gene.* 111:229–233.

Renard, J.P. (1998). Chromatin remodelling and nuclear reprogramming at the onset of embryonic development in mammals. *Reprod. Fertil. Dev* 10:573–580.

Robertson, E.J. (1987). *Embryo-derived stem cell lines. Teratocarcinomas and embryonic stem cells: a practical approach.* Oxford: IRL Press Limited, Oxford pp. 71–112.

Roe, T.Y., Reynolds, T.C., Yu, G., and Brown, P.O. (1993). Integration of murine leukemia virus DNA depends on mitosis. *EMBO J.* 12:2099–2108.

Rottmann, O.J., Antes, R., Hoefer, P., and Maierhofer, G. (1991). Liposomes mediated gene transfer via spermatozoa into avian eggs cells. *J. Anim. Breed. Genet.* 109:64–70.

Rubinson, D.A., Dillon, C.P., Kwiatkowski, A.V., Sievers, C., Yang, L., Kopinja, J., Rooney, D.L., and Ihrig, M.M. (2003). A lentivirus-based system to functionally silence genes in primary mammalian cells, stem cells and transgenic mice by RNA interference. *Nat. Genet.* 33:401–406.

Rucker, E.B., and Piedrahita, J.A. (1997). Cre-mediated recombination at the murine whey acidic protein (mWAP) locus. *Biol. Reprod.* 48:324–331.

Sanes, J.R., Rubenstein, J.L.R., and Nicolas, J.F. (1986). Use of a recombinant retrovirus to study postimplantation cell lineage in mouse embryos. *EMBO J.* 5:3133–3142.

Schellander, K., Peli, J., Schmall, F., and Brem, G. (1995). Artificial insemination in cattle with DNA-treated sperm. *Anim. Biotechnol.* 6:41–50.

Schnieke, A.E., Kind, A.J., Ritchie, W.A., Mycook, K., Scott, A.R., Ritchie, M., Wilmut, I., Colman, A., and Campbell, K. H.S. (1997). Human factor IX transgenic sheep produced by transfer of nuclei from transfected fetal fibroblasts. *Science.* 278:2130–2133.

Simerly, C., Navara, C., Hyun, S.H., Lee, B.C, Kang, S.K., Capuano, S., Gosman, G., Dominko, T., Chong, K.Y., Compton, D., Hwang, W.S., and Schatten, G. (2004). Embryogenesis and blastocyst development after somatic cell nuclear transfer in nonhuman primates: overcoming defects caused by meiotic spindle extraction. *Dev Biol.* 276:237–252.

Sims, M., and First, N.L. (1994). Production of calves by transfer of nuclei from cultured inner cell mass cells. *Proc. Natl. Acad. Sci.* USA. 91:6143–6147.

Spadafora, C. (1998). Sperm cells and foreign DNA: a controversial relation. *BioEssays.* 20:955–964.

Sperandio, S., Lulli, V., Bacci, M.L., Forni, M., Maione, B., Spadafora, C., and Lavitrano, M. (1996). Sperm-mediated DNA transfer in bovine and swine species. *Anim. Biotech.* 7:59–77.

Takada, T., Iida, K., Awaji, T., Itoh, K., Takahashi, R., Shibui, A., Yoshida, K., Sugano, S., and Tsujimoto, G. (1997). Selective production of transgenic mice using green fluorescent protein as a marker. *Nat. Biotechnol.* 15:458–461.

Temin, H.M. (1989). Retrovirus variation and evolution. *Genome.* 31:17–22.

Thomson, J.A., and Marshall, V.S. (1998). Primate embryonic stem cells. *Curr. Top. Dev. Biol.* 38:133–165.

Vernet, M., Bonnerot, C., Briand, P., and Nicolas, J.F. (1993). Application of lacZ gene fusions to preimplantation development. *Methods Enzymol.* 225:434–451.

Wacker, I., Kaether, C., Migala, A., Almers, W., and Gerdes, H.H. (1997). Microtubule-dependent transport of secretory vesicles visualized in real time with a GFP-tagged secretory protein. *J. Cell. Sci.* 110:1453–1463.

Wakayama, T., Kishikawa, H., Kasai, T., Okabe, M., Toyoda, Y., and Yanagimachi, R. (1999). Mammalian transgenesis by intracytoplasmic sperm injection. *Science.* 284:1180–1183.

Wall, R.J., and Seidel, G.E. Jr. (1992). Transgenic farm animals—a critical analysis. *Theriogenology.* 38:337–357.

Wall, R.J., Kerr, D.E., and Bondioli, K.R. (1997). Transgenic dairy cattle: Genetic engineering on a large scale. *J. Dairy Sci.* 80:2213–2224.

Whitelaw, C.B., Radcliffe, P.A., Ritchie, W.A., Carlisle, A., Ellard, F.M., Pena, R.N., Rowe, J., Clark, A.J., King, T.J., and Mitrophanous, K.A. (2004). Efficient generation of transgenic pigs using equine infectious anaemia virus (EIAV) derived vector. *FEBS Lett.* 30(571):233–236.

Wilmut, I., Schinieke, A.E., Mowhir, J., Kind, A.J., and Campbell, K.H.S. (1997). Viable offspring derived from fetal and adult mammalian cells. *Nature.* 385:810–813.

Wolf, D.P., Kuo, H.C., Pau, K.Y., and Lester, L. (2004). Progress with nonhuman primate embryonic stem cells. *Biol. Reprod.* 71:1766–1771.

Wolf, D.P., Meng, L., Ouhibi, N., and Zelinski-Wooten, M. (1999). Nuclear transfer in the rhesus monkey: practical and basic implications. *Biol Reprod.* 60:199–204.

Wolfgang, M.J., Eisele, S.G., Browne, M.A., Schotzko, M.L., Garthwaite, M.A., Durning, M., Ramezani, A., Hawley, R.G., Thomson, J.A., and Golos, T.G. (2001). Rhesus monkey placental transgene expression after lentiviral gene transfer into preimplantation embryos. *Proc. Natl. Acad. Sci.* USA. 98:10728–10732.

Yoder, J.A., and Bestor, T.H. (1996). Genetic analysis of genomic methylation patterns in plants and mammals. *Biol Chem.* 377:605–610.

Zani, M., Lavitrano, M.L., French, D., Lulli, V., Maione, B., Sperandio, S., and Spadafora, C. (1995). The mechanism of binding of exogenous DNA to sperm cells: factors controlling the DNA uptake. *Exp. Cell Res.* 217:57–64.

Chapter 6

Gender Selection in Mammalian Semen and Preimplantation Embryos

Yuksel Agca and Hongsheng Men

Introduction and Background

During the last two decades both the agricultural and biomedical communities have witnessed important advancements in gamete and embryo biotechnologies. Artificial insemination (AI) and embryo transfer (ET) techniques were two of the earliest and most commonly used means of assisted reproductive technologies (ART), and both greatly impacted animal production systems and the treatment of human infertility.

Since the introduction of AI and ET, more sophisticated ART have been developed and widely used in basic and applied research within both veterinary and human medicine. Some of these more sophisticated techniques include transvaginal aspiration of oocytes, *in vitro* oocyte maturation and fertilization, embryo culture and transfer, micromanipulation of gametes and preimplantation embryos, and cryopreservation of germplasm. The incorporation of molecular biological techniques [i.e. polymerase chain reaction (PCR) and florescence in situ hybridization (FISH)] and high-speed, flow cytometric, cell-sorting techniques have further enhanced the agricultural and veterinary and human clinical applications of ART.

For centuries there has been great interest in gender pre-selection for the offspring of domestic animals, as well as humans. However, all such efforts were based on myths or superstitions until the scientific basis for sex determination in mammals was discovered in the early 20th century (Betteridge et al., 1981; Guyer, 1910).

Significant progress has been made in gender pre-selection based on the understanding that "accessory" or "sex" chromosomes control mammalian gender determination. The use of cutting-edge technologies has been critical to the development of future animal production systems, as well as the facilitation of family planning decisions through the diagnosis of X-linked genetic diseases prior to embryo formation or implantation. In this context, gender pre-selection for offspring has been a long sought after technology. Although other methods have been suggested, two reliable and highly repeatable techniques have been developed and widely used for gender pre-selection in mammals. The first is the separation of X and Y chromosome-bearing sperm, and the second is the amplification, using PCR, of a male-specific Y chromosome sequence in cellular material obtained from a preimplantation embryonic biopsy.

Both currently used methods of gender pre-selection have advantages and limitations in terms of their practical use. To date, flow cytometric sorting of X and Y chromosome-bearing sperm in combination with AI, IVF, or intracytoplasmic sperm injection (ICSI) has resulted in production of offspring from a wide range of mammalian species. Similarly, offspring of the desired sex have been obtained following embryonic biopsy and sexing prior to ET. However, the ultimate goal in gender pre-selection is the development of a safe, convenient, and accurate sexing procedure resulting in acceptable pregnancy rates after AI, *in vitro* fertilization (IVF), and/or subsequent ET.

Regardless of the method, a sexing procedure should not adversely affect sperm or embryonic viability and must be rapid, efficient, accurate, and economically feasible to be accepted by the agricultural and biomedical communities. In this chapter, we will first provide a historical overview of the currently used, state-of-the-art techniques for gender pre-selection in domestic animals, and then we will discuss the overall impact of these methods on animal management systems and veterinary and human medicine.

Genetic Basis of Sex Determination in Mammals

In mammals, the gender of offspring is primarily determined by the sex chromosome (i.e., X or Y chromosome) transferred from the male parent. X- and Y-bearing spermatozoa are produced in equal numbers by the testis during mammalian spermatogenesis, and there is generally an equal chance of X- or Y-bearing spermatozoa being involved in the fertilization process. Ovulated oocytes only contain an X-chromosome, so if a sperm with an X chromosome fertilizes the oocyte, the resulting embryo is genetically female (XX). Conversely, the resulting embryo will be male (XY) if a sperm with a Y chromosome fertilizes the oocyte.

During the later stages of normal development, embryos with XY chromosome constitution will develop into a phenotypic male by the action of sex-determining genes on the

Y chromosome, whereas embryos with XX chromosomes will develop into a female by default. Based on the genetics of sex determination, various methods have been developed during the past several decades to pre-select gender in mammalian offspring, especially in livestock. The efforts have primarily focused on either the separation of X- and Y-bearing spermatozoa or gender identification in pre-implantation embryos.

Sperm Sexing by Flow Cytometry

Based on potential density and/or mass differences between X- and Y-bearing spermatozoa, methods of sperm sexing have been developed which involve differential density gradient centrifugation and albumin centrifugation (Windsor et al., 1993). Other approaches, such as electrophoresis, flow fractionation, and laminar flow, have been based on the potential differences on surface charges or swimming behavior (Gledhill, 1988) between sperm containing an X chromosome vs. a Y chromosome. All the above-mentioned approaches, however, have proven to be of little practical value because of non-repeatability, low efficiency, or impaired sperm viability.

An accurate and efficient flow cytometric sperm-sorting method based on differences in DNA content between X and Y chromosome-bearing spermatozoa was introduced in the early 1980s (Garner et al., 1983). This technique, referred to as the "Beltsville sperm sexing technology" because of its development at Beltsville Laboratories in the United States, is the most widely used sperm sexing procedure in the world. It uses flow cytometers that are commonly used for cell-sorting in many fields of science (see Figure 6.1), and several modifications have been made to the standard flow cytometer to make sperm sorting more accurate, repeatable, and efficient (Johnson and Pinkel, 1986).

First, a forward fluorescence detector has replaced the light scatter detector which is standard in the orthogonally configured flow system. In addition, a way of orienting the sperm to the laser beam has been incorporated to collect the fluorescent light from both the edge of the sperm (90° detector) as well as from the side (0° detector) of the sperm. The cylindrical sample injection needle was replaced by a beveled sample injection needle that was designed to create a flat ribbon-type sample-sheath stream, which orients the paddle-shaped head of single spermatozoa to align within the stream. This modification allows a high proportion of sperm face to the beam in a proper plane as they pass the laser beam.

The principle of sperm sexing using flow cytometry is based on detecting the difference in DNA content between X and Y chromosome-bearing spermatozoa. The Y chromosome is smaller and thus carries less DNA than the X chromosome (see Table 6.1). This is valid for almost all mammalian species including bulls, boars, rams, and humans (see Figure 6.2). On the other hand, the autosomes

Table 6.1. Flow cytometric analysis of X- and Y-bearing sperm for DNA difference.

Species	Percent difference
Cattle	3.8%
Sheep	4.2%
Pig	3.6%
Dog	3.9%
Horse	4.1%
Rabbit	3.0%
Human	2.9%
Turkey	0%
Ram	4.2%

carried by X- or Y-bearing sperm are identical in DNA content.

Sperm sexing using flow cytometry requires initial incubation of sperm with a plasma membrane permeable viable dye which strongly interacts with sperm DNA. The Hoechst

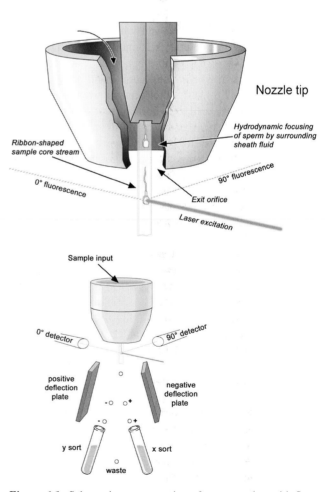

Figure 6.1. Schematic representation of sperm sexing with flow cytometric method.

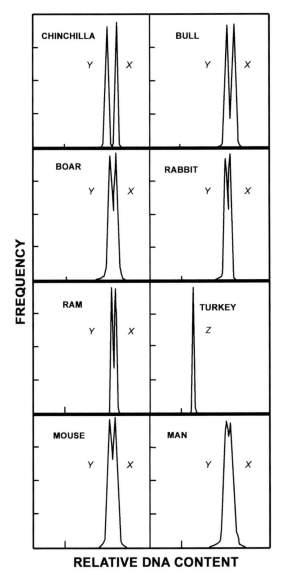

Figure 6.2. Schematic flow cytometric histograms showing the difference in DNA content between X- and Y-chromosome bearing spermatozoa.

field of about 2,000 volts. Both the charged droplets containing sperm and uncharged droplets containing no sperm pass through the electrostatic field. If the system does not make any determination, the spermatozoa are not given any electrical charge, and they are simply discarded. The droplets carrying X and Y chromosome-bearing sperm are electrically charged based on their DNA content. While X chromosome-bearing sperm are positively charged, Y chromosome-bearing sperm are negatively charged. The droplets carrying no sperm are not given any electrical charge. The brightest peak is associated with those sperm whose edge is toward the 90° detector. Thus, the droplets containing miss-oriented sperm emit less light toward the 90° detector and are discarded by the system. In general, 70 percent to 95 percent of the sperm heads are properly oriented in any given sample (Johnson, 1994; Johnson and Welch, 1999).

Factors Affecting the Efficiency of Sperm Sexing Using Flow Cytometry

The current challenge with flow cytometric sperm sexing is to sort sufficient numbers of X or Y chromosome-bearing spermatozoa to impregnate the female following routine AI without the use of more sophisticated ART such as IVF and ICSI. Several important factors influence the accuracy of flow cytometric sperm sexing (Suh et al., 2005), including intensity of the laser, sensitivity of the fluorescence detectors, and optical quality of the system. All of these parameters have to be optimal to detect differences between X and Y chromosome-bearing sperm.

The morphology of the sperm head also influences the accuracy of flow cytometric sperm sexing because the shape of the head affects the orientation of sperm as they pass the laser beam by proper plane (see Figure 6.3). Fortunately, spermatozoa from most domestic livestock have flattened, oval-headed sperm that can be easily oriented within a sorter using hydrodynamic forces. Bull and boar sperm are particularly well-suited for separation using flow cytometry (Johnson and Welch, 1999).

Sorting conditions must be optimized for each species to achieve an acceptable (90 percent or better) sperm sexing accuracy. With the currently used sorting systems, it is possible to sort around 7×10^6 live bull or boar spermatozoa per hour with at least 90 percent accuracy (Seidel and Garner, 2002). However, it should be noted that conventional AI in swine and cattle requires about 1×10^9 and 15×10^6 motile spermatozoa, respectively. It was found that 3×10^5 fresh motile sexed spermatozoa were required to obtain acceptable pregnancy rates which did not differ from pregnancy rates (about 50 percent) obtained from standard AI under the same conditions (Schenk et al., 1999). On the other hand, the number of sexed spermatozoa has to be at least 15×10^6 to compensate for motility loss following cryopreservation, and one study determined that deep uterine insemination of swine with 50×10^6 fresh sex-sorted

33342 is the most commonly used dye known to have a strong affinity to adenine- and thymine-rich sites of the sperm DNA. The flouresencently stained sperm heads are then introduced under pressure into the flow cytometer in liquid suspension. The fluorescence detectors measure the intensity of fluorescence resulting from excitation of the DNA-bound dye molecules by laser. The level of the fluorescence signals depends on the number of florescence molecules bound to sperm DNA. Because X chromosome-bearing spermatozoa contain more DNA than Y chromosome-bearing spermatozoa, it emits a higher level of signals than Y chromosome-bearing spermatozoa when they are excited by laser. The emission signals are then amplified and analyzed to determine the sex of the sperm.

Sperm cells are then electrically charged and deflected to a collection tube as they pass through an electrostatic

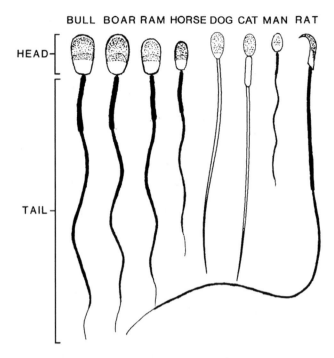

BULL BOAR RAM HORSE DOG CAT MAN RAT

HEAD

TAIL

Figure 6.3. Diagrammatic representation of the morphology of spermatozoa from various mammalian species.

sperm resulted in only a 33% pregnancy rate after deep uterine insemination (Grossfeld et al., 2005). Post-sorting and post-thawing viability of sexed sperm will need to be significantly increased to meet the commercial demand.

Efficient low-dose insemination methods are also essential for the use of sex-sorted sperm (see Figure 6.4). Insemination techniques such as IVF and ICSI require expensive equipment and are labor intensive, but these techniques use significantly fewer sperm to achieve fertilization than standard AI procedures. For example, viable ET offspring were obtained following the IVF of pig and cattle oocytes using a few thousand sorted sperm (Abeydeera et al., 1998; Lu et al., 1999; Rath et al., 1999; Zhang et al., 2003). ICSI procedures require injection of only a single sperm into the cytoplasm of the oocytes to achieve fertilization. Hamano

et al., (1999) transferred blastocyst stage cattle embryos that were produced by ICSI of sex-sorted bull sperm and obtained two healthy calves of the desired gender. Probst and Rath (2003) later described a similar protocol for swine, in which pregnancies delivered a total of 13 male piglets. Although the ability to have sex-sorted and cryopreserved sperm for later AI is an ultimate goal, other insemination methods, particularly IVF, could serve as a powerful bioassay for improving sperm-sorting procedures before their use with conventional AI (Flint et al., 2003). It is foreseeable that IVF procedures in cattle breeding programs will increase considerably, if cryopreserved sex-sorted sperm become commercially available in the near future.

Preimplantation Embryo Sexing

To date, various cytogenetic, immunological, and molecular biological approaches have been investigated to determine the sex of preimplantation embryos. These methods are based on the identification of X or Y chromosomes in whole embryos or in a few biopsied embryonic cells. Embryo sexing was initially done by simple karyotyping in murine (King et al., 1979) and bovine preimplantation embryos (Hare et al., 1976; Sighn and Hare, 1980; Torres and Popescu, 1980; Picard et al., 1985). However, these studies were performed in such a way that embryos could not be recovered after karyotyping and, thus, were of little value to animal breeding programs. A high percentage of the examined embryos have to be recovered after biopsy for an embryonic sex-determination method to be acceptable.

Identification of a Barr Body
Normal mammalian females have two X chromosomes, whereas male mammals have only one X chromosome. For dosage compensation in gene expression, an X chromosome is randomly inactivated during the early stage of embryonic development, and this inactive X chromosome is termed Barr body (Gartler and Riggs, 1983). A few embryonic cells can be biopsied and stained for the identification of a Barr body. This approach in blastocyst stage embryos resulted in the live birth of rabbits of the diagnosed gender (Gardner

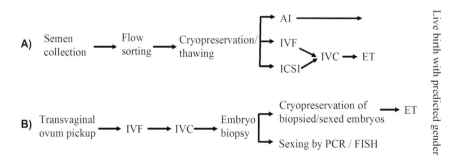

Figure 6.4. Potential use of sex-sorted semen (**A**) and biopsied and sexed embryos (**B**) with the incorporation of currently available assisted reproductive technologies. AI: artificial insemination; IVF: in-vitro fertilization; IVC: in-vitro culture; ICSI: intracytoplasmic sperm injection; ET: embryo transfer; PCR: polymerase chain reaction; FISH: fluorescence in situ hybridization.

and Edwards, 1968). However, the granular nature of embryonic nuclei from domestic animals limits the application of this approach to preimplantation embryo sexing.

Identification of Sex Chromosomes on Metaphase Chromosome Preparations

Similar to the identification of a Barr body, this method also involves a biopsied sample of embryonic cells. However, instead of direct staining, these cells are cultured for several hours in the presence of colchicine or related drugs to arrest them in the metaphase portion of a mitotic division cycle. A metaphase chromosomal spread is made using conventional cytogenetic procedures, and the sex chromosomes are identified with appropriate chromosomal staining techniques.

Detection of Male-Specific Histocompatibility Antigen (H-Y Antigen)

The H-Y antigen was identified following skin graft transplantation incompatibility between male and female in inbred mice (Wachtel, 1984). The expression of H-Y antigen can be detected as early as the 4-cell stage in mouse embryos. Co-culture of murine embryos with H-Y antiserum plus guinea pig complement shifted the female to male ratio in unaffected embryos from 1:1 to 11.5:1, as confirmed by karyotyping (Epstein et al., 1980). Later, White et al. (1983) conducted a similar experiment on a larger scale. Two thousand embryos at the 8- to 16-cell stage were treated for 24 hours, and the unaffected embryos were then transferred into pseudopregnant recipients, resulting in 58 offspring with a high (86 percent) female ratio. H-Y antigen can also be detected by a noninvasive method involving the use of an indirect immunofluorescent assay (i.e., the use of secondary antibody conjugated with a fluorochrome

to detect binding of H-Y antigen to male embryos). This approach was only 80 percent accurate in the identification of the sex in murine, porcine, ovine, and bovine embryos (Jafar and Flint, 1996).

Unfortunately, none of the aforementioned cytogenetic and immunological approaches has found widespread applications in domestic animals. Very recently, more advanced molecular approaches such as PCR and FISH methods have been developed and successfully used for greater than 90 percent accurate sex determination in livestock and humans. Similar to cytogenetic methods, these methods involve preimplantation embryonic biopsy techniques to get a few cells/blastomeres for sex determination (see Figure 6.5).

Polymerase Chan Reaction

Since the realization that physical removal of a single blastomere from a 4-cell mouse embryo via micromanipulation does not appear to affect continued *in vitro* development to the blastocyst and offspring viability, rapid progress has been made in developing embryo sexing techniques using sex-specific gene amplification by PCR (Wilton and Trounson, 1989). A PCR-based method has been developed for the amplification of a Y chromosome-specific sequence obtained from preimplantation bovine embryos (Aasen and Medrano 1990). Kirkpatrick and Monson (1993) have developed a rapid and sensitive method of sex determination which uses nested, allele-specific amplification of bovine zfx (female) and zfy (male). A nested PCR protocol is used to amplify zinc finger protein Y-linked (zfy) and X-linked (zfx). The first primer set was used for amplification of both zfy and zfx. For allele-specific amplification, these mismatches are incorporated into the nested primers. The product of first PCR reaction is used in a nested PCR reaction where the nested primer sets amplify 247 bp of zfx or 167 bp of zfy

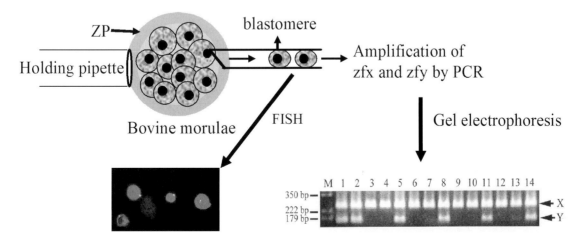

Figure 6.5. Schematic representation of bovine embryo biopsy and sexing with PCR and FISH analysis. Double bands (lanes 1, 2, 5, 8, 11, and 14) indicate male embryos; the single band (lanes 3, 4, 7, 9, 10, 12, and 13) indicates female embryos. FISH using blastomere derived from IVF bovine embryos. Interphase nuclei of male-putative blastomeres and the detection of BtY2-L1 by FITC-conjugated anti-avidin antibody.

gene. Thus, a single band at 247 bp indicates female embryo, and double bands at 247 and 167 bp indicate male embryo (see Figure 6.5).

Using the same zfy/zfx primers and other PCR primers derived from an ovine-specific, randomly amplified polymorphic DNA marker for the Y chromosome (UcdO43), Gutierrez-Adan (1997) has developed an accurate (100 percent), sensitive, and quick (about three hours) method for determining the sex of ovine embryos. Mara et al. (2004) have used the PCR method with a primer pair recognizing a bovine Y chromosome-specific sequence (sex-determining region Y; SRY). The PCR-based embryo sexing method has also been used successfully in swine (Pomp et al., 1995).

Although the previously described PCR-based methods have been applied successfully in livestock breeding programs to manipulate sex ratio of offspring, all of these methods used gel electrophoresis of PCR product. Bredbacka (1998) has developed a simple PCR-based sexing assay for cattle embryos which does not require gel electrophoresis. It uses primers that bind a highly repeated (60,000 times) bovine sequence of Y-chromosome. When the Y chromosome is present, the PCR reaction yields large quantities of PCR product; whereas when the embryo is female, no PCR product is amplified. The reactions are observed under UV light after ethidium bromide has been added to PCR reactions. Pink reactions show the presence of the Y chromosome (male embryo) and colorless reactions demonstrate the absence of the Y chromosome (female embryo).

Hasler et al. (2002) have used this alternative sexing protocol for *in vitro* and *in vivo* derived bovine embryos in a large scale commercial ET program. Biopsies of blastocyst stage embryos are obtained using a steel blade attached to a mechanical micromanipulator. The PCR results have shown that males constituted 49 percent of 3,964 *in vivo* and 53 percent of 1,181 *in vitro* derived embryos. Postpartum sexing revealed the accuracy of the embryonic sex determination to be 98.7 percent and 94.4 percent for male and females embryos, respectively.

Fluorescence in situ Hybridization

Recently, another highly sensitive, molecular cytogenetic method of embryo sexing has been developed. Similar to other previously described cytogenetic methods, this involves embryonic biopsy techniques to obtain a few cells for sex identification. FISH has been successfully used in sex identification for embryos from cattle, pigs, and humans with an accuracy rate greater than 90 percent (Kobayashi et al., 1998; Kawarasaki et al., 2000; Lee et al., 2004; Thornhill and Monk, 1996). Besides gender determination, FISH has also been used extensively to diagnose genetic defects such as X-linked recessive disease in humans (Pettigrew et al., 2000; Li et al., 2005). The principle of this method of embryo sexing is based on the complementary hybridization of a Y-specific DNA probe to the Y chromosome of one or more biopsied cells from an embryo. The

Y-specific DNA is usually labeled with biotin, and avidin-conjugated with a fluorochrome (i.e., FITC) is used visualize the specific hybridization on the Y chromosome (see Figure 6.5).

For sex determination in swine, Kawarasaki et al. (2000) have performed FISH using digoxigenin (dig)-labeled chromosome Y-specific DNA, and a total of 12 piglets of the expected sex have been obtained after ET. Lee et al. (2004) have recently validated embryo sexing by FISH in bovine embryos. In their study bovine Y chromosome-specific PCR product derived from BtY2 sequences was labeled with biotin-16-dUTP (BtY2-L1 probe), and FISH was performed on karyoplasts of biopsed blastomeres (see Figure 6.5). The FISH assay gave high accuracy (96 percent) biopsied blastomeres.

Although the PCR and FISH methods allow for sex determination in a relatively short time and with high reliability, they also present some drawbacks. Non-specific sequences or contaminants can be amplified, and skilled micromanipulation is required to biopsy preimplantation embryos. In addition, the biopsy procedure damages the zona pellucida (egg shell) and can impair its function as a natural barrier against potential microbial pathogens (Thibier, 2001) (see Figure 6.6). It is likely gender determi-

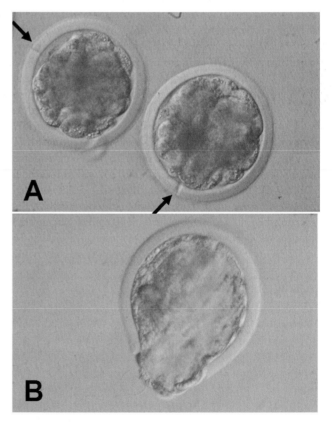

Figure 6.6. **(A)** a biopsied bovine morulae (**arrows** indicate the breached zona pellucida), and **(B)** a hatching blastocyst after morulae biopsy.

nation from biopsied preimplantation embryos will be used less commonly as sperm sexing techniques improve.

Cryosurvival and Fertility of Flow-Sorted Sperm and Biopsied Embryos

Cryopreservation and cryostorage of sex-sorted sperm or biopsied embryos are often required until the results of molecular or cytogenetic analyses (i.e, PCR and FISH) are available. The ability to cryopreserve sex-sorted sperm or biopsied and sexed embryos allow for the wider application of gender pre-selection techniques. National and international transport of frozen sperm and embryos, sample exchange between remotely located research institutes and medical centers, as well as the elimination of some of the logistical problems associated with ovulation synchronization in livestock and humans are all facilitated by cryopreservation of germplasm.

Sperm and preimplantation embryos from different mammalian species demonstrate varying degrees of sensitivity to *in vitro* manipulations. The physical intervention during handling, centrifugation, and the multiple steps involved in cryopreservation procedures have cumulative detrimental affects on sperm and embryos. It has been reported that flow cytometric sperm sexing adversely affects sperm viability. It causes about 30 percent reduction in motility and impaired plasma membrane and acrosome integrity and fertility due to high pressure laser illumination and staining with Hoechst 33342 (Lu et al., 2001).

For optimal sexing efficiency, the relative susceptibilities of sperm and embryos from each mammalian species to the physical stresses that occur during sexing and cryopreservation procedures must be considered. To date, flow cytometrically sorted sperm from cattle, swine, and sheep have been successfully cryopreserved, and live births have been obtained with various methods of AI (Hollinshead et al., 2002; Johnson et al., 2005; Morton et al., 2004; Seidel et al., 1999). One study conducted with sex-sorted bull sperm showed that despite reduced sperm viability, a pregnancy rate of 50 percent was achieved with no abnormalities noted

with respect to the birthweights of offspring, gestation length, and calving ease (Tubman et al., 2003).

The protocols used for the cryopreservation of sexed spermatozoa are based on modifications of existing protocols for the cryopreservation of unsorted spermatozoa (Morton et al., 2004; Schenk et al., 1999). However, the AI of the sexed spermatozoa requires special techniques or equipment due to the limited number of sexed sperm available. The sperm are usually delivered either into the oviduct, utero-oviductal junction, or deep within the uterus to allow sperm easier access to the site of fertilization. Grossfeld et al. (2005) have recently performed non-surgical AI in swine using sex-sorted semen and a specially designed catheter for the deposition of 5×10^6 sperm into the tip of the uterine horns. A pregnancy rate of 33 percent was achieved with sexed sperm, while inseminations with non-sexed spermatozoa resulted in a pregnancy rate of 54 percent. All but one piglet born as a result of the sexed semen were of the predicted sex. Table 6.2 summarizes some of the results representing the recent live births from sexed spermatozoa across several livestock species.

Preimplantation embryo sexing methods require embryonic biopsy techniques which can be detrimental to embryonic development. Depending on one's technical skills, 60 percent to 70 percent of biopsied cleavage stage embryos can develop to the blastocyst stage. Lehn-Jensen and Greve (1978) punctured *in vivo* derived expanded bovine blastocysts and then slowly froze them. They were able to obtain live calves following thawing and ET. Moreover, the biopsy procedure appears to have 10 percent fewer detrimental effects on expanded blastocysts (Agca et al., 1998; Tominaga and Hamada, 2004).

Until 1989, attempts to freeze embryos without an intact zona pellucida were met with little success in cattle (Kanagawa et al., 1979), mice (Bielansk et al., 1987; Wilton et al., 1989), and humans. Niemann et al. (1987) have achieved pregnancy rates of 61 percent and 43 percent from frozen intact and biopsied *in vivo* derived blastocysts, respectively. Another study by Nibart et al., (1989) compared the pregnancy rates after transfer of fresh and

Table 6.2. Pregnancy rates and live births that resulted from artificial insemination using cryopreserved unsorted and sex-sorted spermatozoa in various domestic species.

Species	Frozen sperm	Dosage ($\times 10^6$)	AI sites	Pregnancy rate (%)	Average live births	References
Bovine	Unsorted	20	Uterus	~80%	1	DeJarnette et al., 2004
	Sorted	0.2	Uterine horns	51.0%	1	Seidel et al., 1999
Porcine	Unsorted	1,000	DUI*	72.5%	9.25	Roca et al., 2003
	Sorted	0.2	Oviduct	N/A	6.8	Johnson et al., 2005
Ovine	Unsorted	200	Vaginal or cervical	73.43%	2.15	Paulenz et al., 2005
	Sorted	2–4	Utero-tubal junction	14.6–25%	1.5	Hollinshead et al., 2002

*DUI: deep intrauterine insemination.

frozen biopsied bovine embryos. While fresh, biopsied embryos resulted in a pregnancy rate of 55 percent, transferring frozen biopsied embryos resulted in a pregnancy rate of 41 percent. Agca et al. (1998) biopsied and sexed *in vitro* derived bovine morulae and subsequently cryopreserved these embryos using a vitrification (ultra-rapid cooling) protocol. Those results did not show any significant difference in pregnancy rates between freshly transferred and vitrified biopsied embryos (50 percent vs. 44 percent, respectively). Furthermore, the calves produced as a result of biopsied-sexed and vitrified embryos had normal gestation length, birthweight, and calving ease compared to calves that resulted from routine AI in the same study.

Multiple interventions, such as physical manipulations, biopsy techniques, and cryopreservation, cause a slight, but not a marked, reduction in the developmental competence of pre-implantation bovine and human embryos (Agca et al., 1998; Tominaga and Hamada, 2004; Ciotti et al., 2000; Magli et al., 2004).

Potential Applications of Sexed Semen and Embryos

Gender selection in offspring would be useful in dairy and beef production operations, equine athletics, human medicine, and basic research. In dairy cattle operations, it would allow production of more replacement heifer progeny from superior milk-producing cows. In beef operations, controlling offspring would enable new directions for genetic selection and would make sustainable single calving heifer systems feasible (Taylor et al., 1985). The production of more bull calves would be possible, and progeny testing would be more efficient. There would be substantial commercial applications of gender selection techniques in the swine industry. More boars could be produced, and split-sex feeding could be eliminated. There could also be a significant interest in sex pre-determination in horses, such as when a certain gender is preferred for specific sporting events (Lindsey et al., 2002a and 2002b; Buss et al., 2005).

Embryonic biopsies for preimplantation genetic diagnosis have been widely used in human medicine during the last decade. The successful applications of embryo biopsy techniques, PCR for the amplification of DNA, and FISH analysis have allowed an increasing number of couples to identify sex-linked diseases such as hemophilia or muscular dystrophy (Handyside et al., 1990; Chong et al., 1993; Thornhill and Monk, 1996; Li et al., 2005) and/or autosomal diseases such as cystic fibrosis, Tay-Sachs and sickle cell anemia (Handyside et al., 1992; Lynch and Brown, 1990; Pettigrew et al., 2000) in preimplantation embryos.

Because our current knowledge about sexual dimorphism in mammals is very limited, sexing procedures would be useful in basic research to better understand mammalian sexual dimorphism. With the availability of sexed semen or embryos, many interesting questions may be raised and investigated regarding sexual development of mammalian embryos, even as early as during sperm and egg interactions (Beyhan et al., 1999). Furthermore, studies can be designed to elucidate differential gene expression between male and female embryos under various *in vitro* culture conditions and to determine differences in the developmental kinetics between male and female embryos (Gutierrez-Adan et al., 2001; Peippo et al., 2001).

The current efficiency of the sperm-sorting and embryonic sexing methods of sex determination is somewhat sufficient for experimental studies and human clinical use, but it is not satisfactory for large scale animal production operations. As research to improve the efficiency of sperm sexing progresses and more non-invasive methods of sex determination of preimplantation embryos are developed, the use of gender determination in conjunction with AI, ET, and cryopreservation techniques is expected to have a significant, worldwide impact on livestock production, as well as increased use in veterinary and human medicine.

Acknowledgement

We thank Dr. Tim Evans for his thoughtful comments and critical reading of the manuscript, and Mr. Donald Connor for his assistance with the images.

References

Aasen, E., and Medrano, J.F. (1990). Amplification of the ZFY and ZFX genes for sex identification in humans, cattle, sheep and goats. *Biotechnology* (NY). 8:1279–1281.

Abeydeera, L.R., Johnson, L.A., Welch, G.R., Wang, W.H., Boquest, A.C., Cantley, T.C., Rieke, A., and Day, B.N. (1998). Birth of piglets preselected for gender following in vitro fertilization of in vitro matured pig oocytes by X and Y chromosome bearing spermatozoa sorted by high speed flow cytometry. *Theriogenology.* 50:981–988.

Agca, Y., Monson, R.L., Northey, D.L., Peschel, D.E., Schaefer, D.M., and Rutledge, J.J. (1998). Normal calves from transfer of biopsied, sexed and vitrified IVP bovine embryos. *Theriogenology.* 50:129–145.

Betteridge, K.J., Hare, W.C.D., and Singh, E.L. (1981). Approaches to sex selection in farm animals. In: Brackett, B.G., Seidel, G.E. Jr., and Seidel, S.M. (ds), *New Technology in Animal Breeding.* New York: Academic Press, pp 109–125.

Beyhan, Z., Johnson, L.A., and First, N.L. (1999). Sexual dimorphism in IVM-IVF bovine embryos produced from X and Y chromosome-bearing spermatozoa sorted by high speed flow cytometry. *Theriogenology.* 52:35–48.

Bielanski, A. (1987). Survival in vitro of zona pellucida-free mouse embryos after cooling by conventional two step or vitrification methods. *Cryo Letters.* 8:294–301.

Bredbacka, P. (1998). Recent developments in embryo sexing and its field application. *Reprod. Nutr. Dev.* 38:605–613.

Buss, H., Clulow, J., Sieme, H., Maxwell, W.M., Morris, L.H., Sieg, B., Struckmann, .C, and Rath, D. (2005). Improvement of the freezability of sex-sorted stallion spermatozoa. *Anim. Reprod. Sci.* 89:315–318.

Chong, S.S., Kristjansson, K., Cota, J., Handyside, A.H., and Hughes, M.R. (1993). Preimplantation prevention of X-linked disease: reliable and rapid sex determination of single human cells by restriction analysis of simultaneously amplified ZFX and ZFY sequences. *Hum. Mol. Genet.* 2:1187–1191.

Ciotti, P.M., Lagalla, C., Ricco, A.S., Fabbri, R., Forabosco, A., and Porcu, E. (2000). Micromanipulation of cryopreserved embryos and cryopreservation of micromanipulated embryos in PGD. *Mol. Cell. Endocrinol.* 169:63–67.

DeJarnette. J.M., Marshall, C.E., Lenz, R.W., Monke, D.R., Ayars, W.H., Sattler, C.G. (2004). Sustaining the fertility of artificially inseminated dairy cattle: the role of the artificial insemination industry. *J. Dairy Sci.* 87:E93-E104 (E. Suppl.).

Epstein, C.J., Smith, S., and Travis, B. (1980). Expression of H-Y antigen on preimplantation mouse embryos. *Tissue Antigens.* 15:63–67.

Flint, A.F., Chapman, P.L., and Seidel, G.E. (2003). Fertility assessment through heterospermic insemination of flow-sorted sperm in cattle. *J. Anim. Sci.* 81:1814–1822.

Gardner, R.L., and Edwards, R.G. (1968). Control of the sex ratio at full term in the rabbit by transferring sexed blastocysts. *Nature* 218:346–348.

Garner, D.L., Gledhill, B.L., Pinkel, D., Lake, S., Stephenson, D., Van Dilla, M.A., and Johnson, L.A. (1983). Quantification of the X- and Y-chromosome-bearing spermatozoa of domestic animals by flow cytometry. *Biol. Reprod.* 28:312–321.

Gartler, S.M., and Riggs, A.D. (1983). Mammalian X-chromosome inactivation. *Annu. Rev. Genet.* 17:155–190.

Gledhill, B.L. (1988). Selection and separation of X- and Y-bearing mammalian sperm. *Gamete Res.* 20:377–395.

Grossfeld, R., Klinc, P., Sieg, B., and Rath, D. (2005). Production of piglets with sexed semen employing a non-surgical insemination technique. *Theriogenology.* 63:2269–2277.

Gutierrez-Adan, A., Cushwa, W.T., Anderson, G.B., and Medrano, J.F. (1997). Ovine-specific Y-chromosome RAPD-SCAR marker for embryo sexing. *Anim. Genet.* 28:135–138.

Gutierrez-Adan, A., Granados, J., Pintado, B., and De La Fuente, J. (2001). Influence of glucose on the sex ratio of bovine IVM/IVF embryos cultured in vitro. *Reprod. Fertil. Dev.* 13:361–365.

Guyer, M.F. (1910). Accessory chromosomes in man. *Biol. Bull.* 19:219.

Hamano, K., Li, X., Qian, X.Q., Funauchi, K., Furudate, M., and Minato, Y. (1999). Gender preselection in cattle with intracytoplasmically injected, flow cytometrically sorted sperm heads. *Biol. Reprod.* 60:1194–1197.

Handyside, A.H., Kontogianni, E.H., Hardy, K., and Winston, R.M. (1990). Pregnancies from biopsied human preimplantation embryos sexed by Y-specific DNA amplification. *Nature.* 344:768–770.

Handyside, A.H., Lesko, J.G., Tarin, J.J., Winston, R.M., and Hughes, M.R. (1992). Birth of a normal girl after in vitro fertilization and preimplantation diagnostic testing for cystic fibrosis. *N. Engl. J. Med.* 327:905–909.

Hare, W.C.D., Mitchell, D., Betteridge, K.J., Eaglesome, M.D., and Randall, G.C.B. (1976). Sexing two week old bovine embryos by chromosomal analysis prior to surgical transfer: preliminary methods and results. *Theriogenology.* 5:243–253.

Hasler, J.F., Cardey, E., Stokes, J.E., and Bredbacka, P. (2002). Nonelectrophoretic PCR-sexing of bovine embryos in a commercial environment. *Theriogenology.* 58:1457–1469.

Hollinshead, F.K., O'Brien, J.K., Maxwell, W.M.C., and Evans, G. (2002). Production of lambs of predetermined sex after the insemination of ewes with low numbers of frozen-thawed sorted X- and Y-chromosome bearing spermatozoa. *Reprod. Fert. Dev.* 14:503–508.

Jafar, S.I., and Flint, A.P.F. (1996). Sex selection in mammals: a review. *Theriogenology.* 46:191–200.

Johnson, L.A. (1994) Isolation of X- and Y-bearing sperm for sex pre-selection. *Oxford Reviews of Reproductive Biology.* 16:303–326.

Johnson, L.A., and Pinkel, D. (1986). Modification of a laser-based flow cytometer for high-resolution DNA analysis of mammalian spermatozoa. *Cytometry.* 7:268–73.

Johnson, L.A., Rath, D., Vazquez, J.M., Maxwell, W.M., and Dobrinsky, J.R. (2005). Preselection of sex of offspring in swine for production: current status of the process and its application. *Theriogenology.* 63:615–624.

Johnson, L.A., and Welch, G.R. (1999). Sex preselection: high-speed flow cytometric sorting of X and Y sperm for maximum efficiency. *Theriogenology.* 52:1323–1341.

Kanagawa, H., Frim, J., and Kruuv, J. (1979). The effect of puncturing the zona pellucida on freeze thaw survival of bovine embryos. *Can. J. Anim. Sci.* 59:623–626.

Kawarasaki, T., Matsumoto, K., Chikyu, M, Itagaki, Y., and Horiuchi, A. (2000). Sexing of porcine embryo by in situ hybridization using chromosome Y- and 1-specific DNA probes. *Theriogenology.* 53:1501–1509.

King, W.A., Lineares, T., Gustavasson, I., and Bane, A. (1979). A method for preparation of chromosomes from bovine zygotes and blastocyst. *Vet. Sci. Comm.* 3:51–56.

Kirkpatrick, B.W., and Monson, R.L. (1993). Sensitive sex determination assay applicable to bovine embryos derived from IVM and IVF. *J. Reprod. Fertil.* 98:335–340.

Kobayashi, J., Sekimoto, A., Uchida, H., Wada, T., Sasaki, K., Sasada, H., Umezu, M., and Sato, E. (1998). Rapid detection of male-specific DNA sequence in bovine embryos using fluorescence in situ hybridization. *Mol. Reprod. Dev.* 51: 390–394.

Lee, J.H., Park, J.H., Lee, S.H., Park, C.S., and Jin, D.I. (2004). Sexing using single blastomere derived from IVF bovine embryos by fluorescence in situ hybridization (FISH). *Theriogenology.* 62:1452–1458.

Lehn-Jensen, H., and Greve, T. (1978). Low tempetarure preservation of cattle blastocyst. *Theriogenology.* 9:313–322.

Li, M., DeUgarte, C.M., Surrey, M., Danzer, H., DeCherney, A., and Hill, D.L. (2005). Fluorescence in situ hybridization reanalysis of day-6 human blastocysts diagnosed with aneuploidy on day 3. *Fertil. Steril.* 84:1395–1400.

Lindsey, A.C., Morris, L.H., Allen, W.R., Schenk, J.L., Squires, E.L., and Bruemmer, J.E. (2002a). Hysteroscopic insemination of mares with low numbers of nonsorted or flow sorted spermatozoa. *Equine Vet. J.* 34:128–132.

Lindsey, A.C., Schenk, J.L., Graham, J.K., Bruemmer, J.E., and Squires, E.L. (2002b). Hysteroscopic insemination of low numbers of flow sorted fresh and frozen/thawed stallion spermatozoa. *Equine Vet. J.* 34:121–127.

Lu, K.H., Cran, D.G., and Seidel, G.E. (1999). In vitro fertilization with flow cytometrically-sorted bovine sperm. *Theriogenology.* 52:1393–1405.

Lynch, J.R., and Brown, J.M. (1990). The polymerase chain reaction: current and future clinical applications. *J. Med. Genet.* 27:2–7.

Magli, M.C., Gianaroli, L., Ferraretti, A.P., Toschi, M., Esposito, F., and Fasolino, M.C. (2004). The combination of polar body and embryo biopsy does not affect embryo viability. *Hum. Reprod.* 19:1163–1169.

Mara, L., Pilichi, S., Sanna, A., Accardo, C., Chessa, B., Chessa, F., Dattena, M., Bomboi, G., and Cappai, P. (2004). Sexing of in vitro produced ovine embryos by duplex PCR. *Mol. Reprod. Dev.* 69:35–42.

Morton, K.M., Catt, S.L., Hollinshead, F.K., Maxwell, W.M.C., and Evans, G. (2004). Production of lambs after the transfer of fresh and cryopreserved in vitro produced embryos from prepubertal lamb oocytes and unsorted and sex-sorted frozen-thawed spermatozoa. *Reprod. Dom. Anim* 39:454–461.

Nibart, M., Mechekour, F., Procureur, R., Chense, B., Chupin, D., and Thibier, M. (1989). Pregnancy rates after cervical transfer of biopsied bovine embryos. *Theriogenology.* 311:324–328.

Niemann, H., Pryor, J.H., and Bondioli, K.R. (1987). Effects of splitting the zona pellucida and its subsequent sealing on freeze-thaw survival of day 7 bovine embryos. *Theriogenology.* 28: 675–681.

Paulenz, H., Soderquist, L., Adnoy, T., Nordstoga, A.B., and Andersen Berg, K. (2005). Effect of vaginal and cervical deposition of semen on the fertility of sheep inseminated with frozen-thawed semen. *Vet Rec.* 19:156:372–375.

Peippo, J., Kurkilahti, M., and Bredbacka, P. (2001). Developmental kinetics of in vitro produced bovine embryos: the effect of sex, glucose and exposure to time-lapse environment. *Zygote.* 9:105–113.

Pettigrew, R., Kuo, H.C., Scriven, P., Rowell, P., Pal, K., Handyside, A., Braude, P., and Ogilvie, C.M. (2000). A pregnancy following PGD for X-linked dominant (correction of X-linked autosomal dominant) *incontinentia pigmenti* (Bloch-Sulzberger syndrome): case report. *Hum. Reprod.* 15:2650–2652.

Picard, L., King, W.A., and Betteridge, K.J. (1985). Production of sexed calves from frozen thawed embryos. *Veterinary Record.* 117:603–608.

Pomp, D., Good, B.A., Geisert, R.D., Corbin, C.J., and Conley, A.J. (1995). Sex identification in mammals with polymerase chain reaction and its use to examine sex effects on diameter of day-10 or -11 pig embryos. *J. Anim. Sci.* 73: 1408–1415.

Probst, S., and Rath, D. (2003). Production of piglets using intracytoplasmic sperm injection (ICSI) with flow cytometrically sorted boar semen and artificially activated oocytes. *Theriogenology.* 59:961–973.

Rath, D., Long, C.R., Dobrinsky, J.R., Welch, G.R., Schreier, L. L., and Johnson, L.A. (1999). In vitro production of sexed embryos for gender preselection: high-speed sorting of X-chromosome-bearing sperm to produce pigs after embryo transfer. *J. Anim. Sci.* 77:3346–3352.

Roca, J., Carvajal, G., Lucas, X., Vazquez, J.M., and Martinez, E.A. (2003). Fertility of weaned sows after deep intrauterine insemination with a reduced number of frozen-thawed spermatozoa. *Theriogenology.* 60:77–87.

Schenk, J.L., Suh, T.K., Cran, D.G., and Seidel, G.E. (1999). Cryopreservation of flow-sorted bovine spermatozoa. *Theriogenology.* 52:1375–1391.

Seidel, G.E., and Garner, D.L. (2002). Current status of sexing mammalian spermatozoa. *Reproduction.* 124:733–743.

Seidel, G.E., Schenk, J.L., Herickhoff, L.A., Doyle, S.P., Bink, Z., Green, R.D., and Cran, D.G. (1999). Insemination of heifers with sexed frozen or sexed liquid semen. *Theriogenology.* 51:400.

Singh, E.L., and Hare, W.D.C. (1980). The feasibility of sexing bovine morula stage embryos prior to embryo transfer. *Theriogenology.* 14:421–427.

Suh, T.K., Schenk, J.L., and Seidel, G.E. (2005). High pressure flow cytometric sorting damages sperm. *Theriogenology.* 64:1035–1048.

Taylor, C.S., Moore, A.J., Thiessen, R.B., and Bailey, C.M. (1985). Food efficiency in traditional and sexed controlled systems of beef production. *Anim. Prod.* 40:401–440.

Thibier, M. (2001). Identified and unidentified challenges for reproductive biotechnologies regarding infectious diseases in animal and public health. *Theriogenology.* 56:1465–1481.

Thornhill, A.R., and Monk, M. (1996). Cell recycling of a single human cell for preimplantation diagnosis of X-linked disease and dual sex determination. *Mol. Hum. Reprod.* 2:285–289.

Tominaga, K., and Hamada, Y. (2004). Efficient production of sex-identified and cryosurvived bovine in-vitro produced blastocysts. *Theriogenology.* 61:1181–1191.

Tubman, L.M., Brink, Z., Suh, T.K., and Seidel, G.E. (2004). Characteristics of calves produced with sperm sexed by flow cytometry/cell sorting. *J. Anim. Sci.* 82:1029–1036.

Wachtel, S.S. (1984). H-Y antigen in the study of sex determination and control of sex ratio. *Theriogenology.* 21:19–28.

White, K.L., Lindner, G.M., Anderson, G.B., and Bondurant, R.H. (1983). Cytolytic and fluorescent detection of H-Y antigen on preimplantation mouse embryos. *Theriogenology.* 18:701–705.

Wilton, L.J., Shaw, J.M., and Trounson, A.O. (1989). Successful single-cell biopsy and cryopreservation of preimplantation mouse embryos. *Fertil. Steril.* 51:513–517.

Wilton, L.J., and Trounson, A.O. (1989). Biopsy of preimplantation mouse embryos: development of micromanipulated embryos and proliferation of single blastomeres in vitro. *Biol. Reprod.* 40:145–152.

Windsor, D.P., Evans, G., and White, I.G. (1993). Sex predetermination by separation of X and Y chromosome-bearing sperm: a review. *Reprod. Fertil. Dev.* 5:155–171.

Wintenberger-Torres, S., and Popescu, C.P. (1980). Transfer of cow blastocysts after sexing. *Theriogenology.* 14:309–317.

Zhang, M., Lu, K.H., and Seidel, G.E. (2003). Development of bovine embryos after in vitro fertilization of oocytes with flow cytometrically sorted, stained and unsorted sperm from different bulls. *Theriogenology.* 60:1657–1663.

Chapter 7

Artificial Insemination

Gary Althouse

Artificial insemination (AI), the act of mechanically and unnaturally depositing semen into the female reproductive tract with the goal of achieving conception, was truly the first assisted reproductive technology (ART) to be practiced. As the most frequently used ART procedure today, AI has had and continues to have a tremendous impact on the various animal breeding industries. Driving the implementation of AI are the distinct advantages it brings to each species through the accelerated proof in genetic merit; propagation; and amplification of genetic progress, disease control, delineated reproductive management, and cost savings (i.e., reduced animal transportation, animal inventory, and associated labor costs).

Some of these advantages can also be considered disadvantages, given that this technology can help spread genetic defects and that it requires an increased level of training and intensive breeding management to be successfully integrated into a system.

The majority of breeding in modern dairy cattle, poultry, and swine production systems is performed by AI. Interestingly, early work that was instrumental in the development and application of AI was performed on companion animals. In the scientific literature, the earliest documented study was that of Spallanzani (1784), in which freshly obtained dog semen was inseminated into a bitch which led to the whelping of a litter of three pups. This same scientist (who ironically was a priest by training) also provided insight into the effects of cooling of sperm on viability and longevity. The literature remained devoid of work in AI until a century later, when reports of AI in dogs (Heape, 1897) and horses (for review, see Perry, 1968) surfaced. The Russian scientist Ivanoff (1922) took this knowledge from his initial work in horses and applied it to performing AI in cattle and sheep.

As studies in AI increased in the early 20th century, work also commenced to develop the technology to effectively and efficiently collect semen from the male. From the initial work of Amantea (Bonadonna, 1937), development of the artificial vagina (AV) ensued (Milovanov, 1938). Numerous modifications and novel designs have subsequently occurred within each of the species. Structurally, the AV for most species consists of a firm outside cover with a thin-walled rubber lining housed within. The cavity between the outside cover and rubber liner is filled with tempered water to provide the ideal temperature and pressure conditions to stimulate ejaculation upon penile insertion. The ejaculate is then directed into a collection receptacle, usually by an integrated funnel which is part of the rubber-lined AV.

In addition, methods to analyze, process, and store semen have undergone an immense evolution, much of which is species-specific. The unique physiological attributes of each species have led to species-specific techniques in the application of AI. Fresh-extended and chilled semen is most commonly used by many of the species commercially using AI today. Starting in the mid-1950s, cattle producers made a transition from fresh-extended/chilled semen to frozen-thawed semen. Even with increased frozen-thawed semen use in cattle and other species, in general, overall fertility appears to be slightly lower for frozen-thawed semen than for fresh-extended/chilled semen.

Cattle

Whether dairy or beef cattle, the techniques used to collect and process semen and to breed by AI are essentially the same. Because of the intensive management of today's dairy cattle operations, the majority (more than 70 percent) are bred using AI. Conversely, most beef operations are run under extensive, outdoor management systems. This type of system makes application of AI much more labor-intensive and, thus, today it is only used by about 10 percent of the beef industry.

Bulls are usually housed in dedicated studs, where semen is most commonly collected using an artificial vagina (see Figure 7.1) while mounted and thrusting on a teaser animal. Electroejaculation (see Figure 7.1), a procedure in which electrical stimulations are emitted from a rectal probe eliciting an ejaculate, is used for bulls not trained for routine AV collection.

Ejaculate volume is less than 10 mL (average 4 mL) and contains 2 billion to 12 billion (average of 4 billion) sperm (DeJarnette, 2004; DeJarnette et al., 2004). The ejaculate is assessed for volume and sperm motility, morphology, concentration and total numbers.

Although technology has been available for decades to produce extended-chilled semen, the majority of bull semen

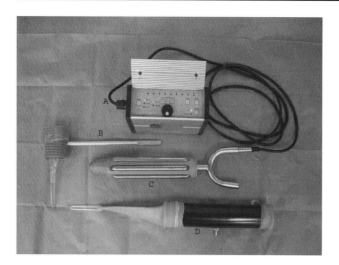

Figure 7.1. Equipment used to collect semen from bulls. **(A):** electroejaculator unit; **(B):** holder with semen collection cone and tube; **(C):** rectal probe; and **(D):** complete artificial vagina.

is processed in a cryoprotectant semen extender and frozen. Frozen doses of semen are packaged into pre-labeled 0.25 or 0.5 mL straws (see Figure 7.2) containing approximately 20 to 40×10^6 sperm, and then frozen and stored at $-196°C$ in liquid nitrogen until it is used.

Appropriate timing for AI in cattle is determined through a systematic estrus detection program and/or pharmacologic (e.g., gonadotropins, prostaglandins, and sex steroid hormones) manipulation to synchronize estrus. Frequent visual assessment (two to three times/day) of the animals for outward signs of estrus is crucial to a breeding program. The primary sign of estrus in cattle is standing to be mounted. Other secondary signs may include vulvar edema, vulvar mucous discharge, frequent urination, vocalization, and a roughened tail head (from being mounted by other animals).

Optimal conception rates are achieved when a cow is inseminated between mid-estrus and estrus termination. As a general rule, a single insemination is performed 10 to 14 hours after first observing clinical signs of estrus. Commonly referred to as the AM/PM rule, cows in which pro-

ducers have identified signs of estrus in either the morning (AM) or evening (PM) are scheduled to be inseminated the following PM or AM, respectively. Alternatively, pharmacologic manipulation programs are available in which a fixed-time insemination can be performed without the need for estrus detection.

Cows are restrained for insemination. Due to their frequent handling, dairy cattle are usually restrained either by tethering or placement in a stanchion. Less frequently handled cattle (e.g., beef) are restrained by a chute.

The dose of semen is then thawed according to manufacturer recommendations, and the thawed straw is placed into an insemination rod (see Figure 7.2). Making sure that the cow is aware of your approach and presence, the vulvar and peri-vulvar regions of the cow are cleaned with a towel or wipe. A sleeved, lubricated hand is then inserted into the rectum. Pushing down on the ventral floor of the rectum, above the vulva, will cause gapping between the labia, allowing for introduction of the insemination rod into the anterior vagina at an angle of about 30°.

Once in the vagina, the insemination rod is repositioned horizontally and directed cranially along the dorsal wall of the vagina toward the cervix. As an aid, the hand in the rectum can be moved cranially along the ventral floor to assist trans-rectally in directing the insemination rod toward the cranial vagina. The hand in the rectum is then used to manually transfix the cervix. Stabilizing the cervix is important in cattle because the cervix protrudes into the vaginal vault, forming a circumferential blind pouch known as the vaginal fornix. Through manual maneuvering of both the cervix and insemination rod, the rod is introduced into the cervix and threaded through it into the uterine body. Once the insemination rod tip is in the uterine body, as determined by transrectal palpation, the dose of semen is deposited. The rod is gently exteriorized from the reproductive tract, and the sleeved hand removed from the rectum.

Although the aforementioned technique is most commonly used for inseminating cattle, other modifications exist. One includes threading the insemination rod into the uterine horn ipsilateral to the ovulating ovary, and depositing the semen in or toward the tip of the horn.

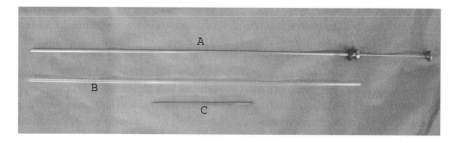

Figure 7.2. Cattle artificial insemination equipment. **(A):** insemination straw gun; **(B):** gun sheath; and **(C):** frozen-thawed semen straw.

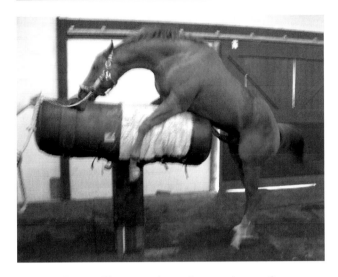

Figure 7.3. A stallion mounting a phantom dummy for semen collection. (Also see color plate)

Equine

Artificial insemination is frequently used in the equine industry. Fresh-extended semen for AI is popular in and between countries where transporting the mare to the stallion is feasible. Shipping of cool-extended semen for AI use at the resident mare's farm is favored when animal transportation is unrealistic or not feasible. The majority of equine AI is performed with extended-chilled semen within 48 to 72 hours of collection and processing. Frozen semen is another option when shipping semen to a mare for AI; however, conception rates can be lower than those from fresh-extended or cool-extended semen. Certain breed registries (i.e., The Jockey Club) do not recognize offspring produced through AI by any means.

Stallions may be housed at dedicated studs or at breeding farms. Stallions are sexually stimulated (e.g., teased) to elicit exteriorization of the penis and tumescence. The penis is washed and cleaned with warm water and disposable wipes. The stallion is then directed toward a mount mare or phantom and allowed to mount (see Figure 7.3). Once mounted, the penis is directed into an artificial vagina (see Figure 7.4). The combination of adequate AV pressure and temperature, sometimes specific to the stallion, stimulates ejaculation.

Stallion ejaculates contain a viscous gel fraction. This is filtered either through an in-line filter in the AV or with a free-standing filter immediately afterward. The gel-free ejaculate is then assessed for volume and sperm motility, morphology, concentration, and total numbers.

For fresh- or cool-extended semen, the semen is diluted with liquid media commonly referred to as an extender. Typically, 500 million to 1 billion total sperm are used as a single dose in a final volume of 50 to 60 mL. In general, the goal is to provide an insemination dose of at least 300 to 500 million progressively motile, morphologically normal sperm at the time of AI (Allen, 2005). If the extended

semen is not immediately used, it is stored at 5°C until use.

For frozen semen, the semen may be centrifuged and then diluted with a cryoprotectant extender, loaded into 0.25, 0.5, or 5 mL pre-labeled straws, and then frozen and stored in liquid nitrogen. Multiple frozen semen straws often are required to produce a single AI dose which consists of more than 300×10^6 motile, frozen-thawed sperm.

Visual signs of an estrous mare are best promoted using a teaser stallion. An estrous mare responds to the stallion by showing interest in his presence, raising her tail, everting her clitoris (e.g., winking), and urinating. In AI programs, it is not uncommon for supplemental diagnostic aids such as rectal palpation of the reproductive tract and/or visualization of the ovaries and uterus using B-mode ultrasonography to be used.

Using these breeding management tools, the goal is to inseminate the mare peri-ovulation (e.g., 48 hours before ovulation to six hours post-ovulation). Estrus can last up to seven to eight days in mares, with ovulation occurring one to two days before the end of estrus. Given the challenges of the lengthy estrus and inappropriate timing of insemination, pharmacologic manipulation to induce estrus and/or ovulation is common in many AI programs.

Once a mare is identified as being in estrus and has a follicle greater than 35 mm in diameter, she is eligible for insemination. For standard insemination, the mare is placed in stocks, her tail is wrapped, and the vulvar/peri-vulvar area is cleaned. The labia are parted, and a sterile sleeved, lubricated hand carrying a pipette is passed through the vagina (see Figure 7.5). The cervix is digitally located, and the pipette introduced into the cervix and gently advanced into the uterine body. A syringe containing the insemination dose is attached to the exteriorized portion of the pipette, and the dose slowly deposited in the uterine body while the hand in the vagina holds the mare's cervix closed around the pipette to minimize loss of semen. The cervix can continue to be held closed as the pipette is withdrawn. Once the pipette is out, the sleeved hand also is withdrawn from the vagina. The mare then is returned to her stall.

For fresh- and cool-extended semen, subsequent inseminations are performed every other day (assuming the

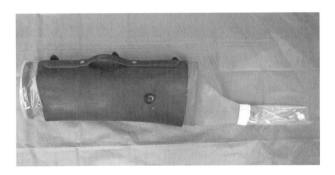

Figure 7.4. A Missouri artificial vagina for stallion semen collection. (Also see color plate)

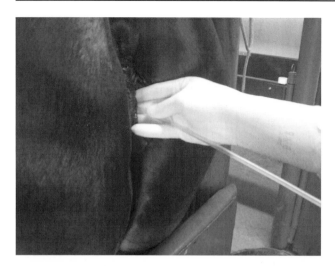

Figure 7.5. A sterile sleeved hand is used to part the mare's labia and introduce the insemination pipette. (Also see color plate)

stallion is of reasonable fertility) until ovulation is detected. Due to the reduced longevity of frozen-thawed semen, mares bred with frozen-thawed semen must be inseminated closer to ovulation (Allen, 2004). In these cases, more frequent monitoring via ultrasonography (up to every six hours) is performed to inseminate her either within six to 12 hours prior to ovulation or within six hours following ovulation, or both (see Figure 7.6). Using pharmacologic manipulation, a fixed-time insemination protocol has also been gaining interest in the industry (Wilsher and Allen, 2004).

Recently, low-dose insemination with less than 50×10^6 motile sperm in no more than 1 mL total volume has been investigated (Katila, 2005). Both transrectal deep intracornual and hysteroscopic insemination techniques have been used to deposit the low-dose inseminates at the tip of the uterine horn ipsilateral to the ovary that contains the dominant follicle. Due to the level of penetration of the reproductive tract and the small amount of inseminate which needs to be deposited at the uterotubal papilla, multiple personnel and sedation of the mare are frequently required. Pregnancy rates of 10 percent to 75 percent have been reported using these techniques (Morris et al., 2000; Morris et al., 2002; Morris et al., 2003; Brinsko et al., 2003; Sieme et al., 2003).

Porcine

Since the early 1990s, the global swine industry has rapidly embraced the use of AI in their reproductive management programs. In developed countries, pig production has evolved from the traditional extensive, outdoor operations to the current and predominant intensive, indoor production systems. It is through this evolution that the majority of piglets born today in developed countries are conceived through AI.

As the industry was making the transition from natural mating to AI, boars frequently were housed and semen collected and processed on-farm. Today, most boars used in AI programs are housed in dedicated studs located off-site from the sow breeding herd. The majority of boars used in commercial breeding operations are crossbred rather than purebred animals.

Young boars are inquisitive and easily trained to mount a stationary dummy (see Figure 7.7). Soon after mounting, the boar begins to thrust, exteriorizing his penis. Using a gloved hand, the semen collector grasps and locks the corkscrew tip portion of the penis in his hand. Applying constant pressure to the penile tip, the boar completes the exteriorization process and commences ejaculation. The boar ejaculate is the most voluminous of the domestic species, usually generating more than 200 mL in volume.

The ejaculate is filtered at the time of collection into a large thermos or cup. Filtering the semen during ejaculation is important in order to separate the bulbourethral gland gel fraction from the remaining ejaculate. The ejaculate is assessed for volume and sperm motility, morphology, concentration, and total numbers. Normal crossbred boar ejaculates generally exhibit more than 80 percent progressively motile sperm and more than 75 percent morphologically normal sperm. A typical ejaculate contains 99.5 billion ±

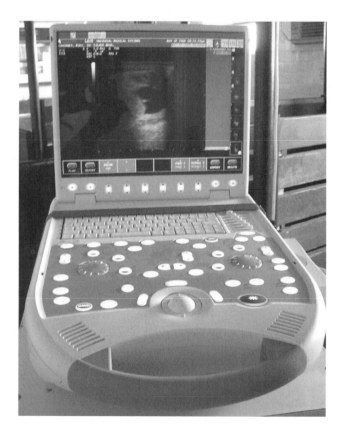

Figure 7.6. Use of transrectal B-mode ultrasonography to visualize a follicle on an equine ovary in situ.

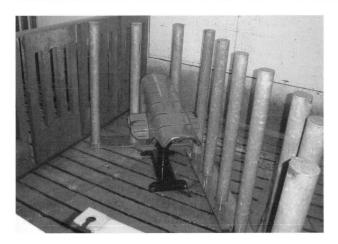

Figure 7.7. A typical boar semen collection pen and phantom mount. Note the spacing of vertical posts to allow the technician easy access and escape from the pen, while yet keeping the boar within the pen. (Also see color plate)

22 billion total sperm (Althouse and Kuster, 2000). If acceptable, the ejaculate is then diluted using a variety of commercially available semen extenders. Extenders are chosen according to the expected shelf life of the product, which can range from a few days to one week.

Unique to the commercial pig industry, many studs frequently pool several (e.g., usually three to six) ejaculates together prior to packaging into doses (Althouse et al., 1998). Pooling semen increases processing efficiency and decreases the effect of any one boar on herd reproductive performance. Understand, though, that semen is only pooled for doses intended to be used for producing slaughter market pigs.

Extended semen is processed into 75 to 90 mL doses of semen which contain 2 billion to 4 billion sperm. Doses are packaged in receptacles (e.g., bottles, tubes, flatpacks) made of a non-leaching plastic material that is non-toxic to spermatozoa. Dose receptacles are specifically designed to be flexible so that they can collapse naturally with the female's uptake of the semen. Extended-chilled semen packaged doses are stored at 15°C to 18°C until used for breeding. Frozen semen is also available for use in swine; however, its use is very limited currently due to its reduced fecundity.

Visual signs of an estrous gilt/sow are best promoted using a teaser boar. Behaviorally, estrus is primarily characterized by eliciting a rigid, immobilized, kyphotic, standing reflex in the gilt/sow. Other signs of estrus may include mounting other females, fence walking, vocalizing, tilted ears, vulvar swelling, and a vulvar discharge. Estrus lasts approximately 36 to 48 hours in gilts (nulliparous females) and 48 to 72-plus hours in sows (pluriparous females), with ovulation occurring mid- to late-estrus. Gilts/sows are teased daily—at a minimum—to determine if they are in estrus. Once identified, they are bred once a day until they no longer exhibit signs of estrus when exposed to a boar.

The goal of a successful AI program is to inseminate the gilt/sow peri-ovulation (e.g., 24 hours before ovulation to six hours post-ovulation). Due to this species' strong signs of estrus and their very predictable return to estrus post-weaning, pharmacological manipulation of the pig's estrus cycle is uncommon.

A single-use, disposable insemination (foam- or spiral-tip) pipette is used for artificial insemination (see Figure 7.8). After eliciting a rigid, standing reflex, the vulvar area is examined and, if soiled, cleaned with a disposable wipe. The vulval lips are parted using the AI technician's thumb and index finger, and the lubricated pipette gently inserted through the parted vulva in a forward and upward motion into the vagina (about 10 to 20 cm). The insemination pipette is then continued forward until it reaches the cervix. Foam-tipped pipettes conform to the cervical rings as it is pushed forward into the cervix, seating the pipette in the cervix. Spiral-tipped pipettes are seated in the cervix by physically rotating the pipette in a counter-clockwise fashion, locking it into the cervix. With either pipette, proper placement of the tip within the cervix is important to prevent leakage back into the vagina during the insemination process.

The extended semen dose is then attached to the exposed end of the pipette and pressure gently applied to the dose to start the flow of semen into the uterus. Once flow has commenced, the sow's uterine motility increases, allowing for passive uptake of the extended semen dose. Semen uptake can be stimulated or enhanced through boar presence and via the technician massaging and placing pressure on the back, flanks, and underline of the gilt/sow. The insemination process may take up to three to five minutes to complete. Transcervical- and deep-uterine insemination techniques have been described in swine (Watson and Behan, 2002; Rath et al., 2003; Vazquez et al., 2005).

Small Ruminants

A large percentage of small ruminant operations (e.g., sheep, goats) are managed as small flocks under free-range, extensive, outdoor systems. Due to this prevailing management style, along with inherent animal value and technical

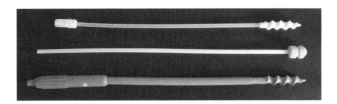

Figure 7.8. Swine artificial insemination pipettes. (**A**): single-use, disposable spiral tip pipette; (**B**): single-use, disposable foam-tip pipette; and (**C**): re-usable Melrose catheter. (Also see color plate)

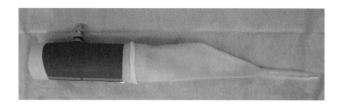

Figure 7.9. A complete ram/buck artificial vagina. (Also see color plate)

difficulty of the technique, AI is currently used by only a very small fraction of the global sheep and goat industries. Small purebred sheep/goat breeders and dairy goat operations are the routine users of AI. Interestingly, these industries may see increased implementation of this assisted reproductive technology as government mandated restrictions of animal movement are implemented to minimize the spread of disease.

Most rams and bucks are kept as flock animals on farms rather than at dedicated studs. Semen collection is performed using an AV designed for use on rams/bucks (see Figure 7.9). The male is allowed to mount a restrained, receptive female or mounting dummy. Once mounted, the AV is placed in front of the prepuce to allow the exteriorized penis to intromit directly into the AV. Rapid pelvic thrusting followed by ejaculation occur quickly, with the male rapidly dismounting post-ejaculation.

The ejaculate is assessed for volume and sperm motility, morphology and concentration. Satisfactory ejaculates exhibit better than 80 percent motility and better than 85 percent normal sperm morphology for the buck, and better than 30 percent motility and better than 51 percent normal sperm morphology for the ram (Bulgin, 1992). The ejaculate is then processed to be used as fresh-extended, cool-extended, or frozen semen. Fresh-extended and cool-extended semen is more commonly used in the goat; whereas, the sheep industry currently prefers the use of frozen semen in their AI programs. A typical intracervical or intrauterine insemination dose contains up to 200×10^6 sperm suspended in no more than 0.25 mL.

In temperate climatic zones both the ewe and doe are seasonally polyestrous, short-day breeders. Natural estrus can last up to 48 hours, with ovulation occurring mid- to late-estrus. Some AI programs employ the use of teaser animals once or twice a day for estrus detection. These teaser males are usually sterilized—either by vasectomy or epididymectomy—with or without penile translocation to prevent intromission. When exposed to a teaser animal, clinical signs of estrus include interest/attractiveness to the male, restlessness, vocalization, tail-flagging, frequent urination, and standing to be mounted. It is important to note that these signs are exhibited more prominently in does than in ewes.

Frequently, and in the absence of teaser males, many small ruminant AI programs employ pharmacologic manip-

ulation (e.g., prostaglandins, progestins, gonadotropins) to synchronize estrus and ovulation for a timed mating during seasonal and non-seasonal use (Baldassarre and Karatzas, 2004; Menchaca and Rubianes, 2004). Many researchers consider pharmacologic manipulation a key component to a successful AI program in small ruminants. The goal of any AI program is to inseminate a good quality dose of semen immediately prior to ovulation. In most situations, this insemination takes place 12 to 24 hours after initiation of standing estrus.

Once identified in natural estrus or after successful application of pharmacologic manipulation, the ewe or doe is prepared for insemination. The animal is restrained and her perineal area cleaned. For intravaginal insemination (IVI), the labia are parted and a pipette passed cranially along the dorsal wall of the vagina. Once resistance to further passage is felt, the pipette is retracted 1 to 2 cm, and the dose (3 billion to 4 billion sperm) deposited in the cranial vagina. In general, fertility rates associated with IVI are poor. As a result, this technique is not favored in sheep; this is true to a lesser extent in goats.

Intracervical insemination (ICI) is the preferred option in small ruminants. With this technique, the ewe/doe is restrained with her hindquarters elevated. After cleaning the perineal area, a lubricated speculum is passed into the vagina (see Figure 7.10). The external cervical os is visualized using illumination. A pipette is then visually passed through the speculum and into the cervix to a depth of 5 to 12 mm. After positioning the pipette in the cervix, the insemination dose is deposited.

Intrauterine insemination (IUI) is also used in small ruminants. Although both non-surgical and surgical techniques have been developed, preference is currently given to the surgical approach (i.e., laparoscopy, laparotomy) due

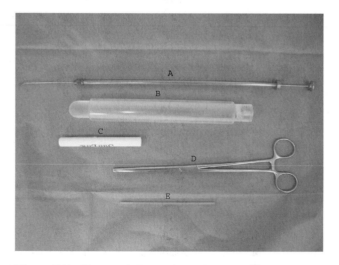

Figure 7.10. Sheep and Goat artificial insemination equipment. **(A):** small ruminant insemination gun; **(B):** vaginal speculum; **(C):** light source; **(D):** cervix holders; and **(E):** frozen-thawed semen straw.

to better success and fecundity results. As with any of our species in which surgical IUI is performed, inherent to the technique are the risks associated with placing an animal under general anesthesia and its concomitant welfare considerations. Conversely, the ewe's unique cervical anatomy makes for difficult catheter passage and possible tissue trauma when using the non-surgical IUI approach (Kershaw et al., 2005). Overall, ICI and IUI are currently the more favored techniques for use in small ruminant AI programs.

Canine

The domestic dog is known to be a fertile species, with the majority of pregnancies achieved under natural mating conditions. Even so, purebred breeders and the racing greyhound industry have embraced AI technologies due to the inherent genetic, economic, and logistical values it can provide. Fresh-unextended, cool-extended, and frozen semen are used in the industry. Fresh-unextended semen is inseminated into a female shortly (e.g., minutes) after collection. Cool-extended semen is typically used when the semen can be delivered and used within 48 to 72 hours of collection and processing. For long-term preservation, convenience, and long-distance shipping durability, frozen semen is the preferred modality.

The male breeding dog is either housed with his owner/guardian or at a mixed-sex kennel. With minimal training, semen is readily collected from most dogs by digital stimulation and application of pressure at the base of the penis. The presence of an estrus bitch can be helpful in stimulating arousal of the dog; however, many have found it unnecessary to obtain an ejaculate.

The dog is taken into a quiet room which has minimal distractions and good footing, and allowed to investigate personnel and surroundings. Once the dog appears relaxed, the handler restrains the dog in the standing position with a lead. The technician approaches and greets the dog and then gently runs his hand along the abdomen. The penis is initially massaged through the prepuce, causing arousal. The prepuce is manually retracted caudally behind the bulbus glandis. If an AV is used (see Figure 7.11), it is then slipped over the penis. Tourniquet digital pressure is applied behind the bulbus glandis, mimicking a "lock." The dog usually initiates pelvic thrusting concomitant with penile engorgement. Once fully engorged, the penis is rotated 180° caudally between the dog's hind legs. Ejaculation soon commences, with the pre-sperm, sperm-rich, and minimal post-sperm rich (e.g., prostatic fluid) fractions collected in the AV receptacle.

A more common alternative to the AV is to perform a free-catch of the sperm-rich fraction of the ejaculate into either a sterile specimen cup or other container. The ejaculate is assessed for volume and sperm motility, morphology, and concentration. Semen intended for extended use is diluted with an extender; with dose volume depends upon

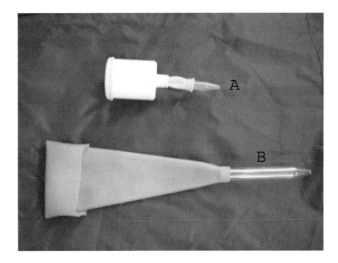

Figure 7.11. Cat (**A**) and dog (**B**) artificial vaginas for the collection of semen.

the number of doses needed and the size of the bitch to be inseminated. Generally, dose volume is between 2 and 10 mL and contains at least 100×10^6 sperm. If it is not used immediately, the extended semen is chilled to 5°C and stored until use. For frozen semen, the semen may be centrifuged and then diluted with a cryoprotectant extender. It is then frozen into pellets or loaded into 0.25 or 0.5 mL pre-labeled straws and frozen. Both pellets and straws are stored in liquid nitrogen. Generally, enough pellets or straws are thawed to obtain a minimum of 100 to 150×10^6 motile sperm for the insemination.

The domesticated bitch is seasonally monoestrous, exhibiting estrous only once or twice a year (for review, see Concannon et al., 1989). The interestrous interval can range from approximately five to 12 months, with an average of seven months. Signs of estrus are best elicited in the presence of an intact teaser dog. Hormonal profiling (e.g., progesterone, LH) and vaginal cytology (see Figure 7.12) can also be used with or without a teaser dog to estimate stage of estrous. Sexual activity is first observed in the proestrus bitch. The presence of a bloody, vulvar discharge (originating from the reproductive tract under estrogen influence) typically characterizes the onset of proestrus. Other signs include vulvar edema, restlessness, excitability, an increase in water intake, and increased urination. During proestrus, the bitch shows interest in the dog but will not stand to be mated. Proestrus can range from two to 15 days, with an average of nine days.

Estrus commences once the bitch accepts mating by assuming a rigid stance, moving her tail to the side and exposing her vulva by arching her back. Estrus can range from three to 12 days, with an average of 10 days. Ovulation generally occurs within five days after the onset of estrus.

Canidae release immature, primary ovocytes at ovulation (Reynaud et al., 2005). First polar body extrusion and subsequent completion of meiosis occur in the oviduct. As

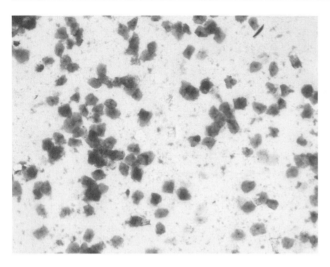

Figure 7.12. Vaginal cytology in a bitch. Sample shows predominantly keratinized epithelial cells, indicative of an estrus bitch. (Also see color plate)

such, dogs are unique in that the oocyte remains viable for days rather than hours, as seen in our other domestic species. Generally, it takes two to three days for ovulated oocytes to become fertilizable. Using a combination of behavioral signs, serial hormonal profiling, and serial vaginal cytology, insemination(s) is targeted an estimated one to five days post-ovulation. Pharmacologic manipulation for induction and synchronization of estrus in the dog is possible (Kutzler, 2005). Variability in treatment efficacy and subsequent fertility, however, have precluded significant clinical use.

Most estrus bitches in AI programs are examined daily to approximate the day of ovulation and, subsequently, the opportune time that fertilizable oocytes are present in the oviduct. For standard intravaginal insemination (IVI), the bitch is restrained and her perineal area cleaned. The vulvae are parted and a plastic pipette (see Figure 7.13) gently inserted and passed cranially along the dorsal vaginal wall. Transabdominal palpation can help to facilitate advancement of the pipette into the cranial vagina. The cervix lies cranio-dorsally from the tip of the vaginal vault. A pseudocervix, approximately 2.5 to 3 cm caudal to the cervix, is present in the cranial vagina and is formed by a distinctive dorsal median fold (Pineda, 1973). This pseudocervix elicits resistance, making further pipette passage difficult.

Many times, the semen dose is deposited at the pseudocervix while still achieving acceptable fertility results. The pipette is withdrawn and the bitch's vestibulum digitally stimulated for a few minutes to elicit strong vaginal contractions to aid in movement of semen up to the site of fertilization. With good quality semen and appropriate AI timing, pregnancy rates can exceed 80 percent. When using frozen semen, a single-timed transcervical (TCI) or surgical insemination are the preferred methods. Poor fertility results are usually achieved with frozen semen if it is used by IVI.

For TCI, a rigid cystoscope, with relay optics, is passed into the cranial vagina as with an IVI pipette (Pretzer et al., 2006). The vaginal vault is visualized as the cystoscope is advanced cranially by both cystoscope manipulation and transabdominal palpation. The cystoscope is passed under the pseudocervix and advanced cranially to visualize and abut the external cervical os. A flexible 8 french urinary catheter is passed through the cystoscope guide and advanced into the cervix. The small dose (less than 2 mL) inseminate is then deposited intrauterine, which is determined by visualizing the insemination process to ensure no backflow has occurred. The cystoscope is removed and the vestibulum digitally stimulated as with IVI.

Surgical insemination is performed under general anesthesia on a dorsally recumbent dog. Either through laparoscopy or by laparotomy, each uterine horn is inseminated via needle puncture, the abdomen closed, and the dog allowed to recover. With good quality semen and appropriate insemination timing, 70 percent or better pregnancy rates can be obtained.

Feline

As with dogs, the cat population has a propensity for excellent reproductive performance. Given this innate attribute as well as the complexities in tom semen collection and overall low client demand, AI is uncommon in cats. Even so, a fair bit of research has been performed on cat AI, with published success. Looking outside its application to the domestic cat population, much of this research has aided in propagating some of our endangered wild cat species.

The behavior and undesirable smell makes a tom unsuitable for a household pet. As such, small numbers of toms are kept in captivity and, if so, usually are housed in a mixed-sex cattery. Semen can be collected using an AV (see Figure 7.11); however, even trained toms can exhibit adverse behavior and temperament when exposed to an estrus queen, making application of the technique difficult.

The most common method of collecting semen from a tom is by electroejaculation (EE). In this method, a probe with electrodes is placed in the rectum of an anesthetized

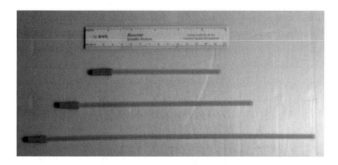

Figure 7.13. Various length artificial insemination pipettes used in inseminating dogs.

tom. The prepuce is retracted to expose the penis. A series of electrical stimulations of various amplitudes and frequencies are then applied to the probe via an electroejaculator unit (Howard et al., 1990). The electrical stimulation elicits muscle contractions in the tom's reproductive tract allowing for emission of an ejaculate which is collected in a small receptacle located at the tip of the penis.

Tom ejaculates are small in volume. If sufficient volume is obtained, sperm motility, morphology, and concentration may be obtained. The semen is then either used immediately unextended or processed for cool-extended or frozen semen. An insemination dose contain 5 to 80×10^6 sperm in less than 1 mL total volume.

Queens are seasonally polyestrous, long-day breeders. Domestic queens are also induced ovulators. That is, ovulation is triggered by mechanical stimulation of the vagina during natural mating. With sufficient vaginal stimulation, ovulation occurs 18 to 24 hours later.

The queen behavior's and vaginal cytology are used to determine if she is in estrus. Behavioral signs are quite obvious, and include increased rolling and rubbing against objects, more frequent and louder vocalization, and induction of lordosis when rubbing the queen's back or when put in the presence of a tom. In AI programs, ovulation is artificially induced using pharmacologic manipulation (e.g., gonadotropins or precursors to) the day before the scheduled AI (Goodrow et al., 1987).

Intravaginal insemination is an option for cats; however, transcervical (TCI) or surgical insemination procedures generally provide for much higher fecundity rates (Zambelli and Cunto, 2005) when using reduced numbers of sperm and/or for frozen semen. For TCI, the queen is heavily sedated or anesthetized. The labia are parted and a lubricated, rigid, small diameter catheter is advanced into the cranial vagina to the cervical os. A flexible 3 french catheter is then threaded through the rigid catheter and through the cervix. Directing both catheters is greatly facilitated by trans-rectal digital manipulation (see Figure 7.14). Once intrauterine, the semen dose is deposited and both the inner and outer catheters withdrawn.

Intrauterine deposition of semen in the anesthetized queen can be performed surgically via laparotomy or laparoscopy. For surgical insemination, the uterus is visualized and semen deposited into either one or both uterine horns via needle puncture. With good quality semen and appropriate technique, a 34 percent to 80 percent pregnancy rate can be attained.

Other Artificial Reproductive Technologies

Artificial insemination (including IVI, TCI, IUI, and low-dose AI) is the most commonly used of the current artificial reproductive technologies. Other important ART exist and are worth a brief discussion. It is important to appreciate that pharmacologic manipulation is an important, if not critical, component (e.g., estrus induction, ovulation, super-

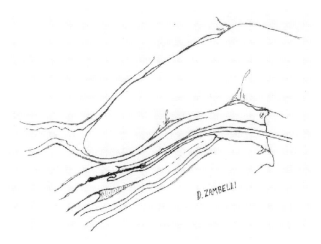

Figure 7.14. Domestic feline artificial insemination technique showing the use of trans-rectal digital manipulation to facilitate AI catheter passage into the uterus.

ovulation, estrus synchronization) in these other ART. Many times these technologies are used as a means of treatment for subfertility or infertility in the animal, but they can also be used simply to propagate desired genetics.

Embryo transfer (ET) is a popular technique used in cattle and horses, and to a lesser extent in the other domestic species. In most species, this procedure requires the surgical/nonsurgical harvesting of preimplantation embryo(s) from the donor animal and transferring this embryo(s) either surgically or nonsurgically into the uterus of a synchronized recipient animal. Embryos can be cooled and stored for short periods of time (preferably less than 24 hours), or frozen if long-term storage is desired.

A newer ART is oocyte transfer (OT), in which oocytes are recovered from mature follicles by laparotomy/laparoscopy or by transvaginal aspiration using ultrasonography. The oocyte(s) is then surgically transferred into the oviduct of the recipient animal, which is then bred naturally or artificially inseminated with the goal of obtaining and carrying this pregnancy to term.

A modification of OT is gamete intrafallopian transfer (GIFT), in which oocytes are harvested as with OT. Matured oocytes and sperm are then transferred together into the oviduct of a recipient animal, with the goal of fertilization, pregnancy, and birth of offspring. A variant of GIFT is zygote intrafallopian transfer (ZIFT), in which a zygote is developed *in vitro* and then transferred to the oviduct of a recipient animal for further development into offspring.

In vitro fertilization (IVF) is an ART which has been applied in practice for a couple of decades. With IVF, harvested, matured oocytes and sperm are placed in media and incubated together *in vitro* in an environmentally controlled chamber. Preimplantation embryos which develop from this union are then transferred to the uterus of a recipient animal to achieve pregnancy and offspring.

A form of IVF is intracytoplasmic sperm injection (ICSI), in which sperm are obtained either from the ejaculate, or via testicular sperm extraction (TESE), or even by microscopic (MESA) or percutaneous (PESA) epididymal sperm aspiration. An individual sperm is then injected directly into a mature oocyte. The sperm-injected oocyte(s) can then be transferred via OT into a recipient or *in vitro* cultured for seven to eight days and then the preimplantation embryo(s) transferred into the recipient's uterus. If mature sperm are unavailable for ICSI, another option is to use round spermatid nucleus injection (ROSNI) or round spermatid injection (ROSI) to try to obtain a zygote or embryo for transfer to a recipient.

References

Allen, W.R. (2005). The development and application of the modern reproductive technologies to horse breeding. *Reprod. Dom. Anim.* 40:310–29.

Althouse, G.C., Levis, D.G., Diehl, J. (1998). Semen collection, evaluation, and processing in the boar. *Pork Industry Handbook,* Purdue University Cooperative Extension Service, West Lafayette, IN: 1–6.

Althouse, G.C., Kuster, C.E. (2000). *A survey of current boar stud practices in USA production.* Paper presented at the 16th International Pig Veterinary Society Congress, Sept. 17–20, in Melbourne, Australia.

Baldassarre, H., Karatzas, C.N. (2004). Advanced assisted reproduction technologies (ART) in goats. *Animal Reproduction Science* 82–83:255–66.

Bonadonna, T. (1937). Le basi scientifiche e le possibilite applicative della fecondazione artificiale neglianimale domestica. Casa Ed. Vannini, Brescia, Italy.

Brinsko, S.P., Rigby, S.L., Lindsey, A.C., Blanchard, T.L., Love, C.C., Varner, D.D. (2003). Pregnancy rates in mares following hysteroscopic or transrectally-guided insemination with low sperm numbers at the utero-tubal papilla. *Theriogenology* 59:1001–09.

Bulgin, M.S. (1992). Ram breeding soundness examination and SFT form. *Proceedings for the Annual Meeting of the Society for Theriogenology,* San Antonio, TX: 210–15.

Concannon, P.W., McCann, J.P., Temple, M. (1989). Biology and endocrinology of ovulation, pregnancy and parturition in the dog. *J. Reprod. Fertil. Suppl.* 39:3–25.

DeJarnette, J.M. (2004). Industry application of technology in male reproduction. *Proceedings from the Applied Reproductive Strategies in Beef Cattle Conference,* Sept 1–2, North Platte, NE: 204–17.

DeJarnette, J.M., Marshall, C.E., Lenz, R.W., Monke, D.R., Ayars, W.H., Sattler, C.G. (2004). Sustaining the fertility of artificially inseminated dairy cattle: the role of the artificial insemination industry. *J. Dairy Sci.* 87:(E. Suppl.):E93-E104.

Goodrowe, K.L., Wildt, D.E. (1987). Ovarian response to human chorionic gonadotropin or gonadotropin releasing hormone in cats in natural or induced estrus. *Theriogenology* 27:811–17.

Heape, W. (1897). The artificial insemination of mammals and subsequent possible fertilization or impregnation of their ova. Proceedings of the Royal Society of London. *Series B, Biological Sciences* 61:52–63.

Heape, W. (1898). On the artificial insemination of mares. *Veterinarian* 71:202–12.

Ivanoff, E.I. (1922). On the use of artificial insemination for zootechnical purposes in Russia. *J. Agric. Sci.* 12:244–56.

Katila, T. (2005). Effect of the inseminate and the site of insemination on the uterus and pregnancy rates of mares. *Animal Reproduction Science* 89:31–38.

Kershaw, C.M., Khalid, M., McGowan, M.R., Ingram, K., Leethongdee, S., Wax, G., Scaramuzzi, R.J. (2005). The anatomy of the sheep cervix and its influence on the transcervical passage of an inseminating pipette into the uterine lumen. *Theriogenology* 64(5):1225–35.

Kutzler, M.A. (2005). Induction and synchronization of estrus in dogs. *Theriogenology* 64(3):766–75.

Menchaca, A., Rubianes, E. (2004). New treatments associated with timed artificial insemination in small ruminants. *Reproduction, Fertility and Development* 16:403–13.

Milovanov, V.K. (1938). Isskusstvenoye ossemenebie selskokhoziasvennykh jivotnykh (The Artificial Insemination of Farm Animals). Seljhozgiz, Moscow.

Morris, L.H.A., Hunter, R.H., Allen, W.R. (2000). Hysteroscopic insemination of small numbers of spermatozoa at the uterotubal junction of preovulatory mares. *J. Reprod. Fertil.* 118:95–100.

Morris, L.H.A., Allen, W.R. (2002). An overview of low dose insemination in the mare. *Reprod. Dom. Anim.* 37:206–10.

Morris, L.H.A., Tiplady, C., Allen, W.R. (2003). Pregnancy rates in mares after a single fixed time hysteroscopic insemination of low numbers of frozen-thawed spermatozoa onto the uterotubal junction. *Equine Vet. J.* 35:197–201.

Perry, Enos J. (1968). The Artificial *Insemination of Farm Animals, 4th revised ed.* New Brunswick: Rutgers University Press.

Pineda, M.H., Kainer, R.A., Faulkner, L.C. (1973). Dorsal median postcervical fold in the canine vagina. *Am. J. Vet. Res.* 34:1487.

Pretzer, S.D., Lillich, R.K., Althouse, G.C. (2006). Single, transcervical insemination using frozen-thawed semen in the greyhound: A case series study. *Theriogenology* 65(2006): 1029–36.

Rath, D., Ruiz, S., Sieg B. (2003). Birth of small piglets following intrauterine insemination of a sow using flow cytometrically sexed boar semen. *Vet Rec.* 152(13):400–1.

Reynaud, K., Fontbonne, A., Marseloo, N., Thoumire, S., Chebrout, M., de Lesegno, C.V., Chastant-Maillard, S. (2005). In vivo meiotic resumption, fertilization and early embryonic development in the bitch. *Reproduction* 130(2): 193–201.

Sieme, H., Bonk, A., Hamann, H., Klug, E., Katila, T. (2004). Effects of different artificial insemination techniques and sperm doses on fertility of normal mares and mares with abnormal reproductive history. *Theriogenology* 62:915–28.

Spallanzani, L. (1784). *Dissertations Relative to the Natural History of Animals and Vegetables.* 2:195–99. Translated. by T. Beddoes.

Vazquez, J.M., Martinez, E.A., Roca, J., Gil M.A., Parrilla I., Carvajal, G., Lucas, X., Vazquez, J.L. (2005). Improving the efficiency of sperm technologies in pigs: the value of deep intrauterine insemination. *Theriogenology* 63(2):536–47.

Watson, P.F., Behan, J.R. (2002). Intrauterine insemination of sows with reduced sperm numbers: results of a commercially based field trial. *Theriogenology* 57(6):1683–93.

Wilsher S., Allen W.R. (2004). Factors controlling micro-cotyledon development and placental efficiency in thoroughbreds: influences of mare age, parity and nutritional insults. *Proceedings from the Workshop on Equine Placenta.* Kentucky Agricultural Experiment Station, Lexington, KY: 58–64.

Zambelli, D., Cunto, M. (2005). Transcervical artificial insemination in the cat. Proceedings of the Annual Conference of the Society for Theriogenology, Charleston, South Carolina. *Theriogenology* 64(3):698–705.

Chapter 8

Embryo Transfer and *In Vitro* Fertilization

John F. Hasler

In its strictest form, embryo transfer (ET) is the process of moving one or more embryos from the reproductive tract of one female to another. Transfers may be conducted by either surgical or nonsurgical procedures and may involve transferring the embryo(s) from either the oviduct or uterus of one female, known as a donor, into the oviduct or uterus of another female, known as a recipient. Embryo transfer also may involve the transfer of laboratory-produced embryo(s), such as those made by *in vitro* or cloning procedures, into the reproductive tract of a recipient.

Embryo transfer procedures are widely used both in commercial programs to produce livestock and in various research contexts. In the human field, all of the reproductive technologies associated with embryo transfer now are grouped in the field of assisted reproductive technology (ART). In fact, it might be appropriate to apply the acronym ART to all the technologies covered in this review.

Commercial embryo transfer has been most widely used in cattle, with millions of animals produced over the past 35 years. The modern livestock ET industry is a result of the pioneering efforts of two groups: the scientists who initially developed the procedures and techniques of ET and, later, the commercial practitioners who modified this technology, making it practical and available first to the cattle industry and then to the livestock industry in general. As used henceforth, ET will refer individually or collectively to the collection, handling, and transfer of embryos.

Historical Background

Credit for the first successful transfer of mammalian embryos is given to Walter Heape, an Englishmen who had an amazingly wide range of interests that included animal breeding. In 1890, Heape transferred two 4-cell Angora rabbit embryos into an inseminated Belgian doe which subsequently gave birth to four Belgian and two Angora young (Heape, 1891). A later paper actually described Heape's technique for handling rabbit embryos, which involved spearing them on the tip of a needle and transferring them to a recipient without an intermediary step of placing them in holding medium (Heape, 1897).

As documented by Betteridge (1981), there is no further record of any successful ETs until the 1920s, when several investigators again reported on transfers in rabbits. During this period, better understanding of the relationship between the pituitary and ovaries led to significant advancements in reproductive technology. Also, development of techniques for superovulation, estrous synchronization, and artificial insemination (AI) set the stage during the 1930s and '40s for successful ET in a number of species—not including cattle, however.

Although Umbaugh (1949) reported four pregnancies in Texas resulting from the transfer of cattle embryos in 1949, all the recipients aborted prior to term. In 1951, the first ET calf was born following the surgical transfer of a slaughter-house-derived day-5 embryo (Willett et al., 1951). It perhaps is unfortunate that most members of the team responsible for this achievement were subsequently directed to pursue development of AI technology, leaving Willett alone to pursue ET research (Betteridge, 2000). Willett moved to Michigan State University in 1956 and died shortly thereafter.

Development of the Modern Commercial Embryo Transfer Industry

Commercial ET started in the early 1970s, in North America, and cattle were the initial focus among farm animals.

Cattle

Commercial ET began in cattle primarily as a result of the high prices being paid for various breeds of so called "exotic" beef cattle that had been imported in small numbers from Europe. Initially, all embryo recoveries and transfers were performed surgically. Although early investigators described nonsurgical embryo recovery techniques (Rowson and Dowling, 1949; Dziuk et al., 1958), these worked rather poorly and few embryos were recovered. As a consequence, the first commercial ET programs during the early 1970s relied on mid-ventral surgical exposure of the uterus and ovaries with the donor under general anesthesia.

Concurrent with the escalating value of exotic cattle, the newly available prostaglandin $F_{2\alpha}$ made synchronization of donors and recipients practical. The necessity for anesthesia and surgery limited most ET to in-house programs with suitable facilities. Another reason that ET was not widely used by the dairy cattle owners at that time was because the udder of dairy cows hindered mid-ventral access to the reproductive tract. The introduction of nonsurgical embryo recovery (flushing) in the mid-1970s and nonsurgical transfer techniques in the late 1970s (for review, see Betteridge, 1977) allowed ET to be practiced on the farm and made it especially attractive to dairy farmers.

The cattle ET industry grew rapidly in the late 1970s, both in the number of practitioners and the number of donors flushed. Prior to the early 1980s, however, the inability to freeze and thaw embryos made it necessary to maintain sufficient numbers of estrous-synchronized recipients so that all embryos could be transferred on any given day. After effective methods of freezing embryos were developed, using either dimethyl sulfoxide or glycerol as cryoprotectants (Wilmut and Rowson, 1973), ET became a much more efficient technology that no longer depended on the immediate availability of suitable recipient cattle. There were no significant additional improvements in ET technology during the 1980s.

A change in the U.S. federal tax regulations in 1986 eliminated the tax advantages of owning cattle as investments and reduced the sale value of many donor cows. This reduced ET activity, at least temporarily, for many ET businesses in the United States. Today, traditional ET technology provides relatively consistent results, and many practitioners have 20 or more years experience in an industry that is mature.

Size of the Cattle ET Industry

The exact size of the cattle ET industry is somewhat difficult to determine. Two statistics can help estimate the scope of ET activity in any given geographical area and/or period of time: practitioners of ET can be polled, or the number of calves that are produced by ET can be determined. Unfortunately, neither of these statistics can be assessed accurately. Not all practitioners belong to an ET organization, and of those who do, a significant percentage do not return questionnaire/census forms (American Embryo Transfer Association, personal communication). Although most ET is conducted on registered rather than grade or commercial cattle, not all breed organizations differentiate between calves that result from ET versus AI or natural breeding. The membership in a number of embryo transfer organizations is shown in Table 8.1.

Founded in 1974 with 82 charter members, the International Embryo Transfer Society (IETS) is the oldest organization of its kind and the only one that is international. Throughout the 1990s, the size of the membership in the IETS has changed very little and currently there are approximately 1,000 members representing 45 countries. There has been a significant change in the vocational composition of the membership, however. With the founding of regional ET organizations, a growing number of commercial ET practitioners have discontinued membership in the IETS in favor of their regional organizations. It appears that after rapid and significant increases in membership during the

Table 8.1. International and national embryo transfer organizations.

Organization	Year founded	Membership
International Embryo Transfer Society (IETS)	1974	~1000
American Embryo Transfer Association (AETA)	1982	340
Canadian Embryo Transfer Association (CETA)	1984	102
Brazilian Society for Embryo Technology (SBTE)	1985	536
European Embryo Transfer Association (AETE)	1986	~170
Japanese Embryo Transfer Society (JETS)	1987	291
Australian Embryo Transfer Society (AETS)	1990	113

1980s, there has been little change in membership of regional ET organizations in the United States, Canada, and Europe. In contrast, the Brazilian society has seen a remarkable increase in membership during the 1990s and currently has more than 500 members.

At the 2006 annual meeting of the IETS, the largest number of abstracts (62) dealt with cloning/nuclear transfer, whereas superovulation and embryo transfer were represented by only 10 and eight abstracts, respectively. Large numbers of abstracts also dealt with developmental biology, *in vitro* procedures, gene expression, transgenesis, and other categories not directly related to ET. Thus, it is clear that a majority of the IETS now is composed of basic researchers representing government and industrial or academic institutions rather than ET practitioners. As a result, the actual processes involved in commercial embryo transfer are now more frequently emphasized in the meetings of the regional associations listed in Table 8.1.

Even within some countries, there are distinctions between organizations that represent the basic sciences related to ET and those that represent commercial practitioners. For example, the Japanese Embryo Transfer Society (JETS), as shown in Table 8.1, has 291 members, most of whom are engaged in basic research (personal communication), whereas most practitioners belong to either the Eastern Japan Embryo Transfer Society (389 members) or the Hokkaido Bovine Embryo Transfer Society (160 members).

In the United States, there have been significant changes—both increases and decreases—in the overall numbers of registrations among different breed associations as well as in the number of calves that are produced by ET and registered yearly. The percentage of all registered Holstein calves produced by ET has exceeded 5 percent for the last 10 years, and the percentage of Angus calves has exceeded 5 percent for the last six years. In contrast, Herefords resulting from ET have never exceeded 2 percent of all registrations. Although they are not illustrated here, a number of other beef breeds have undergone a similar decline. In contrast, the number of Angus, both total registrations and ETs, has steadily increased throughout the last 25 years.

Holstein breeders adopted the use of ET in the early 1970s, with the number of registered calves reaching a peak in the late 1980s. The inability to market all the bulls produced may have depressed the frequency with which dairy farmers have used ET. In 2005, for example, of the approximately 20,000 ET calves registered by the Holstein Association USA, Inc., only 34 percent of total registrations were males.

Another approach to determining the scope of ET activity is to take a census of the members of regional organizations. As noted above, this is a notoriously inaccurate approach because not all practitioners belong to ET organizations and even among the members, only 50 percent comply (AETA, personal communication).

After remaining fairly stable throughout the 1990s, the annual number of cattle embryo recoveries in the United States has increased over the past few years, with more than 42,000 reported for 2005 (AETA, unpublished). Unfortunately, the negative impact during the past few years of bovine spongiform encephalopathy (BSE) on cattle exports from Canada led to a decrease in ET activity, with approximately 11,000 recoveries reported for 2005, compared to more than 14,000 in 2002 (Canadian Embryo Transfer Association, unpublished). The number of cattle embryos recovered in 2004 throughout the world is shown in Figure 8.1.

The largest amount of ET activity was in North and South America. An interesting difference between these two regions is that a majority of embryos are cryopreserved after collection in North America, whereas a majority are transferred fresh in South America. Brazil is the only country in which available data indicate a large increase in ET activity during the past few years. Paralleling the increase in the number of ET practitioners, the number of embryos transferred in Brazil increased from approximately 40,000 in 1995 to 74,000 in 1999 (J.L. Rodrigues, personal communication) and grew to 102,100 in 2004 (Thibier, 2005).

It is even more difficult to determine the scope of ET activity in other species of domestic animals than it is in cattle. Fewer practitioners are involved with ET in pigs, horses, goats, sheep, and dogs and cats, and thus obtaining census information from them is difficult. Furthermore, tabulating ET activity through these species' breed organizations is not productive.

Horses

Embryo transfer in horses has grown substantially in North America in the last few years, due, at least in part, to a change in the regulations of the American Quarter Horse Association (AQHA). The new regulations permit the registration of an unlimited number of ET foals per mare each year, whereas only one per year was previously allowed. The use of frozen semen for insemination in ET procedures was allowed at the same time. In 2006, the AQHA voted to allow the cryopreservation of embryos starting in 2007 (personal communication). Recent reviews of ART procedures in horses include those of Allen (2005), Hinrichs (2005), and Squires (2005).

Pigs

The first ET piglets were produced in 1950 in Ukraine (Kvasnitski, 1950). This led to the slow but steady growth of a commercial pig ET industry in a few countries. It has proven particularly difficult to assess the amount of ET activity in the swine industry. The largest number of transfers in 2004 includes 9,780 in Korea, 2,448 in Canada, and 885 in Taiwan (Thibier, 2005). There are no records for the United States or most other countries. This is partly due to the fact that a large share of pig ET is performed on large, corporate-owned swine production farms and therefore the scope of the work is often confidential. Reviews on the status of ART in the pig include those of Hazeleger and Kemp (1999), Day (2000), Youngs (2001), and Martinez, et al. (2005).

Most of the commercial ET activity in the swine industry involves the movement of genetics between large pathogen-free facilities. Difficulties in the cryopreservation of pig embryos have greatly limited the international movement of embryos from this species. It was recently demonstrated that ET provides a viable method of increasing the numbers of an endangered breed of pigs (Mangalica) that is characterized by small litter sizes (Rátky et al., 2000).

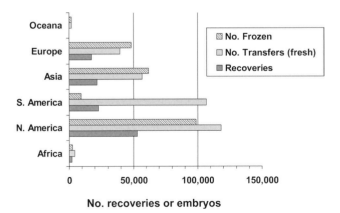

Figure 8.1. The number of cattle donor embryo recoveries and the number of embryos transferred and frozen in major regions of the world in 2004. Courtesy of Thibier, 2005.

Sheep and Goats

Commercial ET in these two species is practiced on a large scale in only a few countries, and the scale of sheep ET is considerably larger than that for goats. Data available to the IETS indicate more than 68,000 transfers of sheep embryos during 2004, primarily in South Africa, Australia, and New Zealand (Thibier, 2005). Fewer than 2,000 goat embryos were transferred, primarily in South Africa. These figures are undoubtedly greatly underreported. Reviews on ART in these species include those of Tibary et al. (2005), Cognié (1999), and Cognié et al. (2003).

Dogs and Cats

"Man's best friend" has merited such close attention throughout recorded history that perhaps it is not surprising that the first known successful artificial insemination was performed in a dog by Spallanzani in 1780 (Heape, 1897). Subsequent progress in knowledge about dog reproduction was slow, however, perhaps due to a lack of commercial value compared to domestic farm animals. Only a few reports on embryo transfer in dogs have been published, and the success was limited (reviewed in Farstad 2000a, 2000b).

In a recent review of ART in dogs and cats, Farstad (2000b) describes as "an understatement" the phrase "cats are not small dogs," and it is clear from the literature that far more progress has been made in understanding basic reproduction in cats compared to dogs. A good deal of the research involving ART and ET in domestic cats has been directed at their use as a model for the numerous species of wild felids that are endangered. ART procedures are more highly developed in cats than in dogs (Farstad, 2000b; Pope, 2000) and, in fact, cryopreservation procedures have resulted in good pregnancy rates following ET (Swanson, et al., 1999).

Superovulation

The species covered in this review include almost exclusively monotocous (horses), usually monotocous (cattle), twin-bearing (sheep and goats), polytocous with small or moderate litters (dogs and cats), and polytocous with large litters (pigs). When females of any of these species are used as embryo donors, *superovulation*, or the induction of the maturation and ovulation of more ova than normal, is usually induced with the injection of a gonadotrophin. The gonadotropin most frequently used is follicle stimulating hormone (FSH) purified from porcine or ovine pituitary glands. In some cases, equine chorionic gonadotropin (eCG), formerly known as pregnant mare serum gonadotropin (PMSG), is used, although it is less popular due to its long half-life.

Cattle

The most frequently reported average number of embryos recovered from superovulated cows is between four and seven. However, the range of response is quite large, with more than 100 ova and as many as 60 or more viable embryos occasionally recovered. It is generally accepted

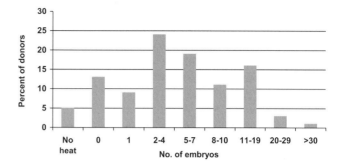

Figure 8.2. The distribution of the number of embryos recovered from each of 984 Holstein cows.

that the observed variation stems more from genetic variation among individual females than factors such as the specific gonadotropin used or the breed of cattle. Many reports indicate that beef breeds of cattle produce slightly more embryos on average than dairy breeds. Although well-controlled comparisons of superovulation among different breeds have not been conducted, data tabulated from the members of the Canadian and American ET associations indicate that beef cattle produced an average of approximately one more embryo per superovulation attempt than did dairy cattle. The distribution of the numbers of embryos recovered from nearly 1,000 Holstein cows, each superovulated once, is shown in Figure 8.2.

The mean number of embryos recovered from this group was approximately six; however, more than 50 percent of them produced fewer than four embryos and nearly 20 percent produced no embryos. Thus, the inconsistency of superovulation, rather than the average number of embryos recovered, is a major factor adding to the expense of embryo transfer in cattle and detracting from the wider application of the technology. Looney (1986) clearly illustrated this problem with the report that in a large commercial cattle ET program, 24 percent of superovulated donors produced no embryos and only 30 percent produced 70 percent of the total number of embryos.

A typical superovulation protocol for cattle involves twice daily injections of FSH for four days. Donors are started in mid-cycle, usually eight to 13 days after a previous estrus (Hasler, et al., 1983; Donalson, 1984) or four days after insertion of a controlled intrauterine drug-releasing devices (CIDR) (reviewed by Bo et al., 2002).

A large body of evidence indicates that the fertility of dairy cattle has significantly declined over the past 20 years on a worldwide basis (Thatcher et al., 2006). Nevertheless, a recent analysis of a large number of superovulation records over a 20-year period did not indicate that response to superovulation in dairy cattle has declined (Hasler, 2006).

Horses

Until recently, single embryo collections were the norm for mares because superovulation usually was not successful. Although it is not clear why, FSH derived from porcine or ovine pituitaries does not reliably induce superovulation in mares, even though it works quite well in cattle, sheep, goats, and pigs. However, an equine FSH pituitary extract (eFSH) first studied at Colorado State University, and now available commercially, has proven to successfully induce superovulation in the mare. Responses to eFSH in mares are not as large as those seen in cattle and other species, and when large responses do occur, embryo collection rates are usually disappointing. This is due to the fact that follicles in the mare can only ovulate and release their oocyte through the ovulation fossa because of the fibrous tunica albuginea that covers the rest of the external surface of the mare ovary (Allen, 2005). Nevertheless, ovulation rates and embryo recovery rates have proven to be about four times greater than single ovulations and the mean of 0.5 embryos per recovery is standard in cycling mares (Squires, et al., 2003).

Pigs

Sows can be successfully superovulated with eCG followed by hCG. However, because sows normally ovulate large numbers of ova, superovulation is less effective than in other species of farm animals and is often not part of pig ET programs (Youngs, 2001). Synchronization of estrus is often achieved by simultaneously weaning groups of sows at three to four weeks of lactation because prostaglandin $F_{2\alpha}$ is much less effective for inducing luteolysis in pigs than in cattle.

Sheep and Goats

Protocols for the superovulation of both sheep and goats usually involve synchronization of the estrous cycle with intravaginal sponges that contain progesterone. The use of a gonadatropin-releasing hormone (GnRH) antagonist, injected three times over a 10-day period to suppress endogenous gonadotropins, has proven efficacious, with an average of 10 embryos per ewe recovered (Cognié et al., 2003). Both multiple injections of FSH and single injections of eCG are used in various commercial superovulation programs in these two species.

As in cattle, there is a high degree of variability in response to superovulation, with a range of zero to 30 transferable embryos recovered. It was estimated that more than 25 percent of superovulated donor goats fail to produce any transferable embryos (Baldassarre, 2004).

Dogs and Cats

Because both of these species are polytocous and there is virtually no commercial application of ET, there are few reports of superovulation. Verstegen et al. (1993) reported recovering an average of nine embryos from cats superovulated with porcine FSH. Superovulation has been used to stimulate follicular growth in the dog so that oocytes can be collected for *in vitro* procedures (Yamada et al., 1993).

Insemination

Donor females are inseminated either artificially (AI) or by natural service, depending on the species and the specific situation. For example, frozen semen is used almost exclusively for transcervical artificial insemination in cattle. In rare cases, however, donor females that proved to be infertile to AI are serviced naturally by a bull. In contrast to cattle, transcervical AI is very difficult in sheep and goats and donors are inseminated primarily by a laparoscopic approach.

Cattle

The fertilization rate after artificial insemination of superovulated cows averages about 65 percent, with about 15 percent of cows having no fertilized ova (Hasler et al., 1983; Donaldson, 1983). Under normal circumstances, embryos from cycling cattle exhibit large numbers of accessory sperm trapped in the zona pellucida. In these embryos, entry of the fertilizing sperm into the vitellus triggers a zona block, trapping sperm that were in the process of penetrating the zona at the time of fertilization. The low numbers of accessory sperm observed in embryos recovered from superovulated cattle suggest that sperm numbers at the site of fertilization are low (Hawk and Tanabe, 1986). Superovulated cattle are often inseminated twice, with one straw at 12 and 24 hours after the onset of estrus.

Sperm numbers affect not only the rate of fertilization; they also are directly associated with embryo quality. DeJarnette et al. (1992) showed that there is a significant and positive correlation between the number of accessory sperm in embryos and the morphological quality of the embryos (reviewed by Saacke et al., 2000). In addition to this phenomenon of an association between sperm numbers and embryo quality, a positive correlation also exists between sperm quality and embryo quality. Evidence for this relationship is supported by data from a commercial ET program, clearly demonstrating that sperm quality not only affects fertilization rate, but also is positively associated with embryo quality (Stroud and Hasler, 2006). It was reported that among more than 9,700 embryos recovered from superovulated cattle, the percentages of those classified as excellent (61 percent), good (56 percent), fair (54 percent), or poor (34 percent) decreased in direct relation to semen quality that was classified as excellent, good, fair, or poor, based on five factors.

Horses

Donor mares are naturally serviced by stallions in some ET programs. Mares inseminated with fresh semen are more likely to achieve fertilization than those inseminated with either cooled or frozen semen (Squires et al., 2003).

Pigs

Donor females are normally bred at 12 and 24 hours after onset of estrus (Youngs, 2001). There have not been any

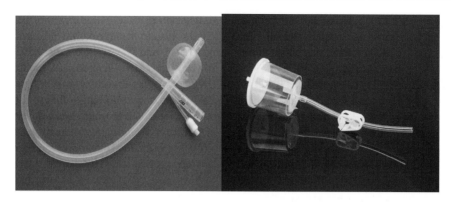

Figure 8.3. Silicone catheter and embryo filter used for bovine embryo collection. Courtesy of Bioniche Animal Health USA, Inc.

definitive studies dealing with the optimization of breeding superovulated gilts and sows.

Sheep and Goats
Natural service by rams or bucks is often used in these two species (Gordon, 1997). However, laparoscopic insemination results in high fertilization rates (Cognié, 2003).

Dogs and Cats
There is simply not enough ET practiced in either of these two species for insemination techniques to have been specifically designed for donors. In one study, the transfer of embryos resulting in pregnancy and delivery of pups involved natural mating (Tsutsui et al., 2001). However, the use of frozen-thawed dog semen in AI is well established (Farstad, 2000). Embryo transfer has been successful with donor cats bred naturally and by AI with frozen semen (Farstad, 2000).

Embryo Recovery

A number of different methods are employed for embryo recovery. Specific methods vary both by necessity among different species and by the preferences of individual practitioners. The use of a catheter inserted transcervically into the uterus is relatively easy and is routine in cattle and horses. Smaller species require either laparoscopic surgery or full surgical exposure to access the uterus.

Cattle
Most embryos are collected six to eight days after estrus. The efficiency of collection by nonsurgical procedures is decreased prior to day 6 because some embryos are still in the oviducts. Cryopreservation and embryo manipulation procedures become less effective after day 8. Bovine embryos also start hatching from the zona on day 8 and become more difficult to locate and recognize in the flush fluid.

Nonsurgical methods for collecting bovine embryos were first developed more than 40 years ago, but because recovery rates were poor, surgical methods continued to be used for many years. However, even under ideal conditions for surgery, scar tissue sometimes forms in the reproductive tract, causing infertility and even sterility in some cases. In addition, surgical collections must be performed in specialized facilities with expensive equipment and supplies. In the mid-1970s much effort was put into improving the nonsurgical methods to avoid damaging valuable donors. Currently, virtually all embryos are collected by the nonsurgical method, which is often referred to as "flushing" embryos.

In preparation for nonsurgically recovering embryos, a local anesthetic is administered by an epidural injection into the tail head. A silicone catheter, temporarily made rigid with a removable metal stylette, is passed through the cervix into the uterus (see Figure 8.3).

Some practitioners pass the catheter and inflate the balloon in one uterine horn, and following embryo collection of that side, deflate the balloon and move the catheter to the other horn, repeating the collection process. This is often referred to as a horn flush; the positioning of the catheter is shown in Figure 8.4.

Other practitioners prefer to inflate the catheter just inside the internal cervical os, thus collecting from both

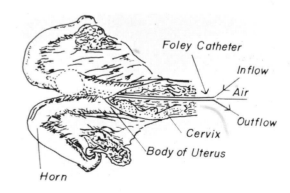

Figure 8.4. Placement of catheter for nonsurgical embryo recovery of uterine horn in bovine. Courtesy of G.E. Seidel, Jr.

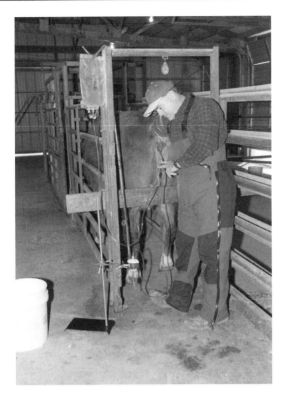

Figure 8.5. Nonsurgical embryo recovery of a donor cow using a gravity flow system for inflow of medium and a filter for collection of embryos. Courtesy of B. Stroud.

uterine horns and the uterine body simultaneously. Flush fluid is introduced into the donor cow either by gravity flow, as seen in Figure 8.5, or by injection with a large syringe. Figure 8.5 also illustrates the use of an embryo filter (see Figure 8.3) held in a ring clamp. In gravity flow collections, flush fluid exiting the uterus passes through a 70 micron stainless steel or nylon mesh in a plastic filter.

All nonsurgical collection procedures involve repeatedly filling and emptying the uterus with flush fluid; some practitioners opt to flush each horn separately, while others flush both horns and the body simultaneously.

A number of isotonic media often based on Dulbecco's PBS, and containing antibiotics and a surfactant such as BSA or polyvinyl alcohol, can be successfully used for recovering embryos of all the species in this review. Embryos usually remain viable in this fluid for at least 24 hours.

Horses

Embryos are recovered quite reliably from mares via nonsurgical flushing of the uterus. The procedure is different from that used in cattle in that a much larger catheter is used, and the cuff is inflated just inside the internal os of the cervix. The uterus is then filled and emptied several times and a total of 2–6 l of medium is used. The outflow medium of the flush is either collected in a vessel or run through an inline embryo filter of the same type used in cattle.

Pigs

Embryos are recovered surgically in commercial ET programs, although there is at least one report of a nonsurgical protocol (Hazelberger et al., 1989). A mid-line incision is performed with the sow on her back under anesthesia. The uterotubal junction in the pig does not allow for retrograde flushing of embryos from the uterus and back through the oviduct. Instead, embryos are flushed out of the uterus through a cannula into a tube or dish (see Figure 8.6).

Sheep and Goats

In commercial situations, embryos are surgically recovered from both of these species via a mid-line incision with the

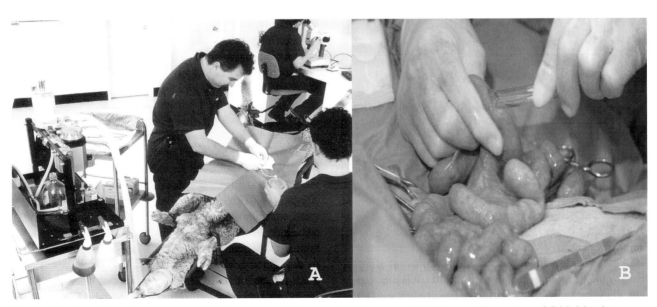

Figure 8.6. Surgical embryo recovery of **(A)** an ewe and **(B)** a sow. (A) Courtesy of D. Osborn, (B) courtesy of C.M. Murphy.

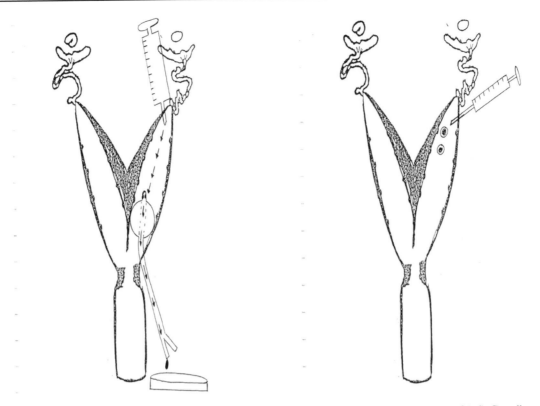

Figure 8.7. Diagram of surgical embryo recovery (left) and transfer (right) in sheep and goats. Courtesy of R.S. Castelberry.

female under anesthesia (see Figure 8.6). In some cases, a laparoscopic approach is used.

The placement of a small catheter and the technique for injecting flush medium are illustrated in Figure 8.7. This approach can be used for both goats and sheep. The method for surgically transferring embryos in these two species is also illustrated.

A nonsurgical, transcervical method was described as satisfactory in goats (Pereira et al., 1998). This method involves the use of a speculum to visualize the cervix in a standing goat. Using forceps, the external os of the cervix was then pulled almost to the vulvar opening so that a small catheter could be introduced and pushed forward into the uterus.

Dogs and Cats

Because maturation of canine oocytes is completed in the oviducts several days after ovulation, embryo recovery is normally not scheduled until eight to 11 days after ovulation or four to seven days after insemination or mating. Based on counts of corpora lutea in one study, 43 percent of potential embryos were recovered by a surgical approach (Tsutsui et al., 2001). Embryo recoveries in these two species are normally performed with the animal under general anesthesia; a mid-line incision is made, the reproductive is exteriorized, and the uterus flushed in a manner similar to that shown for pigs and sheep in Figures 8.6 and 8.7. A cannula rather than a catheter is often used for the outflow.

Embryo Handling and Evaluation

The mammalian oocyte is the largest cell in the body. Oocyte diameters of all the species covered in this review are similar and in the range of 150 to 180 microns. Aside from the similarity in the size of oocytes at ovulation, however, there also are significant differences in early embryonic development among these species. For example, on day 8 after estrus, the cow embryo normally has reached the expanded blastocyst stage, with a diameter of approximately 250 microns, and hatches from the zona pellucida shortly thereafter. The development of cattle embryos from the late morula to the expanded blastocyst stage is shown in Figure 8.8.

The morulae and early blastocysts in Figure 8.8 are typical of the embryos recovered on day 7 post-estrus in cattle. The expanded blastocyst is a typical day-8 embryo. Following the embryo recovery procedure of a donor, embryos are normally located in the flush fluid with the aid of a stereomicroscope at 6× to 10× magnification, transferred to holding medium, and evaluated at 50× magnification. Careful examination with a stereomicroscope of ova/embryos that are recovered from donors is necessary to ensure that viable embryos are not discarded, or on the other hand, unfertilized ova are not transferred or cryopreserved. A highly magnified view of an excellent quality late morula and an unfertilized ovum is shown in Figure 8.9. This is a good example of how these two stages are some-

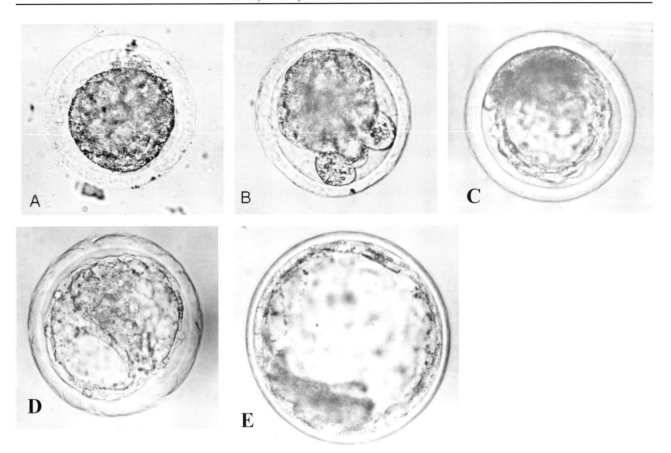

Figure 8.8. *In vivo*-derived cattle embryos. (**A**) Day-7 morula; (**B**) day-7 morula with extruded cells; (**C**) day-7 early blastocyst with extruded material; (**D**) day-7 early blastocyst with two blastocyst carities; (**E**) day-8 expanded blastocyst.

times difficult to differentiate unless they are examined carefully at a magnification of at least 50×.

Following fertilization, horse zygotes increase in size much more rapidly than cattle embryos and may reach 1,000 microns in diameter by day 8. Other differences in embryos among the species in this review include the

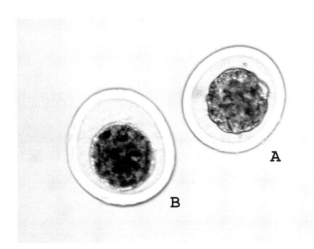

Figure 8.9. (**A**) Day-7 compact bovine morula; (**B**)unfertilized bovine ovum.

amount of lipid, the presence or absence of a capsule, and the time of implantation.

Cattle

Cattle embryos tolerate storage very well at ambient temperature in a variety of holding media. A pH of 7.25 to 7.35 and osmolality of approximately 275 are ideal, although cattle embryos can tolerate rather large deviations from these values for a period of several hours.

It was recently reported that a higher percentage of embryos from lactating dairy cows were classified as poor morphological quality and containing more lipids than embryos from non-lactating dairy heifers (Leroy et al., 2005) Examples of the appearance of some of the embryos from these groups of cows is shown in Figure 8.10.

The dark appearance of one embryo is due to the blockage of the light transmitted from below the embryo as viewed with a stereomicroscope. Leroy et al. (2005) attributed the greater density of this type of embryo to the presence of more than the normal number of lipid droplets in the cytoplasm. It is a widely held view in the ET industry that lipids decrease pregnancy rates and survivability following cryopreservation (personal communication). The differences between the donor groups in this study were dramatic, with only 13 percent of embryos classified as

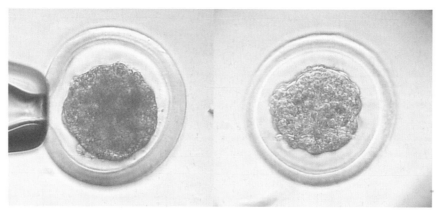

Figure 8.10. Two bovine morulae categorized as pale and dark. Courtesy of Leroy et al., 2005.

excellent and 24 percent with a high lipid content from lactating cows, compared to 63 percent and less than 1 percent, respectively, from the non-lactating group. Unfortunately, pregnancy data following transfer of these embryos into recipients were not included in the study.

Horses

Horse embryos can be maintained at room temperature for a period of several hours in the same media that have proven to work well for cattle embryos. One difference between the two species, however, is that traditional methods for embryo cryopreservation do not work well for horse embryos, especially for those that are greater than 300 microns in diameter (Squires et al., 2003). Horse embryos are often collected at one location and suitable recipients are located elsewhere, often at a distant location. Horse embryos survive cooling very well and thus can be shipped overnight in liquid holding medium in a chilled container (Carney et al., 1991), with high resulting pregnancy rates following ET (Squires et al., 1999). Horse embryos develop a translucent, elastic glycoprotein capsule under the zona starting about day 6 after ovulation (Betteridge, 1989). The capsule remains for approximately 10 days around the blastocyst during its dramatic increase in diameter.

Pigs

Pig embryos are more sensitive to temperature than many other domestic species and cannot be stored at refrigerator temperature (4°C) prior to transfer (Pollard and Leibo, 1994) as can cattle and horse embryos. Unique among the species in this review, it was shown that embryos from superovulated sows vary in rate of development relative to the dosage of eCG used for superovulation (Hazeleger et al., 2000). A dosage of 1,000 IU of eCG resulted in blastocysts with more cells but a similar diameter to blastocysts from sows that received 1,500 IU of eCG.

Sheep and Goats

Sheep and goat embryos tolerate handling and short-term storage similarly to cattle embryos.

Dogs and Cats

The 8-cell dog embryo in Figure 8.11 is characterized by rather dark cytoplasm. Dog embryos develop a capsule-like structure that is similar in appearance to what has been well described in the mare. This structure, evident in the photomicrographs of the blastocysts in Figure 8.11, has not been well-characterized in the literature. The tendency of dog blastocysts to shrink after recovery, also evident in Figure 8.11, has been described (Tsutsui et al., 2001). It has been suggested that the capsule-like structure is, in fact, the zona pellucida and that in the dog it is somehow chemically altered by the embryo; there is an evident change in elasticity so the dog zona does not maintain its shape as do the elastic zonas of most other species (D.C. Kraemer, personal communication). There are no published accounts detailing any specific storage requirements for either dog or cat embryos.

Embryo Transfer

ART procedures for all species that include the transfer of embryos ultimately depend on the availability of suitable recipients. Many factors that influence the suitability of potential recipients have been identified. Methods for preparing females to serve as recipients vary significantly among different species. In cattle, it often is taken for granted that females can be maintained in a group and that estrus, as manifested in mounting behavior, can be easily observed. Mares do not exhibit mounting behavior in a group of females and detection of estrus is much more labor intensive and requires the presence of a stallion.

Induction of estrus in cows and horses is rather easy with the use of prostaglandin (PG). Controlled intrauterine drug-releasing devices (CIDR) frequently are also being used in cows, but rarely in horses, and often this includes treatment with GnRH or estrogen. Synchronization schemes in some of the other species covered in this review are more complicated than in cattle and horses. For example, progesterone and estrogen treatments do not work in pigs as they do in cattle because estrogen may induce pseudopregnancy

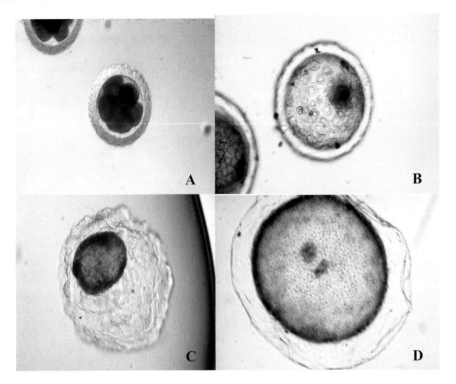

Figure 8.11. *In vivo*-derived dog embryos. **(A)** 8-cell embryo; **(B)** early blastocyst; **(C)** blastocyst that has collapsed inside the capsule-like structure; **(D)** expanded blastocyst. Courtesy of D.C. Kraemer.

(Pusateri et al., 1996). This is because estrogen is the signal for maternal recognition of pregnancy in the pig (Bazar et al., 1986).

Cattle

Today, cattle embryos are nearly always transferred to recipients nonsurgically. A few embryo transfer practitioners still use surgical procedures in rare situations. Before the mid-1970s, most cattle embryos were transferred surgically while the recipients were secured on their backs under general anesthesia in a surgical facility as shown in Figure 8.12.

Embryos were transferred through a mid-line incision made between the udder and navel to expose the uterus. While this procedure resulted in excellent pregnancy rates, it was very labor intensive and required special facilities. A simpler surgical approach, often called a flank transfer, was developed that involved administering a local anesthetic, making a flank incision, slightly exteriorizing the uterine horn, and transferring the embryo through a puncture wound in the uterine wall. This approach was used on cattle and horses, and still is used on horses in some cases.

Nonsurgical transfers in cattle and horses are performed with a special transfer gun, similar to that used for AI. Nonsurgical pregnancy rates in dairy heifers were reported to be similar to those achieved with surgical flank transfers, but pregnancy rates were lower with nonsurgical compared to surgical transfers in diary cows (Hasler, 2006). Most

practitioners administer an epidural injection to relax the rectal muscles.

Although it is similar to artificial insemination, nonsurgical transfer of embryos is a more challenging procedure. First, embryos usually are transferred approximately seven days after estrus. Because the cervix is closed at this stage of the estrous cycle, transversing it with a transfer gun at this time is much more difficult than performing AI when a cow or heifer is in estrus. Sanitation is also more

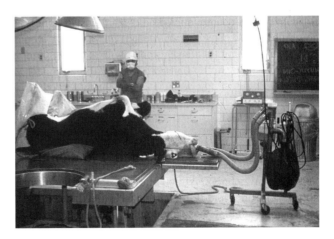

Figure 8.12. Cow under general anesthesia, prepared for mid-ventral surgical embryo recovery or transfer. Courtesy of G.E. Seidel, Jr.

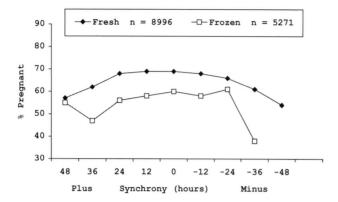

Figure 8.13. Effect of synchrony between bovine embryo age and recipient estrus on the pregnancy rate of recipients following transfer of fresh or frozen-thawed embryos. Plus asynchrony = recipient in estrus before donor; minus asynchrony = recipient in estrus after donor. Courtesy of Hasler, 2001.

important, because penetrating the cervix one week after estrus is more likely to lead to uterine infection. In addition, the embryo is transferred into the uterine horn on the ipsilateral side on which ovulation occurred, whereas semen usually is placed into the body of the uterus. Thus, bovine ET practitioners must be able to palpate the corpus luteum (CL) of the previous estrous cycle.

Both parity and breed affect the pregnancy rate of recipient cattle. Pregnancy rates were much higher in Holstein heifers and heifers and cows representing a variety of beef cattle breeds than in Holstein cows (Hasler, 2001). The degree of estrous synchrony between the donor and recipient has been shown to have a very clear influence on pregnancy rates. The rates did not vary when the degree of estrous asynchrony between donors and Holstein heifers was no more than 24 hours plus or minus (Hasler et al., 1987). Furthermore, there were no differences in pregnancy rates relative to the degree of asynchrony among beef or dairy cows and heifers (Hasler, 2001). Also, as seen in Figure 8.13, although frozen-thawed embryos resulted in a lower pregnancy rate following ET compared to fresh embryos, the influence of synchrony was similar for both fresh and frozen-thawed embryos.

It goes without saying that the quality of embryos that are transferred is a significant factor in determining pregnancy rate. The IETS has adopted a classification of embryo quality that assigns a rating of 1 (excellent/good), 2 (fair) and 3 (poor) (Robertson and Nelson, 1998). In commercial ET programs, some practitioners have further refined this quality scale and separately record excellent and good embryos. An example of this is seen in Table 8.2, which clearly shows that embryo quality influences pregnancy rates. However, the stage of transferred embryos, ranging from late morulae to expanded blastocyts, did not affect pregnancy rates.

Embryo transfer practitioners and scientists long have sought and used various drugs (clenbuterol, ibuprofen, flunixin meglumine) and hormones (progesterone, hCG, eCG, GnRH) in attempts to improve pregnancy rates in recipients. Injection of these products before and/or after transfer has not resulted in consistently higher pregnancy rates in the field trials and experiments that have been conducted thus far. However, a recent field trial, in which flunixin meglumine was administered to recipients a few minutes prior to ET, resulted in higher pregnancy rates compared to controls on two farms but not on a third farm (Purcell et al, 2005).

Horses

A transfer gun holding a one-half cc straw is often used for horse ET, because after day 7, equine embryos are frequently too large to fit in a one–fourth cc straw. Recipients are generally sedated and the perineal area scrubbed prior to transfer. Embryos can be transferred into one of the uterine horns, although results are quite good with transfer into the uterine body. Pregnancy rates following nonsurgical transfer have been reported to be in the range of 70 percent one week after transfer and comparable to those achieved with flank surgical transfer (Squires et al., 1999; Fluery and Alvarenga, 1999; Foss et al., 1999).

As with all species, the health and management of the recipients is probably the single most important factor in

Table 8.2. Effects of embryo grade and stage of development of fresh and frozen-thawed bovine *in vivo*-derived embryos on pregnancy rates of recipients.

Embryo grade	Fresh		Frozen	
	No. transfers	% pregnant	No. transfers	% pregnant
1 (excellent)	4,163	73[a]	2,482	63[a]
2 (good)	3,156	68[b]	2,329	57[b]
3 (fair)	1,641	56[c]	454	44[c]
4 (poor)	61	48[c]	22	36[b,c]
Embryo stage				
M	5,633	67	3,576	58
EB	1,978	70	1140	61
MB	995	71	478	58
XB	391	71	93	51
HB	25	56	—	—

[abc]Values in columns without common superscripts vary significantly (P < 0.05). (Hasler, 2001).
M = morula, EB = early blastocysts, MB = mid blastocyst, XB = expanded blastocyst, HB = hatched blastocyst.

ensuring a high pregnancy rate following ET. Because the CL of horses is not readily discernable by rectal palpation as in cattle, ultrasonography is widely used to determine the suitability of recipient mares. Synchrony between the age of the embryo and the stage of estrus of the recipient is less critical than in cattle. Similar pregnancy rates have been reported for recipients ranging from plus one day (before the donor) to minus three days (after the donor) (McKinnon et al. 1988). The tone of uterus and cervix prior to ET are important in selecting suitable mares (Carnevale et al., 2000). Ovariectomized, progesterone-treated mares have been successfully used as recipients (McKinnon et al., 1988).

Pigs

Most if not all pig embryos are transferred surgically in commercial programs. Experimental nonsurgical procedures have been described, with success rates ranging from poor to moderate (reviewed by Hazeleger and Kemp, 1999, 2001). It was recently reported that 71 percent of sows farrowed an average of 6.9 piglets following nonsurgical transfer into one uterine horn using a catheter specifically designed for the procedure (Martinez et al., 2004). In a commercial application of nonsurgical transfers averaging 28 blastocysts per gilt recipient, 41 percent farrowed an average of 7.2 piglets, compared to 12.8 percent for controls (Ducro-Steverink et al., 2004). In another recent report, success of nonsurgical transfer in gilts was directly related to the number of the estrus, with cervical passage not possible unless gilts had exhibited three or more estrous cycles (Cuello et al., 2005).

More work is needed to clarify whether the pregnancy rate in recipient sows is significantly affected by the location in the uterus of transferred embryos. Youngs (2001) reviewed the literature showing that at least four pig embryos must be transferred to establish pregnancy and that the pregnancy outcome following transfer to one or both uterine horns is not entirely understood. Youngs (2001) also reviewed the literature on estrus synchrony between donors and recipients. More complex than in monotocous species such as cattle and horses, there seems to be an interactive relationship between embryo ages within a group and the synchrony of the recipient in pigs. For example, small blastocysts had a lower pregnancy rate than large blastocysts when transferred to synchronous recipients, while there was no difference in survival in recipients that were one day minus (estrus one day after the donor).

Another apparent anomaly unique to the pig was the report that embryos produced with 1,000 IU of eCG resulted in a 71 percent pregnancy rate following transfer to recipients, compared to only 46 percent for embryos resulting from 1,500 IU of eCG (Hazeleger et al., 2000).

Sheep and Goats

Two embryos are routinely surgically transferred to each recipient of these two species. Pregnancy rates are traditionally high and in the 70 percent range. A diagram illustrating surgical transfer into these species is seen in Figure 8.7.

Dogs and Cats

There are very few reports of ET involving dog embryos. Tsutsui et al. (2001) reported that embryos ranging from 8-cell to blastocysts surgically transferred into three recipients that were between minus four to minus two days of estrous asynchrony did not result in any pregnancies. Of 21 recipients that were minus one to plus two days of synchrony, 12 (57 percent) became pregnant. The number of pups born relative to the number of embryos transferred in this group was 52 percent.

There has been a good deal of attention centered on ET in domestic cats as a model for endangered feline species (Pope, 2000). Successful ETs have been reported by a number of laboratories, but pregnancy rates have been low (Farstad, 2000; Pope, 2000). Because cats are induced ovulators, various hormonal treatments that may be less than optimal have been devised to induce estrus and ovulation in recipients.

Embryo Bisection

Embryos from some mammalian species can be divided in two, and the halves, frequently called *demi embryos*, can potentially develop into identical twins following ET. Embryo bisection, often referred to as splitting, is usually accomplished at the late morula or blastocyst stage prior to hatching from the zona. When bovine embryo bisection was first used commercially in the mid 1980s, it was thought that each demi embryo needed to be placed back into a zona (Williams et al., 1984). Consequently, zonas of unfertilized ova were used to provide a home for the extra demi embryos. This approach to embryo splitting required two micromanipulators: one with an aspiration pipette attached, the other with a microsurgical blade. It was soon discovered, however, that the pregnancy rate of demi embryos was the same whether they were in a zona or not (Seike et al., 1989). In addition, pregnancy rates were similar whether embryos were divided with a glass microneedle or a metal microblade (Kippax et al., 1991). These findings eliminated the need for one micromanipulator and made the procedure simpler and faster.

Embryos can be split while they rest on the bottom of a Petri dish. A metal microsurgical blade used in this approach is shown in Figure 8.14. The photomicrograph in Figure 8.14 shows two bovine demi embryos after the parent embryo was split. The shadow of the microsurgical blade is visible in this view from below the Petri dish. Some practitioners split embryos with a handheld blade without the aid of a micromanipulator.

Cattle

Identical twin Holstein calves derived from a split embryo are shown in Figure 8.15. Because the migration of

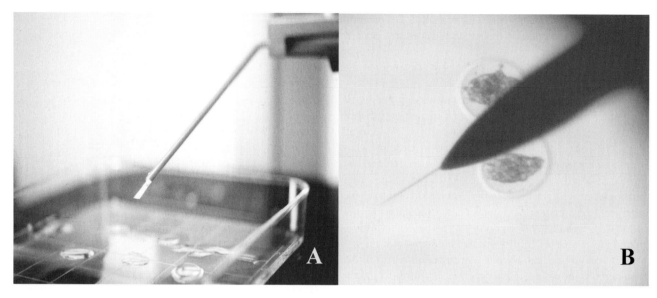

Figure 8.14. (A) Steel microsurgical blade attached to micromanipulator for bisection of embryos held in microdrops of embryo holding medium on the bottom of a Petri dish. (B) Demi embryos after bisection viewed from below with an inverted microscope through the bottom of a Petri dish. Note scratch from blade on the bottom of the Petri dish.

melanocytes is not strictly under genetic control, these calves have slightly different hair color patterns.

A large census of embryo splitting based on a number of different commercial cattle ET operations in the United States showed that pregnancy rates were similar for embryos split at the morula vs. blastocyst stage and at an age ranging from six to seven and a half days (Gray et al., 1991). The overall pregnancy rate following transfer of 1988 demi embryos was 50.2 percent, which translates into a 100.4 percent pregnancy rate had the single intact embryos been transferred. Embryo splitting is used by only a moderate number of ET practitioners; primarily they do not want to

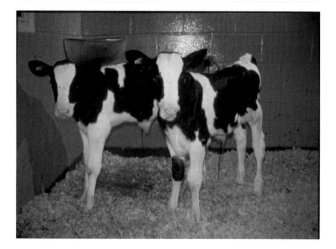

Figure 8.15. Identical twin Holstein calves resulting from transfer of bisected embryo (demi) halves. Courtesy of R.E. Mapletoft.

develop the necessary skills, expend the time, or invest in the equipment.

Between 1982 and 2006 a total of only 2,664 Holstein calves resulting from bisected embryos were registered by the (Holstein Association USA, Inc., personal communication). This is an average of just over 100 calves a year, compared to 15,000–20,000 Holstein calves registered yearly from intact embryos during this period. Numbers of calves of other breeds resulting from transfer of demi embryos are not available.

Horses

Two sets of identical horse twins were produced from demi embryos that resulted from the separation of 8-cell embryos recovered from the oviducts of donor mares (Allen and Pashen, 1984). The demi embryos were produced with the aid of a micromanipulator and each demi was imbedded in an agar chip to prevent the blastomeres from dispersing. The demis were then temporarily cultured in sheep oviducts and, after three and a half to five days, recovered and transferred to recipient mares. Obviously, this approach to embryo splitting is labor intensive and expensive. The presence of the capsule inside the zona of developing horse embryos interferes with conventional splitting as practiced in cattle, and there is currently no commercial activity involving equine embryo splitting.

Pigs

Normal piglets have been produced following transfer of demi embryos that were split by either a glass microneedle (Nagashima et al., 1988) or a steel microblade (Ash et al., 1989). In addition, it has been demonstrated that pregnancy rates are similar whether or not demi embryos are transferred within a zona (Nagashima et al., 1988). This technology has been used as a research tool in swine, but there is currently no commercial application for it.

Sheep and Goats

Because two embryos are usually transferred into recipients of these two species, embryo splitting would appear to have a very practical application. Pregnancy rates following transfer of zona-free goat (Nowshari and Holtz, 1993) and sheep (Chesné et al., 1987) demi embryos, two per recipient, were reported to be high. Udy (1987) reported that a commercial goat embryo splitting project, in which the demis were in zonas, resulted in 59 percent fetal survival at eight weeks of gestation. Nevertheless there is apparently little or no commercial use of embryo splitting in these two species. Pregnancies from IVF-derived sheep embryos that were split and transferred zona-free into recipients were reported recently (Morton et al., 2006).

Dogs and Cats

There are no published reports of embryo splitting in these two species.

In Vitro Fertilization

From its Latin origin, *in vitro* fertilization (IVF) means "fertilization in glass," although today it could more accurately be described as "fertilization in polystyrene." IVF has been adopted as a generic phrase that often includes the procedures of *in vitro* maturation (IVM) and *in vitro* culture (IVC). All three procedures usually are conducted in sequence to produce embryos exclusively *in vitro* (IVP).

In 1959, the rabbit was the first mammalian species in which live offspring were known to have been produced by IVF (Chang, 1968). The next reported success was with laboratory mice in 1968 (Whittingham, 1968). Subsequent progress with *in vitro* technology in mice, however, often did not extend to livestock species, because the mouse did not prove to be a good procedural model.

Cattle

In 1977, *in vitro* fertilization in cattle was first accomplished with semen capacitated in the oviduct or uterus of cows in estrus or the uterus of a rabbit (Iritani and Niwa, 1977). The first live calf resulting from IVF was born in 1981 as the result of the transfer of a 4-cell embryo into the oviduct of a recipient cow (Brackett et al., 1982). Pregnancies were achieved following transfer of IVM-IVF bovine embryos cultured in the oviduct of a sheep for five days (Critser et al., 1986). Two calves were born following transfer of embryos resulting from IVF with sperm capacitated using calcium ionophore and the resulting zygotes cultured in rabbit oviduct (Hanada et al., 1986). The first calves produced entirely from IVM, IVF, and IVC were born in 1987 (Fukuda et al., 1990).

Horses

The first foal born as a result of IVF was matured *in vivo* (Palmer et al., 1991). This was followed by a report of the successful intracytoplasmic sperm injection (ICSI) of equine oocytes after IVM (Squires et al., 1996) and the birth of a foal in 1996 (McCullen, 1996). As noted by Allen (2005), IVF in the horse has been extremely disappointing and only two live foals have been born to date using *in vivo*-matured oocytes recovered by ovum pick-up (OPU).

Pigs

The first birth of piglets resulting from the IVF of oocytes matured *in vivo* occurred 1985 (Cheng et al., 1986). Successful IVM and IVF of pig oocytes with the subsequent birth of piglets were reported in 1989 (Mattioli et al., 1989).

Sheep and Goats

In vitro fertilization in the goat was independently reported in 1984 by Rao et al. (1984) (achieved with xenogenous fertilization in the rabbit oviduct) and Hanada and Pao (1984), who used ionophor-capacitated spermatozoa. The first pregnancies in goats from IVM and IVF were announced by Younis et al. in 1991, followed by the birth of a kid that resulted from *in vivo* culture in 1992 (Crozet et al., 1993). The first documented kid resulting from complete *in vitro* methodology was described in 1994 (Keskintepe et al., 1994), and in 1985 the first lambs resulting from IVM and IVF were reported by Cheng et al. (1986).

Dogs and Cats

The first reported *in vitro* success in cats involved *in vitro* maturation followed by IVF (Goodrowe et al., 1988). The first and only reported pregnancy from IVF oocytes was reported by England et al. (2001).

Research involving *in vitro* procedures has grown dramatically in recent years and there is a very large and rapidly expanding body of literature. For example, even though the first calves resulting entirely IVP were not born until 1987, Ian Gordon's review of laboratory production of cattle embryos (1994) contains more than 170 pages of references on the subject.

Oocyte Collection

There is considerable variation in the methods of collecting oocytes from the species covered in this chapter. Transvaginal aspiration of ovaries manipulated per rectum and guided by a vaginally-inserted ultrasound probe is used in cattle and horses. Smaller species require a laparoscopic approach in which follicles are visibly identified and aspirated.

Cattle

Originally, *in vitro* procedures in cattle primarily were conducted for research purposes and used oocytes collected from superovulated females. When collected either from preovulatory follicles or oviducts 20 to 24 hours after onset of estrus, these oocytes had already undergone maturation and thus were ready for *in vitro* fertilization and *in vitro* culture. Oocytes collected from slaughterhouse-procured ovaries were not useful for studying fertilization and culture until *in vitro* maturation techniques were improved. Consequently, oocytes for research were obtained surgically from superovulated cattle in the 1970s and 1980s (Bederian et al., 1975; Brackett et al., 1980). Although laparoscopic procedures for oocyte retrieval via the paralumbar fossa were developed in the 1980s (Lambert et al., 1986), this approach, like surgical procedures, was expensive, inefficient, and risked the formation of adhesions with subsequent loss of fertility.

The introduction of real-time transrectal ultrasonic imaging (for review, see Griffen and Ginther, 1992) led to the development of techniques for the repeated collection of oocytes from bovine females. Ultrasound-guided collection of oocytes via the paralumbar fossa was described in 1987 (Callesen et al., 1987). The first repeatable, efficient technique involving transvaginal ultrasound-guided aspiration was developed in 1988 (Pieterse et al., 1988) and has become the predominant technique for oocyte collection from living cattle. This technique has become widely known as ovum pick-up (OPU). An ultrasound transducer and attached needle guide of the type used in cattle and horses is shown in Figure 8.16. A diagram of how the transducer is inserted into the vaginal fornix so that a needle can be guided through the vaginal wall and into the ovary is also shown.

Bols et al. (1996a) and Fry et al. (1997) clearly demonstrated that the proportion of oocytes surrounded by a compact cumulus decreased as vacuum pressure increased.

In addition, Bols et al. (1996a) showed that although recovery rates were higher from 18 gauge needles than from 19 or 21 gauge needles, a larger proportion of oocytes with intact cumulus were recovered with the use of the thinner needles. In a comprehensive subsequent study using a disposable needle guidance system, Bols et al. (1997b) proved that aspiration with long-beveled needles resulted in higher oocyte recovery rates than did short-beveled needles.

A significant degree of variation has been reported in the literature regarding the number of oocytes collected via OPU. The number of bovine oocytes ranges from 4.1 (Hasler et al., 1995) and 5.3 (Looney et al., 1994) usable oocytes collected from combined populations of dairy and beef breeds to much higher average numbers. Especially impressive are reports of averages of 17 to 25 oocytes routinely collected in Brazil from Nelore cattle, an indigenous breed of Brahman origin (personal communication). This probably reflects higher numbers of follicles developing in each follicular wave in these cattle.

There have been a number of different approaches to increasing the number of oocytes collected by OPU. Several workers showed that the number of oocytes per collection was similar whether bovine females were collected twice weekly, i.e., every three or four days, or only once weekly (Van der Schans et al., 1991; Gibbons et al., 1994; Broadbent et al., 1997). Hasler (1998) reported that numbers of oocytes per OPU session remained comparable whether donors were collected at three-, four-, or seven-day intervals. At Holland Genetics (Hanenberg and van Wagtendonk-de Leeuw, 1997), the influence of collection interval varied between locations of OPU collection units. In two of three units, three- and seven-day intervals between OPU resulted in significantly more oocytes than a four-day inter-

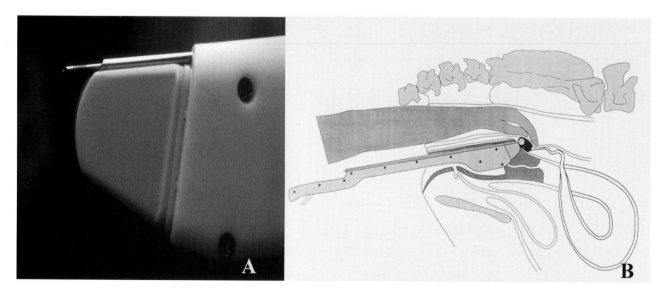

Figure 8.16. **(A)** Ultrasound transducer with oocyte aspiration needle protruding from needle guide. **(B)** Diagram showing position of the ultrasound transducer pressed against vaginal fornix, with ovary manually manipulated per rectum and held up against the vaginal wall.

val. The percentage of oocytes that developed into transferable embryos, however, was significantly higher for three- and four-day collection intervals than for seven-day intervals. Garcia et al. (1996) reported 5.5 oocytes were collected at each OPU session at seven-day intervals on Holstein heifers versus eight oocytes per session when OPU was conducted twice weekly at three- and four-day intervals.

The results of pretreatment of donors with gonadotrophins prior to OPU results in a larger yield of oocytes per OPU session (Bols et al., 1996b; Goodhand et al., 1999; de Ruigh et al., 2000). A so-called "coasting period" involving 48 or 84 hours of FSH starvation was shown to improve oocyte developmental competence as expressed by the rate of development of the 8- and 16-cell stage (Blondin et al., 2002). Recently, this concept has been successfully employed in a commercial bovine IVP business (Durocher et al., 2006).

In a recent, very comprehensive comparison of different OPU intervals with and without FSH, Chaubal et al. (2006) reported that the most productive protocol in terms of oocyte and embryo production involved dominant follicle removal, FSH treatment 36 hours later, and OPU 48 hours after FSH. This treatment was alternated weekly with simple once weekly OPU. The OPU weekly session involving FSH averaged 10.6 oocytes and 2.4 blastocysts, while the alternating weekly OPU with no FSH averaged 4.6 oocytes and 0.9 blastocysts.

Pavlok et al. (1996) injected cows once with recombinantly derived somatotropin (rBST) and noted more good quality oocytes but no difference in follicle numbers compared to control cows. Bols (1997a) treated heifers with rBST on a weekly basis and performed OPU twice weekly for 10 weeks. There was a tendency for the number of follicles to increase over the 20 OPU sessions, with the number of follicles higher in the treated group. However, there was no difference between the treated and control groups in the number of oocytes recovered.

There is little literature regarding the age of bovine donors relative to the number of oocytes collected by OPU. Among Holstein donors that were collected at Em Tran by OPU at least 20 times over a period of four to six months, age was a highly significant ($P < 0.001$) source of variation (Hasler, 1998). However, the only significant difference among groups ($P < 0.05$) was the higher number of oocytes from the six- to nine-year-olds compared to the 14- to 18-year-old age group. A regression analysis showed a linear decrease in oocyte numbers relative to collection session and an interaction of age in the degree of the decline ($P < 0.005$). The number of oocytes decreased between 0.11 and 0.30 per OPU session for cows in the different age groups.

In contrast to these results, Boni et al. (1997) recently showed that although follicle numbers varied, they did not significantly decrease with repeated, twice-weekly OPU sessions over a three- to six-month period. However, the authors did not report on oocyte numbers and, as shown by Bols (1997b), follicle numbers were not always correlated with the number of oocytes retrieved.

There is considerable variation between donors in terms of oocyte production over time. A dramatic example of the relationship between repeated OPU over a long period of time and oocyte recovery and embryo production was described by Hasler (1998). A Holstein donor, eight years of age at the start of OPU, produced a total of 176 embryos by 23 different sires, primarily as a result of weekly OPU collections. Although oocyte numbers clearly decreased relative to OPU session, oocyte viability, as evidenced by embryo production, did not appear to change over time. This clearly shows the potential for production of large numbers of embryos by OPU-IVP methods and the advantage of using different sires weekly or even bi-weekly.

In addition to bovine oocyte retrieval by ultrasound-guided OPU, there are several situations in which oocytes are removed from excised ovaries. When cows either develop terminal diseases or become crippled, ovaries can be removed via a flank laparotomy or through a vaginal incision and the oocytes recovered by follicular aspiration or slicing. Stringfellow et al. (1993) reported collecting an average of 46 oocytes from 18 culled dairy cows by slicing the ovarian cortex. In a highly successful commercial program, Green and McGuirk (1996) reported producing an average of 46 oocytes and nine embryos per donor in more than 100 cases of chronically ill, injured, and senile cows.

A third type of commercial cattle OPU program involves production of valuable embryos from ovaries procured from slaughterhouses. In a mass-production system using ovaries from the slaughterhouse, Lu and Polge (1992) reported producing more than 200,000 *in vitro*-derived blastocysts from approximately 700,000 oocytes in two years. Although this program is no longer in operation, it demonstrated the potential for production of IVP embryos from cattle after slaughter. It has been reported that occasionally between 100 and 200 oocytes can be harvested from one pair of ovaries (Vajta et al., 1996).

In Japan, ovaries from individual Kobi cows are procured at the time of slaughter and sent to an IVP lab for processing. Later in the same day, carcass values of the individually-identified cattle determine which oocytes will be retained and processed through the entire IVP procedure. In Italy, thousands of cattle embryos have been cultured in sheep oviducts for six days following IVM and IVF and then frozen and exported (Lazzari and Galli, 1996).

Horses

Oocytes can be collected from mares via OPU using the same ultrasound equipment that is used in cattle. One difference between the species is that oocytes are usually collected after a specific *in vivo* maturation period in the mare, because complete maturation cannot be successfully achieved *in vitro* with mare oocytes. Mare oocytes also can be collected from slaughterhouse-derived ovaries. However, research with equine oocytes is difficult because there are very few equine slaughterhouses remaining in the United States and ovaries often must be shipped long distances. Storage simulating long-distance shipment of equine ovaries for extended periods of 15 to 18 hours at room temperature or 4°C resulted in significantly lower *in vitro* maturation rates compared to control ovaries (Love et al., 2003). Oocytes transported in CO_2 equilibrated maturation medium achieved maturation equivalent to that for standard incubation.

The large size of pre-ovulatory follicles in the mare and the firm attachment of the cumulus to the follicle wall make recovery more difficult than in cattle (Brück et al., 1999). In fact, successful collection of oocytes from slaughterhouse-derived or excised mare ovaries usually involves scraping the follicle wall.

Other Species

Oocytes from other domestic animals are collected by three general methods:

- Oocytes are obtained from excised ovaries either by follicular aspiration or by slicing or mincing the ovaries.
- Oocytes are aspirated while the ovaries are exposed in situ either via a laparotomy or viewed through a laparoscope.
- Oocytes are aspirated while the ovaries are viewed with the use of a transvaginal ultrasound transducer.

The range in the number of oocytes collected in different species as reported in various studies is extreme (Hasler, 1998). A number of factors may affect the number of oocytes collected from different species, including collection method, animal breed, age and health status, season, reproductive status, and pretreatment with hormones and/or drugs.

Sheep and Goats

OPU in these species generally involves a laparoscopic procedure. In some cases the ovaries are exteriorized and the oocytes collected with a needle connected to a syringe. Treatment of ewes with FSH was shown to increase the numbers of follicles and oocytes collected via OPU (Morton et al., 2005) and to result in a higher percentage of oocytes developing into blastocysts compared to control groups (Berlinguer et al., 2004).

Dogs and Cats

Although preovulatory oocytes can be aspirated from the ovaries of living dogs and cats, most *in vitro* research in these two species has involved the collection of ovulated oocytes from the oviducts or from excised ovaries. Slicing the ovaries has proven to be more efficient at releasing oocytes than aspiration in both species, with an average of 12 oocytes per donor in dogs (Rodrigues and Rodrigues, 2003) and 18.8 in cats (Freistedt et al., 2001).

In Vitro Maturation

In some cases, oocytes are allowed to mature *in vivo* and then are collected via aspiration from Graafian follicles just prior to ovulation. However, this requires very precise timing of the collection and in most cases, immature oocytes are collected and then matured *in vitro*.

Cattle

Because of the interdependence of each step in the IVMFC sequence, there were difficulties in improving the technology in cattle. For example, development of IVC media could not progress rapidly until large numbers of zygotes were available. Production of zygotes, however, depended on the development of semen capacitation procedures and suitable fertilization media as well as the availability of mature oocytes. Except for the small numbers removed from superovulated females, mature oocytes were not readily available until IVM techniques were perfected. Thus, IVF could not be efficiently studied without IVM, but the only definitive proof of complete IVM is fertilization followed by normal cleavage and embryonic development. Such development, however, depends on a suitable IVC system. Currently, the efficiency of IVM is high enough to make feasible extensive research using immature oocytes obtained from slaughterhouse ovaries.

Two aspects of IVM in the bovine are rather remarkable. Oocytes aspirated from a variety of the follicles in any given wave can be induced to mature in approximately 24 hours. Second, maturation can be induced *in vitro* with a wide variety of media. Although it is known that oocytes from follicles less than 2 mm in diameter exhibit lower rates of maturation than oocytes from larger follicles (Schellander et al., 1989; Pavlok et al., 1992), a high percentage of oocytes from larger follicles are competent to undergo IVM.

Not all oocytes collected by OPU from living donors are suitable for processing in an *in vitro* system. The reproductive status of the donor, the size and age of individual follicles, and the OPU technique may affect the type and quality of oocytes that are recovered. In commercial applications of IVF, oocytes usually are categorized in one of four types, of which only types I and II have a realistic possibility of developing into embryos, as shown in Figure 8.17.

The actual rates at which these four types of oocytes developed into blastocysts in a commercial IVP program are shown in Table 8.3. Type III oocytes, often referred to as nude oocytes because they have no cumulus investment, have an extremely low incidence of progressing through IVM and IVF and developing into blastocyts. Type IV oocytes can range from slightly mature to atretic with pycnotic cumulus cells. Type I oocytes have the highest rate of development and are often used exclusively in research.

It has proven to be very feasible to transport bovine oocytes during the maturation process. High rates of embryo development have been routinely achieved from oocytes

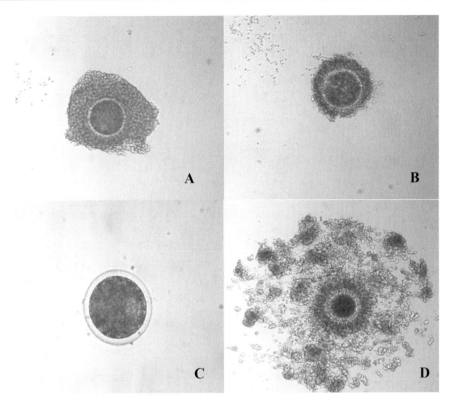

Figure 8.17. Variety of immature bovine oocytes aspirated by OPU. **(A)** Type I oocyte with more than four layers of compact cumulus; **(B)** type II oocyte with one to three layers of cumulus; **(C)** type 3 nude oocyte; **(D)** type 4 oocyte with expanded cumulus.

collected at several locations, placed in CO_2-equilibrated maturation medium in sealed plastic tubes, and transported within a portable incubator by automobile several hundred kilometers (Holland Genetics, Arnhem, The Netherlands, unpublished data). In addition, over a four-year period more than 200,000 oocytes have been placed in CO_2-equilibrated IVM medium within sealed plastic tubes and shipped in a battery-powered incubator (Minitub, Tiefenbach, West Germany) at 39°C by overnight air transportation (Hasler, unpublished data; Stringfellow et al., 1997). In most cases, developmental rates from these oocytes have been similar

Table 8.3. Potential for fertilization and embryonic development in different types of immature bovine oocytes.

Oocyte Type	Cumulus	No. Oocytes	% Cleaved	% Blastocysts	% Hatched
I	>4 layers	571	65[a]	29[a]	19[a]
II	1 to 3 layers	228	40[b]	8[b]	6[b]
III	nude	289	38[b]	<1[c]	<1[c]
IV	expanded	151	38[b]	7[b]	5[b]

[abc]Values within a column with different superscripts differ significantly (P < 0.025) (Hasler, 1994).

to those of control oocytes that underwent IVM in a stationary CO_2-controlled incubator.

Horses

It was initially difficult to determine whether IVM was successful in horses because of the very low rates of IVF and subsequent *in vitro* embryo development. Fulka and Okolski (1981) found that equine oocytes with compact cumulus needed 48 hours of IVM to reach metaphase II. Using TCM-199 containing FSH, LH, estradiol, and fetal calf serum, Del Campo et al. (1995) showed that a maximal percentage (55 percent) of equine oocytes reached metaphase II in 24 hours. Other groups have used 30 to 36 hours for IVM (Alm and Torner, 1994; Choi et al., 1994; Brück et al., 1996). Hinrichs and Williams (1997) recently demonstrated that a larger proportion of horse oocytes with expanded cumulus (74 percent) reached metaphase II during 24 hours of IVM than did oocytes with compact cumulus (30 percent). They noted that oocytes from atretic follicles had greater meiotic competence than did oocytes with compact cumulus from viable follicles at the time of oocyte collection. This is in direct contrast to the bovine situation.

Pigs

It has been well established that nuclear maturation requires significantly more time in pigs than in cattle (for review, see Day and Funahashi, 1996). *In vitro* maturation periods as long as 48 hours in TCM-199 have been used successfully to achieve metaphase II by some workers (Kure-bayashi et al., 1996). Ding and Foxcroft (1992) employed a 47-hour IVM period in TCM-199 and showed that the presence or absence of follicular cells during IVM did not influence the efficiency of nuclear maturation. Oocytes matured in the presence of follicular cells, however, showed a significantly increased rate of male pronuclear formation.

This type of study clearly indicates that traditional methods of assessing IVM, such as the oocyte reaching metaphase II, does not necessarily prove the acquisition of full maturational competence. The use of NCSU 23 medium (Petters and Wells, 1993) with PMSG and hCG for a maturation period of 44 hours proved to be a highly effective IVM system (Koo et al., 1997). However, two-step IVM systems, in which hormonal supplements in NCSU 23, TCM-199, Waymouth's Medium, or Whitten's Medium are present only during the first half of the culture period, have also proven very effective in the pig (Abeydeera et al., 1997; Funahashi et al., 1997b). A high rate of *in vitro* development to blastocysts was achieved with pig oocytes preincubated in NCSU 23 medium supplemented with 10 percent porcine follicular fluid for 12 hours followed by 20 hours incubation with PMSG and hCG and another 20 hours without hormones (Funahashi et al., 1997a).

Sheep and Goats

Based on the percentage of sheep oocytes reaching metaphase II, Yadav et al. (1997) announced that 30 to 32 hours was the optimal duration of IVM. Numerous other workers (Thompson et al., 1995; Baldassarre et al., 1996; Bernardi et al., 1996; Walker et al, 1996; O'Brien et al., 1997; Yadav et al., 1997), however, have employed IVM durations of 22 to 26 hours with quite acceptable results, supported by development of embryos *in vitro*. Almost universally, TCM-199 supplemented with 10 percent or 20 percent serum, FSH, and LH has been used for IVM in sheep.

Recently, acceptable rates of IVM were achieved with ovine oocytes matured in a portable incubator in the absence of continuous CO_2 (Byrd et al., 1997). These authors reported that IVM and IVF rates were similar for oocytes matured in plastic tubes containing either CO_2-equilibrated medium or HEPES buffered medium.

Most of the IVM systems that have been described for goats (Younis et al., 1991; Martino et al., 1994; Crozet et al., 1995; Keskintepe et al., 1997; Mogas et al., 1997; Yadav et al., 1997) are very similar to those commonly used in the bovine and most use TCM-199 supplemented with 20 percent bovine serum, FSH, LH, and estradiol. Most published work also has shown that the optimal time for maturation in the goat appears to be 27 to 30 hours, which is longer than in the bovine. Keskintepe et al. (1996, 1997) conducted IVM cultures in 5 percent O_2, in contrast to the 20 percent O_2 generally used by others.

Dogs and Cats

In contrast to the other species covered in this review, ovarian follicles in canids luteinize prior to ovulation and primary oocytes are ovulated without formation of the first polar body (Holst and Phemister, 1971). Maturation is completed in the oviducts over a period of two to three days (Luvoni, 2000) and, as a consequence, traditional IVM systems have not worked for dogs and other canids. Some success was achieved using synthetic oviduct fluid, a high concentration of BSA, oviductal cell culture, and a very long maturation time of 96 hours (Hewitt and England, 1999). Several different hormone supplementation regimens of IVM systems have been reported to achieve moderate success with dog oocytes. Rodrigues et al. (2004) reported that IVM using TCM-199 supplemented with estradiol and human somatotropin resulted in oocytes that were successfully fertilized *in vitro* and developed to the 8-cell-stage. Kim et al. (2005) added both estrogen (E2) and progesterone (P4) to an IVM system and found that either hormone alone improved the percentage of oocytes undergoing nuclear maturation.

Furthermore, the combination of the two steroids, depending on the concentrations, either decreased or increased maturation. Epididurmal growth factor (EGF) combined with FSH and LH in an IVM system significantly enhanced cumulus cell expansion of dog oocytes (Bolamba et al., 2006). Factors known to be involved in IVM of canine oocytes were recently reviewed in detail (Luvoni et al., 2005).

In vitro maturation has been more successful in the cat than in the dog. Incubation of cat oocytes for 24 hours in TCM-199 supplemented with hormones has reportedly resulted in very satisfactory maturation (Freistedt, 2001; Gomez et al., 2003).

In Vitro Fertilization

Distinct differences among species are perhaps no more apparent than in the IVF of oocytes from the species covered in this chapter. By chance, IVF in cattle is more easily accomplished than in some of the other species discussed here. Other species, especially the mare, have provided real challenges that have not yet been entirely solved.

Cattle

In vitro fertilization in the bovine presents a challenge quite different from that encountered with traditional *in vivo* insemination. As one might expect, IVF rates are low when mature oocytes are exposed to inadequate sperm numbers. In contrast to the situation *in vivo*, however, the use of higher than optimal concentration of *in vitro* sperm numbers results in polyspermy and the production of polyploid zygotes. To determine a suitable concentration for IVF, bulls can be tested at different semen concentrations using slaughterhouse-derived oocytes, which then can be stained

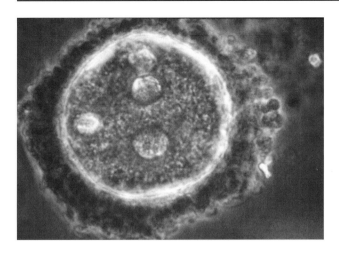

Figure 8.18. Polyspermic bovine zygote stained with orcein 18 hours after *in vitro* exposure to sperm. Note polyspermic fertilization characterized by presence of four pronuclei indicating presence of three sperm.

shortly after IVF and examined for the presence of more than one male pronucleus (see Figure 8.18).

The wide range in the optimal sperm concentrations among bulls used for IVF in one commercial program is shown in Table 8.4. The four Holstein bulls illustrated represent the range of variation observed among many dozens of bulls tested. Some bulls in this example, such as A, worked best at a relatively low sperm concentration, while C worked best at a high concentration. A few bulls, as demonstrated by B, worked well over a wide range of sperm concentrations.

Cleavage rates of inseminated oocytes have traditionally been used as an index of the IVF fertility of bulls. In an experiment using relatively high sperm numbers in all treatments, Kurtu et al. (1996) did not find an influence within sires of sperm concentration on cleavage rate. Others have shown sperm concentration to be significant (Kroetsch and Stubbings, 1992; Hasler, 1994; Brackett and Keskintepe, 1996). Cleavage rates are not always correlated with embryo development rates, however, as illustrated by bulls C and D in Table 8.4.

The relationship between *in vitro* cleavage and embryo development also was demonstrated by data (unpublished) from Holland Genetics, Arnhem, The Netherlands. There was a highly significant difference (P < 0.001) in cleavage rate among 63 sires that were used for IVF on more than 13,000 *in vitro*-matured oocytes obtained by OPU from valuable donor females. The percentage of embryos that developed to a transferable stage, i.e. late morulae or blastocysts, was highly affected by sire (P < 0.001), supporting previous observations (Eyestone and First, 1989a; Shi et al., 1990; Brackett and Keskintepe, 1996).

Holland Genetics also observed a significant correlation between cleavage rate and embryo development rate (P < 0.01) when sufficient numbers of oocytes were employed for the *in vitro* procedures (unpublished, personal communication). There was not a significant correlation between *in vitro* oocyte cleavage and the non-return rates of the bulls when they were used in AI. However, there was a significant correlation (P < 0.05) between the embryo development rate and non-return rates.

These data provide a strong argument for the use of embryo development, and not cleavage alone, as an index of sire fertility. The data also indicate that there is a predictive value for IVF relative to the *in vivo* fertility of bulls used in the field. Interestingly, Schneider et al. (1996) concluded that *in vitro* cleavage and embryo development did not accurately predict fertility of bulls in the field, whereas Marquant-Le Guienne et al. (1990), Bredbacka et al. (1997), and Zhang et al. (1997) reached the opposite conclusion. The non-return rates in the study by Schneider et al. (1996) ranged from an average of 65.8 percent for the low group to 73.2 percent for the high, while only approximately

Table 8.4. Variation among Holstein bulls in the cleavage rate and embryonic development of *in vitro*-fertilized bovine oocytes.

| Bull | No. Oocytes | Sperm concentration (millions/ml) | | | | | |
| | | 0.25 | | 0.5 | | 1.0 | |
		% Cleaved	% Blasts[a]	% Cleaved	% Blasts	% Cleaved	% Blasts
A	1,221	74[b]	34[e]	63[c]	27[f]	54[d]	16[g]
B	720	69	37	72	36	68	34
C	502	37[b]	15[e]	57[c]	24[f]	63[c]	34[g]
D	946	78	45[e]	74	40[e]	74	32[f]

[a]Percentage of blasts (blastocysts) was calculated on day 8 of IVC from the number of oocytes matured. [bcd]Values for percentage cleaved within a row with different superscripts differ significantly (P < 0.05) and [efg]values for percentage of blasts within a row with different superscripts differ significantly (P < 0.05). (Hasler, 1998)

150 oocytes were used for each bull. The high correlation between *in vitro* fertilization and non-return rates (r = 0.82, P = 0.004) found by Bredbacka et al. (1997) may have been related to the wide range (30.2 percent to 73.0 percent) of non-return rates among the sires tested. Zhang et al. (1997) also studied bulls with a wide range (46.2 percent to 74.8 percent) of non-return rates and reported that cleavage rate was more highly related to non-return rate (r = 0.59, P < 0.001) than was embryo development (r = 0.35, P < 0.05).

Horses

Successful *in vitro* fertilization has been very limited in horses. Most studies have used fresh rather than frozen-thawed semen. Capacitation rates much lower than those in cattle were achieved with calcium ionophore (Del Campo et al., 1990; Zhang et al., 1990), while similarly low rates were reported for frozen-thawed semen prepared with swim-up sperm and capacitated with heparin (Dell'Aquila et al., 1996). Fertilization rates of 10 percent and lower were achieved with fresh semen separated from seminal plasma by centrifugation through Percoll™ (Marcos et al., 1996).

ICSI of horse oocytes has proven to work quite well; however, embryo developmental rates in IVC following ICSI have been low. When transferred to the horse oviduct following IVM and ICSI, blastocyst development rates were reported to be 36 percent (Choi et al., 2004) and there are several reports of foals produced by ICSI into horse oocytes matured *in vitro* (Squires et al., 1996; Dell'Aquila et al., 1997; Galli et al., 2002). Although this approach is more technically demanding than conventional IVF, it allows the use of small numbers of fresh sperm, frozen-thawed sperm, or sex-selected sperm. It was recently reported that equine sperm subjected to two freeze cycles were able to initiate embryo blastocyst formation via ICSI and that even non-motile sperm resulted in blastocyst development (Choi et al., 2006).

Another variation of *in vitro* production of horse embryos involves gamete intrafallopian transfer (GIFT), in which oocytes, after undergoing IVM, are transferred to the oviduct of a recipient mare, and then the mare is mated or artificially inseminated. Foals resulting from GIFT have been reported by several research groups (Carnevale et al., 2000; Scott et al., 2001; Hinrichs et al., 2002). A commercial clinical program at Colorado State University has succeeded in producing numerous foals from sub-fertile donor mares using *in vivo* matured oocytes and GIFT (Carnevale et al., 2005).

Pigs

Polyspermic fertilization has proven to be a major problem associated with IVF in pigs (for reviews, see Day and Funahashi, 1996; Day, 2000), and a number of workers have reported that more than 50 percent of IVF zygotes were polyploid. It has been suggested that the block to polyspermy is slower in pigs than in other domestic species (Day and Funahashi, 1996). Capacitation of boar semen does not require the use of glycosaminoglycans such as heparin and, in fact, capacitation can be induced with caffeine (Funahashi and Day, 1993) or by incubating sperm in TCM-199 for approximately 4 hours (Cheng et al., 1986; Rath, 1992; Coy et al., 1993). Treatment of sperm with methyl-β-cyclodextrin compared to caffeine resulted in a lower rate of polyspermia, higher fertilization, and higher blastocyst cell numbers (Mao et al., 2005).

Rath and Niemann (1997) achieved high *in vitro* fertilization rates of *in vivo* matured oocytes with epididymal sperm. These authors hypothesized that epididymal sperm were superior for IVF compared with ejaculated semen due to lack of contact with seminal plasma.

Recently it has been demonstrated that IVF sperm concentration can affect the developmental competence of *in vitro*-matured pig oocytes following IVC (Koo et al., 2005). In this study, structural integrity of blastocysts, based on the ratio of inner cell mass to trophoblast cells, was lower in embryos fertilized by higher sperm concentrations.

Sheep and Goats

Capacitation of ram spermatozoa with heparin for IVF was described by Slavik et al. (1992). Without the use of heparin, however, others have successfully achieved IVF with 2 percent (Walker et al., 1994; O'Brien et al., 1997) or 20 percent (Baldassarre et al., 1996) estrous sheep serum or 20 percent metestrous sheep serum (Pugh et al., 1991) in synthetic oviduct fluid.

In vitro fertilization in goats has been proven to work satisfactorily with techniques very similar to those used in cattle (Younis et al., 1991; Pawshe et al., 1994; Mogas et al., 1997). It has also been shown that caprine blastocysts can be produced following intracytoplasmic sperm injection and *in vitro* culture (Keskintepe et al., 1997).

Dogs and Cats

Rates of IVF in dogs have been low; for example Otoi et al. (2000) reported only one blastocyst developing of 217 inseminated oocytes. *In vitro* fertilization in cats has been more successful than in dogs (reviewed by Luvoni, 2000). In addition, several laboratories have reported successful fertilization via subzonal sperm insertion SUZI in the cat (Farstad, 2000; Luvoni, 2000).

In Vitro Culture of Embryos

Many different types of *in vitro* systems have been designed for the culture of mammalian embryos. Although there is no absolute agreement among researchers, IVC systems are often classified as "defined," "semi-defined," or "non-defined."

Defined culture systems are those in which all of the components can be chemically defined and, as a consequence, products such as serum and BSA are not included. It should theoretically be possible for a defined system to be exactly replicated in any laboratory at any time.

Semi-defined systems are those in which every component is chemically defined with the exception of BSA. Although BSA is obviously more chemically defined than the serum from which it is refined, different lots of BSA have been shown to vary significantly in their ability to support the IVC of embryos, including those of hamsters (McKiernan and Bavister, 1992), cattle (Rorie et al., 1994), and rabbits (Kane, 1983).

Non-defined systems include components such as serum, which contains proteins, hormones, growth factors, vitamins, chelators for heavy ions, and various defined and undefined molecules in varying quantities (Gardner and Lane, 1993; Keskintepe and Brackett, 1996). These systems also have the potential for microbial, especially viral, contamination. In addition, non-defined systems may involve co-culture, in which any of a number of different somatic cells are included in the system or, in the case of conditioned medium, the products of such cells are included in the culture medium.

Not only can the composition of non-defined systems not be characterized, in some cases they cannot be consistently reproduced. Therefore, the use of defined systems is essential for understanding and optimizing the culture requirements of preimplantation embryos of various species. Some very comprehensive and thoughtfully written reviews have been provided by Walker et al. (1992a), Brackett and Zuelke (1993), Gardner and Lane (1993), Bavister (1995), Gordon (1994), and Thompson (1996).

Numerous differences between *in vitro-* and *in vivo-*produced embryos have been described in detail for cattle and other species (Hasler, 1998). The identification of the occurrence of apoptosis, or programmed cell death, has been used to evaluate embryo quality (Maddox-Hyttell et al., 2003). Recently, apoptosis was used to compare *in vitro-* vs. *in vivo-*derived embryos in cattle, horses, pigs, sheep, and goats (Rubio Pomar et al., 2005). Although a higher percentage of apoptotic cells was noted in IVP embryos compared to *in vivo-*produced embryos, the incidence was at a low level that does not reflect the differences described for pregnancy rates achieved with *in vivo* and *in vitro-*produced embryos.

Cattle

An obvious goal in the commercial production of bovine IVF-derived embryos is to produce as many embryos as possible from the original population of immature oocytes. It has been demonstrated that a variety of culture systems are capable of promoting the development of blastocysts from 30 percent to 40 percent of the original oocytes. However, qualitative as well as quantitative characteristics of various IVC systems should be considered.

Using an immunosurgical staining technique, Iwasaki et al. (1990) showed that IVF embryos were composed of fewer cells and had lower proportions of inner cell mass (ICM) to trophoblast cells than did *in vivo* embryos. Others have not reported a difference between IVF and *in vivo*

embryos in overall cell counts (Shamsuddin et al., 1992; Du et al., 1996), but IVF embryos in the Du et al. (1996) study had a lower proportion of ICM cells compared to *in vivo* embryos.

Total cell counts that were produced in different culture systems varied significantly among embryos at the same stage of development (Pinyopummintr and Bavister, 1991; Ectors et al., 1993; Goto et al., 1994; Rieger et al., 1995). However, total cell counts do not necessarily reflect the overall integrity and viability of preimplantation IVF embryos. Van Soom et al. (1996) observed that embryos produced in Menezo's B2 medium had higher cell counts than embryos of the same age produced in TCM-199 and had a larger variation in the number of ICM cells in the B2 embryos. The additional cells in the embryos produced in B2, however, were mainly trophoblast. This finding was based on differential staining of the blastocysts, which is a technically demanding but very useful technique that clearly differentiates between inner cell mass and trophoblast cells. An example of a differentially stained blastocyst is seen in Figure 8.19.

Mucci et al. (2006) showed that inclusion of serum in a bovine IVP system resulted in higher cell counts compared to medium without serum, with an equal yield of blastocysts. Interestingly, the blastocysts resulting from serum IVC did not survive cryopreservation as well as blastocysts produced in the absence of serum.

The rate of embryonic development also varies among IVC systems (Hawk and Wall, 1994; Donnay et al., 1997b; Hasler et al., 1996; Farin et al., 1997). It is clear that within a given IVC system, faster-developing embryos are of higher quality based on cell number (Jiang et al., 1992), end-stage of development (Grisart et al., 1995), and pregnancy rate after transfer (Hasler et al., 1995).

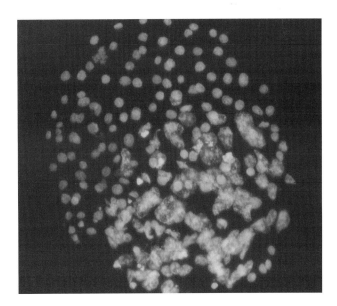

Figure 8.19. Differentially stained bovine IVP-derived blastocyst. The larger cells in the lower part of the blastocyst comprise the inner cells, while the trophoblast cells are the smaller cells in the upper part of the blastocyst.

A study that used fluorescence in situ hybridization showed that a high proportion (72 percent) of bovine embryos cultured in a Menezo's B2 co-culture system were mixoploid, compared to 25 percent of blastocysts developed *in vivo* (Viuff et al., 1999). Of the total number of *in vitro* embryos, 17 percent contained more than 10 percent polyploidy cells. In contrast, all of the *in vivo* embryos contained fewer than 10 percent polyploidy cells. The authors of this study offered a hypothetical link between the polyploidy in *in vitro* embryos and the possibility of polyploidy placental cells developing from them, leading to overactive placentas that in turn are responsible for large calves.

In the past, most commercial *in vitro* production of bovine embryos involved the use of co-culture systems that included a monolayer of somatic cells. Cell types that have been used in the successful co-culture of bovine embryos include primary cells from oviduct (bovine or porcine), mouse oviductal ampullae, cumulus, granulosa, and uterus, as well as established cell lines such as Buffalo Rat Liver (BRL), and Vero cells. These cells have been combined in co-culture systems with a number of different media, including TCM-199, Menezo's B2, and Ham's F-10.

Using a B2-BRL co-culture system, the laboratory at Em Tran, Inc. consistently produced day-8 blastocysts from 40 percent to 45 percent of immature oocytes (Hasler et al., 1996; Farin et al., 1997). Numerous other groups have reported high rates, i.e., more than 30 percent, of blastocyst production from a variety of co-culture systems, including: B2 plus BRLs after IVM in Ham's F-10 (Hawk and Wall, 1994), SOF plus mitomycin-treated Vero cells (Carnegie et al., 1997), TCM-199 plus cumulus cells (Vajta et al., 1996), CR1aa plus BRLs plus 2.5 or 5 percent egg yolk (Elhassan and Westhusin, 1997), CR1aa plus granulosa cells (Palma et al., 1997), TCM-199 plus frozen-thawed cumulus-granulosa cells (Broussard et al., 1994), TCM-199 plus bovine oviductal cells (Rehman et al., 1994), and B2 plus bovine oviductal cells, (Xu et al., 1992).

Excellent rates of embryo development have also been achieved with various media preconditioned by co-culture with a variety of somatic cells. Eyestone and First (1989b) showed that the proportions of oocytes developing to morulae and blastocysts were similar in a co-culture composed of TCM-199 plus oviductal cells compared to TCM-199 conditioned by previous culture with oviductal cells. Eyestone et al. (1991) and Mermillod et al. (1993) proposed that one of the advantages of conditioned medium is that it can be collected, frozen, and stored for future use. Both groups reported high rates of blastocyst development from TCM-199 conditioned for 2 days with bovine oviductal cells. Other reports of successful *in vitro*-conditioned culture systems include TCM-199 or a mixture of Dulbecco's modified Eagle's medium and Ham's F-12 conditioned by BRLs (Vansteenbrugge et al., 1994), and CZB conditioned by either BRLs or oviductal cells (Hernandez-Ledezma et al., 1993).

Moderately successful rates of blastocyst production have been reported with chemically defined, protein-free media (Pinyopummintr and Bavister, 1991; Bavister et al., 1992; Kim et al., 1993). *In vitro* cultures in the three previous studies were conducted in an atmosphere of 5 percent CO_2 in air. However, there is significant evidence that in the absence of co-culture, bovine embryos develop better in a 5 percent CO_2, 5 percent O_2, and 90 percent N_2 atmosphere (Thompson et al., 1990; Fukui et al., 1991). Reducing the oxygen level may be one reason for a recent high level of success with the *in vitro* culture of bovine embryos in defined media without the use of protein.

Keskintepe and Brackett (1996) reported that more than 40 percent of inseminated oocytes developed to the blastocyst stage within 7 days when cultured in synthetic oviduct fluid (SOF) supplemented with citrate, nonessential amino acids, and polyvinyl alcohol (PVA); however, viability of these embryos was not tested by transfer to recipients. Lee and Fukui (1996) used SOF supplemented with essential and nonessential amino acids and PVA incubated in a 7 percent O_2 atmosphere to support more than 30 percent blastocyst development. Gardner et al. (1997) reported similar results with SOF supplemented with Eagle's 20 amino acids and BSA. In the strictest sense, this is not a defined system due to the inclusion of BSA.

Variations of Tervit's (1972) original synthetic oviduct medium, supplemented with amino acids, are now widely used for commercial IVP of cattle embryos (Lane et al., 2003; Wagtendonk-de Leeuw et al., 2000; De La Torre-Sanchez et al., 2006). Although there is no proof that these media have completely eliminated problems with IVP-derived pregnancies, the embryos produced have been characterized as more similar to *in vivo*-derived embryos than those produced in co-culture systems and those containing serum.

Other Species

The emphasis on improving *in vitro* procedures for the oocytes of the other genera in this review has been concentrated primarily on *in vitro* maturation and fertilization. This is logical considering that embryo culture cannot be comprehensively tested without the availability of viable *in vitro*-produced zygotes.

With few exceptions there is nothing remarkably different in the media used to culture embryos from the other species covered in this review compared to media used successfully in cattle. An exception is the NCSU23 medium that was developed specifically for the pig (Petters and Wells, 1993).

Transfer of IVF-Derived Embryos

In most cases, IVF-derived embryos of a given species are transferred in the same manner as *in vivo*-derived embryos. Once removed from the incubator, IVF-derived embryos are usually transferred immediately; whereas, at least with some species, *in vivo*-derived embryos can be held at room temperature for up to 24 hours prior to transfer. Also, as described below for cattle, IVF-derived embryos require that synchrony—the matching of the age of the embryo to the estrous stage of the recipient—be calculated more tightly than is necessary for *in vivo*-derived embryos.

Cattle

Commercial production of bovine embryos through *in vitro* procedures is now successful internationally in a number of laboratories. BOVITEQ Inc. in Quebec (Bousquet et al., 1998), Trans Ova Genetics (Looney et al., 1994; Faber, et al., 2003), and Em Tran, Inc. (Hasler et al., 1995; Hasler, 1998) in the United States are commercial embryo transfer companies that have produced embryos from large numbers of infertile donors. In The Netherlands, IVP embryos are produced from oocytes obtained by OPU from young, reproductively-healthy donors and transferred on-farm around the country (Kruip and den Daas, 1997).

In an Italian commercial program, embryos are produced from slaughterhouse-derived ovaries and frozen for future sale. Published figures from the Italian program include data on more than 12,000 frozen IVF embryos produced from 97,000 oocytes that were recovered from 3,777 donor animals (Lazzari and Galli, 1996). In Japan, the production of IVF-derived embryos from slaughterhouse ovaries is widespread and, in some cases, very large numbers of embryos have been produced. Kuwayama et al. (1996) described the production of more than 150,000 frozen IVP embryos in a one-year period from more than 21,000 ovaries of Japanese Black Cattle. Most of the IVP embryos in Japan are selectively produced from beef donors with high marbling scores for the ribeye area. Although accurate numbers are not available, very large numbers of IVP embryos continue to be produced in this manner in both Japan and South Korea (Thibier, 2005).

The scale of the commercial bovine IVP embryo production is shown in Figure 8.20. The largest numbers of IVP embryos are produced in Japan from oocytes harvested from slaughterhouse material and in Brazil from OPU of living cattle.

In one commercial cattle ET program, the highest pregnancy rate was achieved with grade 1 fresh *in vivo*-derived embryos (Hasler et al., 1995). Significantly lower pregnancy rates were achieved, in order, by *in vivo* frozen, fresh day-7 IVF, fresh day-8 and frozen day-7 IVF, and frozen day-8 IVF embryos. A lower pregnancy rate was also achieved by grade 2 day-8 IVF embryos versus day-7 embryos. In contrast, the transfer of large numbers of *in vivo* embryos, independent of age and grade, demonstrated that early blastocysts (EB) and mid-blastocysts (MB) resulted in higher pregnancy rates than morulae (M), expanded blastocysts (XB), or hatched blastocysts (HB) (Hasler et al., 1987). Transfer of grade 1 day-7 embryos at the EB, MB, or XB stages resulted in higher pregnancy rates ($P < 0.05$) than transfer of corresponding day-8 embryos.

There are few data on the possible effect of the synchrony between the age of the IVF embryos and the day of estrus in the recipients on pregnancy rate. Consequently, in the commercial program at Em Tran, Inc., without regard to their developmental stage or quality, IVF embryos were transferred to zero, plus or minus synchrony recipients (Hasler, 1998). It should be noted that there is a potential for confusion due to the convention of referring to the day of estrus in recipients as day zero (0) whereas in IVF systems the day of fertilization is designated as Day 0 (Hasler et al., 1995; Avery et al., 1995).

For example, early blastocysts first start appearing approximately six days after fertilization both *in vivo* and *in vitro*. However, due to the difference in the designation of day 0 in the two systems, this represents day 6 *in vitro* and day 7 *in vivo*. In determining the degree of synchrony for *in vitro* embryo transfers, zero synchrony involves transferring *in vitro* embryos into recipients whose own embryos would be one day behind in development.

Synchrony data resulting from the transfer of 4,598 seven-day old IVP embryos at Em Tran, Inc., are shown in Figure 8.21. The transfer of IVF embryos into recipients that were plus 12 to 24 hours resulted in a pregnancy rate of 57.6 percent, while zero synchrony resulted in a 55 percent pregnancy rate. The 50.3 percent pregnancy rate that resulted from recipients that were minus 12 to 24 hours was significantly lower than both the zero and plus synchrony.

The explanation for this may be due to the fact that minus synchrony of 24 hours is actually a 48-hour difference between embryo and recipient, as depicted in Figure 8.1. The relationship between embryo-recipient synchrony with IVF embryos is different than that observed in previous studies involving large numbers of surgical transfers in Holstein heifers (Coleman et al., 1987; Hasler et al., 1987).

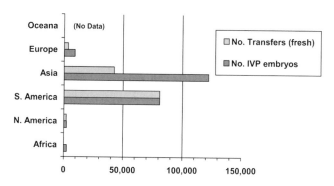

Figure 8.20. The number of IVP embryos produced and transferred (fresh) in major regions of the world in 2004. Courtesy of Thibier, 2005.

Horses

The single IVP foal reported by Palmer et al. (1991) resulted from the transfer of single embryos to eight recipients. This

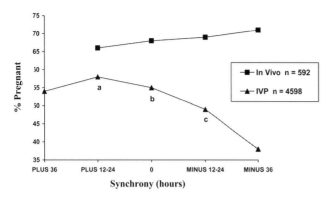

Figure 8.21. Effect of synchrony between bovine embryo age and recipient estrus on the pregnancy rate of recipients following transfer of day-7 *in vivo-* or IVP-derived embryos. Plus asynchrony = recipient in estrus before donor (before day of IVF); minus asynchrony = recipient in estrus after donor (after day of IVF). (a vs. c: P < 0.001; b vs. c: P < 0.025) Courtesy of Hasler, 1998.

foal and the one reported by McCullen (1996) represent the only two foals cited in the literature as having been born as a result of exclusively *in vitro* procedures. This is simply not enough information from which to draw any conclusions regarding embryo quality, interactions between embryo and recipient, or problems with offspring resulting from *in vitro* production.

Pigs

The surgical transfer of swine *in vivo*-derived embryos has been a successful procedure for a number of years. However, following the report of the birth of live piglets resulting from the transfer of *in vitro*-produced embryos in 1989 (Mattioli et al., 1989), there have been few additional published reports of success (Yoshida et al., 1993). Funahashi et al. (1997b) recently reported the birth of 19 live piglets from three recipients. These births resulted from the transfer of 40 early-cleavage stage embryos to the oviducts of four recipients.

Sheep and Goats

Sheep represent the only species of domestic animal, next to cattle, in which large numbers of *in vitro*-derived embryos have been transferred. Walker et al. (1992b) reviewed the older literature on the subject and observed that in the past, pregnancy rates following transfer of cultured sheep embryos were very low. Walker and co-workers transferred multiple *in vivo*-produced and *in vitro*-cultured embryos (cultured from *in vivo*-derived zygotes) to ewes and then flushed the reproductive tracts on day 14. Embryo survival rates were comparable, with 68 percent of the 211 *in vivo* embryos and 66 percent of the *in vitro* embryos developing into elongated conceptuses. The same workers also reported day-50 pregnancy rates of 59 percent versus 48 percent for ewes receiving two *in vivo* or two *in vitro* embryos, respectively.

In contrast, the very low viability of embryos derived from *in vitro*-matured oocytes was clearly demonstrated by the birth of only two lambs following the transfer of 61 day-6 morulae and blastocysts (Pugh et al., 1991). Recently, however, improvements in the efficacy of IVMFC systems (Walker et al., 1996; Bernardi et al., 1996) have resulted in embryo survival rates of 40 percent to 50 percent and pregnancy rates of 60 percent to 70 percent for ewes that received two blastocysts (Thompson et al., 1995; Holm et al., 1996; O'Brien et al., 1997). The transfers in the preceding studies were performed either via midventral laparotomy or with the aid of a laparoscope. The use of a moderately invasive laparoscopic technique involving a modified AI aspic (IMV, L'Aigle, France) allowed the transfer of *in vivo* embryos into 15 to 20 ewes per hour with a high pregnancy rate (McMillan and Hall, 1994). Transcervical transfer of embryos in sheep has not yet proven to be efficacious, with one study producing only one pregnancy following the transfer of 37 embryos into 15 recipients (Buckrell et al., 1993).

Two kids were produced from IVF of *in vivo*-matured goat oocytes (Hanada, 1985), and one kid resulted from an oviduct-cultured oocyte that had been subjected to IVM and IVF (Crozet et al., 1993). The first two kids resulting from IVMFC were the result of the transfer of three embryos at the 4- to 8-cell stage into each oviduct (Keskintepe et al., 1994). A total of six does each received six embryos; two does became pregnant and one subsequently aborted.

Dogs and Cats

There are insignificant data available to merit a discussion on the transfer of IVP embryos in these two species.

Pregnancies and Offspring

Problems with pregnancies resulting from IVP embryos have been described by a number of authors in both cattle (Farin and Farin, 1995; Farin et al., 2006; Kruip and den Daas, 1997; Hasler, 1998; Wagtendonk-de Leeuw et al., 1998, 2000) and sheep (Sinclair et al., 1997; Thompson et al., 1995; Walker et al. 1992b). Although a number of problems with IVP-derived pregnancies and offspring have been described, one of the more obvious is larger-than-normal calves and lambs at birth. As a consequence the syndrome often is referred to as the Large Offspring Syndrome (LOS). Some of the problems associated with this syndrome are shown in Table 8.5. Problems resulting from transfer of IVP embryos have not been reported in the other species covered in this review, perhaps because of the relatively small numbers involved.

A number of reports show that male bovine embryos produced *in vitro* grow more rapidly than female embryos during the first seven to eight days of culture (Avery et al., 1991, 1992; Xu et al., 1992; Carvalho et al., 1996;

Table 8.5. Aberrant characteristics associated with the LOS syndrome of IVP bovine pregnancies and calves.

Large calves

Increased gestation length

Decreased intensity of labor

Increased abortions

Congenital malformations

Increased perinatal mortality

Increased hydroallantois

(Hasler, 1998).

Gutiérrez-Adán et al., 1996; Tocharus et al., 1997). Bovine IVC embryos are usually transferred on day 7 or 8 and the most advanced embryos are usually selected because they tend to be more viable (Hasler et al., 1995; Behboodi et al., 1997). The percentage of male calves born following transfer of *in vitro*-derived embryos has variously been reported as 60 percent (Reichenbach et al., 1992), 62 percent (Guyader-Joly et al., 1993; Massip et al., 1995), 73 percent (Reinders et al., 1995), and 53 percent (Hasler et al., 1995). The 53.4 percent males out of more than 2,000 *in vitro*-derived calves and fetuses reported by Hasler (1998) differed significantly (P < 0.001) from 50 percent and also from the 51.1 percent males reported for 1,751 calves produced from transferred *in vivo*-derived embryos (King et al., 1985) and the 50.5 percent of 24,000 Holstein AI-produced calves that were males (Foote, 1977).

A number of reports indicate that the birthweights of IVF calves often are heavier than those of AI calves (Behboodi et al., 1995; Sinclair et al., 1995; Kruip and den Daas, 1997; Numbabe et al., 1997; Holland Genetics, Arnhem, The Netherlands, unpublished data). Furthermore, Farin et al. (1995) showed that seven-month fetuses derived from IVC embryos were heavier than those from *in vivo* embryos. In 1992 Walker et al. (1992b) reported that lamb birthweights were heavier and gestation lengths longer when ewes carried *in vitro*-cultured embryos than when ewes carried *in vivo*-cultured embryos. Embryos cultured in an *in vitro* system, which was supplemented with 20 percent human serum, were characterized as exhibiting earlier blastocoel formation, increased cyctoplasmic fragmentation, and fewer cells.

The findings of Walker et al. were extended to a study of *in vitro*-culture, with and without serum, of zygotes derived from both *in vivo* and *in vitro* sources (Thompson et al., 1995). Lambs derived from *in vitro* culture containing 20 percent human serum were an average of 20 percent heavier at birth than lambs from the same culture medium containing 0.8 percent BSA and no serum. Thompson et al. (1995) also reported that although gestation length was increased significantly (an average of two days) in the

serum group, gestation length did not account for the heavier birthweights.

Following this study, Holm et al. (1996) reported results from a study that involved *in vivo*- vs. *in vitro*-derived zygotes, *in vivo* vs. *in vitro* embryo culture, and co-culture vs. non-co-culture. Lambs produced from synthetic oviduct fluid medium (SOF) cultures containing 20 percent serum were heavier and had longer gestations than lambs derived from control embryos that were *in vivo*-matured and cultured. Surprisingly, lambs derived from IVM-IVF zygotes *in vivo*-cultured in sheep oviducts were also heavier, with longer gestations, than controls. The authors concluded that IVM-IVF, independent of subsequent culture conditions, was capable of altering birthweight and the duration of gestation.

Culture conditions are not the only reported factors that affect birth-weights in sheep. Alterations of the environment of preimplantation sheep embryos, such as transfer into asynchronous recipients (plus three days), resulted in heavier lambs (Wilmut and Sales, 1981), increased fetal weight that was not based on accelerated development (Young et al., 1996), and increased total muscle fiber number, but not weight, of plantaris muscles (Maxfield et al., 1996). However, exposure of sheep embryos to an asynchronous uterine environment for three days, followed by recovery and transfer to a synchronous uterus, had no effect on fetal growth (Sinclair et al., 1996).

In contrast to their previous study, Maxfield et al. (1997) found that *in vitro* co-culture of sheep embryos produced an increase in the weight of several muscles, including the plantaris; these muscles contained larger primary muscle fibers, but no increase in fiber number (Maxfield et al., 1997). Compared with *in vivo* controls, heavier heart, liver, and kidney weights were also observed in day 61 sheep fetuses derived from *in vitro* embryos cultured in granulosa cell co-culture or SOF supplemented with serum (Sinclair et al., 1997).

Culture studies similar to those in sheep have not been conducted in cattle. The high maintenance costs and longer gestation period makes the bovine a much more expensive model for studying the effects of *in vitro* procedures on subsequent offspring. The preceding studies indicate that serum, co-culture, IVM-IVF, and uterine environment are all capable of influencing fetal development in the sheep. It is not known whether the sheep can be used as a model to study these phenomena in the bovine.

Higher-than-normal abortion rates, ranging from 8 percent to 47 percent, during the first two trimesters of pregnancy were reported for *in vitro*-derived bovine pregnancies (Reichenbach et al., 1992; Reinders et al., 1995; Massip et al., 1995; Hasler et al., 1995). In contrast, abortion rates of 5.3 percent from two to seven months (King et al., 1985), 4.7 percent from two to six months (Hasler et al., 1987), and 4 percent from 40 to 250 days (Callesen et al., 1994) for bovine *in vivo* embryo transfer pregnancies were reported. At Em Tran, abortions among the IVP pregnancies were not randomly distributed among donors and the incidence of abortion was not constant over time (Hasler et al., 1995).

Perinatal and neonatal losses have also been reported as higher in recipients carrying *in vitro*-derived fetuses compared to AI or *in vivo* embryo pregnancies (Van Soom et al., 1994; Hasler et al., 1995; Schmidt et al., 1996; Kruip and den Daas, 1997). There was no difference in the incidence of calf loss at birth between calves produced in the TCM-199 and B2 co-culture systems at Em Tran. However, the overall loss at birth of the IVF calves was 14.9 percent (205/1,376), which is higher than the 9 percent loss previously reported for *in vivo* embryo transfer calves that had also been carried in both cows and heifers (King et al., 1985).

At Em Tran, Inc., an incidence of approximately 1 percent hydrallantois was diagnosed among pregnant Holstein recipients carrying IVF-derived fetuses (Hasler et al., 1995); increased incidence of the problem was also cited by Kruip and den Daas (1997). A frequency of 1 percent is a significantly higher incidence than the frequency of 1 per 7,500 calvings reported in non-IVF pregnancies (Sloss and Dufty, 1980).

Finally, although the data were not quantified, it was reported that labor often was not clearly pronounced in the Holstein heifers used as recipients for IVP embryos (Hasler, 1998). As a result, these recipients often were not observed in labor, and calvings frequently went unassisted, resulting in increased perinatal losses. However, when calves were delivered by scheduled Cesarean section, the survival rate was close to 98 percent.

Because serum has been implicated as a cause of higher birthweights of *in vitro*-derived lambs, (for review, see Young et al., 1998), its use in bovine IVC systems has received a good deal of attention. Deletion of serum during the first four days of co-culture failed to decrease the incidence of problems with *in vitro*-derived pregnancies and calves (Hasler, 2000), whereas Agca et al. (1998) showed that birthweights and gestation lengths were normal for a relatively small number of calves resulting from embryos cultured in serum-free CR1aa (Rosenkrans et al., 1993).

Another study comparing pregnancies resulting from co-cultured embryos versus those produced in SOF containing BSA showed that the use of SOF resulted in lower birthweights and easier calvings (Wantendonk-de Leeuw et al., 2000). Encouraging results were also recently reported from a sheep IVF research program (Sinclair et al., 1999). Pregnancies resulting from the transfer of *in vivo*-derived embryos were compared to those cultured in TCM-199 with granulosa cell co-culture or in SOF with or without human serum. Fetuses were significantly heavier and growth co-efficients for liver and heart for fetuses were greater from co-cultured and serum-supplemented embryos compared to control embryos. The allometric coefficients for liver and heart from fetuses derived from embryos cultured in SOF without serum were not different from controls, however.

The Future of ET and ART

Embryo transfer and ART are well established in a number of countries as commercial procedures in cattle, pigs, sheep, goats, and, to a lesser extent, horses. Millions of cattle have been produced by ET and many thousands of frozen embryos are moved internationally every year. In addition, very large numbers of IVP embryos have been produced from slaughterhouse material in some commercial programs. IVP systems of this type may have the potential for commercial application either where individual identification of the donors is possible or when a unique population of cattle is slaughtered (Kuwayama et al., 1996). Rutledge (1996) described some genetic advantages of producing *in vitro* F_1 hybrid embryos from *Bos taurus* oocytes fertilized with semen from tropical species such as *Bos javanicus* and *Bos gaurus*. The ability to store bovine ovaries for 24 hours without loss of oocyte viability may also make these types of programs more feasible (Schernthaner et al. 1997).

Van Wagtendonk-de Leeuw (2006) recently reviewed the history of OPU and IVP in cattle and offered a view of future applications of IVP technology. She suggested that marker assisted selection or gene assisted selection (Bredbacka, 2001) would be widely incorporated into commercial IVP programs in the future. Another technology that may blend very effectively with IVP of domestic farm animal embryos is the availability of sex-sorted semen (Garner, 2006). It is not clear that sex-sorted semen, as presently produced, is practical for large-scale use in AI programs. However, sex-sorted semen has been successfully used recently for production of IVP cattle embryos resulting in 93 percent heifer calves (Wilson et al., 2006). An extension of this technology is IVF with sex-sorted semen, followed by the use of a microfluidic cumulus cell removal device (Zeringue et al., 2004). This approach reduces the shearing forces exerted on embryos subjected to centrifugation for cumulus removal. The resulting embryos were transferred with a 33 percent pregnancy rate and 95 percent female calves (Wheeler et al., 2006).

There has been no increase during the past 20 years in the average number of embryos produced per superovulated donor. There has, however, been increased embryo production when it is calculated on the basis of embryos per unit time. The use of CIDR allows donors to be superovulated more frequently than in the past, without any obvious problem(s).

The current low success level of superovulation represents a significant obstacle to the future growth of the ET industry. As long as mean embryo production in cattle remains at less than six, with a range of zero to more than 60 and with 20 percent of donors producing no embryos, superovulation will remain an expensive, inefficient procedure. The expense of the gonadotrophins, prostaglandins and/or progesterone implants, the labor involving multiple injections over a period of days, estrus detection, and several inseminations are significant factors in the overall cost of superovulation. Improvements in the efficacy in all species would increase efficiency, both for the donor owner and the ET practitioner, and probably lead to a lowering of the costs of ET.

Ongoing changes in the composition of the beef and dairy cattle industries in North America constitute another factor that will probably influence the volume of conventional ET. A large proportion of beef ET has been used by externally funded hobby farmers, a segment of the beef industry that appears to be in decline. Also in decline is the number of small purebred dairies that have traditionally supplied most of the bull calves purchased by AI studs.

Although it would appear that the greatest opportunity for growth of conventional ET is in less developed countries, this may prove to be a temporary situation. As pointed out by Seidel (1991), due to the cost of animal versus vegetable protein, a decrease in animal agriculture in some countries is likely to occur in the future.

The widespread adoption of freezing embryos in ethylene glycol for direct transfer (DT) after thawing (Voekel and Hu, 1992) has made the transfer of frozen-thawed embryos more practical under a wide variety of conditions in the field. In 2004, 61 percent of all U.S. cattle embryos were frozen following recovery (AETA, personal communication). Ethylene glycol was the cryoprotectant for 89 percent of the embryos that were frozen. Although the skill-level required to transfer these embryos is unchanged from what was needed for transfer of conventionally frozen embryos, no embryologist is needed at thawing. Consequently, a growing number of DT embryos are now being transferred by technicians with experience in AI. There is a growing consensus among veterinary ET practitioners that conventional ET will increasingly become a field staffed by non-veterinarians.

Several authors have directly addressed the question of using IVP as a substitute for the *in vivo* embryos produced by conventional ET procedures (Hasler, 1994; Sinclair et al., 1995; Bousquet et al., 1998; Holm and Callesen, 1998). It is clear from the work at Em Tran and elsewhere (Looney et al., 1994; Hasler et al., 1995; Bols et al., 1996b; Faber et al., 2003) that pregnancies can be produced from donor females that were infertile both to AI and to the application of conventional ET technology. The larger question, however, is whether or not IVP is a realistic alternative to conventional ET for production of embryos from reproductively healthy cattle.

At least one commercial ET unit has provided data comparing the efficacy of conventional ET to IVP in cattle (Bousquet et al., 1998). The success rates quoted in this study (4.7 embryos per OPU session, 48 percent blastocysts from oocytes recovered) greatly exceed the published results of other commercial programs. The authors directly compared the results of IVP and the conventional *in vivo* programs at Boviteq and concluded that IVP would produce about 3.4 times more embryos and 3.2 more pregnancies in

a 60-day period, assuming only one superovulation per donor. In contrast, in a commercial IVF program in Australia, an average of four oocytes suitable for IVM were collected per OPU session and an average of 0.25 normal calves per session resulted (Vivanco-Mackie et al., 2000).

Currently, under commercial conditions in the United States, it is more expensive to produce pregnancies by OPU/IVP than with conventional ET. For most breeders, this technology is an advantage only for extremely valuable cows that are infertile or fail to respond to superovulation. This is likely to change only when the efficiency of IVP improves significantly and the problems with pregnancies and calves are reduced.

The U.S. federal government regulates the movement of live animals across state borders with detailed and strict health regulations. Until now, there has been no federal control of the interstate movement of gametes. It is unlikely that this will continue to be the case indefinitely, however.

Many tens of thousands of frozen cattle embryos have been exported to member countries of the European Union over the past 20 years with no identified cases of pathogen transfer. While individual European countries once required that donor females be tested for as many as 15 pathogens, the current EU regulations require that U.S.-based donors be tested only for epizootic hemorrhagic disease.

Washing procedures suggested by the International Embryo Transfer Society (Stringfellow, 1998) make it possible to safely import *in vivo*-derived embryos originating from donors sero-positive to pathogens such as bovine leukemia and bovine viral diarrhea viruses (BVDV). However, it is a different story with IVF-derived embryos. Because the *in vivo* embryo is exposed to oviductal glycoproteins, the structure of the zona pellucida differs from that of *in vitro*-derived embryos (Wegner and Killian, 1991).

In a recent review, Stringfellow and Givens (2000a) clearly made the case that a number of pathogens are more likely to remain associated with *in vitro*-derived embryos following washing than with *in vivo*-derived embryos. This obviously has potentially serious ramifications for the international movement of IVF-derived embryos. Testing for any microbes in question can be performed on donor cows that produce oocytes via OPU. However, there may be a serious health risk when oocytes are recovered from slaughterhouse-derived ovaries of untested cows. BVDV and BHV-1 viruses were isolated from 0.88 percent and 1.47 percent, respectively, of the batches of oocytes harvested from slaughterhouse ovaries in France (Marquant-Leguienne et al., 2000). Caution also should probably should be observed when using follicle or oviductal cells from slaughterhouse sources (Stringfellow and Givens, 2000b).

Determination of the sex of preimplantation bovine embryos with the use of the polymerase chain reaction (PCR) by conventional (Shea, 1999) or non-electrophoretic protocols (Bredbacka, 1998) is a service offered by a moderate number of ET businesses. When conducted properly, both of these PCR techniques are characterized by high rates of efficiency and accuracy. However, removal of the biopsy from the embryo requires a high level of operator skill. In addition, embryo biopsy is an invasive technique that results in some compromise in the viability of the embryo. Also, the procedure of embryo biopsy and the successful operation of a PCR program necessitate a higher level of hygiene and care than is often practiced in the ET industry. Therefore, although a modest portion of livestock breeders readily accepts sexing embryos with the use of PCR, it is not a technology that will find widespread use throughout the ET industry.

A PCR assay for detection of the bovine leucocyte adhesion deficiency (BLAD) gene was used at Em Tran, Inc. Developed by P. Bredbacka, this assay simultaneously determines the BLAD status and the sex of embryo biopsies. In the near future there will probably be similar PCR assays for bovine genes such as red factor and polled, which will be of interest to a rather limited number of cattle breeders. Genotyping for some of the known alleles, currently conducted only on blood samples, will undoubtedly be adapted for embryo biopsies. The extent of the market for this will depend on the value to cattle breeders of the genes in question.

The flow cytometric technology used to separate X- and Y-bearing sperm into live fractions has been significantly improved over the last 10 years (Johnson, 2000). About 10 million live sperm of each sex can be sorted per hour with a purity of 90 percent (Seidel, 2003). In AI field trials involving approximately 1,000 heifers, pregnancy rates with 1×10^6 sexed, frozen sperm were 70 percent to 90 percent of unsexed controls inseminated with 20 to 40 times as many sperm (Seidel et al., 1999). A recent study involving 574 calves produced from sex-sorted sperm compared to 385 control calves concluded that there were no differences in gestation, neonatal deaths, calving ease, birthweight, or survival rate to weaning (Tubman et al., 2003). The biggest disadvantages of this technique are the slow sorting speed and decreased pregnancy rates.

Due to the time needed for sex sorting semen, straws containing only 2 million total sperm have been used in most field trials. A trial involving the use of sex-sorted semen in superovulated beef heifers and cows was recently reported. A combined group of heifers and cows inseminated twice with 40 million non-sexed sperm per straw produced an average of 8.7 embryos compared to only 3.3 embryos for the donors inseminated with sex-sorted semen (Schenk et al., 2006). The adoption of sexed semen by the ET industry, specifically for superovulated donors, will be affected by the apparent lower fertility, the cost of the semen, and the availability of semen from specific bulls. These factors and other issues on the future of flow-sorted, sexed semen were reviewed by Amann (1999). In addition, Seidel (2003) provided some rather intriguing suggestions as to possible unconventional applications of sexed semen in both beef and dairy programs. The use of this technology currently is limited to licensees of XY, Inc., a company that holds an exclusive license to the patented process that was provided by the U.S. Department of Agriculture (Johnson, 1992).

Summary

Embryo transfer in cattle and, to a smaller extent, pigs, sheep, goats, and horses, has grown into a large international business over the last 25 years. Much of the technology is reasonably well standardized and practitioners have reported that nearly 500,000 embryos are produced from superovulated cows yearly on a worldwide basis. In addition, thousands of frozen cattle, sheep, and goat embryos are routinely sold and moved between countries. However, without improvements in technology, especially superovulation, the ET industry may have a reduced opportunity for growth. It should not be overlooked that animal rights organizations, government regulations, and patents all potentially present negative influences on the ET industry.

Acknowledgements

The author is very thankful to all former staff members of Em Tran, Inc. for their contributions to the long-term success of the ET program at that company. Some of the IVF data generated at Em Tran, Inc. presented here resulted from research that was financially supported by Holland Genetics, Arnhem, The Netherlands.

Bibliography

Abeydeera, W.W., Prather, R.S., and Day, B.D. (1997). In vitro penetration and subsequent development of pig oocytes matured in serum-free culture media. *Biol. Reprod.* 56:215 (Abstract).

Allen, W.R. (2005). The development and application of the modern reproductive technologies to horse breeding. *Reprod. Dom. Anim.* 40:310–329.

Allen, W.R., and Pashen, R.L. (1984). Production of monozygotic (identical) horse twins by micromanipulation. *J. Reprod. Fertil.* 71:607–613.

Alm, H., and Torner, H. (1994). In vitro maturation of horse oocytes. *Theriogenology.* 42:345–349.

Amann, R.P. (1999). Issues affecting commercialization of sexed semen. *Theriogenology.* 52, 1441–1457.

Ash, K., Anderson, G.B., BonDurant, R.H., Pashen, R.L., Parker, K.M., and Berger, T. (1989). Competition between split and nonmicromanipulated embryos in the production of identical piglets. *Theriogenology.* 31:903–910.

Avery, B., Brandenhoff, H.R., and Greve, T. (1995). Development of in vitro matured and fertilized bovine embryos, cultured from days 1–5 post insemination in either Menezo-B2 medium or in HECM-6 medium. *Theriogenology.* 44:935–945.

Avery, B., Jorgensen, C.B., Madison, V., and Greve, T. (1992). Morphological development and sex of bovine in vitro-fertilized embryos. *Mol. Reprod. Dev.* 32:265–270.

Avery, B., Madison, V., and Greve, T. (1991). Sex and development in bovine in-vitro fertilized embryos. *Theriogenology.* 35:953–963.

Baldassarre, H. (2004). State of assisted reproduction technologies in goats. Proc. Joint Conf. AETA/CETA, Tampa, Florida. pp. 25–30.

Baldassarre, H., Furnus, C.C., de Matos, D.G., and Pessi, H. (1996). In vitro production of sheep embryos using laparoscopic folliculocentesis: alternative gonadotrophin treatments for stimulation of oocyte donors. *Theriogenology.* 45:707–717.

Bavister, B.D. (1995). Culture of preimplantation embryos: facts and artifacts. *Human Reprod.* Update 1:91–148.

Bavister, B.D., Rose-Hellekant, T.A., and Pinyopummintr, T. (1992). Development of in vitro matured/in vitro fertilized bovine embryos into morulae and blastocysts in defined culture media. *Theriogenology.* 37:127–146.

Bazer, F.W., Vallet, J.L., Roberts, R.M., Sharp, D.C., and Thatcher, W.W. (1986). Role of conceptus secretory products in establishment of pregnancy. *J. Reprod. Fertil.* 76:841–850.

Bederian, K.N., Shea, B.F., and Baker, R.D. (1975). Fertilization of bovine follicular oocytes in bovine and porcine oviducts. *Can. J. Anim. Sci.* 55:251–256.

Behboodi, E., Anderson, G.B., BonDurant, R.H., Cargill, S.L., Kreuscher, B.R., Medrano, J.F., and Murray, J.D. (1995). Birth of large calves that developed from in vitro-derived bovine embryos. *Theriogenology.* 44:227–232.

Behboodi, E., Gutierrez-Adan, A., and Anderson, G.B. (1997). Inadvertent sex selection in a protocol of in vitro bovine embryo production. *Theriogenology.* 47:265 (Abstract).

Berlinguer, F., Leoni, G., Bogliolo, L., Pintus, P.P., Rosati, I., Ledda, S., and Naitana, S. (2004). FSH different regimes affect the developmental capacity and cryotolerance of embryos derived from oocytes collected after ovum pick up in donor sheep. *Theriogenology.* 61:1477–1486.

Bernardi, M.L., Fléchon, J.-E., and Delouis, C. (1996). Influence of culture system and oxygen tension on the development of ovine zygotes matured and fertilized in vitro. *J. Reprod. Fertil.* 106:161–167.

Betteridge, K.J. (2000). Reflections on the golden anniversary of the first embryo transfer to produce a calf. *Theriogenology.* 53:3–10.

Betteridge, K.J. (1989). The structure and function of the equine capsule in relation to embryo manipulation and transfer. *Equine Vet. J.* 8(Suppl.):92–100.

Betteridge, K.J. (1977). *Embryo transfer in farm animals.* Canada Department of Agriculture, Monograph 16.

Betteridge, K.J. (1981). An historical look at embryo transfer. *J. Reprod. Fert.* 62:1–13.

Blondin, P., Bousquet, D., Twagiramungu, H., Barnes, F., and Sirard, M.A. (2002). Manipulation of follicular development to produce developmentally competent bovine embryos. *Biol. Reprod.* 66:38–43.

Bo, G.A., Baruselli, P.S., Moreno, D., Cutaia, L, Caccia, M., and Tribulo, R. (2002). The control of follicular wave development for self-appointed embryo transfer programs in cattle. *Theriogenology.* 57:53–72.

Bolamba, D., Russ, K.D., Harper, S.A., Sandler, J.L., and Durrant, B.S. (2006). Effects of epidermal growth factor and hormones on granulose expansion and nuclear maturation of dog oocytes in vitro. *Theriogenology.* 65:1037–1047.

Bols, P.E.J., Van Soom, A., Ysebaert, M.T., Vandenheede, J.M.M., and de Kruif, A. (1996a). Effects of aspiration vacuum and needle diameter on cumulus oocyte complex morphology and development capacity of bovine oocytes. *Theriogenology.* 45:1001–1014.

Bols, P.E.J., Van Soom, A., Vanroose, G., and de Kruif, A. (1996b). Transvaginal oocyte pick-up in infertile Belgian blue donor cows: preliminary results. *Theriogenology.* 45:359 (Abstract).

Bols, P.E.J., Lein, A., Ysebaert, M.T., Van Soom, A., and de Kruif, A. (1997a). Effects of long term treatment with bovine somatotropin on oocyte and blastocyst yield after OPU/IVF. *Theriogenology.* 47:315 (Abstract).

Bols, P.E.J., Ysebaert, M.T., Van Soom, A., and de Kruif, A. (1997b). Effects of needle tip bevel and aspiration procedure on the morphology and developmental capacity of bovine compact cumulus oocyte complexes. *Theriogenology.* 47:1221–1236.

Boni, R., Relafen, M.E., Pieterse, M.C., Knout, J., and Kruip, Th. A. M. (1997). Follicular dynamics, repeatability of follicular recruitment in cows undergoing repeated follicular puncture. *Theriogenology.* 48:277–289.

Bousquet, D., Twagiramungu, H., Morin, N., Bryson, C., Charbonneau, G., and Durocher, J. (1998). In vitro embryo production in the cow: an effective alternative to the conventional embryo production approach. *Theriogenology.* 51:59–70.

Brackett, B.G., Bousquet, D., Boice, M.L., Donawick, W.J., Evans, J.F., and Dressel, M.A. (1982). Normal development following in vitro fertilization in the cow. *Biol. Reprod.* 27:147–158.

Brackett, B.G., and Keskintepe, L. (1996). Defined sperm treatments and insemination conditions enable improved bovine embryo production in vitro. *Theriogenology.* 45:259 (Abstract).

Brackett, B.G, Oh, Y.K., Evans, J.F., and Donawick, W.J. (1980). Fertilization and early development of cow ova. *Biol. Reprod.* 23:189–205.

Brackett, B.G., and Zuelke, K.A. (1993). Analysis of factors involved in the in vitro production of bovine embryos. *Theriogenology* 39:43–64.

Bredbacka, P. (2001). Progress on methods of gene detection in preimplantation embryos. *Theriogenology.* 55:23–34.

Bredbacka, P. (1998). Recent developments in embryo sexing and its field application. *Reprod. Nutr. Dev.* 38, 605–613.

Bredbacka, K., Andersson, M., and Bredbacka, P. (1997). The use of in vitro fertilization and sperm assay to evaluate field fertility of bulls. *Theriogenology.* 47:253 (Abstract).

Broadbent, P.J., Dolman, D.F., Watt, R.G., Smith, A.K., and Franklin, M.F. (1997). Effect of frequency of follicle aspiration on oocyte yield and subsequent superovulatory response in cattle. *Theriogenology.* 47:1027–1040.

Broussard, J.R., Thibodeaux, J.K., Myers, M.W., Roussel, J.D., Prough, S.G., Blackwell, J., and Godke, R.A. (1994).

Frozen-thawed cumulus-granulosa cells support bovine embryo development during coculture. *Fertil. Steril.* 62:176–180.

Brück, I., Greve, Z.T., and Hyttel, P. (1999). Morphology of the oocyte-follicular connection in the mare. *Anat. Embryol.* 199:21–28.

Brück, I., Grøndahl, C., Høst, T., and Greve, T. (1996). In vitro maturation of equine oocytes: effect of follicular size, cyclic stage and season. *Theriogenology.* 46:75–84.

Brück, I., Synnestvedt, B., and Greve, T. (1997). Repeated transvaginal oocyte aspiration in unstimulated and FSH-treated mares. *Theriogenology.* 47:1157–1167.

Buckrell, B.C., Gartley, C.J., Buschbeck, C., Jordan, P., and Walton, J.W. (1993). Evaluation of a transcervical AI technique for transferring embryos in sheep. *Theriogenology.* 39:197 (Abstract)

Byrd, S.R., Flores-Foxworth, G., Applewhite, A.A., and Westhusin, M.E. (1997). In vitro maturation of ovine oocytes in a portable incubator. *Theriogenology.* 47:857–864.

Callesen, H., Bak, A., and Greve, T. (1994). Embryo recipients: dairy cows or heifers. *Proceedings of the 10th Scientific Meeting of the AETE*, Lyon, France:125–135.

Callesen, H., Greve, T., and Christensen, F. (1987). Ultrasonically guided aspiration of bovine follicular oocytes. *Theriogenology.* 27:217 (Abstract).

Carnegie, J.A., Durnford, R., Algire, J., and Morgan, J. (1997). Evaluation of mitomycin-treated vero cells as a co-culture system for IVM/IVF-derived bovine embryos. *Theriogenology.* 48:377–389.

Carnevale, E.M., Coutinho da Silva, M.A., Panzani, D., Stokes, J.E., and Squires, E.L. (2005). Factors affecting the success of oocyte transfer in a clinical program for subfertile mares. *Theriogenology.* 64:519–527.

Carnevale, E.M., Maclellan, L.J., Coutinho, S., Scott, T.J., and Squires, E.L. (2000). Comparison of culture and insemination techniques for equine embryo transfer. *Theriogenology.* 54:981–987.

Carnevale, E.M., Ramirez, R.J., Squires, E.L., Alvarenga, M.A., and McCue, P.M. (2000). Factors affecting pregnancy rats and early embryonic death after equine embryo transfer. *Theriogenology.* 54:965–979.

Carney, N.J., Squires, E.L., Cook, V.M., Seidel, G.E. Jr., and Jasko, D.J. (1991). Comparison of pregnancy rates from transfer of fresh versus cooled, transported equine embryos. *Theriogenology.* 36:23–32.

Carvalho, R.V., Del Campo, M.R., Palasz, A.T., Plante, Y., and Mapletoft, R.J. (1996). Survival rates and sex ratio of bovine IVF embryos frozen at different developmental stages on day 7. *Theriogenology.* 45:489–498.

Chang, M.C. (1968). In vitro fertilization of mammalian eggs. *J. Anim. Sci.* 27(Suppl.1):15–22.

Chaubal, S.A., Molina, J.A., Ohlrichs, C.L., Ferre, L.B., Faber, D.C., Bols, P.E.J., Riesen, J.W., Tian, X. and Yang, X. (2006). Comparison of different transvaginal ovum pick-up protocols to optimize oocyte retrieval and embryo production over a 10-week period in cows. *Theriogenology.* 65:1631–1648.

Cheng, W.T.K., Moor, R.M., and Polge, C. (1986). In vitro fertilization of pig and sheep oocytes matured in vivo and vitro. *Theriogenology.* 25:146 (Abstract).

Chesné, P., Colas, G., Cognié, Y., Guérin, Y. and Sévelleo, C. (1987). Lamb production using superovulation, embryo bisection, and transfer. *Theriogenology.* 27:751–757.

Choi, Y.H., Love, C.C., Varner, D.D., and Hinrichs, K. (2006). Equine blastocyst development after intracytoplasmic injection of sperm subjected to two freeze-thaw cycles. *Theriogenology.* 65:808–819.

Choi, Y.H., Okada, Y., Hochi, S., Braun, J., Sato, K., and Oguri, N. (1994). In vitro fertilization rate of horse oocytes with partially removed zonae. *Theriogenology.* 42:795–802.

Choi, Y.H., Roasa, L.M., Love, C.C., Varner, D.D., Brinsko, S.P., and Hinrichs, K. (2004). Blastocyst formation rates in vivo and in vitro of in vitro-matured equine oocytes fertilized intracytoplasmic sperm injection. *Biol. Reprod.* 70:1231–1238.

Coleman, D.A., Dailey, R.A., Leffel, R.E., and Baker, R.D. (1987). Estrous synchronization and establishment of pregnancy in bovine embryo transfer recipients. *J. Dairy Sci.* 70:858–866.

Cognié, Y. State of the art in sheep-goat embryo transfer. *Theriogenology.* 51:105–116.

Cognié, Y., Baril, G., Poulin, N., and Mermillod, P. (2003). Current status of embryo technologies in sheep and goats. *Theriogenology.* 59:171–188.

Coy, P., Martínez, E. Ruiz, S. Vázquez, J.M. Roca, J. and Matas, C. (1993). Sperm concentration influences fertilization and male pronuclear formation in vitro in pigs. *Theriogenology.* 40:539–546.

Critser, E.S., Liebfried-Rutledge, M.L., Eyestone, W.H., Northey, D.L., and First, N.L. (1986). Acquisition of developmental competence during maturation in vitro. *Theriogenology.* 25:150 (Abstract).

Crozet, N., De Smedt, V., Ahmed-Ali, M., and Sevellec, C. (1993). Normal development following in vitro oocyte maturation and fertilization in the goat. *Theriogenology.* 39:206 (Abstract).

Crozet, N., Ahmed-Ali, M., and Dubos, M.P. (1995). Developmental competence of goat oocytes from follicles of different size categories following maturation, fertilization and culture in vitro. *J. Reprod. Fertil.* 103:293–298.

Cuello, C., Berthelot, F., Martinat-Botté, F., Ventrui, E., Guillouet, P., Vásquez, J.M., Roca, J., and Martinez, E.A. (2005). Piglets born after non-surgical deep intrauterine transfer of vitrified blastocysts in gilts. *Anim. Reprod. Sci.* 85:275–286.

Day, B.N. (2000). Reproductive biotechnologies: current status in porcine reproduction. *Anim. Reprod. Sci.* 60–61:161–172.

Day, B.N., and Funashashi, H. (1996). In vitro maturation and fertilization of pig oocytes. In: Miller, R.H., Pursel, V.G., and Normal, H.D. (eds.) *Beltsville Symposium in Agricultural Research XX, Biotechnology's Role in the Genetic Improvement of Farm Animals.* American Society of Animal Science, IL. p 125.

De La Torre-Sanchez, J.F., Preis, K., and Seidel, G.E. Jr. (2006). Metabolic regulation of in vitro-produced bovine embryos. I. Effects of metabolic regulatorsat different glucose concentrations with embryos produced by semen from different bulls. *Reprod. Fertil. Develop.* (In press)

de Ruigh, L., Mullaart, E. and Wagtendonk-de Leeuw, A.M. van. (2000). The effect of FSH stimulation prior to ovum pick-up on oocyte and embryo yield. *Theriogenology.* 53:359 (Abstract).

DeJarnette, J.M., Saacke, R.G., Bame, J. and Vogler, C.J. (1992). Accessory sperm: their importance to fertility and embryo quality, and attempts to alter their numbers in artificially inseminated cattle. *J. Anim. Sci.* 70:484–491.

Del Campo, M.R., Donoso, M.X., Parish, J.J., and Ginther, O.J. (1990). In vitro fertilization of in vitro-matured equine oocytes. *Equine Vet. Sci.* 10:18–22.

Del Campo, M.R., Donoso, X. Parrish, J.J. and Ginther, O.J. (1995). Selection of follicles, preculture oocyte evaluation, and duration of culture for in vitro maturation of equine oocytes. *Theriogenology.* 43:1141–1153.

Dell'Aquila, M.E., Cho, Y.S., Minoia, P., Traina, V., Fusco, S., Lacalandra, G.M., and Maritato, F. (1997). Intracytoplasmic sperm injection (ICSI) versus conventional IVF on abattoir-derived and in vitro-matured equine oocytes. *Theriogenology.* 47:1139–1156.

Dell'Aquila, M.E., Fusco, S., Lacalandra, G.M., and Maritato, F. (1996). In vitro maturation and fertilization of equine oocytes recovered during the breeding season. *Theriogenology.* 45:547–560.

Ding, J., and Foxcroft, G.R. (1992). Follicular heterogeneity and oocyte maturation in vitro in pigs. *Biol. Reprod.* 47:648–655.

Donaldson, L.E. (1983). The effect of prostaglandin F_2 alpha treatments in superovulated cattle on estrus response and embryo production. *Theriogenology.* 20:279–285.

Donaldson, L.E. (1984). The day of the estrous cycle that FSH is started and superovulation in cattle. *Theriogenology.* 22:97–99.

Donnay, I., Van Langendonckt, A., Auquier, P., Grisart, B., Vansteenbrugge, A., Massip, A., and Dessy, F. (1997). Effects of co-culture and embryo number on the in vitro development of bovine embryos. *Theriogenology.* 47:1549–1561.

Du, F., Looney, C.R., and Yang, X. (1996). Evaluation of bovine embryos produced in vitro vs. in vivo by differential staining of inner cell mass and trophectoderm cells. *Theriogenology.* 45:211 (Abstract).

Durocher, J., Morin, N., and Blondin, P. (2006). Effect of hormonal stimulation on bovine follicular response and oocyte developmental competence in a commercial operation. *Theriogenology.* 65:102–115.

Ducro-Steverink, D.W.B., Peter, D.G.W., Mater, C.C., Hazeleger, W., and Merks, J.W.M. (2004). Reproduction results and offspring performance after non-surgical embryo transfer in pigs. *Theriogenology.* 62:522–531.

Dziuk, P.J., Donker, F.D., Nichols, J.P., Petersen, J.E. (1958). Problems associated with the transfer of ova between cattle. *Univ. Minn. Agric. Exp. Sta. Tech. Bull.* 222:1–75.

Ectors, F.J., Thonon, F., Delval, A., Fontes, R.S., Touati, K., and Beckers, J.-F. (1993). Comparison between in vitro culture of bovine embryos in conditioned medium and in presence of bovine oviductal cells versus development in vivo and in rabbit oviducts. *Theriogenology.* 39:211 (Abstract).

Elhassan, Y.M., and Westhusin, M.E. (1997). In vitro development of preimplantation bovine embryos in a coculture system supplemented with egg yolk. *Theriogenology.* 47:288 (Abstract).

England, G.C.W., Verstegen, J.P., and Hewitt, D.A. (2001) Pregnancy following in vitro fertilization of canine oocytes. *Vet. Rec.* 148:20–22.

Eyestone, W.H., and First, N.L. (1989a). Variation in bovine embryo development in vitro due to bulls. *Theriogenology.* 31:191 (Abstract).

Eyestone, W.H., and First, N.L. (1989b). Co-culture of early cattle embryos to the blastocyst stage with oviductal tissue or in conditioned medium. *J. Reprod. Fertil.* 85:715–720.

Eyestone, W.H., Jones, J.M., and First, N.L. (1991). Some factors affecting the efficacy of oviduct tissue-conditioned medium for the culture of early bovine embryos. *J. Reprod. Fertil.* 92:59–64.

Faber, D.C., Molina, J.A., Ohlrichs, C.L., Vander Zwaag, D.F., and Ferré, L.B. (2003). Commercialization of animal biotechnology. *Theriogenology.* 59:125–138.

Farin, C.E., Hasler, J.F., Martus, N.S., and Stokes, J.E. (1997). A comparison of Menezo's B2 and Tissue Culture Medium-199 for in vitro production of bovine blastocysts. *Theriogenology.* 48:699–709.

Farin, P.W., and Farin, C.E. 1995. Transfer of bovine embryos produced in vivo or in vitro: survival and fetal development. *Biol. Reprod.* 52:676–682.

Farin, P.W., Piedrahita, J.A., and Farin, C.E. (2006). Errors in development of fetuses and placentas from in vitro-produced bovine embryos. *Theriogenology.* 65:178–191.

Farstad, W. (2000a). Assisted reproductive technology in canid species. *Theriogenology.* 53:175–186.

Farstad, W. (2000b). Current state of biotechnology in canine and feline reproduction. *Anim. Reprod. Sci.* 60–61:375–387.

Fleury, J.J. and Alvarenga, M.A. (1999). Effects of collection day on embryo recovery and pregnancy rates in a nonsurgical equine embryo transfer program. *Theriogenology.* 51:261 (Abstract).

Foote, R.H. (1977). Sex ratios in dairy cattle under various conditions. *Theriogenology.* 8:349–356.

Foss, R., Wirth, N., and Schiltz, P. (1999). Nonsurgical embryo transfer in a private practice (1998). In: *Proceedings of the Am. Assoc.* Equine Pract. 45:210–212.

Freistedt, P., Stojkovic, M., and Wolf, E. (2001). Efficient in vitro embryo production of cat embryos in modified synthetic oviduct fluid medium: effects of season and ovarian status. *Biol. Reprod.* 65:9–13.

Fry, R.C., Niall, E.M., Simpson, T.L., Squires, T.J., and Reynolds, J. (1997). The collection of oocytes from bovine ovaries. *Theriogenology.* 47:977–987.

Fukuda, Y., Ichikawa, M., Naito, K., and Toyoda, Y. (1990). Birth of normal calves resulting from bovine oocytes matured, fertilized, and cultured with cumulus cells in vitro up to the blastocyst stage. *Biol. Reprod.* 42:114–119.

Fukui, Y., McGowan, L.T., James, R.W., Pugh, P.A., and Tervit, H.R. (1991). Factors affecting the in-vitro development to blastocysts of bovine oocytes matured and fertilized in vitro. *J. Reprod. Fertil.* 92:125–131.

Fulka, J. Jr., and Okolski, A. (1981). Culture of horse oocytes in vitro. *J. Reprod. Fertil.* 61:213–215.

Funahashi, H., Cantley, T.C., and Day, B.N. (1997a). Preincubation of cumulus-oocyte complexes before exposure to gonadotrophins improves the developmental competence of porcine embryos matured and fertilized in vitro. *Theriogenology.* 47:679–686.

Funahashi, H., Cantley, T.C., and Day, B.N. (1997b). Synchronization of meiosis in porcine oocytes by exposure to dibutyryl cyclic adenosine monophosphate improves developmental competence following in vitro fertilization. *Biol. Reprod.* 57:49–53.

Funahashi, H., and Day, B.N. (1993). Effects of follicular fluid on fertilization in vitro on sperm penetration in pig oocytes. *J. Reprod. Fertil.* 99:97–103.

Galli, C., Crotti, G., Turini, P., Duchi, R., Mari, G, Zavaglia, G., Duchamp, G., Daels, P., and Lazzari, G. (2002). Frozen-thawed embryo produced by ovum pick up of immature oocytes and ICSI are capable to establish pregnancies in the horse. *Theriogenology.* 58:705–708 (Abstract).

Garcia, A., Cherdieu, J., Rademakers, A., and Salaheddine, M. (1996). Once versus twice-weekly transvaginal follicular aspiration in the cow. *Proceedings of the 12th Scientific Meeting of the AETE 1996*, Lyon, France :130 (Abstract).

Gardner, D.K., and Lane, M. (1993). Embryo Culture Systems. In: Trounson, A., and Gardner, D.K. (eds.) *Handbook of In Vitro Fertilization.* Boca Raton, FL.: CRC Press, Inc. p 85–114.

Gardner, D.K., Lane, M.W., and Lane, M. (1997). Bovine blastocyst cell number is increased by culture with EDTA for the first 72 hours of development from the zygote. *Theriogenology.* 47:278 (Abstract).

Garner, D.L. (2006). Flow cytometric sexing of mammalian sperm. *Theriogenology.* 65:943–957.

Gibbons, J.R., Beal, W.E., Krisher, R.L., Faber, E.G., Pearson, R.E., and Gwazdauskas, F.C. (1994). Effects of once- versus twice-weekly transvaginal follicular aspiration on bovine oocyte recovery and embryo development. *Theriogenology.* 42:405–419.

Gómez, M.C., Pope, E., Harris, R., Mikota, S., and Dresser, B.L. (2003). Development of in vitro matured, in vitro fertilized domestic cat embryos following cryopreservation, culture and transfer. *Theriogenology.* 60:239–251.

Goodhand, K.L., Watt, R.G., Staines, M.E., Hutchinson, J.S.M. and Broadbent, P.J. (1999). In vivo oocyte recovery and in vitro embryo production from bovine donors aspirated at different frequencies or following FSH treatment. *Theriogenology.* 51:951–961.

Goodrowe, K.L, Wall, R.J., O'Brien, S.J., Schmidt, P.M. and Wildt, D.E. (1988). Developmental competence of domestic cat follicular oocytes. *Biol. Reprod.* 39:355–372.

Gordon, I. (1994). *Laboratory production of cattle embryos.* Wallingford, U.K.: CAB International.

Goto, K., Iwai, N., Ide, K., Takuma, Y., and Nakanishi, Y. (1994). Viability of one-cell bovine embryos cultured in vitro: comparison of cell-free culture and co-culture. *J. Reprod. Fertil.* 100:239–243.

Gray, K.R., Bondioli, K.R. and Betts, C.L. (1991). The commercial application of embryo splitting in beef cattle. *Theriogenology.* 35:37–44.

Green, D., and McGuirk. B.J. (1996). Embryo production from valuable individual salvage cows. *Proceedings of the 12th Scientific Meeting of the AETE*, Lyon, France:134 (Abstract).

Griffen, P.G., and Ginther, O.J. (1992). Research applications of ultrasonic imaging in reproductive biology. *J. Anim. Sci.* 70:953972.

Grisart, B., Massip, A., Collette, L., and Dessy, F. (1995). The sex ratio of bovine embryos produced in vitro in serum-free oviduct cell-conditioned medium is not altered. *Theriogenology.* 43:1097–1106.

Gutiérrez-Adán, A., Behboodi, E., Anderson, G.B., Medrano, J.F. and Murray, J.D. (1996). Relationship between stage of development and sex of bovine IVM-IVF embryos cultured in vitro versus in the sheep oviduct. *Theriogenology.* 46:515–525.

Guyader-Joly, C., Charbonnier, G., Durand, M., Marquant-Le Guienne, B., Humblot, P., Jeanguyot, N., and Thibier, M. (1993). Ability of in vitro produced bovine embryos to develop to term. *Proceedings of the 9th Meeting of the AETE*, Lyon, France:208 (Abstract).

Hanada, A. (1985). In vitro fertilization in goat. *Jpn. J. Anim. Reprod.* 31:21–26.

Hanada, A., and Pao, S. (1984). In vitro fertilization and two-cell embryo transfer in goats. *Jpn. Soc. Zootech. Sci. Annu. Mtg.* 123 (Abstract).

Hanada, A., Enya, Y., and Suzuki, T. (1986). Birth of calves by non-surgical transfer of in vitro fertilized embryos obtained from oocytes matured in vitro. *Jap. J. Anim. Reprod.* 32:208 (Abstract).

Hanenberg, E.H.A.T., and van Wagtendonk-de Leeuw, A.M. (1997). Comparison of 3, 4 or 7 day interval between oocyte collections for in vitro embryo production results. *Theriogenology.* 47:158 (Abstract).

Hasler, J.F. (2006). The Holstein cow in embryo transfer today as compared to 20 years ago. *Theriogenology.* 65:4–16.

Hasler, J.F. (2001) Factors affecting frozen and fresh embryo transfer pregnancy rates in cattle. *Theriogenology.* 56:1401–1415.

Hasler, J.F. (2000). In vitro culture of bovine embryos in Ménézo's B2 medium with or without coculture and serum: the normalcy of pregnancies and calves resulting from transferred embryos. *Anim. Reprod. Sci.* 60–61:81–91.

Hasler, John F. (1998). The current status of oocyte recovery, in vitro embryo production, and embryo transfer in domestic animals, with an emphasis on the bovine. *J. Anim. Sci.* 76(suppl. 3):52–74.

Hasler, J.F. (1994). Commercial applications of in vitro fertilization in cattle. *The Compendium.* 16:1062–1073

Hasler, J.F., Henderson, W.B., Hurtgen, P.J., Jin, Z.Q., McCauley, A.D., Mower, S.A., Neely, B., Shuey, L.S., Stokes, J.E., and

Trimmer, S.A. (1995). Production, freezing and transfer of bovine IVF embryos and subsequent calving results. *Theriogenology.* 43:141–152.

Hasler, J.F., McCauley, A.D., Lathrop, W.F., and Foote, R.H. (1987). Effect of donor-embryo-recipient interactions on pregnancy rate in a large-scale bovine embryo transfer program. *Theriogenology.* 27:139–168.

Hasler, J.F., McCauley, A.D., Schermerhorn, E.C., and Foote, R.H. (1983). Superovulatory responses of Holstein cows. *Theriogenology.* 19:83–99.

Hasler, J.F., Stokes, J.A., and Hurtgen, P.J. (1996). In vitro bovine embryos in BRL co-culture undergo faster early cell cycles in Menezo's B2 than in TCM-199. *Biol. Reprod. 54.* (suppl. 1):89.

Hawk, H.W. and Tanabe, T.Y. (1986). Effect of unilateral corneal insemination upon fertilization rate in superovulating and single-ovulating cattle. *J. Anim. Sci.* 63:551–560.

Hawk, H.W., and Wall, R.J. (1994). Improved yields of bovine blastocysts from in vitro-produced oocytes. II. Media and co-culture cells. *Theriogenology.* 41:1585–1594.

Hazeleger, W., Bouwman, E.G., Noordhuizen, J.P.T.M., and Kemp, B. (2000). Effect of superovulation induction on embryonic development on day 5 and subsequent development and survival after nonsurgical embryo transfer in pigs. *Theriogenology.* 53:1063–1070.

Hazeleger, W., and Kemp, B. (1999). State of the art in pig embryo transfer. *Theriogenology.* 51:81–90.

Hazeleger, W. and Kemp, B. (2001). Recent developments in pig embryo transfer. *Theriogenology.* 56:1321–1333.

Hazeleger, W., Van der Meulen, J., and Van der Lende, T. (1989). A method for transcervical embryo collection in the pig. *Theriogenology.* 32:727–734.

Heape, W. (1891). Preliminary note on the transplantation and growth of mammalian ova within a uterine foster-mother. *Proc. R. Soc. Lond.* 48:457–458.

Heape, W. (1897). Further note on the transplantation and growth of mammalian ova within a uterine foster-mother. *Proc. R. Soc. Lond.* 62:178–183.

Hernandez-Ledezma, J.J., Villanueva, C., Sikes, J.D., and Roberts, R.M. (1993). Effects of CZB versus medium 199 and of conditioning culture media with either bovine oviductal epithelial cells or buffalo rat liver cells on the development of bovine zygotes derived by in vitro maturation-in vitro fertilization procedures. *Theriogenology.* 39:1267–1277.

Hewitt, D.A. and England, G.C.W. (1999). Synthetic oviductal fluid and oviductal cell coculture for canine oocyte maturation in vitro. *Anim. Reprod. Sci.* 55:63–75.

Hinrichs, K. (2005). Update on equine ICSI and cloning. *Theriogenology.* 64:535–541.

Hinrichs, K., and Williams, K.A. (1997). Relationship among oocyte-cumulus morphology, follicular atresia, initial chromatin configuration, and oocyte meiotic competence in the horse. *Biol. Reprod.* 57:377–384.

Hinrichs, K., Love, C.C., Brisko, S.P., Choi, Y.H., and Varner, D.D. (2002). In vitro fertilization of in vitro-matured equine oocytes: effect of maturation medium duration of maturation,

and sperm calcium ionophore treatment, and comparison with rates of fertilization in vivo after oviductal transfer. *Biol. Reprod.* 67:256–262.

Holm, P., Walker, S.K., and Seamark, R.F. (1996). Embryo viability, duration of gestation and birth weight in sheep after transfer of in vitro matured and in vitro fertilized zygotes cultured in vitro or in vivo. *J. Reprod. Fertil.* 107:175–181.

Holst, P.A., and Phemister, R.D. (1971). The prenatal development of the dog. Preimplantation events. *Biol. Reprod.* 5:771–779.

Iritani, A., and Niwa, K. (1977). Capacitation of bull spermatozoa and fertilization in vitro of cattle follicular oocytes matured in culture. *J. Reprod. Fert.* 50:119–121.

Iwasaki, S., Yoshiba, N., Ushijima, H., Watanabe, S., and Nakahara, T. (1990). Morphology and proportion of inner cell mass of bovine blastocysts fertilized in vitro and in vivo. *J. Reprod. Fertil.* 90:279–284.

Jiang, H.S., Wang, W.L., Lu, K.H., Gordon, I., and Polge, C. (1992). Examination of cell numbers of blastocysts derived from IVM, IVF and IVC of bovine follicular oocytes. *Theriogenology.* 37:229 (Abstract)

Johnson, L.A. (1992). Method to preselect the sex of offspring. The United States Dept. of Agriculture, assignee. US Patent No. 5,135,759.

Johnson, L.A. (2000). Sexing mammalian sperm for production of offspring: the state of the art. *Anim. Reprod. Sci.* 60–61, 93–107.

Kajihara, Y., Kometani, N., Kobayashi, S., Shitanaka, Y., and Goto, K. (1991). Pregnancy by bovine blastocysts developed in co-culture with cumulus/uterine endometrial cells after in vitro fertilization. *Jpn. J. Anim. Reprod.* 37:177–184.

Kane, M.T. (1983). Variability in different lots of commercial bovine serum albumin affects cell multiplication and hatching of rabbit blastocysts in culture. *J. Reprod. Fertil.* 69:555–558.

Keskintepe, L., and Brackett, B.G. (1996). In vitro developmental competence of in vitro-matured bovine oocytes fertilized and cultured in completely defined media. *Biol. Reprod.* 55:333–339.

Keskintepe, L., Darwish, G.M., Kenimer, A.T., and Brackett, B. G. (1994). Term development of caprine embryos derived from immature oocytes in vitro. *Theriogenology.* 42:527–535.

Keskintepe, L., Luvoni, G.C., Rzucidlo, S.J., and Brackett, B.G. (1996). Procedural improvements for in vitro production of viable uterine stage caprine embryos. *Small Ruminant Res.* 20:247–254.

Keskintepe, L., Morton, P.C., Smith, S.E., Tucker, M.J., Simplicio, A.A., and Brackett, B.G. (1997). Caprine blastocyst formation following intracytoplasmic sperm injection and defined culture. *Zygote.* 5:261–265.

Kim, J.-H., Niwa, K., Lim, J,-M., and Okuda, K. (1993). Effects of phosphate, energy substrates, and amino acids on development of in vitro-matured, in vitro-fertilized bovine oocytes in a chemically defined, protein-free culture medium. *Biol. Reprod.* 48:1320–1325.

Kim, M.K., Fibrianto, Y.H., Oh, H., Ju Oh, J., Goo, K.H.J., Lee, K.S., Kang, S.K., Lee, B.C., and Hwang, W.S. (2005). Effects of estradiol-17β and progesterone supplementation on in vitro nuclear maturation of canine oocytes. *Theriogenology.* 63:1342–1353.

King, K.K., Seidel, G.E. Jr., and Elsden, R.P. (1985). Bovine embryo transfer pregnancies. I. Abortion rates and characteristics of calves. *J. Anim. Sci.* 61:747–762.

King, W.A., Yadav, B.R., Xu, K.P., Picard, L., Sirard, M-A., Verini-Supplizi, A., and Betteridge, K.J. (1991). The sex ratios of bovine embryos produced in vivo and in vitro. *Theriogenology.* 36:779–788.

Kippax, I.S., Christie, W.B. and Rowan, T.G. (1991). Effects of method of splitting, stage of development and presence or absence of zona pellucida on foetal survival in commercial bovine embryo transfer of bisected embryos. *Theriogenology.* 35:25–35.

Koo, D.B., Kim, N.-H., Lim, J.G., Lee, S.M., Lee, H.T., and Chung, K.S. (1997). Comparison of in vitro development and gene expression of in vivo- and IVM/IVF-derived porcine embryos after microinjection of foreign DNA. *Theriogenology.* 48:329–340.

Koo, D.-B., Kim, Y.-J., Yu, I., Kim, H.-N., Lee, K.-K., and Han, Y.-M. (2005). Effects of in vitro fertilization conditions on preimplantation development and quality of pig embryos. *Anim. Reprod. Sci.* 90:101–110.

Kroetsch, T.G., and Stubbings, R.B. (1992). Sire and insemination does effect in vitro fertilization of bovine oocytes. *Theriogenology.* 37:240 (Abstract)

Kruip, Th.A.M., and den Daas. J.H.G. (1997). In vitro produced and cloned embryos: effects on pregnancy, parturition and offspring. *Theriogenology.* 47:43–52.

Kure-bayashi, S., Miyake, M., Katayama, M., Miyano, T., and Kato, S. (1996). Development of porcine blastocysts from in vitro-matured and activated haploid and diploid oocytes. *Theriogenology.* 46:1027–1036.

Kurtu, J.M., Ambrose, J.D., and Rajamahendran, R. (1996). Cleavage rate of bovine oocytes in-vitro is affected by bulls but not sperm concentrations. *Theriogenology.* 45:257 (Abstract).

Kuwayama, M., Hamano, S., Kolkeda, A., and Matsukawa, K. (1996). Large scale in vitro production of bovine embryos. Proc. 13th Inter. Congr. *Anim. Reprod.* 71 (Abstract).

Kvasnitski, A.V. (1950). The research on interbreed ova transfer in pigs. *Socialist Livestock Breeding Journal, Semi-annual Report of the Ukrainian Ministry of Agriculture*, pp.12–15.

Lambert, R.D., Sirard, M.A., Bernard, C., Béland, R., Rioux, J.E., Leclerc, P., Ménard, D.P., and Bedoya, M. (1986). In vitro fertilization of bovine oocytes matured in vitro and collected at laparoscopy. *Theriogenology.* 25:117–133.

Lane, M., Gardner, D.K., Hasler, M.J., and Hasler, J.F. (2003) Use of G1.2/G2.2 media for commercial bovine embryo culture: equivalent development and pregnancy rates compared to co-culture. Theriogenology 60:407–419.

Lazzari, G., and Galli, C. (1996). In vitro embryo production and its application to cattle breeding. *Proceedings of the 12th Scientific Meeting of the AETE*, Lyon, France:73–82.

Lee, E.-S., and Fukui, J. (1996). Synergistic effect of alanine and glycine on bovine embryos cultured in a chemically defined medium and amino acid uptake by in vitro-produced bovine morulae and blastocysts. *Biol. Reprod.* 55:1383–1389.

Leroy, J.L.M.R., Opsomer, G., De Vliegher, S., Vanholder, T., Goossens, L., Geldhof, A., Bols, P.E.J., de Kruif, A., and Van Soom, A. (2005). Comparison of embryo quality in high-yielding dairy cows, in dairy heifers and in beef cows. *Theriogenology.* 64:2022–2036

Looney, C.R. (1986). Superovulation in beef females. *Proc. 5th Annual Conf. AETA*, Ft. Worth, Texas. pp. 16–29.

Looney, C.R., Lindsey, B.R., Gonseth, C.L., and Johnson, D.L. (1994). Commercial aspects of oocyte retrieval and in vitro fertilization (IVF) for embryo production in problem cows. *Theriogenology.* 41:67–72.

Love, L.B., Choi, Y.H., Love, C.C., Varner, D.D., and Hinrichs, K. (2003). Effect of ovary storage and oocyte maturation method on maturation rate of horse oocytes. *Theriogenology.* 59:765–774.

Lu, K.H. and Polge, C. (1992). A summary of two years' results in large scale in vitro bovine embryo production. *Proceedings of the 12th International Congress on Animal Reproduction*, vol.3, The Hague, The Netherlands, pp. 1315–1317.

Luvoni, G.C. (2000). Current progress on assisted reproduction in dogs and cats: in vitro embryo production. *Reprod. Nutr. Dev.* 40:505–512.

Luvoni, G.C., Chigioni, S., Allievi, E., and Macis, D. (2005). Factors involved in vivo and in vitro maturation of canine oocytes. *Theriogenology.* 63:41–59.

McCullen, K. (1996). CSU produces 'test tube' horse. *Rocky Mountain News*, Science Sect., 10 January.

McKiernan, S.H., and Bavister, B.D. (1992). Different lots of bovine serum albumin inhibit or stimulate in vitro development of hamster embryos. *In vitro Cell. Dev. Biol.* 28A:154–156.

McKinnon, A.O., Squires, E.L., Voss, J.L. and Cook, V.M. (1988). Equine embryo transfer: a review. *Comp. Cont. Educ. Pract. Vet.* 10:343–355.

McKinnon, A.O., Squires, E.L., Carnevale, E.M. and Hermenet, M.J. (1988). Ovariectomized, steroid-treated mares as embryo transfer recipients and as a model to study the role of progestins in pregnancy maintenance. *Theriogenology.* 29:1055–1063.

McMillan, W.H., and Hall, D.R.H. (1994). Laparoscopic transfer of ovine and cervine embryos using the transpic technique. *Theriogenology.* 42:137–146.

Maddox-Hyttell, P., Gjorret, J.L., Vajta, G., Alexopoulos, N.I., Lewis, I., Trounson, A., et al. (2003). Morphological assessment of preimplantation embryo quality in cattle. *Reprod. Suppl.* 61:103–116.

Mao, J., Wu, G.-M., Prather, R.S., Smith, M.F., Cantley, T., Rieke, A., Didion, B.A., and Day, B.N. (2005). Effect of methyl-β-cyclodextrin treatment of pig spermatozoa on in vitro fertilization and embryo development in the absence or presence of caffeine. *Theriogenology.* 64:1913–1927.

Marcos, M.V., Spell, A.R., Butine, M.D., and Arms, M.J. (1996). Influence of cumulus cells on in vitro maturation and fertilization of equine oocytes. *Theriogenology.* 45:263 (Abstract).

Marquant-Le Guienne, B., Humbolt, P., Thibier, M., and Thibault, C. (1990). Evaluation of bull semen fertility by homologous in vitro fertilization tests. *Reprod. Nutr. Dev.* 30:259–266.

Marquant-Leguienne, B., Delalleau, N., Harlay, T., Allietta, M., Diemert, S., LeTallec, B., and Guerin, B. (2000). Results of a four-year survey on viral and bacterial contamination in a bovine embryo production system when using slaughterhouse material. *Theriogenology.* 53, 321 (Abstract)

Martinez, E.A., Caamaño, J.N., Gil, M.A., Rieke, A., McCauley, T.C., Cantley, T.C., Vazquez, J.M., Jordi, R., Vazquez, J.L., Didion, B.A., Murphy, C.N., Prather, R.S., and Day, B.N. (2004). Successful nonsurgical deep uterine embryo transfer. *Theriogenology.* 61:137–146.

Martinez, E.A., Vazquez, J.M., Roca, J., Cuello, C., Gil, M.A., Parrilla, I., and Vazquez, J.L. (2005). An update on reproductive Technologies with potential short-term application in pig production. *Reprod. Dom. Anim.* 40:300–309.

Martino, A., Palamo, M.J., Mogas, T., and Paramio, M.T. (1994). Influence of the collection technique of prepuberal goat oocytes on in vitro maturation and fertilization. *Theriogenology.* 42:859–873.

Massip, A., Mermillod, P., Van Longendonckt, A., Touze, J.L., and Dessy, F. (1995). Survival and viability of fresh and frozen-thawed in vitro bovine blastocysts. *Reprod. Nutr. Dev.* 35:3–10.

Mattioli, M., Bacci, M.L., Galeati, G., and Seren, E. (1989). Developmental competence of pig oocytes matured and fertilized in vitro. *Theriogenology.* 31:1201–1207.

Maxfield, E.K., Sinclair, K.D., Tregaskes, L.D., Christensen, M., Robinson, J.J., and Maltin, C.A. (1996). Asynchronous embryo transfer increases muscle fibre number in ovine fetuses at day 110 of gestation. *Theriogenology.* 45:226 (Abstract).

Maxfield, E.K., Sinclair, K.D., Dolman, D.F., Staines, M.E., and Maltin, C.A. (1997). In vitro culture of sheep embryos increases weight, primary fiber size and secondary to primary fiber ratio in fetal muscle at day 61 of gestation. *Theriogenology.* 47:376 (Abstract).

Meintjes, M., Bellow, M.S., Broussard, J.R., Paul, J.B., and Godke, R.A. (1995). Transvaginal aspiration of oocytes from hormone-treated pregnant beef cattle for in vitro fertilization. *J. Anim. Sci.* 73:967–974.

Mermillod, P., Vansteenbrugge A., Wils, C., Mourmequz, J.-L., Massip, A., and Dessy, F. (1993). Characterization of the embryotrophic activity of exogenous protein-free oviduct-conditioned medium used in culture of cattle embryos. *Biol. Reprod.* 49:582–587.

Mogas, T., Palomo, M.J., Izquierdo, M.D., and Paramio, M.T. (1997). Developmental capacity of in vitro matured and fertilized oocytes from prepuperal and adult goats. *Theriogenology.* 47:1189–1203.

Morton, K.M., de Graaf, S.P., Campbell, A., Tomkins, L.M., Maxwell, W.M.C., and Evan, G. (2005). Repeat ovum pick-up and in vitro embryo production from adult ewes with and without FSH treatment. *Reprod. Dom. Anim.* 40:422–428.

Morton, K.M., Rowe, A.M., Maxwell, W.M.C., and Evans, G. (2006). In vitro and in vivo survival of bisected sheep embryos derived from frozen-thawed unsorted, and frozen-thawed sex-sorted and refrozen-thawed ram spermatozoa. *Theriogenology.* 65:1333–1345.

Mucci, N., Aller, J., Kaiser, G.G., Hozbor, F., Cabodevila, J., and Alberio, R.H. (2006). Effect of estrous cow serum during bovine embryo culture on blastocyst development and cryotolerance after slow freezing or vitrification. *Theriogenology.* 65:1551–1562.

Nagashima, H., Katoh, Y., Shibata, K., and Ogawa, S. (1988). Production of normal piglets from microsurgically split morulae and blastocysts. *Theriogenology.* 29:485–495.

Nowshari, M.A. and Holtz, W. (1993). Transfer of split goat embryos without zonae pellucidae either fresh or after freezing. *J. Anim. Sci.* 71:3403–3408.

Numabe, T., Oikawa, T., Satoh, H., Takada, N., and Horiuchi, T. (1997). Birthweights of calves conceived by transfer of Japanese black cow embryos produced in vitro. *Theriogenology.* 47:378 (Abstract).

O'Brien, J.K., Catt, S.L., Ireland, A., Maxwell, W.M.C., and Evans, G. (1997). In vitro and in vivo developmental capacity of oocytes from prepuberal and adult sheep. *Theriogenology.* 47:1433–1443.

Otoi, T., Murakami, M., Fujii, M., Tanaka, M., Ooka, A., Une, S., and Suzuki, T. (2000). Development of canine oocytes matured and fertilized in vitro. *Vet. Rec.* 146:52–53.

Palma, G.A., Zakhartchenko, V., and Brem, G. (1997). Effect of granulosa cell co-culture in different embryonic stages on the development of in vitro-produced bovine embryos. *Theriogenology.* 47:282 (Abstract).

Palmer, E., Bezard, J., Magistrini, M., and Duchamp, G. (1991). In vitro fertilization in the horse. A retrospective study. *J. Reprod. Fertil.* Suppl. 44:375–384.

Pavlok, A., Koutecka, L., Krejci, P., Slavik, T., Cerman, J., Slaba, J., and Dorn, D. (1996). Effect of recombinant bovine somatotropin on follicular growth and quality of oocytes in cattle. *Anim. Reprod. Sci.* 41:183–192.

Pavlok, A., Lucas-Hahn, A., and Niemann, H. (1992). Fertilization and developmental competence of bovine oocytes derived from different categories of antral follicles. *Mol. Reprod. Dev.* 31:63–67.

Pawshe, C.H., Totey, S.M., and Jain, S.K. (1994). Methods of recovery of goat oocytes for in vitro maturation and fertilization. *Theriogenology.* 42:117–125.

Pereira, R.J.T.A., Sohnrey, B., and Holtz, W. (1998). Nonsurgical embryo transfer collection in goats treated with prostaglandin F_2 and oxytocin *J. Anim. Sci.* 76:360–363.

Petters, R.M., and Wells, K.D. (1993). Culture of pig embryos. *J. Reprod. Fert.* Suppl. 48:61–73.

Pieterse, M.C., Kappen, K.A., Kruip, Th.A.M., and Taverne, M.A.M. (1988). Aspiration of bovine oocytes during transvaginal ultrasound scanning of the ovaries. *Theriogenology.* 30:751–762.

Pinyopummintr, T., and Bavister, B.D. (1991). In vitro-matured/in vitro-fertilized bovine oocytes can develop into morulae/blastocysts in chemically defined, protein-free culture media. *Biol. Reprod.* 45:736–742.

Pollard, J.W., and Leibo, S.P. (1994). Chilling sensitivity of mammalian embryos. *Theriogenology.* 41:101–106.

Pope, C.E. (2000). Embryo technology in conservation efforts for endangered felids. *Theriogenology.* 53:163–174.

Pugh, P.A., Fukui, Y., Tervit, H.R., and Thompson, J.G. (1991). Developmental ability of in vitro matured sheep oocytes collected during the nonbreeding season and fertilized in vitro with frozen ram semen. *Theriogenology.* 36:771–778.

Purcell, S.H., Beal, W.E., and Gray, K.R. (2005). Effect of a CIDR insert and flunixin meglumine, administered at the time of embryo transfer, on pregnancy rate and resynchronization of estrus in beef cattle. *Theriogenology.* 64:867–878.

Pusateri, A.E., Smith, J.M., Smith, J.W. II, Thomford, P.J., and Diekman, M.A. (1996). Maternal recognition of pregnancy in swine. I. Minimal requirement for exogenous estradiol-17β to induce either short or long pseudopregnancy in cycling gilts. *Biol. Reprod.* 55:582–589.

Rao, V., Samah, B.C., and Bhattacharyya, N.K. (1984). Xenogenous fertilization of goat ova in the rabbit oviduct. *J. Reprod. Fertil.* 71:377–379.

Rath, D. (1992). Experiments to improve in vitro fertilization techniques for in vivo-matured porcine oocytes. *Theriogenology.* 37:885–896.

Rath, D., and Niemann, H. (1997). In vitro fertilization of porcine oocytes with fresh and frozen-thawed ejaculated or frozen-thawed epididymal semen obtained from identical boars. *Theriogenology.* 47:785–793.

Rátky, J., Brüssow, K.-P., Solti, L., Torner, H., and Sarlos, P. (2000). Ovarian response, embryo recovery and results of embryo transfer in a Hungarian native pig breed. *Theriogenology.* 56:969–978.

Rehman, N., Collins, A.R., Suh, T.K., and Wright, R.E. Jr. (1994). Development of in vitro matured and fertilized bovine oocytes co-cultured with buffalo rat liver cells. *Theriogenology.* 41:1453–1462.

Reichenbach, H.D., Liebrich, J., Berg, U., and Brem, G. (1992). Pregnancy rates and births after unilateral transfer of bovine embryos produced in vitro. *J. Reprod. Fertil.* 95:363–370.

Reinders, J.M.C., Wurth, Y.A., and Kruipm Th. A.M. (1995). From embryo to calf after transfer of in vitro produced bovine embryos. *Theriogenology.* 43:306 (Abstract).

Rieger, D., Grisart, B., Semple, E., Van Langendonckt, A., Betteridge, K.J., and Dessy, F. (1995). Comparison of the effects of oviductal cell co-culture and oviductal cell-conditioned medium on the development and metabolic activity of cattle embryos. *J. Reprod. Fertil.* 105:91–98.

Robertson, I., and Nelson, R.E. Certification and Identification of the embryo. (1998). In: Stringfellow D.A., and Seidel, S.M. (eds), *Manual of the International Embryo Transfer Society.* Savoy, IL: IETS, pp 103–134.

Rodrigues, B. de á., Carboneiro Dos Santos, L., and Rodrigues, J.L. (2004). Embryonic development of in vitro matured and in vitro fertilized dog oocytes. *Mol. Reprod. Dev.* 67:215–223.

Rodrigues, B. de á., and Rodrigues, J.L. (2003). Influence of reproductive status on in vitro oocyte maturation in dogs. *Theriogenology.* 60:59–66.

Rorie, R.W., Miller, G.F., Nasti, K.B., and McNew, R.W. (1994). In vitro development of bovine embryos as affected by different lots of bovine serum albumin and citrate. *Theriogenology.* 42:397–403.

Rosenkrans, J.F., Zeng, G.Q., McNamara, G.T., Schoff, P.K., and First, N.L. (1993). Development of bovine embryos in vitro as affected by energy substrates. *Biol. Reprod.* 49:459–462.

Rowson, L.E.A., and Dowling, D.F. (1949). An apparatus for the extraction of fertilized eggs from the living cow. *Vet. Rec.* 61:191.

Rubio Pomar, F.J., Teerds, K.J., Kidson, A., Colenbrander, B., Tharasanit, T., Aguilar, B., and Roelen, B.A.J. (2005). Differences in the incidence of apoptosis between in vivo and in vitro produced blastocysts of farm animal species: a comparative study. *Theriogenology.* 63:2254–2268.

Rutledge, J.J. (1996). Cattle production systems based on in-vitro embryo production. *J. Reprod. Dev.* 42:18–22

Saacke, R.G., Dalton, J.C., Nadir, S., Nebel, R.L., and Bame, J.H. (2000). Relationship of seminal traits and insemination time to fertilization rate and embryo quality. *Anim. Reprod. Sci.* 60–61:663–677.

Schellander, K., Brackett, B.G, Keefer, C.L. and Fayrer-Hosken, R.A. (1989). Testing capacitation of bull sperm with zona-free hamster ova. *Anim. Reprod. Sci.* 18:95–104.

Schenk, J.L., Suh, T.K., and Seidel Jr., G.E. (2006). Embryo production from superovulated cattle following insemination of sexed semen. *Theriogenology.* 65:299–307.

Schernthaner, W., Schmoll, F., Brem, G., and Schellander, K. (1997). Storing bovine ovaries for 24 hours between 15 and 21°C does not influence in vitro production of blastocysts. *Theriogenology.* 47:297 (Abstract).

Schmidt, M., Greve, T., Averym B., Beckers, J.F., Sulon, J., and Hansen, H.B. (1996). Pregnancies, calves, and calf viability after transfer of in vitro produced bovine embryos. *Theriogenology.* 46:527–539.

Schneider, C.S., Ellington, J.E., and Wright, R.W. Jr. (1996). Effects of bulls with different field fertility on in vitro embryo cleavage and development using sperm co-culture systems. *Theriogenology.* 45:262 (Abstract)

Scott, T.J., Carnevale, E.M., Maclellan, L.J., Scoggin, C.F., and Squires, E.L. (2001). Embryo development rates after transfer of oocytes matured in vivo, in vitro or within oviducts of mares. *Theriogenology.* 55:705–715.

Seidel, G.E. Jr. (2003). Economics of selecting for sex: the most important genetic trait. *Theriogenology.* 59:585–598.

Seidel, G.E. Jr. (1991). Embryo Transfer: the next 100 years. *Theriogenology.* 35:171–180.

Seidel, G.E. Jr., Schenk, J.L., Herickhoff, L.A., Doyle, S.P., Brink, Z., Green, R.D., and Cran, D.G. (1999). Insemination of heifers with sexed semen. *Theriogenology.* 52:1407–1420.

Seike, N., Saeki, K., Utaka, K., Sakai, M., Takakura, R., Nagao, Y., and Kanagawa, H. (1989). Production of bovine identical twins via transfer of demi-embryos without zonae pellucidae. *Theriogenology.* 32:211–220.

Shamsuddin, M., Larsson, B., Gustafsson, H., Gustari, S., Bartolome, J., and Rodriquez-Martinez, H. (1992). Comparative morphological evaluation of in vivo and in vitro produced bovine embryos. *Proc. 12th Int. Congr. Anim. Reprod.* 3:1333–1335.

Shea, B.F. (1999). Determining the sex of bovine embryos using polymerase chain reaction results: a six-year retrospective study. *Theriogenology.* 51:841–854.

Shi, D.S., Lu, K.H., and Gordon, I. (1990). Effects of bulls on fertilization of bovine oocytes and their subsequent development in vitro. *Theriogenology.* 33:324 (Abstract).

Sinclair, K.D., Broadbent, P.J., and Dolman, D.F. (1995). In vitro produced embryos as a means of achieving pregnancy and improving productivity in beef cows. *Anim. Sci.* 60:55–64.

Sinclair, K.D., McEvoy, T.G., Maxfield, E.K., Maltin, C.A., Young, L.E., Wilmut, I., Broadbent, P.J., and Robinson, J.J. (1999). Aberrant fetal growth and development after in vitro culture of sheep zygotes. *J. Reprod. Fertil.* 116:177–186.

Sinclair, K.D., Maxfield, E.K., Robinson, J.J., Maltin, C.A., and McEvoy, T.G. (1997). Culture of sheep zygotes can alter fetal growth and development. *Theriogenology.* 47:380 (Abstract).

Sinclair, K.D., Tregaskes, L.D., Maxfield, E.K., Robinson, J.J., Broadbent, P.J., and Maltin, C.A. (1996). Fetal growth following temporary exposure of day 3 ovine embryos to an advanced uterine environment. *Theriogenology.* 45:223 (Abstract).

Slavik, T., Fulka, J., and Goll, I. (1992). Pregnancy rate after the transfer of sheep embryos originated from randomly chosen oocytes matured and fertilized in vitro. *Theriogenology* 38:749–756.

Sloss, V., and Dufty, J.H. (1980). *Handbook of Bovine Obstetrics.* Baltimore: Williams and Wilkins.

Squires, E.L. (2005). Integration of future biotechnologies into the equine industry. *Anim. Reprod. Sci.* 89:187–198.

Squires, E.L., Carnevale, E.M., McCue, P.M., and Bruemmer, J.E. (2003). Embryo technologies in the horse. *Theriogenology.* 59:151–170.

Squires, E.L., McCue, P.M., and Vanderwall, D. (1999). The current status of equine embryo transfer. *Theriogenology.* 51:91–104.

Squires, E.L., McCue, P.M., Niswender, K., and Alvarenga, M. (2003). A review on the use of eFSH to enhance reproductive performance. *Proceedings of the American Association of Equine Practitioners* 49:360–362.

Squires, E.L., Wilson, J.M., Kato, H., and Blaszczyk, A. (1996). A pregnancy after intracytoplasmic sperm injection into equine oocytes matured in vitro. *Theriogenology.* 45:306 (Abstract).

Squires, E.L., Wilson, J.M., Kato, H., and Blaszczyk, A. (1996). A pregnancy after intracytoplasmic sperm injection into equine oocytes matured in vitro. *Theriogenology.* 45:306 (Abstract).

Stringfellow, D.A., and Givens, M.D. (2000a). Epidemiologic concerns relative to in vivo and in vitro production of livestock embryos. *Anim. Prod. Sci.* 50–61:629–642.

Stringfellow, D.A., and Givens, M.D. (2000b). Infectious agents in bovine embryo production: hazards and solutions. *Theriogenology.* 53:85–94.

Stringfellow, D.A., Riddell, K.P., Brock, K.V., Riddle, M.G., Galik, P.K., Wright, J.C., and Hasler, J.F. (1997). In vitro fertilization and in vitro culture of bovine embryos in the presence of noncytopathic bovine viral diarrhea virus. *Theriogenology.* 48:171–183.

Stringfellow, D.A., Riddell, M.G., Riddell, K.P., Carson, R.L., Smith, R.C., Gray, B.W., and Wright, J.C. (1993). Use of in vitro fertilization for production of calves from involuntary cull cows. *J. Assist. Reprod. Genet.* 10:280–285.

Stroud, B., and Hasler, J.F. (2006). Dissecting why superovulation and embryo transfer usually work on some farms and not on others. *Theriogenology.* 65:65–76.

Swanson, W.F., McRae, M.A., Wildt, D.E., and Rall, W.F. (1999). Cryoprotectant toxicity and cryopreservation success in IVF-derived domestic cat embryos after embryo transfer. *Theriogenology.* 51:174 (Abstract).

Tervit, H.R., Whittingham, D.G., and Rowson, L.E.A. (1972). Successful culture in vitro of sheep and cattle ova. *J. Reprod. Fertil.* 38:177–179.

Thatcher, W.W., Bilby, T.R., Bartolome, J.A., Silvestre, F., Staples, C.R., and Santos, J.E.P. (2006). Strategies for improving fertility in modern dairy cows. *Theriogenology.* 65:30–44.

Thibier, M. (2005). Significant increases in transfers of both in vivo derived and in vitro produced embryos in cattle and contrasted trends in other species in 2004. A report from the IETS Data Retrieval Committee. *Embryo Transfer Newsletter.* 23(4):11–17.

Thompson, J.G. (1996). Defining the requirements for bovine embryo culture. *Theriogenology.* 45:27–40.

Thompson, J.G., Gardner, D.K., Pugh, P.A., McMillan, W.H., and Tervit, H.R. (1995). Lamb birth weight is affected by culture system utilized during in vitro pre-elongation development of ovine embryos. *Biol. Reprod.* 53:1385–1391.

Thompson, J.G.E., Simpson, A.C., Pugh, P.A., Donnelly, P.E., and Tervit, H.R. (1990). Effect of oxygen concentration on in-vitro development of preimplantation sheep and cattle embryos. *J. Reprod. Fertil.* 89:573–578.

Tibary, A., Anouassi, A., and Khatir, H. (2005). Update on reproductive biotechnologies in small ruminants and camelids. *Theriogenology.* 64:618–638.

Tocharus, C., Sukbunteung, J., Jarauansuwan, M., Chuangsoongneon, U., Kitiyanant, Y., and Pavasuthipaisit, K. (1997). Different developmental stages of bovine embryos produced in vitro: their sex ratio and survival rates. *Theriogenology.* 47:330 (Abstract).

Tsutsui, T., Hori, T., Okazaki, H., Tanaka, A., Shiono, M., Yokosuka, M., and Kawakami, E. (2001). Transfer of canine embryos at various developmental stages recovered by hysterectomy or surgical uterine flushing. *J. Vet. Med. Sci.* 63:401–405.

Tubman, L.M., Brink, Z., Suh, T.K., and Seidel, G.E. Jr. (2003). Normality of calves resulting from sexed sperm. *Theriogenology.* 59:517 (Abstract)

Udy, G.B. (1987). Commercial splitting of goat embryos. *Theriogenology.* 28:837–847.

Umbaugh, R.E. (1949). Superovulation and ovum transfer in cattle. *Am J. Vet. Res.* 10:295–305.

Vajta, G., Holm, P., Greve, T., and Callesen, H. (1996). Overall efficiency of in vitro embryo production and vitrification in cattle. *Theriogenology.* 45:683–689.

Van der Schans, A., van der Westerlaken, L.A.J., de Wit, A.A.C., Eyestone, W.H., and de Boer, H.A. (1991). Ultrasound-guided transvaginal collection of oocytes in the cow. *Theriogenology.* 35:288 (Abstract).

Van Soom, A., Boerjan, M., Ysebaert, M.-T., and De Kruif, A. (1996). Cell allocation to the inner cell mass and the trophectoderm in bovine embryos cultured in two different media. *Mol. Reprod. Dev.* 45:171–182.

Van Soom, A., Mijten, P., Van Vlaenderen, I., Van den Branden, J., Mahmoudzadeh, A.R., and de Kruif, A. (1994). Birth of double-muscled Belgian blue calves after transfer of in vitro produced embryos into dairy cattle. *Theriogenology.* 41:855–867.

Vansteenbrugge, A., Van Langendonckt, A., Scutenaire, C., Massip, A., and Dessy, F. (1994). In vitro development of bovine embryos in buffalo rat liver-or bovine oviduct-conditioned medium. *Theriogenology.* 42:931–940.

Verstegen, J.P., Onclin, K., Silva, L.D., Donnay, I., Mettens, P., and Ectors, F. (1993). Superovulation and embryo culture in vitro following treatment with ultra-pure follicle-stimulating hormone in cats. J. Reprod. Fertil. Suppl. 47:209–218.

Viuff, D., Rickords, L., Offenberg, H., Hyttel, P., Avery, B., Greve, T., Olsaker, I., Williams, J.L., Callesen, H., and Thomsen, P.D. (1999). A high proportion of bovine blastocysts produced in vitro are mixoploid. *Biol. Reprod.* 60:1273–1278.

Vivanco-Mackie, H.W. (2000). Development and application of ovum pick up (OPU) and in vitro embryo production in the bovine. A view to arTech experiences. *Proc. of the Australian Embryo Transfer Society.* Perth, Australia, p 29–48.

Voeklel, S.A., Hu, Y.X. (1992). Direct transfer of frozen-thawed bovine embryos. *Theriogenology.* 37:23–37.

Wagtendonk-de Leeuw, van A.M. (2006). Ovum pick up and in vitro production in the bovine after use in several generations: A 2005 status. *Theriogenology.* 65:914–925.

Wagtendonk-de Leeuw, van A.M., Aerts, B.J.G., and Den Daas, J.H.G. (1998). Abnormal offspring following in vitro production of bovine pre-implantation embryos: a field study. *Theriogenology.* 49:883–894.

Wagtendonk-de Leeuw, van A.M., Mullaart, E.R., de Roos, A.P.W., Merton, J.S., den Daas, J.H.G., Kemp, B., and de Ruigh, L. (2000). Effects of different reproduction techniques: AI, MOET, or IVP, on health and welfare of bovine offspring. *Theriogenology.* 53:575–597.

Walker, S.K., Heard, T.M., Bee, C.A., Frensham, A.B., Warnes, D.M., and Seamark, R.F. (1992a). Culture of embryos of farm animals. In: Lauria, A., and Gandolfi, F. (eds.) *Embryonic Development and Manipulation in Animal Production.* London, United Kingdom: Portland Press, pp 77–92.

Walker, S.K., Heard, T.M., and Seamark, R.F. (1992b). In vitro culture of sheep embryos without coculture: successes and perspectives. *Theriogenology* 37:111–126.

Walker, S.K., Hill, J.L., Bee, C.A., and Warnes, D.M. (1994). Improving the rate of production of sheep embryos using in vitro maturation and fertilization. *Theriogenology.* 41:330 (Abstract).

Walker, S.K., Hill, J.L., Kleemann, D.O., and Noncarrow, C.D. (1996). Development of ovine embryos in synthetic oviductal fluid containing amino acids at oviductal fluid concentrations. *Biol. Reprod.* 55:703–708.

Wegner, C.C., and Killian, G.J. (1991). In vitro and in vivo association of an oviduct estrus-associated protein with bovine zona pellucida. *Mol. Reprod. Dev.* 29:77–84.

Watson, A.J., Watson, P.H., Warnes, D., Walker, S.K., Armstrong, D.T., and Seamark, R.F. (1994). Preimplantation development of in vitro-matured and in vitro-fertilized ovine zygotes: comparison between coculture on oviduct epithelial cell monolayers and culture under low oxygen atmosphere. *Biol. Reprod.* 50:715–724.

Wheeler, M.B., Rutledge, J.J., Fischer-Brown, A., VanEtten, T., Malusky, S., and Beebe, D.J. (2006). Application of sexed semen technology to in vitro embryo production in cattle. *Theriogenology.* 65:219–227.

Whittingham, D.G. (1968). Fertilization of mouse eggs in vitro. *Nature.* 220:592–593.

Wilmut, I., and Rowson, L.E.A. (1973). Experiments on the low-temperature preservation of cow embryos. *Vet. Rec.* 92:686–690.

Wilmut, I., and Sales, D.I. (1981). Effect of an asynchronous environment on embryonic development in sheep. *J. Reprod. Fertil.* 61:179–184.

Wilson, R.D., Fricke, P.M., Leibfried-Rutledge, M.L., Rutledge, J.J., Syverson Penfield, C.M., and Weigel, K.A. (2006). In vitro production of bovine embryos suing sex-sorted sperm. *Theriogenology.* 65:1007–1015.

Willett, E.L., Black, W.G., Casida, L.E., Stone, W.H., and Buckner, P.J. (1951). Successful transplantation of a fertilized bovine ovum. *Science, N.Y.* 113:247.

Williams, T.J., Elsden, R.P., and Seidel, G.E. Jr. (1984). Pregnancy rates with bisected bovine embryos. *Theriogenology.* 22:521–531.

Xu, K.P., Yadav, B.R., King, W.A., and Betteridge, K.J. (1992). Sex-related differences in developmental rates of bovine embryos produced and cultured in vitro. *Mol. Reprod. Dev.* 31:249–252.

Yadav, B.R., Katiyar, P.K., Chauhan, M.S., and Madan, M.L. (1997). Chromosome configuration during in vitro maturation of goat, sheep and buffalo oocytes. *Theriogenology.* 47:943–951.

Yamada, S., Shimazu, Y., Kawano, Y., Nakazawa, M., Naito, K., and Toyoda, Y. (1993). In vitro maturation and fertilization of preovulatory dog oocytes. *J. Reprod. Fertil.* Suppl. 47:227–229.

Yoshida, M., Mizoguchiu, Y., Ishigaki, K., Kojima, T., and Nagai, T. (1993). Birth of piglets derived from in vitro fertilization of pig oocytes matured in vitro. *Theriogenology.* 39:1303–1311.

Young, L.E., Butterwith, S.C., and Wilmut, I. (1996). Increased ovine foetal weight following transient asynchronous embryo transfer is not associated with increased placental weight at day 21 of gestation. *Theriogenology.* 45:231 (Abstract).

Young, L.E., Sinclair, K.D., and Wilmut, I. (1998). Large offspring syndrome in cattle and sheep. *Reviews of Reproduction* 3:155–163.

Youngs, C.R. (2001). Factors influencing the success of embryo transfer in the pig. *Theriogenology.* 56:1311–1320.

Younis, A.I., Zuelke, K.A., Harper, K.M., Oliveira, M.A.L., and Brackett, B.G. (1991). In vitro fertilization of goat oocytes. *Biol. Reprod.* 44:11771182.

Zeringue, H.C., Rutledge, J.J., and Beebe, D.J. (2004). Early mammalian development depends on cumulus removal technique. *Lab Chip* 5:86–90.

Zhang, B.F., Larsson, B., Lundeheim, N., and Rodriguez-Martinez, H. (1997). Relationship between embryo development in vitro and 56-day nonreturn rates of cows inseminated with frozen-thawed semen from dairy bulls. *Theriogenology.* 48:221–231.

Zhang, J.J., Muzs, L.Z., and Boyle, M.S. (1990). In vitro fertilization of horse follicular oocytes matured in vitro. *Mol. Reprod. Dev.* 26:361–365.

Chapter 9

The Comparative Cryobiology of Preimplantation Embryos from Domestic Animals

Steven F. Mullen and John K. Critser

Introduction

Methods for cryopreserving mammalian preimplantation embryos have been available for about 35 years (Whittingham et al., 1972; Wilmut, 1972b), although success has only been achieved for embryos from some taxonomic groups. For example, while frozen and thawed embryos from cows and pigs have developed into live offspring (Massip, 2001), not a single live birth of a domestic dog resulting from the transfer of a frozen-thawed embryo has been reported (Farstad, 2000). There are varying reasons for this discrepancy, ranging from the current status of *in vitro* embryo manipulation (Bavister, 1995; Thompson, 2000), to vast differences in the ability of embryos across taxa to tolerate the various nonphysiological stresses imposed upon them during freezing and thawing (Massip, 2001).

Numerous benefits of embryo cryopreservation can be cited. From the practical standpoint of animal agriculture, being able to freeze embryos from superior females facilitates dispersion of superior genetics from dams, allowing improvements in the genetic quality of herds (Lohuis, 1995) as has resulted with artificial insemination using cryopreserved semen from superior bulls (Barber, 1983). Cryopreservation also facilitates international transport of embryos as a means of infusing genetic variation into indigenous populations (Gunasena and Critser, 1997; Wildt et al., 1997).

In many instances, proper handling (e.g. extensive washing coupled with trypsin treatment) has been shown to remove contaminating pathogens from the surface of embryos (e.g. Akabane virus, bovine leukemia virus, bluetongue virus, bovine viral diarrhea virus, foot-and-mouth disease virus, and bovine herpes virus 1 and 4 (Chemineau et al., 1986; Philpott, 1993 reviewed in Stringfellow, 2000). Therefore, applying proper precautions can allow the creation of a bank of "clean" embryos as a means to regenerate a disease-free herd in the event that a disease outbreak results in the contamination of healthy animals.

Cryopreservation has the potential to eliminate the international transport of diseases with embryo exchange programs (Thibier and Nibart, 1987). However, it should be noted that the effectiveness of these treatments can vary across taxa (Guerin et al., 1997; Stringfellow and Givens, 2000), and there is evidence that some infectious organisms persist after such treatments (Bane et al., 1990; Riddell et al., 1989). In addition, effective measures for *in vivo* derived embryos have been shown to be less effective when applied to *in vitro* derived embryos after experimental contamination (Bielanski and Jordan, 1996; Bielanski and Surjujballi, 1996; Marguant-Le Guienne et al., 1998; Stringfellow et al., 2000; Trachte et al., 1998). Therefore, care must be taken in the development of embryo banks in regard to the potential for disease transmission.

Finally, embryo cryopreservation procedures allow the creation of a bank of frozen material as a back-up in the event of a catastrophic failure with the possibility of eliminating small, isolated populations of either valuable domestic (Critser and Russell, 2000; Glenister et al., 1990; Whittingham, 1974) or exotic animals (Ballou, 1992; Holt et al., 2003; Wildt, 2000).

In this chapter, we review the field of cryobiology and provide an overview of the historical development of preimplantation embryo cryopreservation from several domestic taxa. The literature on embryo cryopreservation for some groups is vast. Here we will only highlight the major points which have allowed the science to advance to its current state. In the section on cryobiology fundamentals, we provide an overview of the many facets of this science, and the place that the mammalian preimplantation embryo has had in its development. We hope this provides insight into the approaches taken to freeze embryos, and the reasons why embryos from some mammals can be cryopreserved relatively easily, while others remain recalcitrant. To provide a proper context, we will begin with a brief overview of preimplantation embryology in mammals.

An Overview of Preimplantation Mammalian Embryology

Development of the mammalian embryo begins with successful fertilization of the mature oocyte (see review by Yanagimachi, 1994). Many events occur in the oocyte after sperm entry, including sperm head decondensation, sperm nuclear reorganization, nuclear reprogramming, and completion of maternal meiosis (Fan and Sun, 2004; Garagna and Redi, 1988; Hartmann, 1983; Kim et al., 1996; McLay

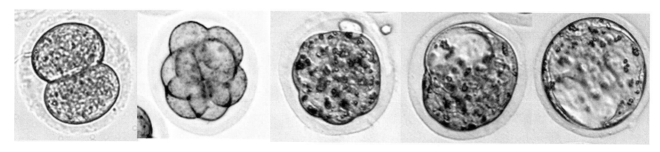

Figure 9.1. Images showing the progression of the preimplantation embryo from the 2-cell stage to the blastocyst stage in the mouse. A 2-cell embryo is shown in panel 1. About two days later the embryo progresses to the 8-cell stage (panel 2). Note that the individual cells are still discernable. The following day, the embryo undergoes compaction and becomes a morula (panel 3), and the individual cells are no longer evident. In panel 4, the early formation of the blastocoel cavity is evident, and by the fifth day, a fully-formed blastocoel cavity has formed (panel 5). In embryos from livestock species, it is more difficult to discern individual cells at the 8-cell stage, due to the significantly higher cytoplasmic lipid content.

and Clarke, 2003; Schatten and Schatten, 1987; Schatten et al., 1988; Schatten et al., 1986; Shimada et al., 2000; Sutovsky et al., 1996; Wassarman et al., 2001). Eventually, a maternal and paternal pronucleus form and the pronuclei are brought into apposition via microtubules (Schatten et al., 1985). The pronuclear membranes break down, and the chromosomes align on the metaphase plate (termed "syngamy") in preparation for the first mitotic cleavage division resulting in a 2-cell embryo.

During the first couple of cell divisions (see Figure 9.1), the embryonic cells, referred to as *blastomeres*, remain as independent entities from the standpoint of their developmental fate. Embryos have been produced by allowing one of the two blastomeres from 2-cell embryos to develop independently (Nicholas and Hall, 1942; Pincus, 1936; Rands, 1986). However, differences have been reported between such embryos and normal embryos, and term development differs across species (Tsunoda and McLaren, 1983 and references therein).

One important developmental event occurs around this time in the progression of the embryo, however. Stockpiling of resources such as mRNA and proteins occurs during maturation of the oocyte, and the early embryo relies on these resources for its support (Capco, 2001; Smith, 1972). There is a transition to genomic control of development at a certain stage of early development, whereby gene products from the embryo are required to direct further developmental fate of the embryo (Nothias et al., 1995; Schultz, 2002).

This approximate temporal transition can be determined by several methods, including incorporation of ^{3}H-Uridine into mRNA, monitoring degradation of maternal messenger RNAs, or culturing embryos with α-amanitin to inhibit gene transcription and then following embryo development in culture. Such studies have determined the temporal events in embryos from different mammals, and have shown that the time at which embryos require embryonic transcription occurs around the 2-cell stage in the mouse (Schultz, 1993), although differences between strains have

been shown (Rambhatla and Latham, 1995), the 4-cell stage in the pig (Tomanek et al., 1989), and the 9- to 16-cell stage in the cow (Memili and First, 1998). It should be noted that upregulation of embryonic transcription is not an all or nothing event, and levels of transcription have been detected as early as the zygote (Bouniol et al., 1995; Tesarik and Kopecny, 1989; reviewed in Memili and First, 2000).

The embryo undergoes compaction—the first noticeable morphological change in its development—around the 8-cell stage. Up to this point, contacts between the blastomeres are tenuous. During compaction, cell-to-cell interactions become more prominent, with tight junctions becoming established between the blastomeres (Pratt et al., 1982). Upon completion of compaction, the embryo becomes a morula, with individual blastomeres no longer discernable.

Tight junctions are essential for continued differentiation of the embryo (Fleming et al., 2001). The next stage of development is marked by the first cell differentiation event (Fleming et al., 2004), culminating in the development of the blastocyst. The blastomeres, up to this stage, remain totipotent (Kelly, 1977; Tarkowski and Wroblewska, 1967). At the early stage of blastocyst development, the cells become irreversibly committed to their developmental fate (Gardner et al., 1973; Rossant, 1976; Ziomek et al., 1982) and differentiate either into cells of the trophectoderm or inner cell mass. The cells of the trophectoderm eventually form the placental tissues, while the majority of the cells in the inner cell mass form the embryo proper. This stage of development is also marked by the formation of a fluid-filled cavity termed the *blastocoel*. The blastocoel develops as a result of the action of several gene products, including the sodium-potassium-ATPase enzyme which pumps sodium ions into the inner space of the embryo, with water following via osmosis (Biggers et al., 1977; Overstrom et al., 1989; Watson and Barcroft, 2001). As cell division continues, the blastocoel cavity eventually constitutes the majority of the volume of the embryo.

After development into the blastocyst, the embryo "hatches" from its glycoprotein shell (the zona pellucida), migrating out of a small crack in its structure. During development of the blastocyst, an acellular, proteinaceous capsule is produced by the trophectoderm and is deposited between the embryo and zona pellucida. An interesting difference is seen in embryos from horses, however (Ginther, 1992). In equine embryos, the zona pellucida peels away from the embryo, leaving the blastocyst encased by the capsule (see discussion in Betteridge, 1989).

In some mammals, such as the mouse and human, the embryo establishes intimate contact with the uterus shortly after hatching from the zona. In others, such as the pig and cow, implantation occurs at a later time, after continued cell division and greater enlargement of the embryo (Dey et al., 2004). Implantation, the mechanisms of which vary widely across mammalian taxa (Lee and DeMayo, 2004; Ramsey, 1975), allows the embryo to acquire nutrients directly from the mother's bloodstream. Without this nutritional support, continued growth and differentiation of the embryo would not be possible.

Cryobiology

While the effects of cold temperatures on biological systems and attempts to preserve cells and tissues through freezing have been investigated for several centuries (Luyet and Gehenio, 1940; Parkes, 1957; Walters and Critser, in press), it is only within the last few decades that reliable methods to cryopreserve some cell types have become available. As will be discussed in more detail below, research using preimplantation embryos has contributed significantly to our understanding of many of the fundamental principles of cryobiology. Cryobiology is a broad discipline, encompassing aspects of physics, chemistry, engineering, mathematics, and cellular and molecular biology.

What follows is a general overview of the more important aspects of the effects of freezing on cells and our current understanding of how to overcome some of these challenges. Interested readers are referred to classic texts such as *Life and Death at Low Temperatures* (Luyet and Gehenio, 1940), *Cryobiology* (Meryman, 1966), and the very recently published *Life in the Frozen State* (Fuller et al., 2004) if more detailed information on the subject is desired.

To truly cryopreserve cells, they must be held at very low temperatures. Liquid nitrogen is the medium most often used to store frozen material (−196°C), because it is relatively easy to generate yet cold enough to prevent the decay of cells during storage. Once cells reach this temperature, it is believed that they can be held indefinitely (Fogarty et al., 2000; Leibo et al., 1994; Mazur, 1970). Consequently, it is the means of getting cells to such temperatures, and equally important, getting them back to physiologic temperature, that constitutes the challenge for effective cell preservation (see Mazur, 2004 for a more thorough discussion of these principles).

Prior to the late 1940s, success with cellular cryopreservation was limited, and the few methods claimed to succeed were often difficult to replicate (Parkes, 1985). It is frequently said that cryobiology as a science was born in 1949 with the report of the serendipitous discovery of the cryoprotective properties of glycerol (Polge et al., 1949). During the ensuing years, it was established that a high degree of cell survival during freezing is only possible if the cells are frozen in solutions containing one or more compounds generically referred to as cryoprotective agents (CPAs). These compounds are often categorized into two classes—permeating, or those which freely diffuse through the plasma membrane, and non-permeating. Common permeating cryoprotectants include glycerol, ethylene glycol (EG), propylene glycol (PG) and other low molecular weight polyols, and dimethylsulfoxide (DMSO). Common non-permeating cryoprotectants include saccharides such as sucrose, fructose, trehalose, and raffinose.

The mechanism of protection of cryoprotectants has often been attributed to several causes, including:

- direct interaction with cell membranes and other macromolecules acting to stabilize their structure (Anchordoguy et al., 1987)
- suppression of the intracellular nucleation temperature (Rall et al., 1983)
- dilution or colligative effects by reducing the ionic concentration in the cytoplasm or suspending medium or the amount of ice formed in the solution (Lovelock, 1953a, 1953b; Mazur et al., 1981; Meryman et al., 1977; Santarius and Giersch, 1983).

While the presence of these compounds is usually necessary for cell survival during freezing, as mentioned above, exposing cells to solutions that contain cryoprotectants is not necessarily benign. For example, in their original 1949 report, Polge et al. showed that rooster sperm maintained a degree of motility comparable to unfrozen sperm after rapid freezing in the presence of glycerol. However, only after the glycerol removal procedure was modified according to a similar method developed for leukocytes (Sloviter, 1951) were the sperm able to fertilize ova (Polge, 1951).

Today, the potential detriment to cells as a result of anisosmotic exposure has been well documented (Agca et al., 2000; Blanco et al., 2000; Gao et al., 1995; Gilmore et al., 1996; Liu et al., 2002; Mazur and Schneider, 1986; Meryman, 1971; Mullen et al., 2004; Pukazhenthi et al., 2000; Williams and Shaw, 1980; Zieger et al., 1999). Mathematical models describing the osmotic response of cells to anisosmotic solutions were developed many years ago (Jacobs and Stewart, 1932; Kedem and Katchalsky, 1958). Often, an early step in optimizing cryopreservation procedures involves determining the limits to which cells can tolerate cell volume excursions, and using this information to develop optimal procedures for the addition and removal of permeating CPAs to cells (Gao et al., 1997; Gao et al., 1995).

After exposure to the cryoprotective solution, cells are cooled progressively until reaching the final storage temperature. The optimal rate of this cooling differs across cell types. Cooling too slowly or quickly can be damaging to the cells for several reasons, including injury due to chilling (see below), intracellular water crystallization, or as a result of exposure to concentrated solutions for extended periods (the so-called "solution effects" injury) (Mazur et al., 1972).

Intracellular ice formation (IIF) is often cited as the primary cause of cell death when supraoptimal cooling rates are used, and is a well-studied phenomenon (Acker et al., 1999; Karlsson et al., 1993; Leibo et al., 1978; McGrath et al., 1975; Muldrew and McGann, 1990; Myers et al., 1989; Pitt, 1992; Pitt and Steponkus, 1989; Ruffing et al., 1993; Toner et al., 1990; Toner et al., 1993; Toner et al., 1991).

Related to understanding the phenomenon of optimal cooling rates during freezing, one of the most influential reports in the field of cryobiology was published in 1963 by Mazur, who proposed a mechanism by which slow cooling prevented IIF. According to his theory, the crystallization of water in the extracellular solution establishes a thermodynamic gradient as a result of the difference in the chemical potential of intracellular and extracellular water. Chemical potential equilibrium can be reestablished by either crystallization of the intracellular water to form ice, or by liquid water flowing out of the cell and joining the extracellular ice phase. The former is often fatal. If the degree of supercooling is low, the probability of intracellular ice formation is reduced, and the second scenario is more likely. If cooling proceeds at a sufficiently slow rate, enough intracellular water can flow out of the cell to prevent excessive supercooling and increase the concentration of the cytoplasm so that damaging ice crystals are not formed upon transfer to liquid nitrogen.

This mechanism explains the different optimal cooling rates for different cell types because it accounts for inherent differences in biophysical characteristics of cells such as water permeability and the surface-to-volume ratio. As a measure of the success of his theoretical work, the procedure that resulted in the best survival for the first successful cryopreservation of mammalian embryos (Whittingham et al., 1972) was similar to that predicted to be effective by the theory put forth nine years earlier.

Intracellular ice formation and the ensuing damage can be prevented by vitrification (Fahy et al., 1984), which is often defined as the transition of a liquid phase to a solid phase without crystallization. Achieving a vitreous state of the cytoplasm requires that cells be equilibrated with intracellular concentrations of solutes at much higher concentrations than those used for slow cooling methods (e.g. >4 M), and also that the cell suspension is cooled quickly (Fahy et al., 1987; Fahy et al., 1984). As mentioned earlier, exposing cells to high solute concentrations can be lethal due to osmotic as well as chemical effects. The higher solute concentrations necessary to achieve vitrification simply exacerbate these problems.

Many methods to reduce the detrimental effects of vitrification solutions have been investigated. To date, these include application of hydrostatic pressure, addition of nonpenetrating agents to the suspension (and a concomitant reduction of the permeating solute concentration), combining different permeating agents to reduce the concentration of each individual agent, and adding compounds to neutralize the toxicity of certain permeating agents (reviewed in Fahy et al., 1984).

The mechanistic explanation of the prevention of intracellular ice formation via slow cooling suggests that there is a cooling rate for each cell type below which survival is predicted to be high. However, empirical studies have shown that there is an optimum cooling rate for different cells, above and below which cell survival diminishes. This observation has been interpreted to mean that two distinct mechanisms of injury occur to cells during freezing (Mazur et al., 1972): intracellular ice formation at supraoptimal rates (as just described), and the effects of the solution.

If cells are to be cooled from physiological temperature to liquid nitrogen without being killed, they must traverse this temperature range once again before being used. The rate of warming from −196°C can be as important to cell survival as the rate of cooling. In typical slow cooling procedures used for preimplantation embryos, cooling proceeds at a rate around 0.5°C/minute to about −35°C, at which the sample is transferred to liquid nitrogen. Some of the earliest investigations in mammalian embryo cryobiology (Wilmut, 1972) demonstrated that the warming rate necessary to achieve survival was directly related to the cooling rate (this had also been observed in other cell types; Mazur and Schmidt, 1968) or the temperature to which the cells were cooled prior to being transferred to liquid nitrogen (Rall and Polge, 1984; Willadsen, 1977).

This outcome has been interpreted as follows: When cooling is hastened (either by applying faster rates or interrupting the cooling at higher temperatures), more water remains in the cells than if cooling was prolonged. This water either forms small ice crystals or vitrifies upon transfer to liquid nitrogen. This state of water is thermodynamically unstable. Rapid warming in this instance would be necessary to maintain cell viability by preventing lethal IIF via devitrification—the transformation of vitreous water into ice (Rall et al., 1984)—or recrystallization—the amalgamation of smaller ice crystals into larger, more damaging ice crystals (Bank, 1973).

One possible explanation for the sensitivity to rapid warming after slow cooling to lower temperatures (which causes more osmotic dehydration than cooling to higher temperatures) is that an excessive osmotic differential is created across the cytoplasmic membrane as the extracellular ice suddenly melts and the cytoplasm remains concentrated (Farrant and Morris, 1973), resulting in damage to the plasma membrane.

The first report on the achievement of vitrification with mammalian (mouse) embryos appeared in 1985 (Rall and

Fahy, 1985). Subsequently, numerous papers describing mammalian embryo vitrification have appeared, and this approach has proven more effective for cryopreserving chilling sensitive embryos than more traditional slow cooling methods (see below).

While there are many factors to consider in developing appropriate cryopreservation methods, success should be achievable for embryos of all organisms given more thorough understanding of their cryobiological properties and further investigations into fundamental cryobiology.

The Sensitivity of Mammalian Preimplantation Embryos to Cooling

Cold shock injury, the detrimental response to a rapid reduction in temperature, has been the subject of investigations for many years (Morris and Watson, 1984). Several factors can affect the response of cells to cold exposure, including the rate of cooling and the time to which the cells are exposed to the temperature.

The plasma membrane is one of the primary sites of injury resulting from cold shock (De Leeuw et al., 1990). During rapid cooling, membrane lipids undergo a transition from a liquid crystalline phase to a gel phase. It is thought that this transition is the cause of the injury, which results in the loss of the selective permeability (Drobnis et al., 1993). Other responses of cold shock damage have been attributed to protein denaturation, metabolic disturbances, and damage to the cytoskeleton and cytoskeletal-membrane attachments (reviewed in Watson and Morris, 1987).

Because cooling to subphysiological temperatures is required for cryopreservation, it is not surprising that many investigations have been conducted in an effort to understand the effects of cold but non-freezing temperatures on preimplantation embryo development. It has been shown that embryos from some species are quite tolerant of cooling, while those from other species are very sensitive to cold temperatures. These factors, which will be discussed in more detail below, have contributed to the evolution of cryopreservation methods for embryos across various taxa. The idea of designing cryopreservation methods to "out race" chilling injury has been applied to embryos from organisms as diverse as pigs and flies (Dobrinsky, 2001; Mazur et al., 1992; Steponkus et al., 1990) and is one of the primary reasons that vitrification methods have been most successful for porcine embryos.

Two of the earliest reports on the developmental effect of cooling mammalian embryos *in vitro* were published in 1947 and 1948 by M.C. Chang. In the first paper, he documented the effects of cooling 2-cell rabbit embryos to 0° or 5°C on their further development. He noted several important factors, including the benefit of slow cooling (four- or five-hour transition from 25°C to 5°C or 0°C, respectively), and that these embryos could be held for 24 hours at 0°C to 15°C with 63 percent to 85 percent continuing development. He also showed that 23 percent of embryos held for

144 hours at 10°C could develop in culture (colder temperatures were more detrimental at these times). He documented several live births from embryos stored at temperatures between 0°C and 15°C, but only one embryo held for 120 to 144 hours at 0°C and 5°C developed to term, and the offspring was smaller than normal.

In his second study, Chang showed that 2-cell and morula stage embryos are more tolerant of cooling and holding at 10°C compared to blastocysts (37 percent, 37 percent, and 19 percent of embryos developed to term, respectively). He also showed that some embryos held at 0°C for 24 and 96 hours can develop to term (11 percent and 6 percent, respectively).

The following year, Pincus (1949) reported on the effects of cooling *in vivo*-derived cattle embryos. He demonstrated that cleavage-stage embryos could develop further *in vitro* after exposure to 10°C for up to 24 hours. However, when the exposure was extended (72 hours) or the temperature was reduced (0°C for 24 or 72 hours), the developmental progression was reduced.

In 1959, Averill and Rowson reported on the effects of cooling, and perhaps the earliest attempt at cryopreservation, on sheep embryos. In this report, they cooled embryos slowly (about 0.5°C/minute) to 5°C to 8°C and stored them for six to nine hours in serum or Ringers solution. Nine of 12 embryos cooled in serum continued development in utero, while zero of five cooled in Ringers developed. They went on to show that storage up to 24 hours was possible (seven of 15 normal embryos), but further storage (48 to 72 hours) was lethal. Storage below 4°C was invariably fatal. Further cooling (down to −79°C) in the presence of 12.5 percent glycerol and storage for 24 hours also proved fatal. In the last experiment, they performed embryo transfer using embryos previously cooled to 4.5°C to 7°C, or below 4°C, for 24 or 72 hours. Of the six embryos cooled to 4.5°C to 7°C, held for 24 hours, and re-warmed, four developed to term (all recipients became pregnant). Two of the five embryos held for 72 hours developed to term. However, none of the embryos cooled below 4°C developed fully.

Several reports were published in the early to mid 1970s documenting the effects of cooling on cattle, pig, and sheep embryos. From these reports, several common themes appear, including the differential cooling sensitivity of embryos across taxa, sensitivity differences at different developmental stages, and embryo source (*in vivo*- versus *in vitro*-derived).

Wilmut (1972a) showed that there is a decrease in *in vivo* derived porcine embryo tolerance to cooling below 15°C. Eight-cell embryos were cooled to 20°C, 15°C, 10°C, or 5°C. None of the embryos cooled to 10°C or 5°C developed either *in vitro* or *in vivo*. This effect was not seen with embryos cooled to the higher temperatures. In 1974, Polge et al. described differences in cooling sensitivity of embryos from cattle, sheep, and pigs. When sheep embryos from 8-cell to the blastocyst stage were cooled to 0°C, all developed normally in rabbit oviducts. The majority of cattle morula also developed, but most of the 8-cell embryos from cattle and all of the pig embryos (8-cell to the blastocyst stage) were killed by this treatment.

In 1975, Wilmut et al. demonstrated a stage-dependent tolerance to chilling of *in vivo* derived cattle embryos. Early stage embryos, up through the early morula stage, demonstrated sensitivity to chilling down to 0°C. However, late morula embryos were more tolerant. For cattle embryos, one might speculate that an effect of the transition to embryonic genome control of development is responsible for this sensitivity because this transition occurs around the morula stage. If this is the case, however, the same mechanism does not appear to be responsible for conferring chilling tolerance to porcine embryos, because they undergo this transition at an earlier stage than cattle embryos.

In 1976, Trounson et al. described a similar stage dependence on chilling tolerance of bovine embryos. Their data also suggested that the cooling rate can affect chilling tolerance as well, with slow cooling conferring a benefit. Time of exposure also seemed to affect on survival, but this depended upon the final storage temperature.

In two other reports that same year, the same group reported on the stage-dependence of tolerance to cooling of cattle (Trounson et al., 1976) and sheep (Willadsen et al., 1976) embryos. The first report demonstrated that bovine blastocysts produced by culturing morulae *in vitro* are more tolerant of cooling than morulae produced *in vivo* (from their previously published study). However, the developmental rate was better for *in vivo*-produced embryos versus *in vitro*-produced embryos (60 percent versus 38 percent). The second study showed that the tolerance of sheep embryos to 0°C exposure increased from the 2- to 4-cell stage (8 percent further cleavage) to the morula stage (71 percent).

Several years later, Pollard and Leibo (1994) designed experiments to determine more precisely the temperature and time effects on bovine and porcine embryos. They showed that while 90 percent of *in vivo*-derived porcine morula cooled to 15°C progressed to the blastocyst stage, only 5 percent of those cooled to 14°C did, and none cooled to 13°C survived. It should be noted that in this first experiment, the embryos were cooled at a rate of 1°C/minute. When embryos were abruptly cooled from 30°C, 80 percent survived exposure to 20°C, but tolerance to 10°C was only possible if the exposure was restricted to 30 seconds.

These authors also demonstrated the differential sensitivity of *in vivo*-derived compared to *in vitro*-derived bovine embryos at the morula and blastocyst stage. *In vitro* blastocysts were shown to be fairly tolerant of cooling to 5°C (80 percent survival) and 0°C (60 percent survival). Similar to the *in vivo*-derived bovine morula in the studies described above, *in vitro*-derived morula were shown to be more temperature sensitive, with only 65 percent surviving exposure to 15°C, and exposure to 10°C could only be tolerated (>60 percent survival) if the exposure lasted for one minute or less.

Similar to the tolerance of bovine blastocysts, equine blastocysts (day 7) can tolerate cooling to 5°C (Carnevale et al., 1987). In fact, in this report, 55 percent of the embryos exposed to this temperature for 24 hours developed in utero for at least 35 days. Cook et al. described successful embryo transfer after cooling and transporting equine embryos by air freight (Cook et al. 1989). The pregnancy rates were no different for control, transported, and cooled-transported embryos. It was later shown that, contrary to the results for freezing discussed below, larger equine blastocysts appear to be more tolerant of cooling compared to smaller blastocysts (Moussa et al., 2003).

One of the more interesting reports to be published recently on chilling injury to embryos demonstrated that the intracellular lipids can have a significant effect on cold exposure to early porcine embryos (see Figure 9.2).

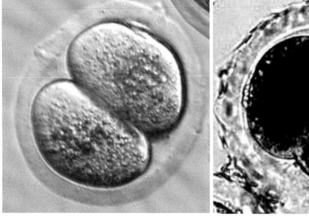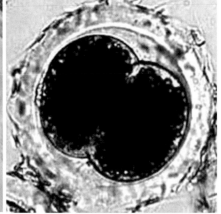

Figure 9.2. Embryos from mammals have varying degrees of cytoplasmic lipids. The left panel shows a 2-cell embryo from a rat and the right panel shows a 2-cell embryo from a pig. The high concentration of lipids makes the pig embryo very dark, whereas a relatively lower lipid concentration makes the rat embryo more transparent. Mammals with embryos of low lipid content include rats, mice, and humans. Pigs, sheep, goats, horses, cats, and dogs have embryos with high lipid content.

Nagashima et al. (1994) demonstrated, by centrifugation and micro-manipulation techniques, that removal of the lipids from 1-cell embryos allows a proportion of the embryos (about 20 percent cooled at the 1-cell stage and about 45 percent cooled at the 2- to 4-cell stage) to tolerate one hour of exposure to 4°C as measured by *in vitro* development to at least the 8-cell stage. This is in contrast to the lethal effects of cooling on non-manipulated embryos.

As will be discussed below, the investigations into cooling tolerance had practical implications to the successes of experiments designed to cryopreserve livestock embryos. Far less work has been done to understand the effects of cooling on embryos from other domestic animals.

The Development of Cryopreservation Procedures for Domestic Animal Embryos

Since the first reports of successful mouse embryo cryopreservation in 1972 (Whittingham et al., 1972; Wilmut, 1972), hundreds of other studies designed to examine factors associated with cryosurvival of mammalian embryos have followed. Below, we will attempt to highlight what we feel are the more important developments in this field for several domesticated animals. We also provide examples using relevant publications that either pioneered the work or provide good examples of the main principles described. It is difficult to provide the details for each report, particularly for the bovine, on which several hundred publications on embryo cryopreservation have appeared. Over the years, several well written reviews have been published. We will refer to many of these to provide the reader with a starting place if there is a desire to gain further knowledge.

Cattle

It likely comes as no surprise that work on cattle embryo cryopreservation followed shortly after the initial reports for the mouse (see Figure 9.3), given the economic incentive to advance cattle embryo transfer (Wilmut and Hume, 1978). Using a method similar to that shown to be effective with mouse embryos, Wilmut and Rowson documented the first birth of a healthy calf derived from frozen and thawed embryos in 1973 (Wilmut and Rowson, 1973).

Not surprisingly, given the stage-specific tolerance of bovine embryos to cooling, they used late-stage (day 10–11) *in vivo*-produced blastocysts for their work. In their first experiment using 2.0 M DMSO as a cryoprotectant, they determined that slow cooling to −70°C (at 0.22°C/minute) was superior to more rapid cooling (0.67°C or 23°C/minute). In the second experiment, they determined that rapid warming (360°C/minute) was favorable to slower warming (60°C/minute). It was the combination of favorable cooling and warming rates that led to the first successful pregnancy. It should be noted that the success rate was quite low, however, with only one of 11 heifers delivering a calf.

For the next several years, many groups began to investigate the effects of the various factors, such as cryoprotectant type and concentration, embryo stage, and cooling and warming rates. Fahning and Garcia (1992) provide an overview of this time period in the early part of their review, and Gordon (1995) provides a nice overview of the development of cattle embryo cryopreservation in his recently revised text as well.

The desire to incorporate practicality into embryo freezing methods drove much of the research during the late 1970s and early 1980s. Following the earlier work of Utsumi and Yuhara (1975) and Tsunoda and Sugie (1977), Massip et al. (1979) reported on a direct comparison of one-fourth

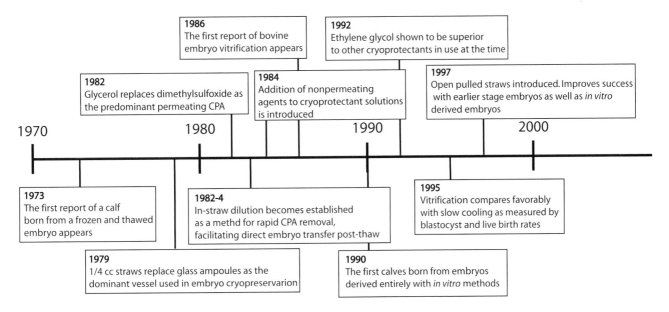

Figure 9.3. Timeline showing the major developments in bovine embryo cryopreservation.

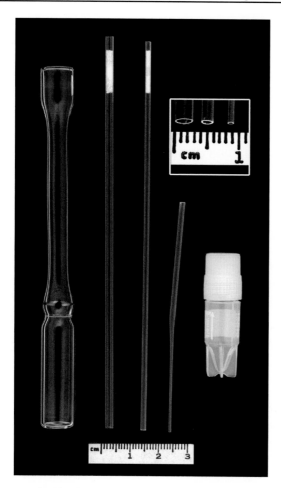

Figure 9.4. Examples of the various types of freezing vessels used to cryopreserve cells. From left to right: glass ampoule, one-half cc straw, one-fourth cc straw, open-pulled straw, and 1.5 ml cryovial. The inset shows the different diameters of the straws for comparison. The smaller diameter straws increase the surface area-to-volume ratio, allowing higher rates of cooling.

cc French straws, typically used for semen freezing, to glass ampoules which, along with glass test tubes, were commonly used as the freezing vessels in preceding research (see Figure 9.4). While the embryos frozen with ampoules generally had a higher development rate *in vitro*, those frozen in straws outperformed their counterparts *in vivo*. The net result was that the pregnancy rates using the two methods were similar. Straw freezing has a marked practical advantage over glass ampoules, in that it facilitates directly transferring embryos into a recipient post-thaw.

Work ensued to develop freezing in straws during the early 1980s, and Stanley Leibo, who had become noteworthy as a contributor to the first report on mouse embryo freezing, took a principle lead with this approach. He showed how cryoprotectant dilution could be achieved within the straws by combining different solutions in the freezing straw (being separated by air bubbles) and mixing them immediately after thawing without removing the embryos from the straw. A 1984 report documented the

effectiveness of this "in straw dilution" method in several field trials, with pregnancy rates typically ranging between 20 percent and 45 percent (Leibo, 1984).

At about the same time, a report by Massip and van der Zwalman (1984) appeared, describing how adding sucrose to the freezing medium could preclude dilution steps after thawing. As a testament to this development, nearly all modern cryopreservation procedures incorporate non-permeating compounds as cryoprotectants in the freezing medium.

The comparisons made by Fahning and Garcia in Table 1 of their review show some of the progressive changes that occurred to bovine embryo cryopreservation methods during the late 1970s through mid-1980s. Glycerol became more commonly used in place of DMSO, and propylene glycol began to be used shortly thereafter. It also became more common for sucrose to be used in the freezing medium after the report by Massip and van der Zwalman appeared, and stepwise CPA removal was superseded by the use of sucrose as an osmotic buffer shortly after it was first described in this context.

In 1992, a detailed report was published on the efficacy of several permeating cryoprotectants, describing the superiority of EG to PG, DMSO, and glycerol when used in a standard slow cooling procedure (Voelkel and Hu, 1992). These authors reported the 72-hour post-thaw viability for frozen *in vivo*-produced embryos as 70 percent for EG, compared to 11 percent, 25 percent, and 30 percent for the others, respectively. They also showed that embryos frozen with EG could be directly transferred to a holding medium after thawing, without the necessary multi-step cryoprotectant removal process or using sucrose as an osmotic buffer, as was typically done with other compounds.

This report went on to show that the optimal concentration for EG was in the range of 1.25 to 1.75 M, with viability dropping off with higher or lower concentrations. Finally, a comparison of direct uterine transfer of embryos frozen in straws with EG and an additional column of just holding medium as a diluent (no sucrose) was made to the traditional freezing method using glycerol and the multi-step dilution procedure *in vitro* followed by transfer. The pregnancy rates (about 50 percent) were comparable using each method, demonstrating the greater efficacy of the EG method given the increased simplicity.

As described above, a major change occurred in the field of cryobiology with the 1985 report in *Nature* by Rall and Fahy (1985). While this initial report used mouse embryos as the model, the demonstration opened the way to applying vitrification procedures for embryos from other species.

In the first report, published in the journal *Cryo-Letters* (Massip et al., 1986), and subsequently reported in a review in *Theriogenology* (Massip et al., 1987), Massip et al. described the use of a combination of glycerol and propylene glycol in one-fourth cc straws to vitrify *in vivo*-derived late morula and blastocysts. This method used a small column of the freezing solution with a larger column of a dilution solution containing sucrose (1 M) in phosphate-buffered saline. Surprisingly, given the results from slow freezing methods, the late morula and early blastocysts survived the process better than late blastocysts, with nine of 23 recipients maintaining pregnancy at 60 days.

Again, as with the slow cooling methods, several reports on embryo vitrification appeared shortly thereafter, describing results with various methods attempting to vitrify bovine embryos.

In 1995, the results of experiments designed to directly compare slow cooling and vitrification methods were published in the journal *Cryobiology* (Van Wagtendonk-De Leeuw et al., 1995). The slow cooling treatments consisted of a method with *in vitro* CPA dilution and another method with in-straw dilution. The vitrification treatments compared just glycerol (6.5 M) and a combination of 25 percent glycerol and 25 percent propylene glycol. The *in vitro* development results showed that the slow cooling with *in vitro* dilution was as good as the two vitrification methods (53 percent, 44 percent, and 51 percent expanded blastocyst development, respectively). The in-straw dilution method was more damaging to the embryos, with only 33 percent expanded blastocyst development. The three superior methods were then compared by embryo transfer, and the slow cooling method was similar in outcome to the vitrification method using only glycerol (59 percent vs. 43 percent pregnancy); the CPA combination method only yielded 24 percent pregnancy. The vitrification method is generally faster than the slow cooling method, making it more efficient. Shortly thereafter, this group compared pregnancy rates with slow-cooling or vitrification in a field trial (van Wagtendonk-de Leeuw et al., 1997), and showed that the methods were comparable in this setting (44.5 percent pregnancy with vitrified embryos versus 45.1 percent with a slow-cooling method).

In 1997, Vajta introduced the method of open pulled straw (OPS) vitrification (Vajta et al., 1997). For this method, a standard one-fourth cc freezing straw is heated and pulled, making the straw narrower and the wall thinner, allowing greater cooling rates (see Figure 9.2). In a 1998 report, this group demonstrated successful cryopreservation of earlier stage embryos (day 3) compared to later stage embryos, as measured by *in vitro* development. Perhaps even more remarkable is the fact that good results were obtained with *in vitro*-produced embryos. The authors attributed the success to several factors, including the increased cooling rate obtainable with the OPS and the ability to immediately dilute the CPA by simply placing the open end of the straw, which contains the vitrified solution, into a diluent contained in a dish, and allowing the vitrified solution to thaw and the embryos to flow out into the solution. Normal calves were born from this method when it was applied to blastocysts.

Significant progress has been made during the past two decades in the ability to mature oocytes from immature cumulus-oocyte complexes *in vitro*, resulting in high levels

of blastocyst formation *in vitro* and live births after embryo transfer (Ball et al., 1984; Nagai, 2001). Such methods will facilitate advances in research (Eyestone, 1994) and human medicine (Menezo and Herubel, 2002). Much of the work on bovine embryo cryopreservation during the past 10 years has been devoted to studies aimed at improving the cryo-survival of *in vitro*-produced embryos.

The first report of calves born from *in vitro* embryos was published in 1990 (Fukuda et al.), although the calves were born three years prior to the appearance of this publication. The authors reported 32 percent survival of the embryos after slow cooling with glycerol, and two of three recipients became pregnant, with one delivering twin calves.

Not surprisingly, both pre- and post-thaw culture conditions have profound effects on the developmental competence of embryos (Leibo and Loskutoff, 1993). Many of the factors that determine success described for *in vivo* embryos have been shown to be similar for *in vitro*-derived embryos, including developmental stage (Zhang et al., 1993) and method of cryopreservation (Mahmoudzadeh et al., 1994). In this last report, vitrification was shown to be superior to slow cooling, both in post-thaw survival and hatching rates.

In 1998, Agca et al. published two reports on cryopreservation of bovine embryos. In the first report (Agca et al., 1998), the authors also showed that vitrification was superior to slow cooling, with 100 percent of the vitrified embryos maintaining morphological integrity deemed acceptable for transfer, contrary to only 36 percent of the embryos frozen with a slow cooling method. The pregnancy rate was nearly twice as high for the recipients that received vitrified embryos (44 percent vs. 23 percent). The pregnancy rate for non-frozen embryos was 50 percent. However, in their second study (Agca et al., 1998) they showed that the calving rates for vitrified and frozen embryos were similar (67 percent vs. 77 percent per recipient; the calving rate for control embryos was about 90 percent). Taken together, however, vitrification is still superior according to their results due to the higher post-thaw survival.

Numerous other reports have appeared in the literature describing efforts to better understand the response of *in vitro*-produced embryos to cryopreservation. If effective methods for *in vitro* embryo production and cryopreservation are developed such that the developmental competence of these embryos is similar to their *in vivo*-derived counterparts, increased potential of embryo technologies will be realized (Hasler, 1992; Kane, 2003).

Pigs

Given the extreme sensitivity of porcine embryos to cooling, it is not surprising that cryopreserving pig embryos was unsuccessful until nearly two decades after methods to cryopreserve cattle embryos had been described (see Figure 9.5). In 1988, Nagashima et al. (1988) reported that hatched blastocyst could survive cooling down to 6°C as measured by *in vitro* culture and embryo transfer (only fetal

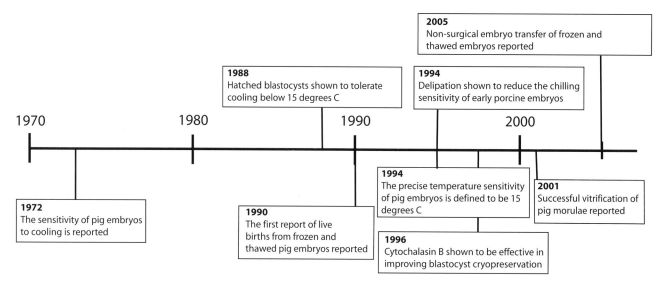

Figure 9.5. Timeline showing the major developments in porcine embryo cryopreservation. Note the lag in time for the first report of a live piglet born from a frozen and thawed embryo compared to Figure 9.1.

development was reported). The following year, Hayashi et al. (1989) published results describing successful late-stage pig blastocysts after freezing to −35°C. A standard slow-cooling approach to freezing with 1.5 M glycerol as the cryoprotectant was used in this report. However, none of the embryos that had been cooled to liquid nitrogen temperatures that were used in this set of experiments developed to term.

In 1990, a report a describing what may be the first successful cryopreservation of pig embryos (as cited in Kashiwazaki et al., 1991) appeared in a Japanese journal. The following year, Kashiwazaki (Kashiwazaki et al., 1991) published results describing successful cryopreservation down to −196°C of pig-hatched blastocysts using methods similar to those described in Hayashi's paper. While survival was still quite low (only 10 percent of the thawed embryos were of the quality deemed appropriate for transfer), four piglets were born from 32 embryos transferred to a recipient.

For the next several years, there was little improvement in pig embryo freezing. In the mid 1990s, a group from the United States reported on results of vitrifying *in vivo*-derived pig blastocysts after exposure to cytochalasin b (CB) used to intentionally depolymerize the actin cytoskeleton (Dobrinsky, 1996, 1997). These authors showed that when CB pretreated expanded blastocysts and early hatched blastocysts were vitrified and subsequently thawed, washed free of the CB, and cultured, their survival was markedly improved. This effect was not seen when applied to morula or expanded hatched blastocysts, however.

A full report on the effects of CB was published a short time later (Dobrinsky et al., 2000), and included the results of embryo transfers. Nearly 40 normal piglets were born after applying their method (approximately 13 percent of the embryos that were transferred developed into normal

offspring). Several of these offspring were retained as breeders and subsequently matured and proved fertile, and a review (Dobrinsky, 2001) reported that three generations of pigs had been raised from the original founders.

In this report the authors also describe live births resulting from embryos that have been pretreated with CB and subsequently had their zonae pellucidae removed after thawing. They concluded this review with a very optimistic tone, saying: "It is now time for breeders and producers to adopt cryopreservation and transfer of pig embryos into pig production for propagating select genetic traits and maintaining germplasm resources for the future." Clearly, the authors were pleased with the progress that was made after decades of struggle and disappointment.

Over the past five years, several groups have continued to publish data on pig embryo cryopreservation, with some reports describing *in vitro* survival data and others describing successful embryo transfers. The factors that show potential include base media used in the cryoprotectant solutions (PBS vs. Hepes-buffered TCM-199; no difference detected) (Berthelot et al., 2000), different vitrification procedures with differing cooling rates (no difference in outcome detected) (Cuello et al., 2004), and different dilution methods (direct vs. three-step; direct dilution as good as three-step dilution) (Cuello et al., 2004). High proportions of embryo survival, as measured by continued *in vitro* development, were reported in all of these studies. However, in those in which embryo transfers were performed, the success was still fairly low, remaining around 13 percent of the total embryos transferred. However, in many instances, high proportions of recipients became pregnant.

Two of these later reports stand out. In 2001, Berthelot et al. reported successful vitrification of compact morula-stage embryos as measured by embryo transfer. While the overall live birth success was still similar to other reports (13 percent), the importance of cryopreservation of morula-stage embryos is due to the zona pellucida remaining intact, which facilitates international embryo transportation. In 2005, Cuello et al. reported on non-surgical embryo transfer in pigs using vitrified embryos. While the success was still 12 percent as measured by the proportion of transferred embryos surviving to term, the method of transfer is much less demanding given that surgery is unnecessary, which makes future studies more practical.

Clearly the numerous reports of live births from cryopreserved pig embryos represent a major accomplishment given the difficulties that have been encountered with porcine embryos. However, there is still room for improvement. In addition, cryopreservation of *in vitro*-produced embryos is still a significant challenge, as are methods simply to mature oocytes and maintain developmentally-competent embryos *in vitro*. Nevertheless, continued work directed at understanding the mechanisms of failure should eventually provide the clues necessary to develop improved methods for these important technologies. Given the recent developments in porcine transgenic technology (Prather et al., 2003) and continued use of pigs as models for human disease (Turk and Laughlin, 2004), ensuring the preservation of rare and valuable porcine genotypes is becoming even more important.

Sheep

As mentioned above, one of the earliest reports of an attempt to freeze sheep embryos, if not the earliest report, appeared in 1959 (Averill and Rowson, 1959). These authors unsuccessfully attempted to freeze embryos to –79°C in the presence of 12.5 percent glycerol for 24 hours or more.

In 1976, Willadsen et al. reported on cooling tolerance, DMSO tolerance, and successful freezing of sheep embryos to temperatures of –60°C. Similar to results in other species, the cooling tolerance (to 0°C in this case) increased with increasing developmental stage. This was also true for the tolerance to DMSO. The authors went on to investigate the ability of embryos to tolerate slow cooling (0.3°C per minute) to temperatures between –1°C and –60°C in the presence of 1.5 M DMSO. In this experiment, nearly all of the embryos showed developmental competence when transferred to the oviducts of rabbits. In their final experiment to assess survival to –196°C, they investigated the effects of slow cooling (0.3°C per minute) and three different warming rates (3°C, 12°C, and 360°C per minute) on morula and early blastocysts. The proportion that survived was zero of five, 10 of 43, and one of four for the respective warming rates. They went on to perform embryo transfers, and of 12 embryos with an intact zona pellucida, five developed to term. They also transferred eight zona-free blastocysts; three of those developed to term.

In 1977, Willadesen presented a more thorough report of the results from their earlier studies in a proceedings from a Ciba foundation symposium on mammalian embryo freezing (Willadsen, 1977). From this report, several very important results were discussed, which continue to remain important considerations in devising cryopreservation procedures.

The first of these resulted from investigating the effects of intentional or spontaneous seeding of the extracellular solution on cell survival. When embryos were cooled slowly (1°C or 0.3°C per minute) to temperatures between –23°C and –30°C, and seeding was either initiated manually at –7°C or –10°C or allowed to occur spontaneously (at approximately –20°C), survival depended upon seeding. Thirteen of 14 embryos frozen with manual seeding survived, but only three of 10 survived spontaneous seeding. It is now generally understood that seeding at temperatures slightly below the melting point of the solution is critical for high cell survival, because this allows osmotic dehydration to occur as described above. At temperatures where spontaneous seeding occurs, the cytoplasmic water is highly supercooled when external water crystallization commences, and is therefore much more likely to nucleate.

The second experiment investigated interactions between the initial concentrations of permeating CPA, cooling rates, and warming rates. The important results from this study were that 1.5 M DMSO was superior to 1 M, and the thawing rate (4°C, 10°C, or 360°C per minute) could affect the survival, but appeared to depend on the cooling rate (0.3°C or 1°C per minute). In this experiment, the cells were cooled to –120°C prior to plunging into liquid nitrogen.

The final experiment investigated the effect of temperature attained prior to liquid nitrogen exposure (from –30°C to –60°C at 6°C intervals) and the thawing rate (4°C or 360°C per minute up to –10°C). The results suggested that interruption of cooling at higher temperatures required faster thawing to achieve high survival, and the opposite was also true; survival was higher after cooling to lower temperatures with slow warming. This relationship between temperature of liquid nitrogen transfer and warming rate is now well established as discussed earlier.

In the report's appendix, the authors describe the births of several lambs resulting from cryopreserving sheep late morula embryos using the best methods determined from their previous experiments. The success was about 30 percent as measured by the number of live offspring per embryo frozen.

Many reports in the 1980s and early 1990s described investigations on the effects of minor changes to the traditional slow-cooling procedure such as changes in cooling rate, stepwise addition and removal of cryoprotectants, and the temperature at which plunging into liquid nitrogen occurred, on both *in vitro* and *in vivo* survival of sheep embryos (see Fahning and Garcia, 1992, for more details). Pregnancy and birth rates were generally high (often greater than 50 percent).

A few generalizations can be made which are applicable across embryos from several taxa. It is apparent that survival increases with later developmental stage embryos, and ethylene glycol appears to confer better protection to embryos than DMSO or glycerol. For example, Heyman et al. (1987) achieved a 54 percent live birth rate using *in vivo*-derived embryos and a slow-cooling procedure with EG as the cryoprotectant (1.5 M final concentration) and an in-straw dilution technique with immediate transfer. Even greater success was achieved by McGinnis et al. (1993), with eight lambs resulting from the transfer of 11 embryos. Similar results were determined by Cocero et al. (1996), with a significant interaction between cryoprotectant and embryo stage (EG was better than glycerol, and the effect was greatest among morula stage embryos). In this report, birth rate ranged from about 35 percent to 45 percent. Song-sasen et al. (1995), taking a more fundamental approach, determined EG to be superior to propylene glycol and DMSO. They achieved success rates of 15 percent (births per embryo frozen) and 21 percent (births per embryo transferred).

Vitrification methods began to be tested with sheep embryos around 1990, also with noteworthy success. Frequently, these methods were similar or identical to methods tested with cattle or pig embryos. Ethylene glycol and glycerol, usually at a final concentration of 25 percent each, were frequently used as the cryoprotectants. Open-pulled straws and standard one-fourth cc straws were used in different studies, with no major difference in outcome.

In 1993, Ali and Shelton compared the post-vitrification viability of day 6 *in vivo* produced sheep embryos using one of three vitrification solutions (VS1: 5.5 M EG plus 2.5 M glycerol; VS11: 6 M EG plus 1.8 M glycerol; and VS14: 5.5 M EG plus 1 M sucrose). They showed that survival was 0 percent with VS1. However, use of VS11 resulted in relatively good *in vitro* survival, and both VS11 and VS14 resulted in high pregnancy rates (50 percent to 100 percent) in most instances.

A 1998 study (Martinez and Matkovic, 1998) compared slow-cooling and vitrification methods using morula and blastocyst-stage embryos. Similar to the study mentioned above, ethylene glycol proved better than glycerol for slow-cooling, and the effect was more pronounced with morula-stage embryos compared to blastocysts (as measured by pregnancy rates). They went on to show that a single-step method of ethylene glycol removal post-thaw worked equally as well as a three-step method (48 percent pregnancy for each method). In their final experiment, the authors compared two solutions for vitrification, one containing propylene glycol and glycerol (final concentration of 25 percent each), and the other containing ethylene glycol (40 percent) plus Ficoll 70 (18 percent) plus sucrose (0.3 M; all final concentrations). While the differences were noticeable (28 percent vs. 40 percent pregnancy), these results were not statistically significant. The pregnancy rate with vitrified morula embryos using the EG plus Ficoll plus sucrose solution was quite high (55 percent), with an equally high weaning rate. This was very similar to the weaning rate for freshly transferred embryos. The surprising result from this study was that the weaning rate for vitrified morulae was higher than that for blastocysts when using the EG-based solution (55 percent vs. 26 percent).

In 2002, a study (Papadopoulos et al., 2002) was published on the differences in pregnancy rates and fetal measurements from *in vitro*- vs. *in vivo*-produced embryos and non-frozen vs. vitrified embryos. The fetuses were measured for weight and crown rump lengths at day 42 of gestation. While there was not a significant interaction between the effects, *in vivo*-produced embryos as well as non-frozen embryos had better outcomes. The measured parameters for the fetuses were slightly higher for non-frozen *in vitro*-produced embryos compared to non-frozen *in vivo*-produced embryos (6.4 grams vs. 5.8 grams; 5.2 cm vs. 4.8 cm). Interestingly, vitrification only affected *in vivo*-produced embryos, with fetuses from vitrified embryos being heavier (6.6 grams vs. 5.8 grams) and having a longer crown rump measurement (5.2 cm vs. 4.8 cm) compared to those transferred fresh.

Recently, Dattena et al. (2004) determined that different vitrification methods (comparing factors such as glycerol and DMSO as cryoprotectants, open-pulled straws and one-fourth cc straws, and single vs. multi-step CPA dilution) worked equally well. However, they also showed that *in vivo*-produced embryos tend to survive vitrification better than their *in vitro* counterparts. They achieved very high lambing rates (about 60 percent per vitrified embryo) for *in vivo*-derived embryos, and significantly lower rates for *in vitro*-derived embryos (about 20 percent).

Horses

Assisted reproduction in horses lags behind that of many other domestic animals. This is likely due to fewer economic incentives to develop these technologies, because horses are not used as food animals nearly to the same degree as cattle, pigs, and sheep. Regarding embryo cryopreservation per se, most equine breed registers have not approved the registration of foals born from frozen and thawed embryos (Squires et al., 2003).

To date, the majority of studies on equine embryo cryopreservation have used slow cooling methods developed for use with embryos from other domesticated animals. It is typical for embryos to be cooled at rates around 1°C to 4°C per minute to −6°C, and then to be cooled at a rate around 0.3°C to −30°C prior to plunging into liquid nitrogen (reviewed in Seidel, 1996). More recently, vitrification methods have been tested against more traditional approaches. This will be further discussed below.

The first report of a live foal born from a cryopreserved embryo appeared in the literature in 1982 (Yamamoto et al.). An interesting fact about this article is that two of the major themes that have emerged from all of the later studies on equine embryo cryopreservation were first reported there. In this report, the authors noted that later-stage embryos (day 8) appeared more susceptible to cryoinjury compared to day-6 embryos, although they apparently were fairly tolerant of cooling, at least to 0°C. Furthermore, they showed that only embryos frozen in glycerol were able to develop to term; DMSO apparently was not protective under their conditions.

From the literature to date, there is significant evidence that glycerol is a superior permeable cryoprotectant for equine embryos, particularly compared to DMSO, PG, and EG. In 1993, Meira et al. showed that embryo morphology was better preserved with glycerol as the cryoprotectant, and pregnancy rates from embryos frozen with glycerol were markedly higher (33 percent) than those frozen with PG (0 percent). In that same year, Landin e Alvarenga et al. (Landin e Alvarenga et al., 1993) showed that ultrastructural preservation was superior in slowly frozen embryos in the presence of glycerol compared to PG. In embryos frozen with PG, it was noted that almost no cellular organelles were intact post-thaw, whereas the morphology of the embryonic cells frozen with glycerol were very similar to those that were not frozen. In this study, the authors noted a difference in morphological characteristics between the inner-cell mass cells and the trophectoderm, with the later having fewer disruptions (this is another general theme that has arisen in several studies and will be discussed further). The pregnancy rates using glycerol were also superior in this study (40 percent) compared to the use of PG (0 percent). Additional studies drew the same conclusion regarding the failure of PG (Bruyas et al., 1997; Seidel et al., 1989) and EG (Huhtinen et al., 2001) to cryoprotect equine embryonic cells compared to glycerol.

As was mentioned, several studies have shown that the blastocyst becomes much less tolerant to freezing at it progressively develops. This result has been determined using various measures including pregnancy rates (Czlonkowska et al., 1985; Eldridge-Panuska et al., 2005; Slade et al., 1985), and post-thaw embryo morphology (Seidel et al., 1989). As mentioned above, an acellular, proteinacious capsule develops subjacent to the zona pellucida around the mid-blastocyst stage of equine development (Betteridge, 1989). The results from the studies investigating the temporal sensitivity of equine blastocysts to freezing suggest that this structure acts as a permeability barrier to the cryoprotectants, effectively preventing these substances from getting into the embryonic cells and preserving them during freezing.

In 1993, Pfaff et al. reported on the qualitative permeability of different stages of equine blastocysts to EG and glycerol. They noted that the permeability, as measured by embryo shrinking and re-swelling upon exposure to cryoprotectants, decreased as the embryonic stage increased. Furthermore, they noticed that as the embryo developed to the latest stages, the volumetric response suggested that the embryo became impermeable to these compounds, as significant re-swelling was not apparent. This was particularly true for glycerol. This observation was supported by Bass et al. (2004), who noted that late-stage blastocysts continued to shrink after being exposed to 1.5 M glycerol for 15 minutes.

In 2001, Legrand et al. looked at the effects of capsule thickness on cell damage as a result of exposure to glycerol. They found a positive correlation of cell damage to capsule thickness, but only up to the point of a fully formed capsule, where cell damage (measured by nuclear morphology) was not apparent. The authors interpreted these results as evidence of osmotic damage, because the glycerol penetration decreased with capsule thickening. They speculated that the fully-formed capsule was completely impenetrable to water and glycerol, thus the cells did not respond osmotically to the hypertonic extracellular solution and were not damaged. However, this interpretation is incongruous with the studies mentioned earlier in which noticeable embryo shrinking occurred in later stage blastocysts when placed into glycerol solutions. However, in these studies, capsule thickness was not quantified.

One obvious way to test whether the capsule represents a contributing factor to cryoinjury is to remove it from the embryo prior to freezing. Legrand et al. (2001) conducted this experiment by digesting the capsule with a 15-minute exposure to various concentrations of trypsin or collagenase. They showed that typsin treatment was superior to collagenase, and a concentration of 0.2 percent allowed successful cryopreservation, with six of eight embryo transfers resulting in pregnancies. A study published a short time later by the same group confirmed this effect, but with reduced success (Legrand et al., 2002).

As mentioned above, several studies have shown that cells from the inner cell mass often suffer more damage post-thaw than those of the trophectoderm. This has been determined using several methods, including vital dye staining (Barry et al., 1989; Huhtinen et al., 2001) and nuclear morphology (Bruyas et al., 1993). These results are consistent with the interpretation that embryo penetration by cryoprotectants is incomplete, resulting from poor permeability of the embryo to these compounds. These results are not necessarily consistent with the interpretation that the capsule itself is responsible for the poor permeability, because many of these studies were performed with earlier embryos (day 6) where, presumably, the capsule was absent or incompletely formed.

In many ways, the evolution of research on equine embryo cryopreservation followed a similar pattern to that described above for the work on cow, pig, and sheep embryos. Initially, traditional slow-cooling protocols were attempted, similar to the one shown to be successful with mouse embryos. Subsequently, minor modifications were applied and tested (Seidel, 1996). Early on, one-fourth cc straws were compared to glass ampoules and found to work equally well, and because of the convenience they offered for embryo transfer, were quickly adopted. Frozen samples briefly exposed to air prior to being plunged into water baths for final thawing proved superior (Squires et al., 1989). Incorporation of sucrose into the CPA removal media proved beneficial with equine embryos, as had been shown with embryos from other taxonomic groups (Huhtinen et al., 1997). The efficacy of direct transfer of embryos from straws into recipient mares was also tested (Eldridge-Panuska et al., 2005), with beneficial results.

Also similar to the history of cattle, sheep, and pig embryo freezing, vitrification methods were tested on equine embryos after the first report with mouse embryos. In 2001, Oberstein et al. tested two vitrification methods against a traditional slow cooling method. While the results from this study showed that the post-thaw embryo score was similar across treatments, the proportion of live cells as measured by vital dye staining was higher for the slow cooling method. These differences in proportions were not statistically significant, however.

This last point is important for further discussion when reviewing equine embryo cryopreservation studies. The results from many of the studies reviewed here are somewhat difficult to interpret due to factors such as a small sample size and confounding of variables in treatments. This is not the first time this critique has been raised regarding studies on equine embryo cryopreservation (Seidel, 1996) and fertility (Amann, 2005) studies. Statistically significant differences across treatments were not determined in many of the studies, when in fact the differences in the treatment means were fairly large. In the defense of the authors of these studies, obtaining equine embryos in large numbers is challenging, and housing large numbers of recipient mares is expensive. Nevertheless, for the field to move forward, it is imperative that studies are well designed with sufficient power to detect treatment effects. One could even argue that this is more important with equine embryo studies, because the time and expense to conduct them makes it less likely that experiments will be repeated to confirm or refute the results.

Goats

The first article describing kids born from frozen embryos was published in 1976 (Bilton and Moore). The authors studied the effects of cooling and freezing on the viability of *in vivo*-produced morula and blastocyst-stage embryos. In the cooling experiment, they investigated the effects on day-5 (morula) embryos. They used a slow-cooling procedure (1°C/minute) to bring the embryos to 5°C, and held them for one or two days before warming them slowly (0.6°C/minute) to 37°C. They cultured these embryos for two days and recorded the development. Of the embryos held for one day, 50 percent (8 of 16) showed normal development to blastocysts *in vitro*. A similar proportion (12 of 22; 55 percent) of the embryos held for two days also developed to blastocysts *in vitro*. This represents about a 35 percent reduction in the developmental potential due to extended cooling, because 13 of 15 embryos not having been cooled developed *in vitro*. However, it is much better that the results from cooling pig embryos, as previously discussed.

These authors also froze day-7 blastocysts using a traditional slow-cooling technique. They tested several variables, including two CPAs (glycerol, 1 M final) or DMSO (2 M final), and two cooling rates between the temperatures of 6°C and −60°C (either 0.2°C or 1.4°C per minute). They seeded external ice at −2.5°C, and plunged the glass test tubes into liquid nitrogen after reaching −60°C. They warmed slowly to 37°C, first with a warming rate of 1.4°C, 2.2°C, 4.6°C, or 8°C/minute up to 0°C, then at a rate of 0.6°C up to 37°C. They proceeded to slowly dilute the cryopreservation media by adding a holding medium in a dropwise fashion over 25 minutes until the CPA was diluted to 25 percent of the initial concentration. The embryos were then washed in a holding medium and cultured for one day prior to embryo transfer.

Only two of the 23 embryos frozen in DMSO developed in culture, one from each of the two cooling rates and one each from the 2.2°C and 8.0°C warming rate. Neither of these embryos developed in utero. Five of 25 embryos frozen in glycerol developed in culture. All five were cooled at the 0.2°C/minute rate; two and three were warmed at 1.4°C and 2.2°C, respectively. All five of these were transferred to recipients, and three developed into live young, two from the first warming rate, and one from the second.

The historical progress of embryo cryopreservation in goats is similar to that for the other taxa described above. Several papers were published describing experiments that tested different cryoprotectants. There were conflicting results in some of the reports (e.g. Bilton and Moore, 1976; Mani and Vadnere, 1988); however, the treatment effect in these two papers was confounded by other variables. In 1993, Le Gal et al. investigated glycerol and ethylene glycol as cryoprotectants with both morula and blastocyst-stage embryos, and found EG to be superior to glycerol, both by *in vitro* and *in vivo* measurements. They also showed that blastocysts tended to survive better than morulae, particularly when measured by live birth rate.

Further reports substantiated the claim of superiority for EG as a cryoprotectant. Fiéni et al. (1995) showed that EG was superior to DMSO and glycerol, particularly with morula stage embryos (the proportion of viable blastocysts was higher using EG than DMSO, but the difference was not statistically significant). Ethylene glycol was also shown to be superior to glycerol in a study published two years later (HanChi et al., 1997).

In the studies by Le Gal and Fiéni, the effect of stepwise dilution vs. a single-step dilution of the cryoprotectants was also investigated. In both of these studies, they tested three dilution methods: stepwise dilution of the CPA, stepwise dilution of the CPA with 0.25 M sucrose added to the dilution media, and one-step removal of the CPAs using 0.25 M sucrose only. In both of these studies, stepwise removal proved superior, with the inclusion of sucrose generally working better. In the study published by Le Gal et al., the live birth rate using EG and the best stepwise removal procedure was high, with seven of the 12 transferred blastocysts developing to term.

The first report of successful goat embryo vitrification appeared in the literature in 1990 (Yuswiati and Holtz). Both morula and blastocysts were vitrified with a combination of glycerol and PG (25 percent each). The cryoprotectants were diluted from the embryos in 1 M sucrose for 10 minutes. The morula and blastocysts (57 percent and 76 percent were deemed transferable, respectively) were kept separate and transferred to recipients. Two does each gave birth to a single kid, one receiving an embryo vitrified at the morula stage, and the other receiving an embryo after having been vitrified as a blastocyst.

Further research into vitrification was conducted during the next several years. Two reports, testing different vitrification methods, were published more recently (Begin et al., 2003; El-Gayar and Holtz, 2001). In the 2001 report, the authors investigated the OPS method, and compared the results to a conventional slow-cooling method using glycerol. For the OPS vitrification, the embryos were vitrified in 20 percent each of EG and DMSO. The embryos were initially washed in a step-wise series of solutions containing sucrose (0.33 M then 0.2 M for one minute each). The embryos were then washed in an isotonic solution and held in culture medium for two hours prior to transfer. Within two hours post-thaw, the morphology of all of the vitrified embryos was similar to those having no treatment. The rate of re-expansion for the slowly cooled group was not as fast, however. The pregnancy rate for vitrified-thawed embryos was 100 percent, and the kidding rate was 93 percent. This is markedly better that the results using the conventional cryopreservation method (58 percent and 50 percent respectively). Sixty-four percent of the vitrified embryos developed into live offspring compared to only 42 percent of those that were cryopreserved with the slow cooling method.

In the 2003 report, Begin et al. investigated two vitrification methods, the solid surface vitrification method (SSV) and the cryoloop (CL) method, using 2- and 4-cell embryos. In the SSV method, 35 percent EG, 5 percent polyvinylpyrrolidone, and 0.4 M trehalose were used as cryoprotectants. In the CL method, 20 percent each of DMSO and EG plus 10 mg/ml ficoll and 0.65 M sucrose were used as cryoprotectants. Immediate survival of 72 percent and 100 percent of the embryos was recorded from each respective method. After a two-hour culture period, 39 percent and 88 percent of the embryos frozen with the respective methods were considered viable. Long-term culture to the blastocyst stage was poor for all groups, including a control (0 percent for SSV, 13 percent for CL, and 9 percent for control). Even though the culture results were poor, the proportion of embryos developing to blastocysts was similar for the control and CL method. However, because only three replicates were conducted, statistical significance for these treatments was not attained.

Cats

Only a handful of reports on cryopreserving embryos from domestic cats have appeared in the literature.

The first kittens from embryos having been previously frozen and transferred to recipient queens were described in 1988 (Dresser et al.). The investigators adopted a technique used with cattle embryos to achieve their success. They used glycerol as a cryoprotectant at a final concentration of 1.35 M and employed a slow-cooling method. They loaded the embryos into one-fourth cc straws after exposure to the CPA solution, and transferred the straw directly to a freezing machine pre-cooled to −6°C. After seeding ice, they cooled the samples to −32°C at a rate of 0.5°C per minute. They held the samples there for 15 minutes, and then proceeded to cool to −34°C at the same rate. The samples were held again, this time for 30 minutes before plunging into liquid nitrogen.

They tested three different thawing methods in these experiments. One consisted of thawing in ambient air for three minutes. The other two consisted of transferring the straws to water baths, at temperatures of 28°C or 37°C. After thawing, the straw contents were expelled into an isotonic solution supplemented with 0.8 M sucrose at a temperature of 37°C.

In the initial experiments, they cultured some embryos as controls, cultured others and then performed transfers, or performed embryo transfers directly after the washing. They determined that water bath thawing was superior to air thawing, and 18-hour post-thaw culture was superior to direct transfer. Only the combination of warming rate and culture that proved superior resulted in live births. Five litters containing a total of 17 kittens were born from 11 transfer events. One hundred and sixteen embryos were thawed and cultured prior to transfer to achieve these results, giving a success rate of 15 percent.

In 1994, Pope et al. attempted to cryopreserve cat embryos that were derived from *in vivo*-matured oocytes fertilized *in vitro*. They tested two different CPA exposure methods: exposure to 1.4 M PG and 0.125 M sucrose simultaneously, or first exposure to 1.4 M PG then exposure to 1.4 M PG and 0.125 M sucrose. They used a cooling profile similar to the one described in the report above, but they terminated cooling at −30°C and plunged into liquid nitrogen with no holding period. They used a multi-step CPA removal procedure, assessed zona integrity, and then cultured the embryos for six days. The one-step CPA exposure proved superior (68 percent vs. 36 percent *in vitro* development; no difference in zona integrity between the treatments).

They went on to test two different thawing methods using the superior freezing method described in the first experiment. Thawing consisted of either a five-second air thaw followed by immersion into a 37°C water bath or a two- to three-minute air thaw. They determined that neither method appeared superior as measured by zona integrity and *in vitro* culture.

Finally, the authors applied the superior CPA method in their first experiment with the air plus water bath thawing method and performed transfer with surviving embryos. Half of the recipient queens (two of four) littered, with a total of three kittens born from 58 embryos transferred.

In 1997, the same group attempted to freeze embryos after maturing the oocytes *in vitro* and performing IVF and culture. They froze embryos at the 2-, 4-to-8-, or 16-to-30-cell stage using either a procedure similar to the one described in their previous report or another in which cooling proceeded down to –150°C at a rate of 10°C per minute after slow cooling to –30°C. The overall development rates of the embryos at the respective stages were 77 percent, 85 percent, and 69 percent. Fewer (2 percent) of the embryos cooled to –150°C exhibited zona damage compared to those cooled only to –30°C (11 percent). Of the embryos cooled to –30°C, 78 percent developed to morula or blastocysts on day 7, 85 percent of those cooled to –150°C proceeded similarly, and more than 90 percent of the unfrozen embryos developed to this stage. None of these differences were statistically significant. In this report, no transfers occurred with frozen thawed embryos.

In 2003, Gómez et al. reported on embryo transfers from a freezing procedure similar to that described in Pope (1997). While none of the embryos frozen at the 4-to-8-cell stage resulted in pregnancies after transfer, two kittens were born from transfer of embryos frozen at the morula stage. However, only two healthy kittens were born from 187 embryos transferred to 15 recipients. One kitten died during parturition, but post-mortem analysis did not result in any unusual findings.

Dogs

In general, assisted reproductive technologies are poorly developed for domestic dogs in comparison to other domesticated animals (Farstad, 2000). Many investigations into the cryobiology of spermatozoa in dogs have been reported (Bouchard et al., 1990; Farstad, 1996; Hay et al., 1997; Okano et al., 2004; Rota et al., 1995; Songsasen et al., 2002; Thirumala et al., 2003). In addition, reports on oocyte maturation, *in vitro* fertilization, and embryo culture have been published (Renton et al., 1991; Yamada et al., 1992; Yamada et al., 1993). However, to our knowledge there are no reports in the literature describing experiments on embryo cryopreservation from domestic dogs.

Summary

Many similarities have been shown across taxa, including stage-specific tolerance of cooling and freezing. On the contrary, significant differences have also been determined in embryos from different taxa, including chilling sensitivity and tolerance to different types of cryoprotectants. While significant progress has been made, further improvements are needed. This is particularly true for *in vitro*-produced embryos.

Not only are there many avenues for study available for young investigators interested in embryo cryopreservation, but in some animals the entire field of assisted reproduction is in its infancy. This is truly an exciting time for the field of assisted reproductive technology.

Bibliography

Acker, J.P., Larese, A., Yang, H., Petrenko, A., and McGann, L.E. (1999). Intracellular ice formation is affected by cell interactions. *Cryobiology.* 38:363–71.

Agca, Y., Liu, J., Rutledge, J.J., Critser, E.S., and Critser, J.K. (2000). Effect of osmotic stress on the developmental competence of germinal vesicle and metaphase II stage bovine cumulus oocyte complexes and its relevance to cryopreservation. *Mol. Reprod. Dev.* 55:212–19.

Agca, Y., Monson, R.L., Northey, D.L., Mazni, O.A., Schaefer, D.M., and Rutledge, J.J. (1998). Transfer of fresh and cryopreserved IVP bovine embryos: normal calving, birth weight and gestation lengths. *Theriogenology.* 50:147–62.

Agca, Y., Monson, R.L., Northey, D.L., Peschel, D.E., Schaefer, D.M., and Rutledge, J.J. (1998). Normal calves from transfer of biopsied, sexed and vitrified IVP bovine embryos. *Theriogenology.* 50:129–45.

Ali, J., and Shelton, J.N. (1993). Successful vitrification of day-6 sheep embryos. *J. Reprod. Fertil.* 99:65–70.

Amann, R.P. (2005). Weaknesses in reports of "fertility" for horses and other species. *Theriogenology.* 63:698–715.

Anchordoguy, T.J., Rudolph, A.S., Carpenter, J.F., and Crowe, J.H. (1987). Modes of interaction of cryoprotectants with membrane phospholipids during freezing. *Cryobiology.* 24:324–31.

Averill, R.L.W., and Rowson, L.E.A. (1959). Attempts at storage of sheep ova at low temperatures. *J. Agric. Sci.* 52:392–395.

Ball, G.D., Leibfried, M.L., Ax, R.L., and First, N.L. (1984). Maturation and fertilization of bovine oocytes in-vitro. *Journal of Dairy Science.* 67:2775–85.

Ballou, J.D. (1992). Potential contribution of cryopreserved germ plasm to the preservation of genetic diversity and conservation of endangered species in captivity. *Cryobiology.* 29:19–25.

Bane, D.P., James, J.E., Gradil, C.M., and Molitor, T.W. (1990). In-vitro exposure of preimplantation porcine embryos to porcine parvovirus. *Theriogenology.* 33:553–561.

Bank, H. 1973. Visualization of freezing damage. II. Structural alterations during warming. *Cryobiology.* 10:157–70.

Barber, K.A. 1983. Maximizing the impact of dairy and beef bulls through breeding technology. *J. Dairy Sci.* 66:2661–71.

Barry, B.E., Thompson, D.L. Jr., White, K.L., Wood, T.C., Hehnke, K.E., Rabb, M.H., and Colborn, D.R. (1989). Viability of inner cell mass versus trophectodermal cells of frozen-thawed horse embryos. *Equine. Vet. J.* Suppl. 8:82–3.

Bass, L.D., Denniston, D.J., Maclellan, L.J., McCue, P.M., Seidel, G.E. Jr., and Squires, E.L. (2004). Methanol as a cryoprotectant for equine embryos. *Theriogenology.* 62:1153–9.

Bavister, B.D. (1995). Culture of Preimplantation Embryos: Facts and Artifacts. *Human Reproduction Update.* 1:91–148.

Begin, I., Bhatia, B., Baldassarre, H., Dinnyes, A., and Keefer, C.L. (2003). Cryopreservation of goat oocytes and in-vivo derived 2- to 4-cell embryos using the cryoloop (CLV) and solid-surface vitrification (SSV) methods. *Theriogenology.* 59:1839–1850.

Berthelot, F., Martinat-Botte, F., Locatelli, A., Perreau, C. and Terqui, M. (2000). Piglets born after vitrification of embryos using the open pulled straw method. *Cryobiology.* 41:116–24.

Berthelot, F., Martinat-Botté, F., Perreau, C. and Terqui, M. (2001). Birth of piglets after OPS vitrification and transfer of compacted morula stage embryos with intact zona pellucida. *Reproduction, Nutrition, Development.* 41:267–272.

Bielanski, A., and Jordan, L. (1996). Washing or washing and trypsin treatment is ineffective for removal of non-cytopathic bovine viral diarrhea virus from bovine oocytes or embryos after experimental viral contamination of an in-vitro fertilization system. *Theriogenology.* 46:1467–1476.

Bielanski, A., and Surjujballi, O. (1996). Association of Leptospira borgpetersenii serovar hardjo type hardjobovis with bovine ova and embryos produced by in-vitro fertilization. *Theriogenology.* 46:45–55.

Biggers, J.D., Borland, R.M., and Powers, R.D. (1977). Transport mechanisms in the preimplantation mammalian embryo. *Ciba Found. Symp.* 129–53.

Bilton, R.J., and Moore, N.W. (1976). In-vitro culture, storage, and transfer of goat embryos. *Aus. J. Biol. Sci.* 29:125–9.

Blanco, J.M., Gee, G., Wildt, D.E., and Donoghue, A.M. (2000). Species variation in osmotic, cryoprotectant, and cooling rate tolerance in poultry, eagle, and peregrine falcon spermatozoa. *Biol. Reprod.* 63:1164–71.

Bouchard, G.F., Morris, J.K., Sikes, J.D., and Youngquist, R.S. (1990). Effect of storage temperature, cooling rates and two different semen extenders on canine spermatozoal motility. *Theriogenology.* 34:147–157.

Bouniol, C., Nguyen, E., and Debey, P. (1995). Endogenous transcription occurs at the 1-cell stage in the mouse embryo. *Exp. Cell. Res.* 218:57–62.

Bruyas, J.F., Bézard, J., Lagneaux, D. and Palmer, E. (1993). Quantitative analysis of morphological modifications of day 6.5 horse embryos after cryopreservation: differential effects on inner cell mass and trophoblast cells. *Journal of Reproduction and Fertility.* 99:15–23.

Bruyas, J.F., Martins-Ferreira, C., Fieni, F., and Tainturier, D. (1997). The effect of propanediol on the morphology of fresh and frozen equine embryos. *Equine Vet. J.* Suppl. 80–4.

Capco, D.G. (2001). Molecular and biochemical regulation of early mammalian development. *Int. Rev. Cytol.* 207:195–235.

Carnevale, E.M., Squires, E.L., and McKinnon, A.O. (1987). Comparison of Ham's F10 with CO2 or Hepes buffer for storage of equine embryos at 5 C for 24 h. *Journal of Animal Science.* 65:1775–1781.

Chang, M.C. (1947). Normal development of fertilized rabbit ova stored at low temperatures for several days. *Nature.* 159:602–3.

Chang, M.C. (1948). Transplantation of fertilized rabbit ova: the effect on viability of age, in-vitro storage period, and storage temperature. *Nature.* 161:978.

Chemineau, P., Procureur, R., Cognié, Y., Lefèvre, P.C., Locatelli, A., and Chupin, D. (1986). Production, freezing and transfer of embryos from a bluetongue-infected goat herd without bluetongue transmission. *Theriogenology.* 26:279–290.

Cocero, M.J., Sebastian, A.L., Barragan, M.L., and Picazo, R.A. (1996). Differences on post-thawing survival between ovine morulae and blastocysts cryopreserved with ethylene glycol or glycerol. *Cryobiology.* 33:502–7.

Cook, V.M., Squires, E.L., McKinnon, A.O., Bailey, J., and Long, P.L. (1989). Pregnancy rates of cooled, transported equine embryos. *Equine Vet. J.* Suppl. 8:80–1.

Critser, J.K., and Russell, R.J. (2000). Genome resource banking of laboratory animal models. *Ilar. J.* 41:183–6.

Cuello, C., Berthelot, F., Martinat-Botte, F., Venturi, E., Guillouet, P., Vazquez, J.M., Roca, J. and Martinez, E.A. (2005). Piglets born after non-surgical deep intrauterine transfer of vitrified blastocysts in gilts. *Anim. Repr. Sci.*

Cuello, C., Gil, M.A., Parrilla, I., Tornel, J., Vazquez, J.M., Roca, J., Berthelot, F., Martinat-Botte, F., and Martinez, E.A. (2004). In-vitro development following one-step dilution of OPS-vitrified porcine blastocysts. *Theriogenology.* 62:1144–52.

Cuello, C., Gil, M.A., Parrilla, I., Tornel, J., Vazquez, J.M., Roca, J., Berthelot, F., Martinat-Botte, F., and Martinez, E.A. (2004). Vitrification of porcine embryos at various developmental stages using different ultra-rapid cooling procedures. *Theriogenology.* 62:353–61.

Czlonkowska, M., Boyle, M.S., and Allen, W.R. (1985). Deep freezing of horse embryos. *Journal of Reproduction and Fertility.* 75:485–490.

Dattena, M., Accardo, C., Pilichi, S., Isachenko, V., Mara, L., Chessa, B., and Cappai, P. (2004). Comparison of different vitrification protocols on viability after transfer of ovine blastocysts in-vitro produced and in-vivo derived. *Theriogenology.* 62:481–93.

De Leeuw, F.E., Chen, H.C., Colenbrander, B., and Verkleij, A.J. (1990). Cold-induced ultrastructural changes in bull and boar sperm plasma membranes. *Cryobiology.* 27:171–83.

Dey, S.K., Lim, H., Das, S.K., Reese, J., Paria, B.C., Daikoku, T., and Wang, H. (2004). Molecular cues to implantation. *Endocr. Rev.* 25:341–73.

Dobrinsky, J.R. (1996). Cellular approach to cryopreservation of embryos. *Theriogenology.* 45:17–26.

Dobrinsky, J.R. (1997). Cryopreservation of pig embryos. *J. Reprod. Fertil.* Suppl. 52:301–12.

Dobrinsky, J.R. (2001). Cryopreservation of pig embryos: adaptation of vitrification technology for embryo transfer. *Reprod. Suppl.* 58:325–33.

Dobrinsky, J.R. (2001). Cryopreservation of swine embryos: a chilly past with a vitrifying future. *Theriogenology.* 56:1333–44.

Dobrinsky, J.R., Pursel, V.G., Long, C.R., and Johnson, L.A. (2000). Birth of piglets after transfer of embryos cryopreserved by cytoskeletal stabilization and vitrification. *Biology of Reproduction.* 62:564–570.

Dresser, B.L., Gelwicks, E.J., Wachs, K.B., and Keller, G.L. (1988). First successful transfer of cryopreserved feline (*Felis catus*) embryos resulting in live offspring. *J. Exp. Zool.* 246:180–6.

Drobnis, E.Z., Crowe, L.M., Berger, T., Anchordoguy, T.J., Overstreet, J.W., and Crowe, J.H. (1993). Cold shock damage is due to lipid phase transitions in cell membranes: a demonstration using sperm as a model. *J. Exp. Zool.* 265:432–7.

El-Gayar, M., and Holtz, W. (2001). Technical note: vitrification of goat embryos by the open pulled-straw method. *Journal of Animal Science.* 79:2436–2438.

Eldridge-Panuska, W.D., di Brienza, V.C., Seidel, G.E. Jr., Squires, E.L., and Carnevale, E.M. (2005). Establishment of pregnancies after serial dilution or direct transfer by vitrified equine embryos. *Theriogenology.* 63:1308–19.

Eyestone, W.H. (1994). Challenges and progress in the production of transgenic cattle. *Reprod. Fertil. Dev.* 6:647–52.

Fahning, M.L., and Garcia, M.A. (1992). Status of cryopreservation of embryos from domestic animals. *Cryobiology.* 29:1–18.

Fahy, G.M., Levy, D.I., and Ali, S.E. (1987). Some emerging principles underlying the physical properties, biological actions, and utility of vitrification solutions. *Cryobiology.* 24:196–213.

Fahy, G.M., MacFarlane, D.R., Angell, C.A., and Meryman, H.T. (1984). Vitrification as an approach to cryopreservation. *Cryobiology.* 21:407–26.

Fan, H.Y. and Sun, Q.Y. (2004). Involvement of mitogen-activated protein kinase cascade during oocyte maturation and fertilization in mammals. *Biol. Reprod.* 70:535–47.

Farrant, J., and Morris, G.J. (1973). Thermal shock and dilution shock as the causes of freezing injury. *Cryobiology.* 10:134–40.

Farstad, W. (2000). Current state in biotechnology in canine and feline reproduction. *Anim. Reprod. Sci.* 60–61:375–87.

Farstad, W. (1996). Semen cryopreservation in dogs and foxes. *Animal Reproduction Science.* 42:251–260.

Fiéni, F., Beckers, J.P., Buggin, M., Bruyas, J.F., Perrin, J., Daubié, M., and Tainturier, D. (1995). Evaluation of cryopreservation techniques for goat embryos. *Reproduction, Nutrition, Development.* 35:367–373.

Fleming, T.P., Sheth, B., and Fesenko, I. (2001). Cell adhesion in the preimplantation mammalian embryo and its role in trophectoderm differentiation and blastocyst morphogenesis. *Front. Biosci.* 6:D1000–7.

Fleming, T.P., Wilkins, A., Mears, A., Miller, D.J., Thomas, F., Ghassemifar, M.R., Fesenko, I., Sheth, B., Kwong, W.Y. and Eckert, J.J. (2004). Society for Reproductive Biology Founders' Lecture (2003). The making of an embryo: short-term goals and long-term implications. *Reprod. Fertil. Dev.* 16:325–37.

Fogarty, N.M., Maxwell, W.M., Eppleston, J., and Evans, G. (2000). The viability of transferred sheep embryos after long-term cryopreservation. *Reprod. Fertil. Dev.* 12:31–7.

Fukuda, Y., Ichikawa, M., Naito, K. and Toyoda, Y. (1990). Birth of normal calves resulting from bovine oocytes matured, fertilized, and cultured with cumulus cells in-vitro up to the blastocyst stage. *Biol. Reprod.* 42:114–9.

Gao, D., Mazur, P., and Critser, J.K. (1997). Fundamental Cryobiology of Mammalian Spermatozoa. In: Karow, A.M., and Critser, J.K. (eds) *Reproductive Tissue Banking, Scientific Principles.* San Diego: Academic Press, pp263–328.

Gao, D.Y., Liu, J., Liu, C., McGann, L.E., Watson, P.F., Kleinhans, F.W., Mazur, P., Critser, E.S., and Critser, J.K. (1995). Prevention of osmotic injury to human spermatozoa during addition and removal of glycerol. *Hum. Reprod.* 10:1109–22.

Garagna, S,. and Redi, C.A. (1988). Chromatin topology during the transformation of the mouse sperm nucleus into pronucleus in-vivo. *J. Exp. Zool.* 246:187–93.

Gardner, R.L., Papaioannou, V.E., and Barton, S.C. (1973). Origin of the ectoplacental cone and secondary giant cells in mouse blastocysts reconstituted from isolated trophoblast and inner cell mass. *J. Embryol. Exp. Morphol.* 30:561–72.

Gilmore, J.A., Du, J., Tao, J., Peter, A.T., and Critser, J.K. (1996). Osmotic properties of boar spermatozoa and their relevance to cryopreservation. *J. Reprod. Fertil.* 107:87–95.

Ginther, O.J. (1992). *Reproductive Biology of the Mare*, 2nd ed. Cross Plaines: Equiservices.

Glenister, P.H., Whittingham, D.G., and Wood, M.J. (1990). Genome cryopreservation: a valuable contribution to mammalian genetic research. *Genet. Res.* 56:253–8.

Gómez, M.C., Pope, E., Harris, R., Mikota, S., and Dresser, B.L. (2003). Development of in-vitro matured, in-vitro fertilized domestic cat embryos following cryopreservation, culture and transfer. *Theriogenology.* 60:239–251.

Gordon, I. (1995). Preservation of embryos and oocytes. *Laboratory Production of Cattle Embryos, 2nd Edition*; Cambridge, USA: CABI Publishing.

Guerin, B., Nibart, M., Marquant-Le Guienne, B., and Humblot, P. (1997). Sanitary risks related to embryo transfer in domestic species. *Theriogenology.* 47:33–42.

Gunasena, K.T., and Critser, J.K. (1997). Utility of viable tissues ex vivo: banking of reproductive cells and tissues. In Karow, A.M., and Critser, J.K. (eds) *Reproductive Tissue Banking Scientific Principles.* San Diego: Academic Press pp 472.

HanChi, H., JennRong, Y., and ReyChun, H. (1997). Effects of diluents and cryoprotectants on cryopreservation of semen and embryos in Taiwan black goats. *Journal of Taiwan Livestock Research.* 30:371–7.

Hartmann, J.F. (1983). Mammalian fertilization: gamete surface interactions in-vitro. In: *Mechanism and Control of Animal Fertilization*, New York: Academic Press, 325–364.

Hasler, J.F. (1992). Current status and potential of embryo transfer and reproductive technology in dairy cattle. *J. Dairy Sci.* 75:2857–79.

Hay, M.A., King, W.A., Gartley, C.J., Leibo, S.P., and Goodrowe, K.L. (1997). Effects of cooling, freezing and glycerol on penetration of oocytes by spermatozoa in dogs. *J. Repro. Fertil.* Suppl. 51:99–108.

Hayashi, S., Kobayashi, K., Mizuno, J., Saitoh, K., and Hirano, S. (1989). Birth of piglets from frozen embryos. *Vet. Rec.* 125:43–4.

Heyman, Y., Vincent, C., Garnier, V., and Cognie, Y. (1987). Transfer of frozen-thawed embryos in sheep. *Vet. Rec.* 120: 83–5.

Holt, W.V., Abaigar, T., Watson, P.F., and Wildt, D.E. (2003). Genetic resource banks for species conservation. In: Holt, W.V., Pickard A.R., Rodger. J.C., and Wildt, D.E. (eds) *Reproductive Science and Integrated Conservation*, Cambridge: Cambridge University Press, pp 267–280.

Huhtinen, M., Lagneaux, D., Koskinen, E., and Palmer, E. (1997). The effect of sucrose in the thawing solution on the morphology and mobility of frozen equine embryos. *Equine Vet. J.* Suppl. 94–7.

Jacobs, M.H., and Stewart, D.R. (1932). A simple method for the quantitative measurement of cell permeability. *J. of Cel. and Comp. Physiol.* 1:71–82.

Kane, M.T. (2003). A review of in-vitro gamete maturation and embryo culture and potential impact on future animal biotechnology. *Anim. Reprod. Sci.* 79:171–90.

Karlsson, J.O., Cravalho, E.G., Borel Rinkes, I.H., Tompkins, R.G., Yarmush, M.L., and Toner, M. (1993). Nucleation and growth of ice crystals inside cultured hepatocytes during freezing in the presence of dimethyl sulfoxide. *Biophys. J.* 65:2524–36.

Kashiwazaki, N., Ohtani, S., Miyamoto, K., and Ogawa, S. (1991). Production of normal piglets from hatched blastocysts frozen at −196 degrees C. *Vet. Rec.* 128:256–7.

Kedem, O., and Katchalsky, A. (1958). Thermodynamic analysis of the permeability of biological membranes to non-electrolytes. *Biochimica et Biophysica Acta.* 27:229–246.

Kelly, S.J. (1977). Studies of the developmental potential of 4- and 8-cell stage mouse blastomeres. *J. Exp. Zool.* 200:365–76.

Kim, N.H., Simerly, C., Funahashi, H., Schatten, G., and Day, B.N. (1996). Microtubule organization in porcine oocytes during fertilization and parthenogenesis. *Biol. Reprod.* 54:1397–404.

Landin e Alvarenga, F.C., Alvarenga, M.A. and Meira, C. (1993). Transmission electron microscopy of equine embryos cryopreserved by different methods. *Equine Vet. J.* Suppl. 15:67–70.

Le Gal, F., Baril, G., Vallet, J.C., and Leboeuf, B. (1993). In-vivo and in-vitro survival of goat embryos after freezing with ethylene glycol or glycerol. *Theriogenology.* 40:771–777.

Lee, K.Y. and DeMayo, F.J. (2004). Animal models of implantation. *Reproduction.* 128:679–95.

Legrand, E., Bencharif, D., Barrier-Battut, I., Delajarraud, H., Corniere, P., Fieni, F., Tainturier, D., and Bruyas, J.F. (2002). Comparison of pregnancy rates for days 7–8 equine embryos frozen in glycerol with or without previous enzymatic treatment of their capsule. *Theriogenology.* 58:721–3.

Leibo, S.P. 1984. A one-step method for direct nonsurgical transfer of frozen-thawed bovine embryos. *Theriogenology* 21:767–790.

Leibo, S.P., McGrath, J.J. and Cravalho, E.G. (1978). Microscopic observation of intracellular ice formation in unfertilized mouse ova as a function of cooling rate. *Cryobiology.* 15:257–71.

Leibo, S.P., Semple, M.E., and Kroetsch, T.G. (1994). In-vitro fertilization of oocytes by 37-year-old cryopreserved bovine spermatozoa. *Theriogenology.* 42:1257–1262.

Liu, J., Christian, J.A., and Critser, J.K. (2002). Canine RBC osmotic tolerance and membrane permeability. *Cryobiology.* 44:258–68.

Lohuis, M.M. (1995). Potential benefits of bovine embryo manipulation technologies to genetic improvement programs. *Theriogenology.* 43:51–60.

Lovelock, J.E. (1953a). The haemolysis of human red blood cells by freezing and thawing. *Biochim. Biophys. Acta.* 10:414–426.

Lovelock, J.E. (1953b). The mechanism of the protective action of glycerol against haemolysis by freezing and thawing. *Biochim. Biophys. Acta.* 11:28–36.

Luyet, B.J., and Gehenio, P.M. (1940). *Life and Death at Low Temperatures*, Normandy, Missouri: Biodynamica.

Mahmoudzadeh, A.R., Soom, A. van, Ysebaert, M.T., and Kruif, A. de. (1994). Comparison of two-step vitrification versus controlled freezing on survival of in-vitro produced cattle embryos. *Theriogenology.* 42:1389–1397.

Mani, I., and Vadnere, S.V. (1988). Cryoprotective effect of different concentrations of dimethylsulfoxide (DMSO) and glycerol on freezing of goat embryos. *Indian Journal of Animal Reproduction.* 9:136–137.

Marguant-Le Guienne, B., Remond, M., Cosquer, R., Humblot, P., Kaiser, C., Lebreton, F., Cruciere, C., Guerin, B., Laporte, J., and Thibier, M. (1998). Exposure of in-vitro-produced bovine embryos to foot-and-mouth disease virus. *Theriogenology.* 50:109–16.

Martinez, A.G., and Matkovic, M. (1998). Cryopreservation of ovine embryos: slow freezing and vitrification. *Theriogenology.* 49:1039–49.

Massip, A. (2001). Cryopreservation of embryos from farm animals. *Reprod. Dom. Anim.* 36:49–55.

Massip, A., and van der Zwalmen, P. (1984). Direct transfer of frozen cow embryos in glycerol-sucrose. *Vet. Rec.* 115:327–8.

Massip, A., Van der Zwalmen, P., Scheffen, B., and Ectors, F. (1986). Pregnancies following transfer of cattle embryos produced by vitrification. *Cryo-Letters.* 7:270–73.

Massip, A., Zwalmen, P. van der, and Ectors, F. (1987). Recent progress in cryopreservation of cattle embryos. *Theriogenology.* 27:69–79.

Massip, A., Zwalmen, P. van der, Ectors, F., Coster, R. de, D'Ieteren, G., and Hanzen, C. (1979). Deep freezing of cattle embryos in glass ampules or French straws. *Theriogenology.* 12:79–84.

Mazur, P. (1970). Cryobiology: the freezing of biological systems. *Science.* 168:939–49.

Mazur, P. (1963). Kinetics of water loss from cells at subzero temperatures and the likelihood of intracellular freezing. *Journal of General Physiology.* 47:47–69.

Mazur, P. (2004). Principles of cryobiology. In: Fuller, B.J., Lane, N., and Benson, E.E. (eds) *Life in the Frozen State*, Boca Raton: CRC Press, pp 672.

Mazur, P., Cole, K.W., Hall, J.W., Schreuders, P.D., and Mahowald, A.P. (1992). Cryobiological preservation of Drosophila embryos. *Science*. 258:1932–5.

Mazur, P., Leibo, S.P. and Chu, E.H. (1972). A two-factor hypothesis of freezing injury. Evidence from Chinese hamster tissue-culture cells. *Exp. Cell. Res.* 71:345–55.

Mazur, P., Rall, W.F., and Rigopoulos, N. (1981). Relative contributions of the fraction of unfrozen water and of salt concentration to the survival of slowly frozen human erythrocytes. *Biophys. J.* 36:653–75.

Mazur, P., and Schmidt, J.J. (1968). Interactions of cooling velocity, temperature, and warming velocity on the survival of frozen and thawed yeast. *Cryobiology*. 5:1–17.

Mazur, P., and Schneider, U. (1986). Osmotic responses of preimplantation mouse and bovine embryos and their cryobiological implications. *Cell. Biophys.* 8:259–85.

McGinnis, L.K., Duplantis, S.C. Jr.. and Youngs, C.R. (1993). Cryopreservation of sheep embryos using ethylene glycol. *Animal Reproduction Science*. 30:273–280.

McGrath, J.J., Cravalho, E.G. and Huggins, C.E. (1975). An experimental comparison of intracellular ice formation and freeze-thaw survival of HeLa S-3 cells. *Cryobiology*. 12: 540–50.

McLay, D.W., and Clarke, H.J. (2003). Remodelling the paternal chromatin at fertilization in mammals. *Reproduction*. 125: 625–33.

Meira, C., Alvarenga, M.A., Papa, F.O., Obe, E., and Landin e Alvarenga, F.C. (1993). Cryopreservation of equine embryos using glycerol and 1,2-propanediol as cryoprotectants. *Equine Vet. J.* Suppl. 15:64–6.

Memili, E., and First, N.L. (1998). Developmental changes in RNA polymerase II in bovine oocytes, early embryos, and effect of alpha-amanitin on embryo development. *Mol. Reprod. Dev.* 51:381–9.

Memili, E., and First, N.L. (2000). Zygotic and embryonic gene expression in cow: a review of timing and mechanisms of early gene expression as compared with other species. *Zygote*. 8:87–96.

Menezo, Y.J., and Herubel, F. (2002). Mouse and bovine models for human IVF. *Reprod. Biomed. Online*. 4:170–5.

Meryman, H.T. (1971). Osmotic stress as a mechanism of freezing injury. *Cryobiology*. 8:489–500.

Meryman, H.T., Williams, R.J., and Douglas, M.S. (1977). Freezing injury from "solution effects" and its prevention by natural or artificial cryoprotection. *Cryobiology*. 14:287–302.

Morris, G.J., and Watson, P.F. (1984). Cold-Shock injury—a comprehensive bibliography. *Cryo-Letters*. 5:352–72.

Moussa, M., Duchamp, G., Mahla, R., Bruyas, J.F., and Daels, P.F. (2003). In-vitro and in-vivo comparison of Ham's F-10, Emcare holding solution and ViGro holding plus for the cooled storage of equine embryos. *Theriogenology*. 59:1615–1625.

Muldrew, K., and McGann, L.E. (1990). Mechanisms of intracellular ice formation. *Biophys. J.* 57:525–32.

Mullen, S.F., Agca, Y., Broermann, D.C., Jenkins, C.L., Johnson, C.A., and Critser, J.K. (2004). The effect of osmotic stress on the metaphase II spindle of human oocytes, and the relevance to cryopreservation. *Hum. Reprod.* 19:1148–54.

Myers, S.P., Pitt, R.E., Lynch, D.V., and Steponkus, P.L. (1989). Characterization of intracellular ice formation in Drosophila melanogaster embryos. *Cryobiology*. 26:472–84.

Nagai, T. (2001). The improvement of in-vitro maturation systems for bovine and porcine oocytes. *Theriogenology*. 55:1291–301.

Nagashima, H., Kashiwazaki, N., Ashman, R.J., Grupen, C.G., Seamark, R.F., and Nottle, M.B. (1994). Removal of cytoplasmic lipid enhances the tolerance of porcine embryos to chilling. *Biol. Reprod.* 51:618–22.

Nagashima, H., Kato, Y., Yamakawa, H., and Ogawa, S. (1988). Survival of pig hatched blastocysts exposed below 15 deg C. *Theriogenology*. 29:280.

Nicholas, J.S., and Hall, B.V. (1942). Experiments on developing rats II. The development of isolated blastomeres and fused eggs. *Journal of Experimental Zoology*. 90:441–459.

Nothias, J.Y., Majumder, S., Kaneko, K.J., and DePamphilis, M.L. (1995). Regulation of gene expression at the beginning of mammalian development. *J. Biol. Chem.* 270:22077–80.

Okano, T., Murase, T., Asano, M., and Tsubota, T. (2004). Effects of final dilution rate, sperm concentration and times for cooling and glycerol equilibration on post-thaw characteristics of canine spermatozoa. *J. Vet. Med. Sci.* 66:1359–64.

Overstrom, E.W., Benos, D.J., and Biggers, J.D. (1989). Synthesis of Na+/K+ ATPase by the preimplantation rabbit blastocyst. *J. Reprod. Fertil.* 85:283–95.

Papadopoulos, S., Rizos, D., Duffy, P., Wade, M., Quinn, K., Boland, M.P., and Lonergan, P. (2002). Embryo survival and recipient pregnancy rates after transfer of fresh or vitrified, in-vivo or in-vitro produced ovine blastocysts. *Animal Reproduction Science*. 74:35–44.

Parkes, A.S. (1957). Introductory Remarks. *Proceedings of the Royal Society of London*, 147:424–553.

Parkes, A.S. (1985). *The Rise of Cryobiology*, Cambridge: Cambridge University Press.

Pfaff, R., Seidel, G.E., Squires, E.L., and Jasko, D.J. (1993). Permeability of equine blastocysts to ethylene glycol and glycerol. *Theriogenology*. 39:284.

Philpott, M. (1993). The dangers of disease transmission by artificial insemination and embryo transfer. *Br. Vet. J.* 149: 339–69.

Pincus, G. (1936). *The Eggs of Mammals*, New York: Macmillan.

Pitt, R.E. (1992). Thermodynamics and intracellular ice formation. In: Steponkus, P.L. (ed) *Advances in Low-temperature Biology*, London: JAI Press.

Pitt, R.E., and Steponkus, P.L. (1989). Quantitative analysis of the probability of intracellular ice formation during freezing of isolated protoplasts. *Cryobiology*. 26:44–63.

Polge, C., Smith, A.U., and Parkes, A.S. (1949). Revival of spermatozoa after vitrification and dehydration at low temperatures. *Nature*. 164:666.

Polge, C., Wilmut, I., and Rowson, L.E. (1974). The low temperature preservation of cow, sheep, and pig embryos. *Cryobiology.* 11:560.

Pollard, J.W., and Leibo, S.P. (1994). Chilling sensitivity of mammalian embryos. *Theriogenology.* 41:101–106.

Pope, C.E., McRae, M.A., Plair, B.L., Keller, G.L., and Dresser, B.L. (1994). Successful in-vitro and in-vivo development of in-vitro fertilized two- to four-cell cat embryos following cryopreservation, culture and transfer. *Theriogenology.* 42:513–525.

Prather, R.S., Hawley, R.J., Carter, D.B., Lai, L., and Greenstein, J.L. (2003). Transgenic swine for biomedicine and agriculture. *Theriogenology.* 59:115–23.

Pratt, H.P., Ziomek, C.A., Reeve, W.J., and Johnson, M.H. (1982). Compaction of the mouse embryo: an analysis of its components. *J. Embryol. Exp. Morphol.* 70:113–32.

Pukazhenthi, B., Noiles, E., Pelican, K., Donoghue, A., Wildt, D., and Howard, J. (2000). Osmotic effects on feline spermatozoa from normospermic versus teratospermic donors. *Cryobiology.* 40:139–50.

Rall, W.F., and Fahy, G.M. (1985). Ice-free cryopreservation of mouse embryos at −196 degrees C by vitrification. *Nature.* 313:573–5.

Rall, W.F., Mazur, P., and McGrath, J.J. (1983). Depression of the ice-nucleation temperature of rapidly cooled mouse embryos by glycerol and dimethyl sulfoxide. *Biophys. J.* 41:1–12.

Rall, W.F. and Polge, C. (1984). Effect of warming rate on mouse embryos frozen and thawed in glycerol. *J. Reprod. Fertil.* 70:285–92.

Rall, W.F., Reid, D.S., and Polge, C. (1984). Analysis of slow-warming injury of mouse embryos by cryomicroscopical and physiochemical methods. *Cryobiology.* 21:106–21.

Rambhatla, L., and Latham, K.E. (1995). Strain-specific progression of alpha-amanitin-treated mouse embryos beyond the two-cell stage. *Mol. Reprod. Dev.* 41:16–9.

Ramsey, E.M. (1975). *The placenta of laboratory animals and man*, USA: Holt, Rinehart, and Winston, Inc.

Rands, G.F. (1986). Size regulation in the mouse embryo. II. The development of half embryos. *J. Embryol. Exp. Morphol.* 98:209–17.

Renton, J.P., Boyd, J.S., Eckersall, P.D., Ferguson, J.M., Harvey, M.J., Mullaney, J., and Perry, B. (1991). Ovulation, fertilization and early embryonic development in the bitch (*Canis familiaris*). *J. Reprod. Fertil.* 93:221–31.

Riddell, K.P., Stringfellow, D.A., Wolfe, D.F., and Galik, P.K. (1989). Seroconversion of recipient ewes after transfer of embryos exposed to Brucella ovis in-vitro. *Theriogenology.* 31:248.

Rossant, J. (1976). Investigation of inner cell mass determination by aggregation of isolated rat inner cell masses with mouse morulae. *J. Embryol. Exp. Morphol.* 36:163–74.

Rota, A., Strom, B.L., and Linde-Forsberg, C. (1995). Effects of seminal plasma and three extenders on canine semen stored at 4 degrees C. *Theriogenology.* 44:885–900.

Ruffing, N.A., Step022onkus, P.L., Pitt, R.E., and Parks, J.E. (1993). Osmometric behavior, hydraulic conductivity, and incidence of intracellular ice formation in bovine oocytes at different developmental stages. *Cryobiology.* 30:562–80.

Santarius, K.A., and Giersch, C. (1983). Cryopreservation of spinach chloroplast membranes by low-molecular-weight carbohydrates. II. Discrimination between colligative and noncolligative protection. *Cryobiology.* 20:90–9.

Schatten, G., and Schatten, H. (1987). Cytoskeletal alterations and nuclear architectural changes during mammalian fertilization. *Curr. Top. Dev. Biol.* 23:23–54.

Schatten, G., Simerly, C., Palmer, D.K., Margolis, R.L., Maul, G., Andrews, B.S., and Schatten, H. (1988). Kinetochore appearance during meiosis, fertilization and mitosis in mouse oocytes and zygotes. *Chromosoma.* 96:341–52.

Schatten, G., Simerly, C., and Schatten, H. (1985). Microtubule configurations during fertilization, mitosis, and early development in the mouse and the requirement for egg microtubule-mediated motility during mammalian fertilization. *Proc. Natl. Acad. Sci. USA.* 82:4152–6.

Schatten, H., Schatten, G., Mazia, D., Balczon, R., and Simerly, C. (1986). Behavior of centrosomes during fertilization and cell division in mouse oocytes and in sea urchin eggs. *Proc. Natl. Acad. Sci. USA.* 83:105–9.

Schultz, R.M. (2002). The molecular foundations of the maternal to zygotic transition in the preimplantation embryo. *Hum. Reprod. Update.* 8:323–31.

Schultz, R.M. (1993). Regulation of zygotic gene activation in the mouse. *Bioessays.* 15:531–8.

Seidel, G.E. Jr. (1996). Cryopreservation of equine embryos. *Veterinary Clinics of North America, Equine Practice.* 12:85–99.

Seidel, G.E. Jr., Squires, E.L., McKinnon, A.O., and Long, P.L. (1989). Cryopreservation of equine embryos in 1,2 propanediol. *Equine Vet. J. Suppl.* 8:87–8.

Shimada, A., Kikuchi, K., Noguchi, J., Akama, K., Nakano, M., and Kaneko, H. (2000). Protamine dissociation before decondensation of sperm nuclei during in-vitro fertilization of pig oocytes. *J. Reprod. Fertil.* 120:247–56.

Slade, N.P., Takeda, T., Squires, E.L., Elsden, R.P., and Seidel, G.E. Jr. (1985). A new procedure for the cryopreservation of equine embryos. *Theriogenology.* 24:45–58.

Sloviter, H.A. (1951). Recovery of human red blood-cells after freezing. *Lancet.* 260:823–4.

Smith, L.D. (1972). Protein synthesis during oocyte maturation. In Biggers, J.D., Schuetz, A.W. (eds) Oogenesis, Baltimore: Baltimore University Park Press.

Songsasen, N., Buckrell, B.C., Plante, C., and Leibo, S.P. (1995). In-vitro and in-vivo survival of cryopreserved sheep embryos. *Cryobiology.* 32:78–91.

Songsasen, N., Yu, I., Murton, S., Paccamonti, D.L., Eilts, B.E., Godke, R.A., and Leibo, S.P. (2002). Osmotic sensitivity of canine spermatozoa. *Cryobiology.* 44:79–90.

Squires, E.L., Carnevale, E.M., McCue, P.M., and Bruemmer, J.E. (2003). Embryo technologies in the horse. *Theriogenology.* 59:151–70.

Squires, E.L., Seidel, G. E. Jr., and McKinnon, A.O. (1989). Transfer of cryopreserved equine embryos to progestin-treated ovariectomised mares. *Equine Vet. J. Suppl.* 89–91.

Steponkus, P.L., Myers, S.P., Lynch, D.V., Gardner, L., Bronshteyn, V., Leibo, S.P., Rall, W.F., Pitt, R.E., Lin, T.T., and MacIntyre, R.J. (1990). Cryopreservation of Drosophila melanogaster embryos. *Nature.* 345:170–2.

Stringfellow, D.A., and Givens, M.D. (2000). Epidemiologic concerns relative to in-vivo and in-vitro production of livestock embryos. *Anim. Reprod. Sci.* 60–61:629–42.

Stringfellow, D.A., Riddell, K.P., Galik, P.K., Damiani, P., Bishop, M.D., and Wright, J.C. (2000). Quality controls for bovine viral diarrhea virus-free IVF embryos. *Theriogenology.* 53:827–39.

Sutovsky, P., Navara, C.S., and Schatten, G. (1996). Fate of the sperm mitochondria, and the incorporation, conversion, and disassembly of the sperm tail structures during bovine fertilization. *Biol. Reprod.* 55:1195–205.

Tarkowski, A.K., and Wroblewska, J. (1967). Development of blastomeres of mouse eggs isolated at the 4- and 8-cell stage. *J. Embryol. Exp. Morphol.* 18:155–80.

Tesarik, J., and Kopecny, V. (1989). Nucleic acid synthesis and development of human male pronucleus. *J. Reprod. Fertil.* 86:549–58.

Thibier, M., and Nibart, M. (1987). Disease control and embryo importations. *Theriogenology.* 27:37–47.

Thirumala, S., Ferrer, M.S., Al-Jarrah, A., Eilts, B.E., Paccamonti, D.L., and Devireddy, R.V. (2003). Cryopreservation of canine spermatozoa: theoretical prediction of optimal cooling rates in the presence and absence of cryoprotective agents. *Cryobiology.* 47:109–24.

Thompson, J G. (2000). In-vitro culture and embryo metabolism of cattle and sheep embryos—a decade of achievement. *Anim. Reprod. Sci.* 60–61:263–75.

Tomanek, M., Kopecny, V., and Kanka, J. (1989). Genome reactivation in developing early pig embryos: an ultrastructural and autoradiographic analysis. *Anat. Embryol. (Berl)* 180:309–16.

Toner, M., Cravalho, E.G., and Huggins, C.E. (1990). Thermodynamics and kinetics of intracellular ice formation during freezing of biological cells. *Journal of Applied Physiology.* 69:1582–1593.

Toner, M., Cravalho, E.G., and Karel, M. (1993). Cellular response of mouse oocytes to freezing stress: prediction of intracellular ice formation. *J. Biomech. Eng.* 115:169–74.

Toner, M., Cravalho, E.G., Karel, M., and Armant, D.R. (1991). Cryomicroscopic analysis of intracellular ice formation during freezing of mouse oocytes without cryoadditives. *Cryobiology.* 28:55–71.

Trachte, E., Stringfellow, D., Riddell, K., Galik, P., Riddell, M. Jr., and Wright, J. (1998). Washing and trypsin treatment of in-vitro derived bovine embryos exposed to bovine viral diarrhea virus. *Theriogenology.* 50:717–26.

Trounson, A.O., Willadsen, S.M., and Rowson, L.E.A. (1976). The influence of in-vitro culture and cooling on the survival and development of cow embryos. *Journal of Reproduction and Fertility.* 47:367–70.

Trounson, A.O., Willadsen, S.M., Rowson, L.E., and Newcomb, R. (1976). The storage of cow eggs at room temperature and at low temperatures. *J. Reprod. Fertil.* 46:173–8.

Tsunoda, Y., and McLaren, A. (1983). Effect of various procedures on the viability of mouse embryos containing half the normal number of blastomeres. *J. Reprod. Fertil.* 69:315–22.

Tsunoda, Y., and Sugie, T. (1977). Survival of rabbit eggs preserved in plastic straws in liquid nitrogen. *J. Reprod. Fertil.* 49:173–4.

Turk, J.R., and Laughlin, M.H. (2004). Physical activity and atherosclerosis: which animal model? *Can. J. Appl. Physiol.* 29:657–83.

Utsumi, K., and Yuhara, M. (1975). Survival of rat eggs after freezing and thawing. *Jap. J. Fert. and Ster.* 20:102.

Vajta, G., Booth, P.J., Holm, P., Greve, T., and Callesen, H. (1997). Successful vitrification of early stage bovine in-vitro produced embryos with the open pulled straw (OPS) method. *Cryo-Letters.* 18:191–195.

van Wagtendonk-De Leeuw, A.M., Den Daas, J.H., Kruip, T.A., and Rall, W.F. (1995). Comparison of the efficacy of conventional slow freezing and rapid cryopreservation methods for bovine embryos. *Cryobiology.* 32:157–67.

van Wagtendonk-de Leeuw, A.M., den Daas, J.H.G., and Rall, W.F. (1997). Field trial to compare pregnancy rates of bovine embryo cryopreservation methods: vitrification and one-step dilution versus slow freezing and three step dilution. *Theriogenology.* 48:1071–1084.

Voelkel, S.A., and Hu, Y.X. (1992). Direct transfer of frozen-thawed bovine embryos. *Theriogenology.* 37:23–37.

Walters, E., and Critser, J.K. (In Press). History of sperm cryopreservation. In: Pacey, A., and Tomlinson, M.J. (eds) *Practical Guide for Sperm Banking*, Cambridge: Cambridge University Press.

Wassarman, P.M., Jovine, L., and Litscher, E.S. (2001). A profile of fertilization in mammals. *Nat. Cell. Biol.* 3:E59–64.

Watson, A.J., and Barcroft, L.C. (2001). Regulation of blastocyst formation. *Front. Biosci.* 6:D708–30.

Watson, P.F., and Morris, G.J. (1987). Cold shock injury in animal cells. In: Bowler, K., and Fuller, B.J. (eds) *Temperature and Animal Cells*, Cambridge: The Company of Biologist Limited, pp 311–340.

Whittingham, D.G. (1974). Embryo banks in the future of developmental genetics. *Genetics.* 78:395–402.

Whittingham, D.G., Leibo, S.P., and Mazur, P. (1972). Survival of mouse embryos frozen to −196 degrees and −269 degrees C. *Science.* 178:411–4.

Wildt, D.E. (2000). Genome resource banking for wildlife research, management, and conservation. *Ilar. J.* 41:228–34.

Wildt, D.E., Rall, W.F., Critser, J.K., Monfort, S.L., and Seal, U.S. (1997). Genome Resource Banks. *Bioscience.* 47:689–698.

Willadsen, S.M. (1977). Factors affecting the survival of sheep embryos during freezing and thawing. *Ciba Found. Symp.* 175–201.

Willadsen, S.M., Polge, C., Rowson, L.E., and Moor, R.M. (1976). Deep freezing of sheep embryos. *J. Reprod. Fertil.* 46:151–4.

Williams, R.J., and Shaw, S.K. (1980). The relationship between cell injury and osmotic volume reduction: II. Red cell lysis correlates with cell volume rather than intracellular salt concentration. *Cryobiology.* 17:530–9.

Wilmut, I. (1972a). The effect of cooling rate, warming rate, cryoprotective agent and stage of development on survival of mouse embryos during freezing and thawing. *Life Sci. II.* 11:1071–9.

Wilmut, I. (1972b). The low temperature preservation of mammalian embryos. *J. Reprod. Ferti.* 31:513–4.

Wilmut, I., and Hume, A. (1978). The value of embryo transfer to cattle breeding in Britain. *Vet. Rec.* 103:107–10.

Wilmut, I., Polge, C., and Rowson, L.E. (1975). The effect on cow embryos of cooling to 20, 0 and −196c. *J. Reprod. Fertil.* 45:409–11.

Wilmut, I., and Rowson, L.E. (1973). Experiments on the low-temperature preservation of cow embryos. *Vet. Re.* 92:686–90.

Yamada, S., Shimazu, Y., Kawaji, H., Nakazawa, M., Naito, K., and Toyoda, Y. (1992). Maturation, fertilization, and development of dog oocytes in-vitro. *Biol. Reprod.* 46:853–8.

Yamada, S., Shimazu, Y., Kawano, Y., Nakazawa, M., Naito, K., and Toyoda, Y. (1993). In-vitro maturation and fertilization of preovulatory dog oocytes. *J. Reprod. Fertil.* Suppl. 47: 227–9.

Yamamoto, Y., Oguri, N., Tsutsumi, Y., and Hachinohe, Y. (1982). Experiments in the freezing and storage of equine embryos. *J. Reprod. Fertil. Suppl.* 32:399–403.

Yanagimachi, R. (1994). Mammalian fertilization. In: Knobil, E., and Neill, J.D. (eds) *The Physiology of Reproduction*, New York: Raven Press.

Yuswiati, E., and Holtz, W. (1990). Work in progress: successful transfer of vitrified goat embryos. *Theriogenology.* 34:629–632.

Zhang, L., Barry, D.M., Denniston, R.S., Bunch, T.D., and Godke, R.A. (1993). Birth of live calves after transfer of frozen-thawed bovine embryos fertilised in-vitro. *Veterinary Record.* 132: 247–249.

Zieger, M.A., Woods, E.J., Lakey, J.R., Liu, J., and Critser, J.K. (1999). Osmotic tolerance limits of canine pancreatic islets. *Cell. Transplant.* 8:277–84.

Ziomek, C.A., Johnson, M.H., and Handyside, A.H. (1982). The developmental potential of mouse 16-cell blastomeres. *J. Exp. Zool.* 221:345–55.

Chapter 10

Animal Cloning

Liangxue Lai and Randall S. Prather

Definition of Animal Cloning

Cloning is making a biological copy of another organism with the identical genetic makeup of the founding individual. It is an asexual method of reproduction. Natural examples of cloning include organisms such as bacteria, yeast, and some snail and shrimp species. The two bacteria that result from asexual reproduction are genetically identical; they are clones of each other.

Specifically, animal cloning refers to the creation of a new genetic replica of an original living or dead animal. The only clones produced naturally in mammals are identical twins. These are formed when cells produced by the early divisions of the fertilized egg separate and independently develop into new individuals. They are therefore genetically identical to each other but not identical to their parents. Cloned animals can be created by three processes:

Cloning by embryo splitting involves the division of the preimplantation embryo into equal halves, which produce two genetically identical embryos. It has been used predominantly in sheep and cattle.

Cloning by blastomere dispersal begins with the mechanical separation of individual cells prior to the formation of the blastocyst.

Cloning by nuclear transfer (NT) is a delicate series of events that take place in a short period of time but have long-lasting effects on development. The procedures involve the complete removal of genetic material (chromosomes) from a matured oocyte or an egg to produce an enucleated cell (cytoplast). It is replaced by a nucleus containing a full complement of chromosomes from a suitable donor cell (karyoplast), which is introduced into the recipient cytoplast by direct microinjection or by fusion of the donor and recipient cells. The egg is then implanted in another adult female for normal gestation and delivery. Depending on the source of donor nuclei, cloning by nuclear transfer can be classified into embryonic cell (unspecialized) NT and somatic cell (differentiated) NT. Somatic cell NT is the most important process used for animal cloning and has most potential applications.

This chapter focuses on somatic cell NT.

History of Animal Cloning

The first successful cloning experiments in vertebrates arose from the desire of embryologists to know whether the process of cell differentiation from an egg involved permanent or stable changes in the genome. One idea was that as cells differentiate, the genes no longer needed (such as skin genes in intestinal cells) could be lost or permanently repressed. The other idea was that all genes are present in all cell types, and that cell differentiation involved the selective activation and repression of genes appropriate to the cell type. To answer this question, in 1938, Hans Spemann proposed a "fantastical experiment" of cloning.

In 1952, the first successful transplantation of nuclei from early embryo cells was achieved by Briggs and King working with the American frog *Rana pipiens*. When they took nuclei from more advanced embryos they found they could no longer obtain normal development in the way that they could from early cell nuclei. This led to the view that some loss or permanent inactivation of genes might accompany development and cell differentiation. Later, in the 1960s and '70s, John Gurdon could transplant the nucleus from the cells of tadpoles and get these cells to grow all the way to adult frogs. But when he transplanted the nucleus from a cell of an adult frog he couldn't get the same degree of development.

Scientists took it to the next stage in the late 1980s by cloning mammalians. Success in nuclear transfer, that is, the birth of live mammalian offspring, was achieved primarily with preimplantation embryonic nuclei in several species, including sheep, cattle, pigs, and rabbits. Cloning in mice followed later. Those pioneers limited themselves to using the early unspecialized embryo cells, but not adult mammal cells.

While this work appeared to be accumulating more and more evidence to support the view that some loss or permanent inactivation of genes might accompany development and cell differentiation, it was establishing the background leading up to the birth of Dolly, the first mammal to develop from the nucleus of an adult somatic cell in 1997. Wilmut and colleagues took fetal fibroblast cells and cells derived from the mammary gland of an adult sheep and reported successful production of live offspring from both cell types. Despite its long history, the cloning of animals by nuclear transplantation is undergoing a "renaissance" after the birth of Dolly. The amount of work and achievements in the last nine years are probably greater than those obtained in the half century of earlier research.

Applications of Somatic Nuclear Transfer

Somatic cell nuclear transfer has many applications beyond simply making animals that are genetically identical and expanding desirable genotypes. While genetic copies of animals for research breeding can be constructed, the technique can also be used to create transgenic as well as knock-out animals, and possibly be used to save endangered species.

Making Clones for Animal Research Purposes

When the animals used in experiments are exactly the same physiologically, the experiments are much easier to control and fewer animals are needed. Inbred strains of animals have been a mainstay of biological research for years. These animals have been bred by brother-sister mating for many generations until they are essentially all genetically identical and homozygous (i.e., they carry two identical copies of most genes). Experimental analysis is then simplified, because variations in response to experimental treatment due to variations in genetic background can be eliminated. Clearly, generating homozygous inbred lines in larger animals with long generation times and small numbers of offspring is not readily achievable. By somatic cell nuclear transfer, we can produce a large number of genetically identical animals, which may reduce variability in experiments. This process can be carried on indefinitely, in theory. Although some scientists believe that animals may be more susceptible to disease if they are part of herds with genetically identical genes, cells are also capable of being genetically engineered to root out diseases that the donor animal may have carried.

Propagating Desirable Stocks

In animal breeding strategies, rapid spread of desirable traits within stocks of domestic animals is of obvious commercial importance. Nuclear transfer cloning, especially from adult nuclei, could provide an additional means of increasing the average "genetic merit" of a given generation of animals. The ability to make identical copies of adult prize cows, sheep, and pigs is a feature unique to nuclear transfer technologies and may well be used in livestock production if the efficiencies of adult nuclear transfer can be improved.

Improving Generation and Propagation of Transgenic Livestock

Transgenic technology developed to add genes has been widely applied to livestock species because it is technically simple. Transgenesis by zygote injection is inefficient. Not all injected eggs develop into transgenic animals, and then not all transgenic animals express the transgene in the desired manner. Characterizing a transgenic line of livestock is a slow and expensive business. Nuclear transfer would speed up the expansion of a successful transgenic line, but, perhaps more important, it would allow more efficient generation of transgenic animals in the first place. Foreign DNA could be introduced into cell lines in culture, and cells containing the transgene in the right configuration could be grown and used as a source of nuclei for transfer, ensuring that all offspring are transgenic. Transgenic cattle, goats, and pigs have been successfully produced by somatic cell cloning.

Generating Targeted Gene Alterations

The most powerful technology for genetic manipulation in mammals—gene targeting—was developed in mice, and depends on the ability of mammalian DNA, when added to cells in culture, to recombine homologously with identical DNA sequences in the genome and replace them.

In mice, this can be achieved in embryonic stem (ES) cells. The combination of homologous recombination and ES cell technology has been responsible for the explosive generation of knock-out mice, in which specific genes have been deleted from the genome. These mice enhance understanding of normal gene function and allow generation of accurate models of human genetic disease. Gene targeting approaches can also be used to ensure correct tissue-specific expression of foreign transgenes and to misexpress genes in inappropriate tissues. If applied to domestic animals, this technology could increase the efficiency of transgene expression by targeting transgenes to appropriate regions of the genome for expression. It could also be used to mutate endogenous genes to influence animal health and productivity or to help prevent rejection of xenografts.

There are no validated ES cell lines in domestic animals to date. Nuclear transfer from non-pluripotent cell lines provides a possible alternative to the ES cell route for introduction of targeted gene alterations into the germ line. McCreath et al. reported the first success of obtaining gene-targeting sheep by using gene-targeted fibroblasts as a source of donor nuclei for NT. Successful production of cloned pigs for xenotransplantation resulting from combination of somatic nuclear transfer with specific modification (knock out) of fetal fibroblasts has also been reported.

Repopulating Endangered Animals and Bringing Animals Back from Extinction

An interesting possibility offered by the nuclear transfer procedure is the making of interspecific hybrids, that is, the use of oocytes (recipient cytoplasts) and donor cells from different species. Endangered species such as the bald eagle and giant panda that have difficulty reproducing in zoos may be preserved using interspecific nuclear transfer technology. This is an important option for the cloning of endangered species where the lack of significant number of oocytes is a major limit, but also for the study of nuclear cytoplasmic interaction with particular reference to mitochondria.

A considerable number of interspecific cloned embryos were produced using bovine oocytes as recipient cytoplasts although they had severely limited developmental capacity. Better results have been obtained with very close species such as the domestic sheep and the muflon (or the cow and the gaur). This underscores the importance in conservation efforts of preserving cells of animals that are in danger of extinction to create a "genetic trust" for future cloning. Furthermore, cross-species nuclear transfer technology confers certain advantages over traditional conservation efforts, such as the possibility of cloning extinct animals such as the wooly mammoth. It may be possible to clone already extinct animals when sufficient nuclear information from the animals is available.

Factors Affecting Efficiency of Somatic Nuclear Transfer

One of the most difficult challenges is cloning's low efficiency and high incidence of developmental abnormalities. The efficiency of somatic cell nuclear transfer, when measured as development to term as a proportion of oocytes used, has been very low (1 percent to 2 percent). Developmental defects, including abnormalities in cloned fetuses and placentas, and high rates of pregnancy loss and neonatal death have been encountered by every research team studying somatic cloning.

A number of variables influence the ability to reproduce a specific genotype by cloning. These include species, source of recipient ova, cell type of nuclei donor, treatment of donor cells prior to NT, the method of artificial oocyte activation, embryo culture, possible loss of somatic imprinting in the nuclei of reconstructed embryos, failure to remodel and reprogram the transplanted nucleus adequately, and the techniques employed for NT. Some of the variables are discussed below.

Clonability of Different Species

So far, sheep, mice, cattle, goats, pigs, cats, mules, horses, rats, ferrets, and dogs have been successfully produced by somatic nuclear transfer cloning. However, we have seen that the published data suggest that some species are more amenable to cloning than others in nuclear transfer.

Part of this difference may reflect the intensity of research in certain species. Ruminants and mice are the mammalian species in which most of the initial work on somatic cell nuclear transfer was initiated, with reasonably good results judging from the number of offspring obtained. Although NT of pigs once lagged behind that of mice, cattle, and sheep, tremendous progress has been made since the first piglet from somatic cell NT was reported in 2000. Successful production of pigs resulting from random genetic modification *in vitro* followed by NT as well as those with a specific modification (knockout) have been reported by

several groups in a short period. The production of cloned transgenic pigs is now in the transition from investigation to practical use. Cloning in the cat, horse, mule, ferret, and dog are more difficult mainly due to the limited information on basic reproductive physiology and lack of assisted reproductive techniques.

But part of the reason for different clonability among species may reflect another critical component for the successful reprogramming of the donor nucleus—namely, the time between nuclear transfer and the activation of the embryonic genome. In order for a differentiated nucleus to redirect development in the environment of the egg, its particular constellation of regulatory proteins must be replaced by those of the egg in time for the embryo to use the genome of the donor nucleus to transcribe the genes it needs for normal development. In mammals, the time at which embryonic gene activation occurs varies among species. For example, in the rat, the coordination between nuclear transfer and timing of oocyte activation is hampered because almost all of the oocytes spontaneously, although abortively, activate within 60 minutes of their removal from oviducts. Only after treatment of oocytes with MG132, a protease inhibitor that reversibly blocks the first meiotic metaphase-anaphase transition, were living cloned rats obtained. Another example is the monkey, in which embryonic cloning has been successful, but somatic nuclear transfer has not resulted in offspring. The failure of primate somatic NT appears to be a result of stricter molecular requirements for mitotic spindle assembly than in other mammals.

Source of Oocytes

The cytoplasm of the oocyte is the garage in which the donor nuclei are remodeled. The oocyte cytoplasm contains factors that reprogram the donor cell genome after NT. Because these factors have not yet been molecularly identified, intact oocytes are still needed for NT, and molecular selection of oocytes with high reprogramming potential is currently not possible.

Most of the early cloning work done in the mouse that used fertilized eggs as recipient cytoplasts led to the conclusion that mouse cloning was impossible. It was the discovery by Willadsen that unfertilized eggs were much more efficient for sheep embryo cloning that caused a reinvestigation into cloning in mammals. On the one hand, this important breakthrough simplified the procedures for cloning, but on the other hand it raised the need for an adequate population of competent oocytes.

Matured oocytes are needed in large numbers. *In vivo*-matured oocytes are thought to be the best source from a quality point of view, as judged by their ability to develop into blastocysts following fertilization. For laboratory animals or small mammals, good quality matured oocytes can be recovered *in vivo* from animals which have ovulated, but when it comes to large animals such as cattle, sheep, or pigs, *in vivo*-matured oocytes are very expensive to acquire.

Furthermore, for cattle or horses it is technically feasible but almost impossible economically.

Thus, many have chosen to use *in vitro*-matured oocytes. Immature oocytes are derived from ovaries obtained from the slaughterhouse and subsequently matured *in vitro*. This allows a large number of oocytes to be synchronized in a specific development stage. While *in vitro*-matured oocytes derived from the ovaries of prepubertal animals can result in development to the blastocyst stage and term, oocytes from sexually mature animals may be more suitable. The use of oocytes recovered from slaughtered animals has simplified the cloning protocol and solved the animal welfare issues for animals such as cattle, pigs, sheep, goats, and horses. In companion animals, veterinary clinics can supply ovaries recovered from ovariectomized animals.

In practice, the use of *in vitro*-matured (IVM) oocytes also has some technical advantages, including the possibility of choosing the length of the maturation period, using oocytes at different stages of the meiotic cycle, deferring maturation to appropriate and/or desired times, and even inducing haploidization as a way to generate gamete-like nuclei from somatic nuclei, potentially for those patients that lack gametes.

Donor Cell Type

The origin of the nuclei used in cloning can have profound effects on the developmental potential of reconstructed embryos. Many somatic cell types, including mammary epithelial cells, ovarian cumulus cells, fibroblast cells from skin and various internal organ cells, Sertoli cells, macrophage, and blood leukocytes have been successfully used for nuclear transfer. However, a clear consensus on the superior somatic cell type for nuclear transfer has not yet been reached. This is partly because different laboratories employ diverse procedures, and cell culture, nuclear transfer, and micro-manipulation all require critical technical skills. Cells can be used directly after recovery from the donor animal or following a period in culture or after cryopreservation.

In practice, differences between cell types are not larger than different clonal populations derived from the same tissue sample, indicating that the status of the chromatin is more important than the tissue of origin. Analysis of cells has shown considerable variation in development between individual cell populations, and at present has provided no definitive method for identifying which are best suited for NT. Factors that are thought to influence the suitability include the effects of oxidative damage associated with metabolism, genome instability, and chromosomal pathologies. All of these factors may be influenced by the method of isolation and culture and the number of population doublings in culture. Even different subclones of fibroblasts derived from the same fetus and cultured in the same conditions to the same generation lead to different *in vitro* developmental potential of reconstructed embryos.

Several genome modifications are known to occur to the cell genome; for example, genetic recombination occurring in a B or T lymphocyte could explain the low efficiency of cloning with these cells. Such modifications are not limited to the blood lineage. Chromatin structure and epigenetic modifications are considered the main factor in determining a successful outcome, and the more the cell is differentiated the more difficult it is to reverse the chromatin status back to an embryonic stage. This lack of reversibility has been demonstrated in DNA methylation studies in bovine cloned embryos and with the expression of Oct-4 and Oct-4-related genes in the mouse.

Some scientists speculated that it is possible that the low percentage of nuclei that result in live births are the nuclei of stem cells that are present in the population at a similar percentage. This also explains why blastomere cloning has been much more successful and why, when using embryonic stem cells to clone mice, the development to term of such embryos is close to that of fertilized embryos. This is probably because the pattern of gene expression of embryonic stem cells is closer to embryo cells, and together they are very different from somatic cells. In the mouse, it is also evident as an effect of the genetic background whereby inbred embryos are less viable at birth and beyond.

The cells to be used as a source of donor nuclei for the production of genetically modified animals must meet two criteria: they must be able to direct term development, and they should possess a proliferative ability such that the correct DNA modification can be selected prior to senescence. Fetal-derived fibroblasts are a popular choice of cells to begin studies because they are capable of extensive proliferation. The problem with all somatic cells is that they tend to become senescent before sufficient rounds of gene transfer and/or targeting and selection can be performed. This problem may be overcome by isolating readily transfectable and selectable cells with high proliferative potential and long-term karyotypical normalcy, similar to murine ES and EG cell lines. Primordial germ cell-derived lines have been isolated from pig fetuses, and transfected lines have been shown to contribute to chimera formation when injected into pig blastocysts, but in no case has germ line transmission been demonstrated. Thus, further development is needed to create cells that are developmentally competent and able to proliferate indefinitely *in vitro*.

Cell Cycle Coordination

The cycle phase of donor cells is another factor that affects the efficiency of NT. Wilmut et al. stated that the donor cells for NT must be in G0 of the cell cycle (quiescent phase). But Cibelli et al. showed that cycling cells, which contain cells in different phases of the cell cycle, could be successfully used for NT in cattle. G2/M-stage cells can be another choice, which is proved by some early studies on NT using G2/M stage blastomeres as nuclear donors to produce cloned mice and sheep, and recent successes of using G2/ M-stage (ES) cells as donors to produce cloned mice. We further used fetal fibroblasts treated with colchicines, which theoretically would synchronize the cells into G2/M-cell cycle stage, and produced a live cloned pig. To maintain normal ploidy, the extra chromosomes derived from G2/ M-stage cells probably are expelled by the oocyte as a second polar body. G2/M-stage fibroblast nuclei could direct reconstructed embryos to develop to term. The cell cycle stage preferred for the recipient cytoplast is the metaphase II, where it is believed that the remodeling and reprogramming activity are at a maximum.

Construction of Nuclear Transfer Embryos

Cloning by nuclear transfer includes a series of complex and delicate events including removal of the original chromosomes of an oocyte, insertion of new genetic material into the same oocyte, and artificial activation of the reconstructed oocyte. Although the technique of replacing the nucleus of the oocyte has been substantially the same for many years, we know very little of the underlying mechanisms of genomic reprogramming, and we proceed mainly on an empirical basis by trial and error to achieve a successful endpoint, a live birth and a surviving animal. The technical aspects are still the main players in determining the outcome of the experimental procedure, the repeatability of the experiments in the same laboratory, and the comparison of results between laboratories.

Enucleation of Oocytes

The oocyte is enucleated by using a micropipette to aspirate the chromosomes that are arranged in a metaphase plate in the presence of cytoskeletal inhibitors such as cytochalasin-B. At the same time the DNA can be stained with a fluorescent dye to visualize (in the species with a dark cytoplasm) the metaphase plate and to be certain of the removal. Other approaches have been attempted to scale up this step. For instance, in the frog, ultraviolet irradiation is effective in destroying the metaphase chromosomes. However, similar approaches by physical means have not been successful so far in mammals. Chemical enucleation has been attempted in the mouse and pigs with limited success.

At present, there are no alternatives to the mechanical removal of the metaphase plate, at least in mammals. In the mouse, where the zona is difficult to penetrate, the development of piezo-electric manipulators has improved the enucleation procedure and allowed the direct injection of the donor nucleus. Because the condensed chromosomes are always located in cytoplasm underneath the first polar body, enucleation of *in vitro*-matured metaphase II oocytes can be performed by aspirating the first polar body and adjacent cytoplasm without staining the chromatin. By using this "blind enucleation" method the enucleation rate varies between 85 percent and 90 percent.

Insertion of Donor Nuclei into Cytoplasts

There are two approaches to put the donor nuclei into the cytoplasts: directly injecting donor nuclei into enucleated oocytes and injecting the intact donor cell into the perivitelline space and subsequently fusing the donor cell with the recipient oocytes. Both approaches can work and result in live offspring.

With direct injection, it is essential that the cell membrane of the donor cell be broken to allow the interaction of the nucleus with the host cytoplasm. As a result, the plasma membrane and much of the cytoplasm material of the donor cell is not transferred, and only remnants of cytoplasm are injected with the donor nucleus. This may be an advantage for it can reduce some unknown adverse effects caused by components of donor cytoplasm such as mitochondria. The disadvantage is that the injury caused by penetration of the injection pipette may compromise the developmental ability of NT embryos. The use of a piezoelectric manipulator facilitates the direct injection procedure and also overcomes this disadvantage to some extent, although it is not essential. The use of direct injection also can meet specific needs such as when donor cells are too small in size to be efficiently fused or when cells are not viable or do not have a functional membrane (fixed or lyophilized, for example). The use of experimental conditions such as heat or chemicals to investigate ways of helping the remodeling and reprogramming of the nucleus by altering chromatin structure also precludes the use of cell fusion, thus making direct injection the only option.

In contrast, with cell fusion it is essential that both membranes are intact and viable and all of the components of the donor cell (nuclear, cytoplasmic, and plasma membrane) merge with the enucleated oocytes. This is because the transfer of the nucleus is the result of the fusion of cell membranes of the oocyte and the donor cell. The fusion of donor cells with cytoplast can be mediated by virus in mice, but has not been reported to be as efficient in large animals. So far, electric cell fusion has become the standard both for embryonic and somatic nuclear transfer for all animals. However, in a direct comparison of the two methods in cattle, it was found that fewer blastocysts are obtained after direct injection, but their ability to deliver offspring is similar.

Thus far oocyte enucleation has always preceded nuclear transfer. However, this prevents the exposure of the introduced nucleus to the proteins surrounding the metaphase plate that could have a role in reprogramming. To overcome this limitation, a technique called "reverse-order" nuclear transfer has been developed, whereby the donor nucleus is first transferred and the metaphase plate is removed after activation when it reaches the anaphase-telophase II. Although more blastocysts were obtained, no data are available on the development to term of these embryos.

A completely novel approach for nuclear transfer called "hand made cloning" has been developed recently. It involves the removal of the zona pellucida that simplifies all the manipulation on the oocyte itself and all the work can be done without a micro-manipulator because the oocytes are halved with a hand-held blade. Finally, two halves without metaphase chromosomes are stuck together with the donor cell with phytoemoagglutinin and fused. This new procedure, when oocyte supply is not a limiting factor, can significantly increase the production of blastocysts, but more importantly it requires little training and less capital investment as compared to the conventional micro-manipulation technique. However, this approach is not yet available for other animals.

Activation of Reconstructed Oocytes

Physiologically, oocyte activation is triggered by sperm factors released at sperm entry and followed by repeated calcium oscillations over a period of time. Because no sperm are used for nuclear transfer, after the donor nuclei are transferred into the enucleated oocytes, the reconstructed oocytes must be artificially activated to overcome the meiotic arrest and initiate subsequent development. Activation of oocytes can be induced artificially by a variety of physical and chemical agents.

The activation protocols are usually assessed by their ability to induce parthenogenetic activation of the metaphase oocyte and subsequent embryo development. Oocytes can spontaneously activate at aging because of the degradation of M-phase proteins. This event has been exploited in the early embryo cloning days when the electric pulses used for cell fusion were sufficient to activate. However, for somatic cloning, in which high kinase levels are necessary for remodeling and reprogramming, aging of the oocyte and/or repeated pulsing might represent a limitation because the somatic nucleus will be exposed to decreased levels of MPF.

Today the most commonly used protocols are based on physical or chemical means to accomplish the same objective of inducing calcium oscillations to repeatedly degrade cell cycle proteins or block new synthesis. In the mouse, exposure to strontium for a few hours is sufficient to activate oocytes at a high rate. In ruminants, the use of a calcium ionophore (ionomycin) followed by a treatment with kinase inhibitors such as 6-DMAP (dimethyl amino purine) or protein synthesis inhibitors for four to six hours are the most effective treatments available today. In the pig, repeated electrical stimulation alone or in combination with the above-mentioned inhibitors is used.

Insufficient or non-physiological activation could be a cause for failure of development even after implantation. It has been demonstrated that, in rabbit oocytes, adequate electrical stimulation that mimics the calcium oscillations of fertilization can extend post-implantation development of the resulting parthenogenetic embryos. For this reason experiments have been performed that use sperm extracts injected into oocytes at the time of activation, although results were inferior to conventional protocols.

The chronology of the events taking place during nuclear transfer and activation is relevant to the successful outcome. With embryonic nuclei, activation is best before or at the same time as nuclear transfer; with somatic nuclei, activation follows a few hours nuclear transfer and the optimal time window seems to be two to three hours with cycloheximide and two to six hours with 6-DMAP.

Control of ploidy should also be a priority when activation follows nuclear transfer. If the donor nucleus is in G0/G1, then any extrusion of chromosomes should be prevented, either by the use of 6-DMAP or in other protocols by the use of cytoskeletal inhibitors such as cytochalasin-B. In the case of donor cells in G2/M, the extrusion of half of the chromosomes is necessary to re-establish normal ploidy and therefore 6-DMAP or cytochalasin-B should not be used.

Culture of NT Embryos

After embryo reconstruction and activation, the culture requirements of cloned embryos should be the same as for normally fertilized embryos. However, in the mouse, there are indications that early stage cloned embryos develop better in a medium containing glucose. This is not the case for fertilized embryos, however, indicating possible abnormalities. Only a proportion of the manipulated embryos develop to blastocyst, and this proportion is generally lower than in the case of IVF embryos.

The need for an *in vitro* culture system is desirable in any species, but this is especially true for large animals, because of the difficulties of implanting early embryos into the oviducts and the excessive costs of recipients as well as the high rate of early embryo wastage. In the initial experiments, embryo culture was performed *in vivo* to the sheep oviduct after agar embedding. More recently, with the refinement of *in vitro* protocols, the culture is carried out almost exclusively *in vitro*. The use of semi-defined media such as m-SOF in a controlled atmosphere of 5 percent CO_2 and 5 percent O_2 is the most popular system in farm animal species. The exception is the pig, in which the best results were traditionally obtained with NCSU medium and PZM-3.

One of the main contradictions of *in vitro* culture systems is that improvement is usually assessed on the percentage of embryos that develop to blastocyst. This is not necessarily the best indicator of embryo quality, especially for cloned embryos that tend to have lower pregnancy rates and high rates of abortions. Ideally, it would be appropriate to have a culture system permissive for embryos that have higher competence to develop to term. This would reduce the number available for transfer, the number of recipients, and the costs involved. A theoretical possibility exists to determine the best embryos for transfer. In principle it is possible to biopsy developing embryos, as is done for pre-implantation diagnosis, and screen them for the normal expression of developmentally important genes either by

PCR or by using microarrays when a presumptive pattern of normality has been identified. There is now sufficient evidence that the vast majority of somatic cloned embryos have an abnormal pattern of gene expression compared to normal embryos. However, because it is not yet clear what the crucial genes required are and their normal level of expression, it is unknown how much deviation from the average can be tolerated in mammals.

Phenotypes of Cloned Animals

There are high incidences of abnormal phenotypes among the cloned animals in all species. Generally, these aberrant phenotypes are referred to as large offspring syndrome (LOS). They were first described in cattle derived from *in vitro* oocyte maturation, fertilization, and culture to the blastocyst stage before embryo transfer. There is extreme variability in the percentages of apparently healthy offspring produced from study to study. These differences in incidences of abnormalities in clones will generate testable hypotheses that likely will lead to procedures to reduce abnormalities and allow the identification of important variables in methodology, species/strain of animals, source of donor nucleus, and investigator skills.

The most prevalent phenotype was a skewed distribution of birthweights. Some abnormal phenotypes are found in all species, while others tend to be species-specific, e.g. high birthweights are not observed in pigs. Aberrant DNA methylation is clearly implicated in some abnormalities of NT-derived embryos and offspring.

Widespread genome demethylation normally occurs soon after fertilization, followed by de novo methylation as soon as differentiation occurs. One example in pigs is an enlarged tongue (macroglossia), which is consistent with Beckwith-Wiedemann syndrome and aberrant IGF2 gene methylation and expression in humans. The high variation in cloning efficiency observed between embryos generated from clonally derived cells could be attributed to donor cells that have different levels of methylation before the nuclear transfer procedure. Cloned embryos often fail to recapitulate the normal pattern of global demethylation and gene-specific methylation observed during normal embryogenesis.

Even when an animal with an abnormal phenotype is cloned, such abnormalities generally do not appear in the resulting offspring. Presumably, these phenotypes are not transmitted to the next generation because the DNA methylation pattern of the genome is reestablished during gametogenesis or altered during culture of the donor cells or embryo. An extremely high embryonic and fetal attrition (greater than 50 percent in most studies) occurs during gestation of cloned pregnancies. The consensus is that most of the fetuses are normal but malnurtured because of epigenetically abnormal placentas. Many of the stillbirths and neonatal deaths reported are likely due to in part to abnormal placentation.

Mammalian cloning by somatic cell nuclear transfer is now a standard methodology in laboratories in more than 20 countries. About 75 percent of these cloning laboratories work on livestock (cattle, pigs, sheep, and goats), less than 10 percent work on mice, and the rest work on at least 20 other species.

Bovine Cloning

Since the birth of Dolly the sheep, the bovine species is undoubtedly the domestic mammal which is the most studied and advanced for somatic cloning. More than 75 percent of all livestock cloning organizations are involved in bovine cloning; the number of research groups cloning cattle exceeds that of all other mammalian species together. The first calves derived from somatic cell nuclear transfer were born in 1998 nearly simultaneously in the USA and in France. From the different research groups and companies, it can be estimated that up to the 2004, about 1,500 calves have been obtained through somatic nuclear transfer worldwide, mainly in North America, Japan, New Zealand, and Europe, but also in South America or Asia.

Applications of Bovine Cloning

The bovine embryo offers several advantages with relatively late activation of its genome and late implantation compared to the mouse model. The generation of sets of clones can be used as more homogeneous animal models for experimental purposes, permitting a reduction in the number of cattle necessary for long-term studies on pathology or nutrition projects. To really evaluate a treatment effect on the physiology and zootechnical performances of cattle, variability due to genetic difference between animals can be reduced by the use of sets of clones, especially if the trait is highly heritable—milk production for instance.

Somatic cloning may contribute to the preservation of endangered bovine breeds and nuclear transfer can be considered as another tool for the strategy of conservation and use of biodiversity. Many examples are arising in this field and some have proven to be feasible. Recently in New Zealand, nuclear transfer has been used to clone the unique female of the "Enderby Island" cattle. This resulted in the production of more than 20 females, which will be bred by semen from different bulls that were frozen-stored before this breed became extinct.

Furthermore, the bovine oocyte can be used as a recipient of somatic nuclei from other endangered species. Using this approach of inter-specific nuclear transfer, Gaur fibroblasts (*Bos gaurus*) fused to bovine enucleated oocytes (*Bos taurus*) have resulted in an offspring that was born dead of the *Bos gaurus* genotype and chimeric *Bos taurus* mitochondria as an interspecies model.

For cattle breeding and selection, somatic cloning offers several potential advantages to existing breeding schemes, e.g. the use of clones could help to learn more precisely the genetic value of progenitors. Prospective calculations by geneticists indicate that in dairy breeds, genetic value evaluated by milk production of a set of five female clones is as precise as that of milk performance of at least 25 non-cloned daughters of a given bull, and annual genetic progress could be improved by 20 percent. Another example is the fact that genocopies of a highly valuable bull can be obtained through nuclear transfer in case of accidental death or severe disease of this progenitor, provided some cells have previously been frozen and stored. The possibility of securing this risk was first demonstrated in Canada with the birth of the clone bull Starbuck II using donor cells from the original bull when it died.

Multiplication of specific phenotypes by cloning is another possibility, provided the cost of the technique is reduced and its application well-controlled. Cells taken from a small muscle biopsy on slaughtered animals two or three days after death can be used as donor cells for cloning and subsequent widespread dissemination of desirable carcass traits. However, potential applications of bovine cloning go well beyond the replication of valuable genitors.

Because targeted genetic modifications can be made in donor cells prior to nuclear transfer, cloning can be used to more efficiently generate transgenic animals for different purposes: therapeutic protein production in milk and blood for bio-medicine, or genetically modified livestock for improved animal production in which undesirable traits are be eliminated and other positive traits are added. Applications include safer, healthier, and, finally, cheaper cattle products.

Deletion of the PrP (prion protein) gene has been achieved in ovine fibroblasts before cloning, resulting in lambs carrying the gene deletion. The PrP gene is directly associated with BSE in cattle. By knocking-out this gene, the resulting prion-free livestock should resist disease such as BSE. Such projects are currently being developed to increase disease resistance and to improve the safety of products. Other applications, beyond animal food production, include production of biomaterials through improved transgenesis efficiency. One example is spider silk proteins, which are secreted in the milk of transgenic goats. Spider silk is very strong and it is thought that it can be woven together to make items such as bullet-proof vests.

Source of Donor Cells

Cattle can be cloned from cell nuclei of diverse cell and tissue types, including donor cells from female adult cumulus, oviduct, uterus, skin, and newborn skin cells; male adult skin and ear cells; newborn skin and liver cells; and fetal skin cells. Most of the donor cells used were probably fibroblasts, except for the cumulus, oviduct, and uterine cells, the cellular phenotype of which was obvious.

In cattle, a higher proportion of transferred cloned embryos reconstructed from morula stage blastomeres resulted in viable offspring compared to adult fibroblasts (28 percent vs. 5 percent, respectively). Presently, fibroblasts are the most commonly used somatic cells. For some

agricultural applications, such as cloning of progeny-tested bulls, the source of donor cells is usually be restricted to easily accessible adult tissues such as skin, tails, and ears. For transgenic applications, where the cells undergo time-consuming selection steps and extensive propagation *in vitro*, it is beneficial to use cells from fetuses because they have a longer proliferative lifespan before reaching replicative senescence.

Cells after long-term culture or near the end of their replicative life span do not result in significantly reduced cloning efficiencies compared to fresh or short-term culture cells. For transgenic purposes, some adult stem cells might be a better option due their long term proliferative and fast growth ability, such as adult bone marrow mesenchymal stem cells which can result in healthy cloned cattle when they are used as donor cells.

Cell Cycle Coordination

Cloned calves have been generated from serum-starved, proliferating, and mitotically arrested somatic donor cells. For non-transgenic fibroblasts, the overall output of viable calves at term and weaning is significantly higher with G0 than with G1 cells. For transgenic fibroblasts, however, cells selected in G1 show significantly higher development to calves at term and higher postnatal survival to weaning than cells in G0. This suggests it may be necessary to coordinate donor cell type and cell cycle stage to maximize overall cloning efficiency.

Presumptive G0 cells are obtained by either serum deprivation or culture to confluency. Both methods rely on the depletion of essential growth-promoting activities in the culture but may not be functionally equivalent. For serum-starvation, cells are cultured in medium containing 0.5 percent FCS for three to seven days. Because different cell types (for example, bovine cumulus cells and fibroblasts) respond very differently to serum-starvation, it is necessary to check the efficiency of serum-deprivation for every new line. Some cell types need much longer to respond to serum-starvation, while others will not tolerate prolonged serum-withdrawal and die.

G1 donor cell populations are obtained by mitotic selection. This method relies on the positive identification and selection of mitotic cells under the light microscope and avoids potentially cytotoxic cell cycle inhibitors. It is a tedious procedure with much lower throughput than non-selection methods, such as drug-induced G1-arrest, but with the advantage of obtaining a more uniform and defined starting population of donor cells. It takes 15 to 30 minutes to pick about 30 cell doublets, resulting in about 60 individual cells for NT. A similar selection method for larger numbers of mitotic cells is the "shake-off" procedure previously used to generate viable calves. Cells treated with various other "arrest/release" methods rapidly lose their synchrony, and it has been suggested that cells could never be truly synchronized by imposing reversible metabolic blocks.

Collection of Oocytes

The procedures of bovine *in vitro*-matured oocytes have been well established and are used for bovine nuclear transfer in most laboratories.

Slaughterhouse ovaries are collected from mature cows (preferably of the same breed), placed into saline (30°C), and transported into the laboratory within two to four hours. Cumulus-oocyte complexes (COC) are collected by aspirating 3-mm to 12-mm follicles. Oocytes derived from 3-mm follicles are equally developmentally competent for NT but show lower fusion efficiency. Only COC with a compact, non-atretic cumulus oophorus-corona radiata and a homogenous ooplasm should be selected for IVM. After IVM in medium B199–10 for 18 to 20 hours, the cumulus cells are dispersed either by manual pipetting (more suitable for a small number of oocytes) or preferably by vortexing up to 180 oocytes in bovine testicular hyaluronidase.

Enucleation of Oocytes

Oocytes are stained for five minutes in droplets of 5 μg/mL Hoechst 33342. At that point enucleation can be visually confirmed and conducted efficiently.

Insertion of Donor Nuclei into Cytoplasts

Although successful cloning using direct injection is achievable, electrical fusion is easier to master and by far the more widespread method in cattle. One study found no significant effect of piezo-actuated nuclear injection versus cell fusion on calving rate, but the numbers were too low to be conclusive. In most laboratories, the donor cells were injected into the perivitelline space of zona-intact cytoplasts.

Some groups use a zona-free embryo reconstruction system (see Figure 10.1) that is essentially a simplified version of previously described conventional zona-intact procedures. The enucleation is conducted without a zona pellucida. Reconstructed oocytes are created by using the lectin-mediated agglutination to replace the step of microinjecting the donor cell into the perivitelline space of zona-intact cytoplasts. About three times more couplets can be produced per minute, and there is no need for a different set of microinjection pipettes. Furthermore, lectin-attachment prevents the separation between donor cell and cytoplast that sometimes occurs using the zona-intact microinjection method. Although lectin-attachment involves extensive mouth pipetting of zona-free oocytes, there is no major handling problem at this or any other step of the procedure. This zona-free NT protocol effectively doubles the throughput in cloned embryo and cloned offspring production. Due to its increased throughput, ease of operation, and reproducibility, it has virtually replaced zona-intact NT in some laboratories. It is also substantially easier to learn for new staff members, especially for those with no previous micro-manipulation experience.

Activation of Oocytes

An electrical pulse alone is not optimal to induce complete activation of oocytes for bovine nuclear transfer. Two chem-

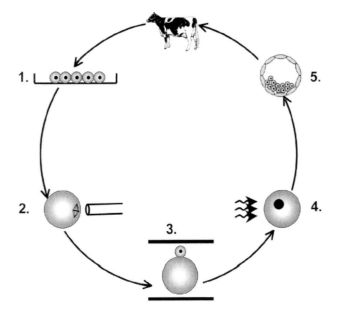

Figure 10.1. Zona-free cloning procedure. (**1**) Isolation and culture of fetal or adult somatic donor cells. (**2**) Removal of zona pellucida from recipient oocytes before aspiration of the meiotic spindle complex. (**3**) NT step: Lectin-mediated attachment of donor cells to cytoplasts followed by automated alignment and bulk electrical cell fusion of donor-cytoplast couplets. (**4**) Chemical activation of fused NT reconstructs by using ionomycin and 6-DMAP. (**5**) Single *in vitro* culture of NT reconstructs to blastocysts and transfer into recipient cows. Courtesy of Oback and Wells, 2003.

ical activation treatments (ionomycin/cycloheximide [CHX] or ionomycin/6-dimethylaminopurine [6-DMAP]) can be used to induce activation of bovine oocytes and there are no significant differences in calving rates. Cell fusion combined with 6-DMAP activation is superior to direct injection or CHX, respectively, for achieving high rates of NT blastocyst development. When using a combination of ionomycin and 6-DMAP, reconstructs are activated three to four hours post-fusion. Activation is induced by incubation in 30 μL drops of 5 μM ionomycin in HSOF +1 mg/mL bovine albumin for four minutes, followed by treatment of 2 mM 6-DMAP for four hours.

Cloned Embryo Culture

Reconstructed embryos are cultured *in vitro* for seven days to the blastocyst stage in SOF containing minimum essential media and essential and non-essential amino acids and 8 mg/mL bovine albumin.

Embryo Transfer and Pregnancy Maintenance

Total embryo development to compacted morula and blastocyst stages is assessed after seven days, and grade 1 and 2 embryos are selected for embryo transfer. Recipient cows are synchronized by a single 10 to 12 day CIDR-B™ treatment. Each cow receives 250 mg cloprostenol four days prior to CIDR withdrawal. The cows are then closely monitored for signs of estrus behavior, which normally peaks 36 to 48 hours later. On day 7 following estrus, a single cloned blastocyst is non-surgically transferred into the uterine lumen ipsilateral to the corpus luteum. The pregnancy status of recipient cows can be determined with ultrasonography on day 35 of gestation.

Development throughout gestation and placentome formation can be monitored daily from day 35 to day 90 by ultrasonography, and after day 90 by palpation per rectum. Clinical hydroallantois (or hydrops) is a frequent complication in cloned pregnancies, in particular between day 120 and day 200 of gestation. Because there is currently no therapy for hydrops, the syndrome is managed through early detection of excess extra-embryonic fluid accumulation, followed by shorter monitoring intervals (every one to two weeks) and, if necessary, Caesarean or induced abortion.

Recipients can receive 20 mg of a long-acting corticosteroid nine days before the planned delivery date (typically on day 270 to day 282 of gestation). Concomitantly, vitamins A, D3, and E are administered to help prevent milk fever and increase resistance to infection after parturition. A short-acting corticosteroid can be administered seven days later. Calving typically commences the following day, peaking around 43 hours after the second corticosteroid injection. Cows are closely monitored and allowed to calve naturally if at all possible or with manual assistance to varying degrees as necessary. Caesarean section is required in less than 10 percent of cases.

Present Success Rates

For agricultural applications, the most practical readout of cloning efficiency is the proportion of transferred embryos resulting in healthy calves at weaning and beyond. Present success rates in cattle cloning range widely. Clones have a three-fold lower success rate than IVF embryos; about 30 percent of fresh IVF embryos transferred develop into healthy calves at weaning.

After transfer of somatic nuclear transfer blastocyts into the uterus of recipient cows, peri-implantation losses are important and the proportion of initiated pregnancies that fail during this period can be estimated to be 50 percent. Late gestation losses between day 90 and calving can be as high as 44 percent among the recipients carrying adult somatic clones, whereas when the rate of abortion in normal bovine sexual reproduction is usually very limited and less than 5 percent after the first trimester. Most cloned embryos are lost throughout gestation due to severe placental abnormalities such as placentome malformation and hydroallantois. The average cattle cloning efficiency to term and weaning is 5.6 percent and 3.7 percent, respectively.

Phenotypes of Offspring

The calving and perinatal periods are critical in the process of obtaining normal live calves through somatic nuclear

transfer. Postnatal losses at birth or during the first few days of life are associated with prolonged gestation, dystocia, or LOS. More than 10 percent of the somatic clone calves born are affected by LOS. This syndrome results from epigenetic modifications arising from imprinted genes such as IGFR2 shown to be associated with fetal overgrowth in sheep. Such epigenetic changes occurring in early embryo development are, in part, the consequences of the different *in vitro* manipulations. These modifications may be propagated throughout development and affect gene expression, not only during gestation or during the postnatal period, but also into adulthood.

Cloned calves can experience a variety of dysfunctions and anomalies at birth, such as respiratory distress, cardiopathology, abnormal kidneys, and hypertrophic liver. Further postnatal mortality occurs after the first week and up to the fourth month. A wide range of other illnesses have been reported in clones, including infections such as ruminitis and abomasomitis, coccidiosis, infection following trauma, and thymic aplasia. Finally, the proportion of somatic cloned calves that are able to develop normally into adults is limited to 50 percent to 70 percent, according to various groups.

Growth rates are reported to be normal. The reproductive characteristics of cloned heifers derived from adult somatic cloning have been evaluated in terms of puberty, follicular dynamics, and hormone profiles, and are no different than those from control noncloned animals. Cloned heifers have proven to be able to reproduce; Lanza et al. reported an 83 percent conception rate on first insemination. Similarly, limited numbers of cloned bulls have been evaluated for libido, semen production quantitatively and qualitatively, and preliminary results suggest that there is no deleterious effect of cloning on the semen parameters of these cloned sires.

Research is being conduced to address potential food safety concerns regarding milk or meat derived from cloned animals. A recent study by Walsh et al. concluded that the gross chemical composition of milk from cloned cows is similar to that of non-cloned cows. Preliminary results on digestibility, composition, feeding value, or allergenicity of meat obtained from somatic cloned animals indicate that the biological/biochemical properties are similar to that of conventional animals, but these results must be confirmed on larger numbers of animals before drawing any conclusions.

Somatic cloned cattle of both sexes have now reached adulthood in different institutes worldwide, and are still being observed for possible long-term effects of NT or longevity of the animals. Data already available indicate they perform similarly to non-cloned controls. In contrast to the cloned generation, the offspring of clones obtained following sexual reproduction are phenotypically and clinically normal. This confirms that the deviations observed in clones are of epigenetic origin and are not transmitted to the progeny, as demonstrated in the mouse model.

Pig Cloning

The first successful cloning experiment in pigs was reported as early as 1989. Prather et al. used blastomeres from 4-cell stage embryos as donor nuclei and *in vivo*-derived metaphase II oocytes as recipient cytoplasts. A total of 88 NT embryos were transferred to recipient gilts for continued development. A single piglet was born.

Similar success was not reported with embryonic cells until more than 10 years later. As a result, pig cloning once was considered difficult. With a similar NT technique that produced Dolly, in which a cultured differentiated somatic cell is fused with a mature egg whose genetic material has been removed, successful cloning of pigs was not reported until three years later.

Polejaeva et al. announced the first successful somatic cell cloning in 2000 with the birth of five healthy cloned piglets. These animals were produced via a different technology from that generally used for NT. The authors first fused porcine granulosa-derived donor cells to enucleated mature oocytes. After 18 hours, the donor nucleus was removed from the first oocyte and transferred to the cytoplasm of an enucleated fertilized egg. The investigators adopted this double NT strategy because they surmised that in the original one-step method, the activation stimulus provided after NT was insufficient to support full-term development of the embryo. This report led the pig cloners to think that the procedures for pig cloning might be more complicated and difficult than those for other animals.

However, almost simultaneously, Onishi et al. reported the birth of a live cloned piglet by directly injecting porcine fetal fibroblast donor nuclei into enucleated oocytes with piezo-actuated microinjection. This was significant because it proved that the two-step NT is unnecessary to make somatic cell NT pigs.

Both groups used mature oocytes collected directly from female pigs rather than culturing immature oocytes *in vitro*. Matured oocytes are needed in large numbers and *in vivo*-matured oocytes are very expensive. Thus, many have chosen to use *in vitro* matured oocytes. Immature oocytes are derived from ovaries obtained from the slaughterhouse and subsequently matured *in vitro*. Betthauser et al. had systematically optimized each step in the NT procedure, including the source of oocytes and their maturation *in vitro*, the culture of donor cells, the activation of oocytes following NT, and the *in vitro* culture of embryos and their transfer to recipient gilts. The result is a more reproducible methodology that enables strategies to genetically modify pigs.

Applications of Swine Cloning

The most important application of pig cloning is in the modification of pig genetics. In the agricultural field, modification of the genome could (1) alter the carcass composition such that it is a healthier product, (2) produce pork faster or more efficiently, (3) create animals that resist specific diseases, (4) reduce the major losses normally observed during the first month of swine embryogenesis, (5) create animals that are more environmentally friendly, and (6) create healthier animals.

In the medical field, specific genetic modifications in the pig provide the possibility of producing recombinant products in animals for biomedical or nutraceutical uses, and the possibility of producing models of human genetic disease for research and drug development. Somatic NT could play important roles in pig genetic modification in the following three ways.

Improving Generation of Transgenic Pigs

We added a gene for the enhanced green fluorescent protein (EGFP) to a fetal-derived cell line by using a replication-defective retrovirus. These cells were then used as donors in an NT scheme that used oocytes that had been matured in a defined system. The genetically marked tissues (EGFP) from the pigs produced from these cells will likely be very useful for basic research in which such marked cells are required. A humanized fat-1 gene, encoding an n-3 fatty acid desaturase, has been introduced into cloned pigs, which are capable of producing high levels of n-3 fatty acids from their n-6 analogs and consequently have a significantly reduced n-6/n-3 ratio in their tissues. The hfat-1 transgenic pigs rich in n-3 fatty acids provide not only an alternative source of n-3 fatty acids but also an excellent large animal model to study the importance of n-3 fatty acids in modern human diseases.

Improving Propagation of Transgenic Pigs

Nuclear transfer would speed up the expansion of a successful transgenic line by using skin cells of the transgenic pigs to make more clones. Ear skin fibroblasts from a transgenic pig produced by oocyte transduction and expressing EGFP were isolated and used as donor nuclei for NT. Four live cloned pigs were born. As in the nuclear donor pig, all of the offspring expressed the EGFP in similar tissues. Bondioli et al. produced cloned pigs from cultured skin fibroblasts derived from an H-transferase transgenic boar. The cells used in these studies were subjected to an extensive culture time, unsuccessful transformation, freezing and thawing, and clonal expansion from single cells prior to NT. One 90-day fetus and two healthy piglets resulted from NT by fusion of these fibroblasts with enucleated oocytes. During the process of generation of fat-1 transgenic pigs, a first generation of transgenic cloned pig with high expression of omega-3 fatty acid died about three weeks after birth. When the ear cells from this dead piglet were used as donor cells for nuclear transfer, we produced eight normal and healthy cloned pigs with the same expression level of omega-3 fatty acid.

Generating Targeted Gene Alterations

The first such example is that of knocking out a gene that is responsible for hyperacute rejection (HAR) when organs from swine are transferred to primates. Fibroblasts generally cannot proliferate indefinitely *in vitro*. Senescence of primary fibroblasts in livestock is generally seen following approximately 30 populations doubling *ex vivo* in non-clonal cultures. In pig fetal fibroblasts, clonal isolates are generally lost at passage following 24 to 28 population doublings *ex vivo*. This presents a technical hurdle as compared to mouse ES cells. However, this problem can be overcome to some extent by using a gene trap strategy which may result in a higher targeting rate.

To target the GGTA1 locus a long region of homology to the GGTA1 locus was used in a vector constructed from the same inbred line of miniature pig from which the fetal fibroblasts were derived, thus providing for isogeneticity to the target locus. A stop codon and selection cassette was inserted into exon 9, upstream of the catalytic domain of the protein. The selection cassette contained no promoter and was preceded by an internal ribosome entry site. Gene trap designs of this nature have been shown to result in relatively high targeting rates, because the vast majority of non-targeted recombination events do not result in transcription. Additionally, transient expression of the selection cassette cannot occur. Furthermore, transfecting the cells as early as possible after isolation (passage 2, or about six population doublings) proved to be another helpful measure to overcome the hurdle.

RT-PCR can be performed on crude cell lysates the day following transfection to quickly identify potentially targeted clones. In our experiments, an absolute targeting of 8×10^{-7} was obtained, which is similar to that in mouse ES targeting (1×10^{-6}), producing enough cells to be used as donor nuclei. However, it is unlikely we could achieve two targeting events in the one primary cell line and still maintain enough cells for NT. Rather, removal of the second allele would be accomplished by breeding or producing a cloned fetus, or piglet, thus providing cells which can be used for a second round of targeting and NT.

To produce homozygous GGTA1 knock-out piglets by natural breeding, assuming both male and female heterozygous knock-out pigs are available at the same time and are fertile, is feasible but takes up to 12 months. However, by using a second-round knockout and cloning strategy, we could save up to six months and all cloned piglets would be GGTA1 double knockout (DKO). Two groups have chosen to use second-round knockout and cloning strategy to produce homozygous GGTA1 knockout piglets and successfully obtained five galactosyltransferase-deficient pigs.

In conclusion, the techniques of NT in pigs, while developed, are not efficient. Nevertheless, the possibility of making specific genetic modifications to pigs offers great potential to both medicine and agriculture.

Source of Donor Cells

In pigs, fibroblast and cumulus cells have been clonable. Fetal fibroblasts derived from day-35 to day-40 fetuses are excellent for use as the nucleus donors to produce cloned pigs because fetal fibroblasts are dispersed in connective tissues throughout the fetal body and they are capable of extensive proliferation, which is an advantage for genetic modification of donor nuclei before nuclear transfer.

Treatment of Donor Cells

If the fetal fibroblast cells have been cultured for a short time (less than 30 days) and passaged a few times (fewer than seven passages) after primary culture, thawed cells are recommended to be cultured further before they are used for nuclear transfer, because freshly cultured cells fuse at a higher rate. For genetically modified cells, which undergo intensive selection and long-term culture, the attachment and proliferative ability becomes very low, thus the thawed cells should be used as donors for nuclear transfer immediately without extensive culture.

Collection of Oocytes

Mature oocytes can be collected from either live animals and used immediately, or from abattoir animals and matured *in vitro*. Both methods result in offspring, but the *in vitro* matured oocytes are much less expensive.

Collection of In Vivo-*matured Oocytes*

Sexually mature gilts must be obtained and they can have their estrous cycle synchronized. Oral administration of 18 mg to 20 mg Regu-Mate mixed into the feed for four to 14 days using a scheme dependent on the stage of estrous cycle can be used. Estrumate is administered intramuscularly on the last day of the Regu-Mate treatment. Superovulation is induced with single i.m. injection of 1,500 IU of pregnant mare serum gonadotropin (PMSG) 15 to 17 hours after the last Regu-Mate feeding. One thousand units of human chorionic gonadotropin are administered i.m. 82 hours after the PMSG injection. Oocytes can be collected 46 to 54 hours after the hCG injection by reverse flush of the oviducts using prewarmed PVA-TL-Hepes containing 0.3 percent BSA.

Collection of In Vitro-*matured Oocytes*

For pig nuclear transfer, matured oocytes are needed in large numbers and *in vivo*-matured oocytes are very expensive to acquire. Thus, many have chosen to use *in vitro*-matured oocytes. Immature oocytes are derived from ovaries obtained from the slaughterhouse and subsequently matured *in vitro*. Recently, progress of *in vitro* production of pig embryos in our laboratory has resulted in a routine, chemically defined system of producing embryos that are developmentally competent. By using this defined system a large number of oocytes can be synchronized in a specific development stage.

Prepubertal porcine ovaries are collected from an abattoir and transported to the laboratory in a thermos filled with saline maintained at 30°C to 35°C within four hours after collection. Follicular fluid from 3 mm to 6 m antral follicles is aspirated by using an 18-gauge needle attached to a 10 ml disposable syringe. Cumulus-oocyte complexes (COCs) with uniform cytoplasm and several layers of cumulus cells are selected and rinsed twice in PVA-TL-Hepes and three times in basic maturation medium. Approximately 50 to 70 COCs are transferred into each well of four-well dishes containing 500 µl maturation medium covered with 100 µl light mineral oil. The oocytes are matured for 42 to 44 hours at 39°C, 5 percent CO_2 in air.

While *in vitro*-matured oocytes derived from the ovaries of prepubertal animals can result in development to the blastocyst stage and term, oocytes from sexually mature pigs may be more suitable. For the maturation of oocytes derived from sows, the procedure is similar to that for the prepubertal pigs. The following maturation medium is recommended: TCM199-Hepes supplemented with 5 µg/ml insulin, 10 ng/ml EGF, 0.6 mM cysteine, 0.2 mM Na-pyruvate, 3 µg/ml FSH, 25 µg/ml gentamicin, and 10 percent porcine follicular fluid, and cultured at 39°C, in air.

After maturation, oocytes are transferred into denuding medium in a 1.5 ml centrifuge tube. Vigorously vortexing oocytes for four to five minutes removes the cumulous cells, and then the oocytes can be transferred into manipulation medium in a 35 mm dish. Oocytes with an intact plasma membrane, round shape, and visible perivitelline space are selected and kept in manipulation medium until use.

Enucleation of Matured Oocytes

The matured oocytes are stained with 5 µg/ml hoechst 33342 in manipulation medium for at least 30 minutes. Oocytes are transferred into the drops of enucleation medium in 100 mm dishes covered with light mineral oil. Five minutes later enucleation is accomplished by aspirating the first polar body and the metaphase II plate in a small amount of surrounding cytoplasm by using a beveled glass pipette with a diameter of 25 µm to 30 µm. Confirmation of successful enucleation is observed by visualizing the karyoplast, while still inside the pipette, under violet light.

The exposure of oocytes to the violet light should be no more than three to five seconds. Exposure to hoechst has deleterious effects on the development of pig oocytes to the blastocyst stage. Because the condensed chromosomes are generally located in the cytoplasm underneath the first polar body in pigs, enucleation of *in vitro*-matured metaphase II oocytes can be performed by simply aspirating the first polar body and adjacent cytoplasm without staining the chromosomes (blind enucleation). This blind enucleation is thought to result in better development after nuclear transfer.

Insertion of Donor Nuclei into Cytoplasts

There are two methods to get the donor nucleus into the cytoplasm of the oocyte. The first is by direct injection in the cytoplasm. The indirect method involves inserting the donor cell under the zona pellucida with the recipient oocyte. The two cells can then be chemically or electrically fused.

Direct Injection of the Donor Nucleus into the Cytoplasm of Enucleated Oocytes

After enucleation, oocytes are transferred to NCSU-23 with BSA medium, and kept at 39°C, 5 percent CO_2 in air. Enucleated oocytes and donor cells are put into the drops of micromanipulation medium in 100 mm dishes covered with light mineral oil. The plasma membrane of the fibroblast cell is broken and visible cytoplasmic material is removed by gently aspirating it in and out of an injection pipette that has a sharp, beveled 10 µm (for G0/G1 stage donors) or 15 µm (for G2/M stage donors) diameter tip. The nucleus and remaining cellular debris are then injected into the cytoplasm of enucleated oocytes using the same slit in the zona pellucida as made during enucleation.

Care should be taken to inject a cell into the cytoplasm with as little medium as possible. Be certain that the membrane of the oocyte is penetrated and the donor nucleus is left inside the oocyte. When the pipette is withdrawn, the puncture in the membrane should automatically seal immediately.

Injection of Donor Cells into the Perivitelline Space of Enucleated Oocytes

The donor cells and unenucleated oocytes are put into the same drop of enucleation medium in 10 mm dishes covered with light mineral oil. The user should enucleate the oocytes as described above. A single donor cell can then be injected into the perivitelline space of enucleated oocytes using the same slit in zona pellucida as made during enucleation. Injected oocytes can be kept in NCSU23 with BSA before fusion and activation. Fusion is achieved with two DC pulses (one-second interval) of 1.2 kV/cm for 30 µsec on a BTX Electro-Cell Manipulator 200 (BTX, San Diego, CA) in a chamber consisting of platinum wire electrodes 1 mm apart. Embryos are kept in NCSU-23 with BSA for another 40 to 60 minutes before the fusion rate is evaluated. Fused embryos are cultured in 500 µl NCSU 23 with BSA overlayed with mineral oil. The surviving embryos (intact plasma membrane) are selected for transfer into surrogates after culture for 18 to 22 hours.

Oocyte Activation

After the donor cells are transferred into the enucleated oocytes, the reconstructed oocytes must be activated to initiate subsequent development similar to fertilization. Activation of oocytes can be induced artificially by a variety of physical and chemical agents.

Electrical Activation

With the above fusion medium (with 1 mM Ca^{2+}) oocyte activation can be accomplished during fusion. If the reconstructed oocytes are made by direct injection of donor nuclei into the cytoplasm, the oocytes can be activated electrically in this fusion medium with the same parameters used for fusion.

Chemical Activation

Combined thimerosal/dithiothreitol (DTT) treatment of the oocytes also can be used to activate oocytes. Oocytes are treated with 200 µM thimerosal for 10 minutes and then washed once with embryo manipulation medium. The oocytes are then treated with 8 mM DTT for 30 minutes.

Electrical Fusion Combined with Chemical Activation

Fusion of the donor cells into the cytoplasm of enucleated oocytes can be accomplished in a chamber consisting of platinum wire electrodes 500 µm apart and SOR2 medium (0.25 M sorbitol, 1 mM calcium acetate, 0.5 mM magnesium acetate, 0.1 percent BSA, pH 7.2, and osmolarity 250 mOsm) with an electrical pulse of 95 volts for 45 µs. The reconstructed oocytes are treated with 15 µm ionomycin for 20 minutes. Then the reconstructed oocytes are treated with 1.9 mM 6-dimethylaminopurine in culture medium for three to four hours.

Culture of Embryos

After activation, embryos are transferred to 500 µL embryo culture medium (NCSU-23 or PZM-3) in a four-well dish and covered with light mineral oil. A pronucleus can be found eight to 15 hours after activation. Cleavage of most oocytes can occur at 24 hours (in PZM-3) or 24 to 36 hours (NCSU-23) after activation. Blastocysts should form on day 6 to day 7 after activation. Platelet activating factor (PAF) is not normally expressed in early embryo development; however, it is aberrantly expressed in SCNT embryos. If PAF were added to NCSU-23 for the entire 168 hours of culture, then the SCNT embryos could develop to the blastocyst stage at a significantly higher rate.

Preparation of Surrogate Gilts

Surrogate gilts or sows can be used that have cycled naturally or have had their estrous cycles synchronized.

Naturally Cycling Surrogate Gilts

Potential surrogates are heat checked twice a day. Depending upon the exact time of estrus, nuclear transfer-derived embryo transfers can be performed five to 36 hours following the onset of estrus.

Estrous Cycle-synchronized Surrogate Gilts

Regu-Mate (18 to 20 mg/hd/day) mixed into the feed is given for 14 days using a scheme dependent on the stage of estrous cycle. This is followed by an injection of 1,000 units of hCG 105 hours after the last Regu-Mate treatment. Embryo transfer is performed 22 to 26 hours after the hCG.

Embryo Transfer

In the pig, there is an additional difficulty of pregnancy recognition by the surrogate that requires a signal from four or more embryos around day 12 of gestation. To minimize any adverse effect on the *in vitro* conditions on the development of NT embryos, transfer to the surrogate is generally at a very early stage. Because the nuclear transfer embryos are generally of a low quality, a large number (more than 100) 1-cell stage embryos cultured 18 to 22 hours with good shape (intact membrane) are surgically transferred into an oviduct of the surrogate. Two different strategies might be employed if there are not enough NT embryos available for transfer. The first is to co-transfer "helper embryos" as an aid to inducing and maintaining pregnancy. These helper embryos may be parthenogenetic embryos that are capable of establishing a pregnancy but degenerate by day 30 of gestation because of genomic imprinting. Alternatively, the helper embryos might be derived from a normal mating. Finally, administration of estradiol, the normal signal for maternal recognition of pregnancy, on day 12 can aid in maintaining the pregnancy of small litters.

Present Success Rates

The fusion rate of donor cells to enucleated cytoplasts is about 70 percent to 90 percent. Premature chromosome condensation occurs in 70 percent to 85 percent of the reconstructed oocytes 0.5 hours after activation. At eight to 15 hours after activation the percentage of embryos that form pronuclei is 60 percent to 75 percent. The developmental competence of nuclear transfer embryos varies greatly by source of oocytes, donor cells, and activation method.

In our lab, if we use the IVM oocytes as recipient cytoplasts, fetal fibroblasts as donor nuclei, and an electrical pulse for activation, the cleavage rate after *in vitro* development for 24 to 36 hours is 60 percent to 80 percent; after a week the blastocyst formation rate is 10 percent to 40 percent with an average nuclear number in those blastocysts of 25 to 35. For *in vivo* development, initial the pregnancy rate at day 25 is 50 percent to 80 percent. Many of the pregnant surrogates will lose their fetuses on day 25 to day 45. Most of the time, the fetuses gradually degenerate in the uterus and finally disappear. In a few cases the surrogates lose their fetuses via abortion rather than resorption. About 20 percent to 30 percent of the surrogates are able to develop to term. One to eight piglets can be produced by each surrogate. Average birthweight is a little smaller than the normal range. No overweight newborn cloned piglets have been observed.

Equine Cloning

Equine cloning is in its infancy; the first equine clones, three mules and one horse foal, were born in 2003. The cloned mules were derived from fetal fibroblast cells and the horse foal from adult somatic cells. Three more cloned horse foals were born in 2005. Progress in equine cloning has been hampered by the fact that attempts at *in vitro* fertilization have been largely unsuccessful. Therefore, little work has been reported on equine *in vitro* oocyte maturation and *in vitro* embryo production.

Applications of Equine Cloning

The potential applications of horse cloning include the following three aspects: (1) the preservation of genetics from individual animals that would otherwise not be able to reproduce, such as geldings; the genetics of exceptional individuals that have been castrated, or die before being able to reproduce, could also be saved; (2) the preservation of genetic material of endangered and/or exotic species, such as the Mongolian wild horse; and (3) because of the companion animal role that horses fill for some individuals, it is likely that some horse owners will have individual animals cloned for emotional fulfillment.

Source of Donor Cells

There is little information about the optimal source of cells for equine cloning. The mule clone that was born was a result of nuclear transfer using fetal fibroblasts. Blastocysts have been produced after nuclear transfer with fetal and adult fibroblasts and with cumulus cells. Pregnancies have been obtained from embryos produced with adult fibroblasts. Fibroblast cells were obtained by biopsy of oral mucosa or skin. Pieces of tissue were minced and placed in a $25 \, cm^2$ tissue culture flask containing DMEM/F-12 supplemented with 10 percent FBS and antibiotics. Cells were cultured in 5 percent CO_2 and air at 37°C to 38.2°C until fibroblast cells became confluent. Cells were then trypsinized and transferred to DMEM/F-12 1 10 percent FBS and 10 percent DMSO for cryopreservation and storage in liquid nitrogen.

Cells were typically passaged two to three times prior to cryopreservation. For nuclear transfer cells were thawed and cultures reestablished in four-well multi-dishes. They were then passaged three to seven times and grown to confluence prior to use for nuclear transfer.

Cell Cycle Coordination

In the horse, G0 and G1 cells have been used, which were from confluent cultures. Frozen-thawed cells were cultured in 4-well multi-dishes with 0.5 mL DMEM/F-12 containing 10 percent FBS at 38.2°C in an atmosphere of 5 percent CO_2 and air. The medium was replaced after three to four hours to remove the DMSO. Cells typically reach confluency by three to five days of culture and are 80 percent G0-G1 as determined by flow cytometric analysis.

When cells are serum starved for three to five days in DMEM with 0.5 percent FBS, more than 90 percent of them can be at the G0 and G1 stage.

Collection of Oocytes

The availability of horse oocytes is a limiting factor. Ovaries from the slaughterhouse are scarce, and the anatomy and physiology of the mare's ovary makes this species a poor oocyte donor as compared with other large domestic species. Oocytes can be harvested from the ovaries of slaughtered mares or from ovum pickup (OPU) of live donors. An average of three to four immature oocytes per ovary can be recovered from the ovaries of slaughtered animals; oocyte retrieval from live donors by OPU is slightly more variable and ranges from three to six oocytes per session. The maturation rate of horse oocytes is also quite variable, averaging between 25 percent and 70 percent in published studies.

Interestingly, in the horse the recovered cumulus-oocyte complexes are a mixed population with either a compact or an expanded cumulus. While expanded cumulus-oocyte complexes are often discarded for *in vitro* embryo production in cattle and pigs, they represent about 40 percent of the total population of recovered oocytes in the horse and seem to have some developmental competence for maturation, cleavage, and blastocyst formation.

There are two methods for oocyte recovery from live mares. If only the dominant preovulatory follicle is to be aspirated, this may be accomplished by follicle puncture through the flank, with the ovary held per rectum. This technique requires minimal instrumentation (equine abdominal trochar, 20 cm 13-gauge needle, connection tubing, and syringe), and the expected oocyte recovery rate from gonadotropin-stimulated preovulatory follicles is about 75 percent. Typically, aspiration is performed two to 12 hours before the expected time of ovulation (expected ovulation is 38 hours after hCG administration or 42 hours after deslorelin administration). The flank technique is made possible by the large size of the preovulatory follicle in the horse (about 40 mm diameter), which makes it easily identified on palpation per rectum and easily located by the needle during aspiration. Detomidine hydrochloride (0.5 mg/mare) and butorphanol (5 mg/mare) is given for tranquilization and analgesia. Probantheline bromide is administered (20 to 30 mg) to the mares to induce relaxation of the rectum.

The skin is anesthetized using 1 mL of a 2 percent lidocaine solution, and a stab incision is made through the skin with a scalpel. An equine trochar-cannula is passed through the skin incision and abdominal musculature into the peritoneal cavity, the trochar removed, and the needle of the aspiration apparatus inserted through the cannula into the dominant follicle. The operator uses one hand to manipulate the ovary per rectum while the other hand is used to direct the needle and puncture the dominant preovulatory follicle. Follicle aspiration is performed by a second person applying slow, gentle suction with the syringe.

The alternative method is transvaginal ultrasound-guided follicle puncture, which is applicable to aspiration both of the preovulatory follicle and of immature follicles. While oocyte recovery from the dominant, gonadotropin-stimulated follicle is similar to that of puncture through the flank (80 percent), recovery of oocytes from immature follicles is low (20 percent to 30 percent). This is attributed to the tighter, broader connection of the equine cumulus-oocyte complex to the follicle wall in the horse, as compared to that in cattle. For this procedure, mares are sedated with 0.02 to 0.04 mg/kg detomidine hydrochloride 15 minutes prior to aspiration. Probantheline bromide

(0.01 mg/kg) is administered to the mares to induce relaxation of the rectum. The transvaginal handle containing a 5 Hz curvilinear transducer and aspiration needle is wrapped with Parafilm-M. The perineal region is washed with providone iodide scrub. The transvaginal handle is lubricated with sterile KY jelly and placed into the vagina alongside the cervix ipsilateral to the ovary containing the follicles to be aspirated. The ovary is brought adjacent to the transvaginal probe via manipulation per rectum. Follicles are punctured and fluid aspirated into a 50 mL tube using a vacuum pump set at 150 mm Hg.

The average number of oocytes recovered per mare per aspiration session is three. If follicle aspiration is performed frequently (e.g., once every four to 12 days), the number of follicles available for aspiration and the number of oocytes recovered decrease in a linear fashion. Only about 50 percent of recovered immature equine oocytes may be expected to mature *in vitro*; thus, only one to two mature oocytes would be expected per 12 to 14 days. Therefore, most people use recovery from the preovulatory follicle after gonadotropin stimulation once per cycle (which may be reduced to 14 days by use of prostaglandin for corpus luteum lysis) rather than aspiration of immature follicles. Unfortunately, it is difficult to use follicle superstimulation to increase the number of preovulatory follicles available for aspiration; mares do not respond well to superstimulation regimens. In addition, if superstimulation does occur, because of the large size of the follicles, once one preovulatory follicle has been aspirated the remaining follicles on that ovary lose their tone and are difficult to puncture.

If mature oocytes are recovered *ex vivo*, they are held in maturation medium with or without gonadotropins at 38.2°C in a humidified atmosphere of 5 percent CO_2 and air until the expected time of ovulation (as predicted from the time of hCG or deslorelin administration). If immature oocytes are recovered, they are matured in maturation medium in microdroplets at a ratio of 10 µL medium per oocyte under similar conditions for 24 to 36 hours.

Recovery of immature oocytes from excised ovaries, followed by maturation of these oocytes *in vitro*, may be performed using ovaries obtained from an abattoir. Methods for recovery and classification of horse oocytes vary substantially from those of other species. Because of the close connection of the horse oocyte to the follicle wall, follicle aspiration, as performed in cattle and pigs, results in a low oocyte recovery rate.

The preferred method for recovering oocytes from horse ovaries is to slice open the follicles and scrape the entire granulosa cell layer from the follicle. Excess tissue is trimmed away from the ovary, then follicles on the surface are located and opened completely with a scalpel blade so that the interiors of both halves are visible. The granulosa layer is scraped from the wall of the follicle using a bone curette. A 0.5 cm curette works for most follicles; however, larger and smaller curettes are useful for larger and smaller follicles. The tissue is washed from the curette into a 35 mm Petri dish using a stream of holding medium from a 20-gauge needle attached to a 10 cc syringe. The contents of each follicle are washed into a separate Petri dish.

Once all of the follicles on the surface of the ovary have been processed, the ovary is sliced in 0.5 cm slices to visualize any follicles. All follicles on the ovary may be processed. While the maturation rate for oocytes from small follicles is lower than that for large follicles, some of these still exhibit developmental competence. As oocytes are located within each Petri dish, the phenotype of both the mural granulosa cells and cumulus cells should be evaluated. Any sign of expansion of either cumulus or granulosa, from cells protruding from a sheet of granulosa to full expansion, results in the oocyte being classified as expanded (Ex). Oocytes having both compact mural and cumulus granulosa may be classified as compact (Cp).

In contrast Ex oocytes from cattle, Ex oocytes from horses should not be discarded. In the horse, Ex oocytes have superior meiotic competence to Cp oocytes, and also appear to have equal if not superior developmental competence.

Classification of the oocytes is important because the two groups appear to have different requirements for maturation. Oocytes showing obvious signs of degeneration should be discarded. Typically, about 60 percent of recovered oocytes are classified as Ex, 30 percent as Cp, and 10 percent or less as degenerated. Horse oocytes may have heterogeneous cytoplasm (segregation of the dark and light cytoplasmic areas); this is a sign of competence for maturation and oocytes showing this trait should not be discarded.

Selected oocytes were matured in microdrops of maturation medium covered in mineral oil and contained in a 35-mm Petri dish at a ratio of 10 µL medium per oocyte. They were incubated at 38.2°C in 5 percent CO_2 in air for 24 hours. Although the optimal duration of oocyte maturation for nuclear transfer has not yet been determined, based on data involving embryo development after intracytoplasmic sperm injection (ICSI), horse oocytes classified as Ex should be cultured for 24 to 30 hours, and those classified as Cp should be cultured for 30 to 36 hours before being used for nuclear transfer and the production of cloned embryos.

Enucleation of Oocytes

For oocyte enucleation the cumulus cells are removed by repeated pipetting in a solution of TCM 199 supplemented with 5 percent FBS and 0.05 percent hyaluronidase. In the horse, the metaphase plate may be some distance from the polar body. This relationship may be closer in *in vivo*-matured oocytes which can be enucleated just by aspirating cytoplasm near the polar body. For enucleation of *in vitro*-matured oocytes, they are first incubated for five to 10 minutes in TCM199 containing 10 percent FBS, 5 µg/mL hoechst 33342, and 5 µg/mL cytochalasin B.

Oocytes are then transferred to a 100 µL manipulation droplet covered with mineral oil and maintained in a Petri dish. Three different methods of oocyte enucleation have been reported for horse oocytes.

The first method is conducted using a beveled glass pipette (around 20 µm outside diameter). The tip can be sharpened to a spike, making it easier to penetrate the zona pellucida. Oocytes are held with a holding pipette (120 to 140 µm outside diameter); an enucleation pipette is then inserted into the oocyte and the polar body is removed along with the adjacent cytoplasm containing the metaphase plate. Removal of both the polar body and metaphase plate are confirmed by observation under UV light. However, the enucleation rates using this method are only 69 percent, because the zona pellucida of horse oocytes is more pliable than that of bovine or porcine oocytes.

The second method is conducted using a glass needle to first make a slit over the polar body, then using a blunt pipette to aspirate the polar body and metaphase plate. If the metaphase plate is separate from the polar body a second slit can be made, or the oocyte cytoplasm rotated to locate the metaphase plate. While this takes extra time, the enucleation rate was 84 percent.

The third method involves using a blunt pipette (10 to 13 µm outside diameter) and drilling out a core of the zona pellucida with the aid of a piezo drill. The blunt pipette is placed next to the polar body and piezo pulses (speed and intensity 3 to 5 in a Prime Tech piezo, respectively) are applied to drill a hole in the zona pellucida. The polar body and metaphase plate can then be removed using the same blunt pipette. The piezo drill speeds up enucleation time compared to the second method. The efficiency of enucleation using this approach was 89 percent.

Insertion of Donor Nuclei into Cytoplasts

After enucleation, cells are transferred into a 100 µL droplet next to enucleated oocytes. Cells are picked up using a 20 µm outside diameter glass pipette and inserted into the perivitelline space of the enucleated oocyte.

Prior to electrical fusion, the oocyte-cell couplets are equilibrated in fusion medium, then gently transferred to a fusion chamber (0.5 mm, BTX, model 450) that also contains fusion medium. Electrical fusion is induced by applying two DC pulses of 1.9 kV/cm for 25 µsec. The fusion rate is 32 percent to 37 percent. A 69 percent fusion rate can be obtained in fusion medium containing 0.3 M mannitol and by applying double DC pulses of 2.4 kV/cm for 30 µsec. When 0.28 M mannitol in a 1-mm fusion chamber and two DC pulses of 2.2–2.5 kV/cm for 30 µsec are used with injection of inactivated Sendai virus into the perivitelline space, fusion rates increase from 49 percent to 57 percent to 81 percent to 82 percent.

When enucleated zona-free oocytes are fused with donor cells using 200 µg/mL of phytohemagglutinin and double DC pulses of 1.2 kV/cm for 30 µsec the fusion rates are 97 percent to 100 percent. When fusion is conducted using enucleated *in vivo*-matured oocytes and fetal fibroblast cells in 3.5 M mannitol with double pulses of 2.25 kV/cm for 15 µsec, the fusion rate can reach 92 percent. Couplets that failed to fuse after the first pulse can be subjected to subsequent electrical pulses until fusion occurs or the enucleated oocyte lyse.

Direct injection of the donor cell into the cytoplasm of horse enucleated oocyte has been conducted using a beveled glass pipette. A piezo drill can be used for direct injection. A blunt pipette with an outside diameter 8 to 9 mm is mounted on the piezo drill. Immediately before injection, cells held in a drop of manipulation medium are gently aspirated in and out of the injection pipette until the cell membrane is broken. The injection pipette carrying three to four cells is then moved into a separate drop of medium that contains the enucleated oocytes. A single cell is then injected into each enucleated oocyte by applying a single pulse, using the piezo drill to break the oocyte's membrane.

Activation of Oocytes

Activation of horse oocytes has been problematic and two approaches have been reported: chemical activation or activation with cytosolic sperm extract. Oocytes can be activated by incubating them in 2 mL of 50 µM calcium ionophore in TCM 199 without serum for 5 minutes. The oocytes are then washed in TCM 199 with 20 percent FBS and cultured for eight to 10 hours in 10 µg/mL cycloheximide in TCM 199. The cleavage rate of oocytes reconstructed with adult somatic cells and activated using this treatment is 0 percent to 9 percent. Activation treatment of reconstructed oocytes with 5 µM ionomycin for four minutes followed by incubation in a mixture of 5 µg/mL cycloheximide and 1 mM 6-DMAP for four hours resulted in high cleavage rates (69 percent to 88 percent).

To use a sperm extract to activate horse oocytes, twice-washed ejaculated stallion sperm (900 g for 10 minutes) are resuspended in nuclear isolation medium. The suspension is then subjected to four cycles of freezing (five minutes per cycle in liquid N2) and thawing (five minutes per cycle at 15°C), then sperm are pelleted at 20,000 g for 50 minutes at 2°C. The resulting supernatant is removed and stored at −80°C until use.

For activation, 2 to 4 pL of sperm extract are injected into horse reconstructed oocytes with a 5 µm inner diameter pipette. Injection volume is controlled by the movement of mercury within the pipette. The cleavage rate when this method is employed for activating reconstructed oocytes was 51 percent; this was higher than with calcium ionophore and cycloheximide. When 2 mM 6-DMAP for four hours was used in combination with sperm extract, the cleavage rate increased to 79 percent. The optimum timing of activation in reconstructed horse oocytes has not been determined. Reconstructed oocytes have been activated at one to two hours, two to four hours, or eight to 10 hours after fusion. There are no significant differences in cleavage rates between activation immediately after donor cell injection or eight to 10 hours afterward.

Embryo Culture

Another peculiar aspect specifically relevant to horse nuclear transfer is the limited developmental competence of nuclear transfer embryos *in vitro*. Very little information on culture systems for horse embryos is available. Several culture systems for horse reconstructed oocytes have been explored. Reconstructed oocytes are co-cultured on a monolayer of oviductal epithelial cells for six to seven days; 53 percent cleavage with 4 percent to 7 percent blastocyst formation rates are obtained.

Reconstructed oocytes cultured in synthetic oviductal fluid with amino acids for eight days yielded 69 percent to 88 percent cleavage and 1 percent to 4 percent blastocyst rates. If reconstructed oocytes are cultured in G1.2 medium at a ratio of $10\,\mu L$ per oocyte they obtained a 51 percent cleavage rate with average 4.4 nuclei at 96 hours. When reconstructed oocytes are cultured in DMEM/F-12 + 10 percent FBS in 5 percent CO_2, 5 percent O_2, and 90 percent N2 for 6.5 to 7.5 days this results in 60 percent cleavage with 5 percent blastocyst formation.

Embryo Transfer and Pregnancy Maintenance/ Present Success Rates

Two laboratories have reported pregnancies from cloned equine embryos. Woods et al. transferred reconstructed embryos (resulting from transfer of a mule fetal fibroblast nucleus to an enucleated, *in vivo*-matured oocyte) to the oviducts of recipient mares immediately after activation. They obtained a pregnancy rate of 6.9 percent (21 of 305). Embryo transfer was performed through a flank laparotomy using a procedure similar to oocyte transfer in the mare. Of the pregnancies, only three (14 percent) were maintained beyond 45 days. All three were carried to term, resulting in the birth of live, healthy mule foals, without need of assistance.

Galli et al. reported the unassisted birth of a live, healthy horse foal. This foal was produced by transfer of an adult somatic cell to an enucleated, *in vitro*-matured oocyte, followed by *in vitro* culture of the resulting embryo to the blastocyst stage. Seventeen blastocysts were transferred nonsurgically, resulting in four pregnancies (24 percent pregnancy rate). Two pregnancies were lost soon after 21 days and one at 187 days. Transfer was performed transcervically using a disposable bovine embryo transfer gun. The gun was passed manually into the vagina and inserted into the external cervical os without cannulating the os digitally. The hand was withdrawn from the vagina and the gun passed through the cervix and into the uterus, where the embryo was expelled. Recipient mares were synchronized by selecting mares with a preovulatory follicle (at least 35 mm in diameter) then administrating hCG or deslorelin (expected ovulation 38 hours after hCG administration or 42 hours after administration of deslorelin). Mares were synchronized to ovulate one to three days after nuclear transfer was performed.

Phenotypes of Cloned Equine

One of the most exciting aspects of the birth of these cloned equids is that all four foals were born without assistance and have been essentially normal from birth. In the case of the mule project, many pregnancies were lost early in gestation, although all pregnancies that were viable after 60 days continued uneventfully to term.

Dog Cloning

There are many applications for cloning canids, as have been described above for other species. Unfortunately, the dog presents challenges that have been surmounted in other species. The major challenge is a source of mature oocytes. While this is difficult, dog cloning is achievable.

Applications of Dog Cloning

Current applications for cloning dogs include genotype replication of pets, conservation of valuable genetics, conservation of endangered species, and production of animals for use as models to study animal and human diseases. There is also considerable interest in cloning service dogs such as search and rescue and seeing eye dogs to determine whether or not these cloned animals would exhibit the same skills (following training) as their original cell donors.

Regardless of the application, dogs, as companion animals, occupy a special place in society and therefore require special considerations when they are involved in a controversial procedure such as cloning. Some of these considerations reduce the efficiency and increase the cost of cloning members of this species. For example, in the United States, dogs enrolled in the cloning project as oocyte donors or embryo recipients could participate for no longer than eight months. The surgical procedures were limited to one to two surgeries per animal, with the final surgery always involving a spay so to prepare the animals for adoption into private homes. The dogs were housed individually but exercised for at least one hour per day in supervised groups. At the end of their involvement in the project, they were moved to special facilities (a training house) where they were prepared for adoption into carefully selected homes. To reduce the likelihood of the animals being abandoned, the new owners were given a 90-day trial period during which they could return the dogs.

Source of Cells

Donor cells can be obtained from biopsies of the skin and oral mucosa of a dog. The tissue samples measure approximately $1 \times 3\,cm$ and $1 \times 2\,cm$ and are collected under light tranquilization and local anesthesia. Sections of the subcutaneous and submucosal tissues are cut into small (approximately $1\,mm^2$) pieces and cultured in tissue culture medium at 37°C in an atmosphere of 5 percent CO_2 and air to obtain fibroblasts. Explants are maintained in culture until they approach 90 percent confluency. Cells are then trypsinized and resuspended at concentrations of approximately 1×10^6 cells per mL, and then are either cryopreserved in cryovials containing DMEM with 10 percent DMSO and 10 percent FBS and stored in liquid nitrogen or returned to culture. Cells are normally passaged every three to four days.

Cell Cycle Coordination

Canine fibroblasts are not specifically treated to regulate the cell cycle. Several days prior to nuclear transfer, the cells are thawed and cultured for three to five days at 37°C in a humidified atmosphere of 5 percent CO_2 in air.

Source of Oocytes

The adaptation of nuclear transfer for application in the canidae involves the management of two reproductive physiological phenomena that are unique among mammals. Canine oocytes are not mature when ovulated, and their reproductive cycle length is 6 to 12 months. Fortunately, the time of ovulation can be accurately estimated by hormone analysis. Canine ovaries are abundantly available from spay clinics, and embryo transfer procedures have been developed for canidae. However, *in vitro* maturation of canine oocytes and induction of synchronized ovulation are very inefficient. Therefore, the most useful current approach appears to be surgically collecting *in vivo*-matured ova and returning the cloned embryos to the oocyte donor, while supplementing this with the relatively infrequent availability of *in vitro*-matured oocytes and synchronized recipients.

The most useful source of oocytes is the oviducts of naturally ovulating female dogs. The timing of ovulation is estimated by using visual observation of proestrus, vaginal cytology for detection of cytological estrus, serum LH assays to detect the LH surge, and progesterone assays to validate the LH surge. The mature oocytes are collected on day 6 or day 7 after the estimated LH surge.

Under general anesthesia, the reproductive tract is exposed by midventral laparotomy using aseptic surgical procedures. The numbers of ovulations on each ovary are estimated by digital palpation and observation of the ovary through the ovarian bursa. The opening of the fimbriated end of the oviduct is located visually and by probing with the collection catheter. The oviduct is then cannulated using a flanged, intramedic catheter (outside diameter 1.27 to 1.57 mm) which is ligated into place using a quick release square knot. The catheter is then retracted until stopped as the flange contacts the ligature. The base of the oviduct, immediately anterior to the uterotubal junction, is visualized by placing digital pressure to blanch the surrounding tissue. The oviductal lumen is then cannulated using a fine (23- to 27-gauge) hypodermic needle attached to a 6 cc syringe filled with oocyte collection medium.

Approximately 4 mL of the collection medium is injected through the lumen of the oviduct and out through the catheter, and collected in a sterile plastic Petri dish. After removing the catheter from the oviduct, the flanged end is rinsed into the collection dish and the lumen of the catheter is flushed using the hypodermic needle. Viable mature ova as indicated by the presence of the first polar body and metaphase II chromosomes are selected and used for nuclear transfer.

In vitro maturation of canine oocytes has been relatively unsuccessful. Although as many as 50 oocytes can be obtained from extirpated ovaries of mature bitches at most any stage of the cycle, or during pregnancy, very few appear to be competent to mature using currently available technology. Reproductive tracts from normal bitches greater than six months of age were collected after routine ovariohysterectomy at private clinics, placed immediately into physiological saline solution (PSS) at 37°C, and transported back to the laboratory for processing within 6 hours. Ovaries were removed from the tract, washed free from blood in fresh (PSS), and then repeatedly slashed with a no. 10 scalpel blade at room temperature in bench medium consisting of TCM-199-Hank's salts and 25 mM Hepes, supplemented with 1 percent fetal calf serum.

Only oocytes with more than two layers of cumulus and a homogenous cytoplasm of 0.100 mm in diameter were selected for use. Oocyte-cumulus complexes were washed three times in bench medium prior to transfer to maturation medium, where they were cultured for approximately 48 hours at 39°C. The rates of maturation to MII obtained were extremely variable and ranged from 1.9 percent to 19 percent. Understanding the mechanisms of oocyte maturation in this species, which possesses the same components as other mammalian species (FSH and LH surges, follicular oestradiol production changing to progesterone production, LH-induced ovulation), but responds to them so differently, continues to present a significant scientific challenge.

Enucleation

Cumulus cells of canine oocytes are denuded by aspirating them in and out of a mouth pipette in 0.5 percent hyaluronidase solution for 5 minutes. The oocytes are then prepared for enucleation by a 15- to 20-minute incubation in enucleation medium containing hoechst .33342. They are then transferred into drops of the same medium within a Petri dish and covered with mineral oil. Enucleation is performed by aspirating the polar body and a small portion of cytoplasm containing the metaphase II chromosomes. During and after enucleation, the oocytes are quickly exposed to UV light and observed by fluorescence microscopy to locate the metaphase II chromosomes and to confirm that they had been removed.

Insertion of Donor Nuclei into Cytoplasts

The nucleus donor cells are placed into the microdrop containing the enucleated oocytes. A single donor cell is then inserted within the perivitelline space of each enucleated oocyte using the micro-manipulators and the same pipette used for enucleation. Care is taken to assure that the plasma membranes of the two cells are in close contact with each other. The oocyte-fibroblast couplets are then washed twice in fusion medium and pipetted onto a fusion chamber that also contains fusion medium. The couplets are aligned manually with the aid of a glass tool fashioned from a capillary tube such that the contact between the donor cell and oocyte are parallel to the electrodes.

Fusion is induced using a BTX Electrocell Manipulator 200 to deliver two electrical pulses, 4 Kv/cm 25 μsec each. Following electrofusion, the couplets are maintained in manipulation medium for 30 to 120 minutes at 39°C.

Activation

Fused 1-celled embryos are activated by removing them from culture, equilibrating in fusion medium, and applying 2×55 μsec 0.5 Kv/cm DC pulses. The embryos are then immediately transferred to 2 mM Hepes-buffered TCM199 supplemented with 10 percent fetal calf serum, 10 μg/mL cyclohexamide and 5 μg/mL cytochalasin B, and cultured for five hours at 39°C.

Embryo Culture

To observe the *in vitro* developmental potential, the cloned embryos are cultured *in vitro* using a B2-Vero cell monolayer co-culture system in an atmosphere of 5 percent CO_2 in humidified air, under oil, at 39°C. For embryo transfer the reconstructed oocytes embryos are transferred in recipients four hours after activation.

Preparation of Embryo Recipients

The GNRH agonist Lupron is useful for induction of fertile estrus in the domestic dog. Of 60 bitches treated with Lupron, 36 exhibited estrus and 26 (43 percent) ovulated, yielding 121 ova (two ova/treated bitch). Several other compounds have been reported to induce estrus in bitches, including human menopausal gonadotropin (HMG), gonadotropin releasing hormone (GNRH), and Cabergoline, but none are as effective as Lupron.

A regimen that appears promising is the deslorelin implant placed beneath the vulvar mucosa, followed by removal on the day after the LH surge. Seven of the eight treated bitches ovulated, and the LH surges occurred on day 9 to day 13 after implant administration, with four occurring on day 9. It should be remembered that for bitches to serve as recipients they must be at least 150 days past their previous ovulation. Also, it is ovulation time that must synchronized, not estrus.

Unfortunately, data are not available for establishing the degree of synchrony required for the transfer of tubal stage canine embryos. A 50 percent conception rate was achieved when 1- to 8-cell naturally fertilized embryos were transferred to the lower uterine tubes of bitches that were synchronized within one day, plus or minus.

Embryo Transfer and Pregnancy Maintenance

Cloned embryos are transferred to naturally or hormonally synchronized recipient bitches, or they can be transferred back into the same animals that have served as donors for recipient oocytes. When the embryos are transferred to the oocyte donors the animals are re-anesthetized and the surgical incision is re-opened. When hormonally or naturally synchronized recipients are used the anesthesia and surgical procedures are the same as described above for ovum collection. In the middle third of the oviduct, through a puncture wound into the lumen of the oviduct made with a 22-gauge hypodermic needle, the embryos are deposited using a 125 or 150 μm diameter flexible catheter and pipette that is marketed for the removal of granulosa cells from mammalian oocytes. The tip of the transfer catheter is directed toward the uterotubal junction, inserted 1.5 to 2 cm, and withdrawn slowly as the plunger is depressed. The puncture wound in the oviduct is not closed. After transfer of the embryos the reproductive tract is gently returned to the abdominal cavity.

Recipients are examined by transabdominal ultrasound for evidence of pregnancy beginning approximately 21 days after transfer.

Present Success Rate

In one group's efforts to make cloned dogs, a total of 259 canine ova were obtained from 54 surgical collections for an average of 4.8 oocytes per collection attempt. Of these, 136 were judged to be viable, thus yielding 2.5 usable oocytes per collection. Fifty-four percent of the viable ova yielded transferable quality embryos following nuclear transfer (n = 74). During this same period, 57 transferable quality embryos were produced using *in vitro*-matured oocytes.

In all, 131 embryos were transferred to 27 recipients. One pregnancy was diagnosed by ultrasound on day 21, but the last detected fetal heartbeat was on day 36. A dead fetus was delivered surgically on day 39 and DNA analysis confirmed that it developed from a cloned embryo. In general, fusion rates using canine oocytes and donor cells are similar to those reported in other species and average 50 percent to 60 percent. Approximately 30 percent of the cloned canine embryos cultured *in vitro* cleaved, but none developed to the blastocyst stage in culture. Successful somatic-cell nuclear transfer (SCNT) depends on the quality, availability, and maturation of the animal's unfertilized oocytes. Unlike other mammals, dogs ovulate at first meiotic prophase, and their oocytes mature for two to three days in the oviduct's distal regions.

Another group reported the birth of two cloned dogs. One is healthy and the other one experienced neonatal respiratory distress during the first week and died 22 days after birth as a result of aspiration pneumonia. They collected an average of 12 oocytes from each female, and achieved a 75 percent fusion rate. A total of 1,095 reconstructed canine embryos were transferred into 123 recipients. Three pregnancies were confirmed by ultrasound scans at 22 days gestation in recipients after transfer of constructs. Pregnancy was established only after embryo transfer of very-early-stage nuclear-transfer constructs (that is, less than four hours after oocyte activation). This transfer of early-stage embryos is a crucial factor in successful assisted reproductive technology for dogs. One fetus miscarried and two others were carried to term.

Bibliography

Abeydeera, L.R., Wang, W.H., Cantley, T.C., et al. (2000). Development and viability of pig oocytes matured in a protein-free medium containing epidermal growth factor. *Theriogenology.* 54, 787–797.

Amano, T., Tani, T., Kato, Y., et al. (2001). Mouse cloned from embryonic stem (ES) cells synchronized in metaphase with nocodazole. *J. Exp. Zool.* 289(2), 139–145.

Baguisi, A., Behboodi, E., Melican, D.T., et al. (1999). Production of goats by somatic cell nuclear transfer. *Nat. Biotechnol.* 17, 456–461.

Baguisi, A., and Overstrom, E.W. (2000). Induced enucleation in nuclear transfer procedures to produce cloned animals. *Theriogenology.* 53, 209.

Betthauser, J., Forsberg, E., Augenstein, M., et al. (2000). Production of cloned pigs from in-vitro systems. *Nat. Biotechnol.* 18, 1055–1059.

Boiani, M., Eckardt, S., Scholer, H.R., et al. (2002). Oct4 distribution and level in mouse clones: consequences for pluripotency. *Genes Dev.* 16, 1209–1219.

Bondioli, K., Ramsoondar, J., Williams, B., Costa, C., Fodor, W. (2001). Cloned pigs generated from cultured skin fibroblasts derived from a H-transferase transgenic boar. *Mol. Reprod. Dev.* 60, 189–195.

Booth, P.J., Tan, S.J., Reipurth, R., et al. (2001). Simplification of bovine somatic cell nuclear transfer by application of a zona-free manipulation technique. *Cloning Stem Cells.* 3, 139–150.

Booth, P.J., Viuff, D., Tan, S., et al. (2003). Numerical chromosome errors in day 7 somatic nuclear transfer bovine blastocysts. *Biol. Reprod.* 68, 922–928.

Bordignon, V., and Smith, L.C. (1998). Telophase enucleation: an improved method to prepare recipient cyto-plasts for use in bovine transfer. *Mol. Reprod. Dev.* 49, 29–36.

Bortvin, A., Eggan, K., Skaletsky, H., et al. (2003). Incomplete reactivation of Oct4-related genes in mouse embryos cloned from somatic nuclei. *Development.* 130, 1673–1680.

Bourc'his, D., Le Bourhis, D., Patin, D., et al. (2001). Delayed and incomplete reprogramming of chromosome methylation patterns in bovine cloned embryos. *Curr. Biol.* 11, 1542–1546.

Bradshaw, J., Jung, T., Fulka, J. Jr., et al. (1995). UV irradiation of chromosomal DNA and its effect upon MPF and meiosis in mammalian oocytes. *Mol. Reprod. Dev.* 41, 503–512.

Briggs, R., and King, T.J. (1952). Transplantation of living nuclei from blastula cells into enucleated frog's eggs. *Zoology.* 38, 455–463.

Bromhall, J.D. (1975). Nuclear transplantation in the rabbit egg. *Nature.* 258, 719–722.

Brück, I., Synnestvedt, B., and Greve, T. (1997). Repeated transvaginal oocyte aspiration in unstimulated and FSH-treated mares. *Theriogenology.* 47, 1157–1167.

Campbell, K.H., McWhir, J., Ritchie, W.A., et al. (1996). Sheep cloned by nuclear transfer from a cultured cell line. *Nature.* 380, 64–66.

Carnevale, E.M., and Ginther, O.J. (1995). Defective oocytes as a cause of subfertility in old mares. *Biol. Reprod. Mono.* 1, 209–214.

Carnevale, E.M., Maclellan, L.J., Coutinho da Silva, M.A., et al. (2000). Comparison of culture and insemination techniques for equine oocyte transfer. *Theriogenology.* 54, 981–987.

Chavatte-Palmer, P., Heyman, Y., Richard, C., et al. (2002). Clinical, hormonal, and hematologic characteristics of bovine calves derived from nuclei from somatic cells. *Biol. Reprod.* 66, 1596–1603.

Cheong, H.T., Takahashi, Y., and Kanagawa, H. (1993). Birth of mice after transplantation of early cell-cycle stage embryonic nuclei into enucleated oocytes. *Biol. Reprod.* 48, 958–963.

Chesne, P., Adenot, P.G., Viglietta, C., et al. (2002). Cloned rabbits produced by nuclear transfer from adult somatic cells. *Nat. Biotechnol.* 20, 366–369.

Cibelli, J.B., Stice, S.L., Golueke, P.J., et al. (1998). Cloned transgenic calves produced from nonquiescent fetal fibroblasts. *Science.* 280, 1256–1258.

Cibelli, J.B., Campbell, K.H., Seidel, G.E., et al. (2002). The health profile of cloned animals. *Nat. Biotechnol.* 20, 13–14.

Cibelli, J.B., Stice, S.L., Golueke, P.J., et al. (1998a). Transgenic bovine chimeric offspring produced from somatic cell-derived stem-like cells. *Nat. Biotechnol.* 16, 642–646.

Cho, J.K., Lee, B.C., Park, J.I., et al. (2002). Development of bovine oocytes reconstructed with different donor somatic cells with or without serum starvation. *Theriogenology.* 57, 1819–1828.

Choi, Y.H., Love, C.C., Love, L.B., et al. (2002). Developmental competence in-vivo and in-vitro of in-vitro–matured equine oocytes fertilized by intracytoplasmic sperm injection with fresh or frozen-thawed sperm. *Reproduction.* 123, 455–465.

Choi, Y.H., Love, C.C., Chung, Y.G., et al. (2002). Production of nuclear transfer horse embryos by Piezo driven injection of somatic cell nuclei and activation with stallion sperm cytosolic extract. *Biol. Reprod.* 67, 561–567.

Choi, Y.H., Shin, T., Love, C.C., et al. (2002c). Effect of coculture with theca interna on nuclear maturation of horse oocytes with low meiotic competence, and subsequent fusion and activation rates after nuclear transfer. *Theriogenology.* 57, 1005–1011.

Choi, Y.H., Love, C.C., Varner, D.D., et al. (2003). Effects of gas conditions, time of medium change, and ratio of medium to embryo on in-vitro development of horse oocytes fertilized by intracytoplasmic sperm injection. *Theriogenology.* 59, 1219–1229.

Choi, Y.H., Chung, Y.G., Walker, S.C., et al. (2003). In-vitro development of equine nuclear transfer embryos: effects of oocyte maturation media and amino acid composition during embryo culture. *Zygote.* 11, 77–86.

Chung, Y.G., Mann, M.R., Bartolomei, M.S., et al. (2002). Nuclear-cytoplasmic "tug of war" during cloning: effects of somatic cell nuclei on culture medium preferences of preimplantation cloned mouse embryos. *Biol. Reprod.* 66, 1178–1184.

Collas, P., and Barnes, F.L. (1994). Nuclear transplantation by microinjection of inner cell mass and granulose cell nuclei. *Mol. Reprod. Dev.* 38, 264–267.

Cook, N.L., Squires, E.L., Ray, B.S., et al. (1993). Transvaginal ultrasound-guided follicular aspiration of equine oocytes. *Equine Vet. J. Suppl.* 15, 71–74.

Cooper, S. (1998). Mammalian cells are not synchronized in G1-phase by starvation or inhibition: considerations of the fundamental concept of G1-phase synchronization. *Cell Prolif.* 31, 9–16.

Dai, Y., Vaught, T.D., Boone, J., et al. (2002). Targeted disruption of the a1,3-galactosyltransferase gene in cloned pigs. *Nat. Biotechnol.* 20, 251–255.

Daniels, R., Hall, V., and Trounson, A.O. (2001). Analysis of gene transcription in bovine nuclear transfer embryos reconstructed with granulosa cell nuclei. *Biol. Reprod.* 63, 1034–1040.

de Matos, D.G., Furnus, C.C., Moses, D.F., et al. (1995). Effect of cysteamine on glutathione level and developmental capacity of bovine oocyte matured in-vitro. *Mol. Reprod. Dev.* 42, 432–436.

De Sousa, P.A., King, T., Harkness, L., et al. (2001). Evaluation of gestational deficiencies in cloned sheep fetuses and placentae. *Biol. Reprod.* 65, 23–30.

De Sousa, P.A., Dobrinsky, J.R., Zhu, J., et al. (2002). Somatic cell nuclear transfer in the pig: control of pronuclear formation and integration with improved methods for activation and maintenance of pregnancy. *Biol. Reprod.* 66, 642–650.

Dean, W., Santos, F., Stojkovic, M., et al. (2001). Conservation of methylation reprogramming in mammalian development: aberrant reprogramming in cloned embryos. *Proc. Natl. Acad. Sci. USA.* 98, 13734–13738.

Dieleman, S.J., Hendriksen, P.J., Viuff, D., et al. (2002). Effects of in-vivo prematuration and in-vivo final maturation on developmental capacity and quality of preimplantation embryos. *Theriogenology.* 57, 5–20.

Dominko, T., Santos-Ramalho, J., Chan, A., et al. (1999). Optimization strategies for production of mammalian embryos by nuclear transfer. *Cloning.* 1, 143–152.

Dominko, T., Mitalipova, M., Haley, B., et al. (1999). Bovine oocyte cytoplasm supports development of embryos produced by nuclear transfer of somatic cell nuclei from various mammalian species. *Biol. Reprod.* 60, 1496–1502.

Dominko, T., Chan, A., Simerly, C., et al. (2000). Dynamic imaging of the metaphase II spindle and maternal chromosomes in bovine oocytes: implications for enucleation efficiency verification, avoidance of parthenogenesis, and successful embryogenesis. *Biol. Reprod.* 62, 150–154.

Du, F., Sung, L.Y., Tian, X.C., et al. (2002). Differential cytoplast requirement for embryonic and somatic cell nuclear transfer in cattle. *Mol. Reprod. Dev.* 63, 183–191.

Duchamp, G., Bézard, J., and Palmer, E. (1995). Oocyte yield and the consequences of puncture of all follicles larger than 8 millimetres in mares. *Biol. Reprod. Mono.* 1, 233–241.

Eggan, K., Akutsu, H., Loring, J., et al. (2001). Hybrid vigor, fetal overgrowth, and viability of mice derived by nuclear cloning and tetraploid embryo complementation. *Proc. Natl. Acad. Sci. USA.* 98, 6209–6214.

Enright, B.P., Taneja, M., Schreiber, D., et al. (2002). Reproductive characteristics of cloned heifers derived from adult somatic cells. *Biol. Reprod.* 66, 291–296.

Fahrudin, M., Otio, T., Murakami, M., et al. (2001). The effects of culture medium on in-vitro development of domestic cat embryos reconstructed by nuclear transplantation. *Theriogenology.* 55:268 (abstract).

Fahrudin, M., Otoi, T., Karja, N.W.K., et al. (2001). The effects of donor cell type and culture medium on in-vitro development of domestic cat embryos reconstructed by nuclear transplantation. *Asian-Aust. J. Anim. Sci.* 14, 1057–1061.

Farstad, W. (2000). Assisted reproductive technology in canid species. *Theriogenology.* 53, 175–186.

Franz, L.C., Squires, E.L., O'Donovan, M.K., et al. (2001). Collection and in-vitro maturation of equine oocytes from estrus, diestrus and pregnant mares. *J. Equine Vet. Sci.* 21, 26–32.

Freshney, R.I. (2000). *Culture of Animal Cells—A Manual of Basic Technique* New York: Wiley-Liss.

Fulka, J. Jr., and Moor, R.M. (1993). Noninvasive chemical enucleation of mouse oocytes. *Mol. Reprod. Dev.* 34, 427–430.

Galli, C., Duchi, R., Moor, R.M., et al. (1999). Mammalian leukocytes contain all the genetic information necessary for the development of a new individual. *Cloning.* 1, 161–170.

Galli, C., Maclellan, L.J., Crotti, G., et al. (2002). Development of equine oocytes matured in-vitro in different media and fertilized by ICSI. *Theriogenology.* 57, 719 (abstract).

Galli, C., Lagutina I., Lazzary G. (2003). Introduction to cloning by nuclear transplantation. *Cloning Stem Cell.* 7, 223–232.

Galli, C., Lagutina, I., Vassiliev, I., et al. (2002). Comparison of microinjection (piezo-electric) and cell fusion for nuclear transfer success with different cell types in cattle. *Cloning Stem Cells.* 4, 189–196.

Galli, C., Duchi, R., Crotti, G., et al. (2003). Bovine embryo technologies. *Theriogenology.* 59, 599–616.

Galli, C., Lagutina, I., Crotti, G., et al. (2003). A cloned horse born to its dam twin. *Nature.* 424, 635.

Galli, C., Lagutina, I., Vassiliev, I., et al. (2002). Comparison of microinjection (piezo-electric) and cell fusion for nuclear transfer success with different cell types in cattle. *Cloning Stem Cells.* 4, 189–196.

Gardner, D.K., Lane, M., Spitzer, A., et al. (1994). Enhanced rates of cleavage and development for sheep zygotes cultured to the blastocyst stage in-vitro in the absence of serum and somatic cells: amino acids, vitamins, and culturing embryos in groups stimulate development. *Biol. Reprod.* 50, 390–400.

Gardner, D.K. (1998). Changes in requirements and utilization of nutrients during mammalian preimplantation embryo development and their significance in embryo culture. *Theriogenology*. 49, 83–102.

Gasparrini, B., Gao, S., Ainslie, A., et al. (2003). Cloned mice derived from embryonic stem cell karyoplasts and activated cytoplasts prepared by induced enucleation. *Biol. Reprod.* 68, 1259–1266.

Gibbons, J., Arat, S., Rzucidlo, J., et al. (2002). Enhanced survivability of cloned calves derived from roscovitine-treated adult somatic cells. *Biol. Reprod.* 66, 895–900.

Gomez, M.C., Pope, C.E., Harris, R., et al. (2000). Birth of kittens produced by intracytoplasmic sperm injection of domestic cat oocytes matured in-vitro. *Reprod. Fertil. Dev.* 12, 423–433.

Gomez, M., Jenkins, J.A., Giraldo, A., et al. (2003). Nuclear transfer of synchronized African wild cat somatic cells into enucleated domestic cat oocytes. *Biol. Reprod.* 69, 1032–1041.

Gurdon, J.B., and Uehlinger, V. (1966). "Fertile" intestine nuclei. *Nature*. 210, 1240–1241.

Gurdon, J.B., and Byrne, J.A. (2003). The first half-century of nuclear transplantation. *Proc. Natl. Acad. Sci. USA*. 100, 8048–8052.

Hagemann, L.J., Weilert, L.L., Beaumont, S.E., et al. (1998). Development of bovine embryos in single in-vitro production (sIVP) systems. *Mol. Reprod. Dev.* 51, 143–147.

Hashizume, K., Ishiwata, H., Kizaki, K., et al. (2002). Implantation and placental development in somatic cell clone recipient cows. *Cloning Stem Cells*. 4, 197–209.

Hawley, L.R., Enders, A.C., and Hinrichs, K. (1995). Comparison of equine and bovine oocyte-cumulus morphology within the ovarian follicle. *Biol. Reprod. Mono*. 1, 243–252.

Heyman, Y., Chavatte-Palmer, P., LeBourhis, D., et al. (2002). Frequency and occurrence of late-gestation losses from cattle cloned embryos. *Biol. Reprod.* 66, 6–13.

Heyman, Y., Zhou, Q., Lebourhis, D., et al. (2002). Novel approaches and hurdles to somatic cloning in cattle. *Cloning Stem Cells*. 4, 47–55.

Hill, J.R., Burghardt, R.C., Jones, K., et al. (2000). Evidence for placental abnormality as the major cause of mortality in first-trimester somatic cell cloned bovine fetuses. *Biol. Reprod.* 63, 1787–1794.

Hinrichs, K. (1991). The relationship of follicle atresia to follicle size, oocyte recovery rate on aspiration, and oocyte morphology in the mare. *Theriogenology*. 36, 157–168.

Hinrichs, K., Matthews, G.L., Freeman, D.A., et al. (1998). Oocyte transfer in mares. *J. Am. Vet. Med. Assoc.* 212, 982–986.

Hinrichs, K., and Schmidt, A.L. (2000). Meiotic competence in horse oocytes: interactions among chromatin configuration, follicle size, cumulus morphology, and season. *Biol. Reprod.* 62, 1402–1408.

Hinrichs, K., Shin, T., Love, C.C., et al. (2001). Comparison of bovine and equine oocytes as host cytoplasts for equine nuclear transfer. *Havemeyer Found. Mono. Ser.* 3, 43–44 (abstract).

Hinrichs, K., Choi, Y.H., Love, L.B., et al. (2002). Effect of holding time and media on meiotic and developmental competence of horse oocytes. *Theriogenology*. 58, 675–678.

Hochedlinger, K., and Jaenisch, R. (2002). Monoclonal mice generated by nuclear transfer from mature B and T donor cells. *Nature*. 415, 1035–1038.

Jaenisch, R., Eggan, K., Humpherys, D., et al. (2002a). Nu-effects of recipient oocyte volume on nuclear transfer in cattle. *Mol. Reprod. Dev.* 50, 185–191.

Jaenisch, R., Eggan, K., Humpherys, D., et al. (2002b). Nuclear cloning, stem cells, and genomic reprogramming. *Cloning Stem Cells*. 4, 389–396.

Inaba, T., Tani, H., Gonda, M., et al. (1998). Induction of fertile estrus in bitches using a sustained-release formulation of a GnRH agonist (leuprolide acetate). *Theriogenology*. 49, 975–982.

Kanitz, W., Alm, H., Becker, F., et al. (1999). Repeated follicular aspiration in mares: consequences for follicle growth and oocyte quality. *J. Reprod. Fertil. Suppl.* 55, 463–472.

Kanitz, W., Becker, F., Alm, H., et al. (1995). Ultrasound guided follicular aspiration in mares. *Biol. Reprod. Mono.* 1, 225–231.

Kasinathan, P., Knott, J.G., Moreira, P.N., et al. (2001a). Effect of fibroblast donor cell age and cell cycle on development of bovine nuclear transfer embryos in-vitro. *Biol. Reprod.* 64, 1487–1493.

Kasinathan, P., Knott, J.G., Wang, Z., et al. (2001b). Production of calves from G1 fibroblasts. *Nat. Biotechnol.* 19, 1176–1178.

Kato, Y., Tani, T., Sotomaru, Y., et al. (1998). Eight calves cloned from somatic cells of a single adult. *Science*. 282, 2095–2098.

Kato, Y., Imabayashi, H., Mori, T., Tetsuya, Tani, T., et al. (2004). Nuclear transfer of adult bone marrow mesenchymal stem cells: developmental totipotency of tissue-specific stem cells from an adult mammal. *Bio. Reprod.* 70:415–418.

Kato, Y., Tani, T., and Tsunoda, Y. (2000). Cloning of calves from various somatic cell types of male and female adult, newborn and fetal cows. *J. Reprod. Fertil.* 120, 231–237.

Katska, L., Bochenek, M., Kania, G., et al. (2002). Flow cytometric cell cycle analysis of somatic cells primary cultures established for bovine cloning. *Theriogenology*. 58, 1733–1744.

Kitiyanant, Y., Saikhun, J., and Pavasuthipaisit, K. (2003). Somatic cell nuclear transfer in domestic cat oocytes treated with IGF-I for in-vitro maturation. *Theriogenology*. 59, 1775–1786.

Kubota, C., Yamakuchi, H., Todoroki, J., et al. (2000). Six cloned calves produced from adult fibroblast cells after long-term culture. *Proc. Natl. Acad. Sci. USA*. 97, 990–995.

Kühholzer, B., Hawley, R.J., Lai, L., et al. (2001). Clonal lines of transgenic fibroblast cells derived from the same fetus result in different development when used for nuclear transfer in pigs. *Biol. Reprod.* 64, 1695–1698.

Kuretake, S., Kimura, Y., Hoshi, K., et al. (1996). Fertilization and development of mouse oocytes injected with isolated sperm heads. *Biol. Reprod.* 55, 789–795.

Kwon, O.Y., and Kono, T. (1996). Production of identical sextuplet mice by transferring metaphase nuclei from four-cell embryos. *Proc. Natl. Acad. Sci. USA.* 93, 13010–13013.

Lagutina, I., Crotti, G., Colleoni, S., et al. (2003). Nuclear transfer in horses. *Theriogenology.* 59, 269 (abstract).

Lai, L., Tao, T., Machaty, Z., et al. (2001). Feasibility of producing porcine nuclear transfer embryos by using G2/M-stage fetal fibroblasts as donors. *Bio. Reprod.* 65, 1558–1564.

Lai, L., Park, K.W., Cheong, H.T., et al. (2000). Transgenic pig expressing the enhanced green fluorescent protein produced by nuclear transfer using colchicine-treated fibroblasts as donor cells. *Mol. Reprod. Dev.*

Lai, L., Kolber-Simonds, D., Park, K.W., et al. (2002). Production of *a*-1,3-galactosyltransferase knockout pigs by nuclear transfer cloning. *Science.* 295, 1089–1092.

Lai, L., Park, K.W., Cheong, H.T., et al. (2002). A transgenic pig expressing the enhanced green fluorescent protein produced by nuclear transfer using colchicine treated fibroblasts as donor cells. *Mol. Reprod. Dev.* 62, 300–306.

Lai, L., and Prather, R.S. (2003). Production of cloned pigs by using somatic cells as donors. *Cloning Stem Cells.* 5, 233–241.

Lai, L., Jing, X., Kang, J.X., Li, R., et al. (2006). Generation of cloned transgenic pigs rich in omega-3 fatty acids. *Nature Biotech.* (In Press).

Lanza, R.P., Cibelli, J.B., Blackwell, C., et al. (2000). Extension of cell life-span and telomere length in animals cloned from senescent somatic cells. *Science.* 288, 665–669.

Lanza, R.P., Cibelli, J.B., Faber, D., et al. (2001). Cloned cattle can be healthy and normal. *Science.* 294, 1893–1894.

Lee, G.S., Kim, H.S., Lee, C.K., et al. (2004). Role of messenger RNA expression of platelet activating factor and its receptor in porcine in-vitro-fertilized and cloned embryo development. *Biol Reprod.* 71, 919–925.

Li, G.P., Tan, J.H., Sun, Q.Y., et al. (2000). Cloned piglets born after nuclear transplantation of embryonic blastomeres into porcine oocytes matured in-vitro. *Cloning.* 2, 45–52.

Li, X., Morris, L.H.A., and Allen, W.R. (2001). Influence of co-culture during maturation on the developmental potential of equine oocytes fertilized by intracytoplasmic sperm injection (ICSI). *Reproduction.* 121, 925–932.

Li, X., Morris, L.H., and Allen, W.R. (2002). In-vitro development of horse oocytes reconstructed with the nuclei of fetal and adult cells. *Biol. Reprod.* 66, 1288–1292.

Li, X., Tremoleda, J.L., and Allen, W.R. (2003). Effect of the number of passage of fetal and adult fibroblasts on nuclear remodeling and first embryonic division in reconstructed horse oocytes after nuclear transfer. *Reproduction.* 125, 535–542.

Long, C.R., Walker, S.C., Tang, R.T., et al. (2003). New commercial opportunities for advanced reproductive technologies in horses, wildlife and companion animals. *Theriogenology.* 59, 139–149.

Liu, L., Dai, Y., and Moor, R.M. (1997). Nuclear transfer in sheep embryos: the effect of cell cycle coordination between nucleus and cytoplasm and use of in-vitro matured oocytes. *Mol. Reprod. Dev.* 47, 255–264.

Machaty, Z., Wang, W.H., Day, B.N., et al. (1997). Complete activation of porcine oocytes induced by the sulfhydryl reagent, thimerosal. *Biol. Reprod.* 57, 1123–1127.

Maclellan, L.J., Sims, M.M., and Squires, E.L. (2000). Effect of oviductal-conditioned medium during maturation on development of equine embryos following intracytoplasmic sperm injection. *Theriogenology.* 53, 396 (abstract).

McCreath, K.L., Howcroft, J., Campbell, K.H., et al. (2000). Production of gene-targeted sheep by nuclear transfer from cultured somatic cells. *Nature.* 405, 1066–1069.

Miyoshi, K., Rzucidlo, S.J., Pratt, S.L., et al. (2003). Improvements in cloning efficiencies may be possible by increasing uniformity in recipient oocytes and donor cells. *Biol. Reprod.* 68, 1079–1086.

Nagashima, H., Fujimura, T., Takahagi, Y., et al. (2003). Development of efficient strategies for the production of genetically modified pigs. *Theriogenology.* 59, 95–106.

Neil, G.A., and Zimmermann, U. (1993). Electrofusion. *Methods Enzymol.* 220, 174–196.

Oback, B., and Wells, D. (2002a). Donor cells for cloning many are called but few are chosen. *Cloning Stem Cells.* 4, 147–169.

Oback, B., and Wells, D. (2002b). Practical aspects of donor cell selection for nuclear cloning. *Cloning Stem Cells.* 4, 169–175.

Oback, B., and Wells, D.N. (2003) Cloning cattle. *Cloning and Stem Cells.* 2003;5(4):243–256.

Oback, B., Wiersema, A.T., Gaynor, P., et al. (2003). Cloned cattle derived from a novel zona-free embryo reconstruction system. *Cloning Stem Cells.* 5, 3–12.

Pace, M.M., Augenstein, M.L., Betthauser, J.M., et al. (2002). Ontogeny of cloned cattle to lactation. *Biol. Reprod.* 67, 334–339.

Park, K.W., Cheong, H.T., Lai, L., et al. (2001). Production of nuclear transfer-derived swine that express the enhanced green fluorescent protein. *Anim. Biotechnol.* 12, 173–181.

Park, K.W., Lai, L., Cheong, H.T., Cabot, R., Sun, Q.Y., Wu, G.M., Rucker, E.B., Durtschi, D., Bonk, A., Samuel, M., Rieke, A., Day, B.N., Murphy, C.N., Carter, D.B., Prather, R.S. (2002) Mosaic gene expression in nuclear transfer-derived embryos and the production of cloned transgenic pigs from ear-derived fibroblasts. *Bio. Reprod.* 66, 1001–1005.

Perry, A.C.F., Wakayama, T., and Yanagimachi, R. (1999). A novel trans-complementation assay suggests full mammalian oocyte activation is coordinately initiated by multiple, sub-membrane sperm components. *Biol. Reprod.* 60, 747–755.

Peura, T.T., Lewis, I.M., and Trounson, A.O. (1998). The effect of recipient oocyte volume on nuclear transfer in cattle. *Mol. Reprod. Dev.* 50, 185–191.

Phelps, C.J., Koike, C., Vaught, T.D., Boone, J., Wells, K.D., Chen, S.H., Ball, S., Specht, S.M., Polejaeva, I.A., Monahan, J.A., Jobst, P.M., Sharma, S.B., Lamborn, A.E., Garst, A.S., Moore, M., Demetris, A.J., Rudert, W.A., Bottino, R., Bertera, S., Trucco, M., Starzl, T.E., Dai, Y.F., Ayares, D.L. (2003). Production of alpha 1,3-galactosyltransferase-deficient pigs. *Science.* 299, 411–414.

Piedrahita, J.A., Wells, D.N., Miller, A.L., et al. (2002). Effects of follicular size of cytoplast donor on the efficiency of cloning in cattle. *Mol. Reprod. Dev.* 61, 317–326.

Polejaeva, I.A., Chen, S.H., Vaught, T.D., et al. (2000). Cloned pigs produced by nuclear transfer from adult somatic cells. *Nature.* 407, 86–90.

Polge, C., Rowson, L.E., and Chang, M.C. (1966). The effect of reducing the number of embryos during early stages of gestation on the maintenance of pregnancy in the pig. *Reprod. Fertil.* 12, 395–397.

Pope, C.E., McRae, M.A., Plair, B.L., et al. (1997). In-vitro and in-vivo development of embryos produced by in-vitro maturation and in-vitro fertilization of cat oocytes. *J. Reprod. Fertil. Suppl.* 51, 69–81.

Pope, C.E. (2000). Embryo technology in conservation efforts for endangered felids. *Theriogenology.* 53, 163–174.

Po Peura, T.T. (2003). Improved in-vitro development rates of sheep somatic nuclear transfer embryos by using a reverse-order zona-free cloning method. *Cloning Stem Cells.* 5, 13–24.

Prather, R.S., Barnes, F.L., Sims, M.M., et al. (1987). Nuclear transplantation in the bovine embryo: assessment of donor nuclei and recipient oocyte. *Biol. Reprod.* 37, 859–866.

Prather, R.S., Sims, M.M., and First, N.L. (1989). Nuclear transplantation in early pig embryos. *Biol. Reprod.* 41, 414–418.

Prather, R.S., Sutovstky, P., Green, J.A. (2004). Nuclear remodeling and reprogramming in transgenic pig production. *Exp. Biol. Med.* 229:1120–1126.

Presicce, G.A., and Yang, X. (1994). Parthenogenetic development of bovine oocytes matured in-vitro for 24 hr and activated by ethanol and cycloheximide. *Mol. Reprod. Dev.* 38, 380–385.

Ptak, G., Clinton, M., Tischner, M., et al. (2002). Improving delivery and offspring viability of in-vitro–produced and cloned sheep embryos. *Biol. Reprod.* 67, 1719–1725.

Ramsoondar, J.J., Machaty, Z., Costa, C., Williams, B.L., Fodor, W.L., Bondioli, K.R. (2003). Production of {alpha}1,3-galactosyltransferase-knockout cloned pigs expressing human {alpha}1,2-fucosylosyltransferase. *Biol Reprod.* 69, 437–445.

Renard, J.P., Chastant, S., Chesne, P., et al. (1999). Lymphoid hypoplasia and somatic cloning. *Lancet.* 353, 1489–1491.

Rieger, D., McGowan, L.T., Cox, S.F., et al. (2002). Effect of 2,4-dinitrophenol on the energy metabolism of cattle embryos produced by in-vitro fertilization and culture. *Reprod. Fertil. Dev.* 14, 339–343.

Robertson, I., and Nelson, R. (1998). Certification and identification of the embryo. In: Stringfellow, D.A., and Seidel, S.M. (eds) *Manual of the International Embryo Transfer Society.* Illinois: International Embryo Transfer Society pp 103–134.

Roth, S., Guo, J., Malakooti, N., et al. (2003). Birth of rats by nuclear transplantation using 2-cell stage embryos as donor nucleus and recipient cytoplasm. *Theriogenology.* 59, 283.

Schnieke, A.E., Kind, A.J., Ritchie, W.A., et al. (1997). Human factor IX transgenic sheep produced by transfer of nuclei from transfected fetal fibroblasts. *Science.* 278, 2130–2133.

Shimozawa, N., Ono, Y., Kimoto, S., et al. (2002). Abnormalities in cloned mice are not transmitted to the progeny. *Genesis.* 34, 203–207.

Shin, T., Kraemer, D., Pryor, J., et al. (2002). A cat cloned by nuclear transplantation. *Nature.* 415, 859.

Sims, M., and First, N.L. (1994). Production of claves by transfer of nuclei from cultured inner cells mass cells. *Proc. Natl. Acad. Sci. USA.* 91, 6143–6147.

Siracusa, G., Whittingham, D.G., Molinaro, M., et al. (1978). Parthenogenetic activation of mouse oocytes induced by inhibitors of protein synthesis. *J. Embryol. Exp. Morphol.* 43, 157–166.

Skrzyszowska, M., Katska, L., Smorag, Z., et al. (2001). In-vitro development of somatic nuclear transferred cat embryos. *Theriogenology.* 55, 292 (abstract).

Smeaton, D.C., McGowan, L.T., Scott, M.L., et al. (2003). Survival of in-vitro produced cattle embryos from embryo transfer to weaning. *Proc. N. Z. Soc. Anim. Prod.* 63, 57–60.

Solter, D. (2000). Mammalian cloning: advances and limitations. *Nat. Rev. Genet.* 1, 199–207.

Stice, S.L., and Robl, J.M. (1988). Nuclear reprogramming in nuclear transplant rabbit embryos. *Biol. Reprod.* 39, 657–664.

Susko-Parrish, J.L., Leibfried-Rutledge, M.L., Northey, D.L., et al. (1994). Inhibition of protein kinases after an induced calcium transient causes transition of bovine oocytes to embryonic cycles without meiotic completion. *Dev. Biol.* 166, 729–739.

Tamashiro, K.L., Wakayama, T., Akutsu, H., et al. (2002). Cloned mice have an obese phenotype not transmitted to their offspring. *Nat. Med.* 8, 262–267.

Tanaka, S., Oda, M., Toyoshima, Y., et al. (2001). Placentomegaly in cloned mouse concepti caused by expansion of the spongiotrophoblast layer. *Biol. Reprod.* 65, 1813–1821.

Tani, T., Kato, Y., and Tsunoda, Y. (2001). Direct exposure of chromosomes to nonactivated ovum cytoplasm is effective for bovine somatic cell nucleus reprogramming. *Biol. Reprod.* 64, 324–330.

Tao, T., Macháty, Z., Boquest, A.C., et al. (1999). Development of pig embryos reconstructed by microinjection of cultured fetal fibroblast cells into in-vitro matured oocytes. *Anim. Reprod. Sci.* 56, 133–141.

Tao, T., Machaty, Z., Abeydeera, L.R., et al. (2000). Optimisation of porcine oocyte activation following nuclear transfer. *Zygote.* 8, 69–77.

Thompson, J.G., Simpson, A.C., Pugh, P.A., et al. (1990). Effect of oxygen concentration on in-vitro development of preimplantation sheep and cattle embryos. *J. Reprod. Fertil.* 89, 573–578.

Thompson, J.G., McNaughton, C., Gasparrini, B., et al. (2000). Effect of inhibitors and uncouplers of oxidative phosphorylation during compaction and blastulation of bovine embryos cultured in-vitro. *J. Reprod. Fertil.* 118, 47–55.

Tian, X.Y. (2004). Reprogramming of epigenetic inheritance by somatic cell nuclear transfer. *Reprod. Biomed. Online.* 8, 501–508.

Tsunoda, Y., Kato, Y. (2002). Recent progress and problems in animal cloning. *Differentiation*. 69, 58.

Tsutsui, T., Hore, T., and Kawakami, E. (2001). Intratubal transplantation of early canine embryos. *J. Reprod. Fertil.* Suppl. 57, 309–314.

Vogelsang, M.M., Kreider, J.L., Bowen, M.J., et al. (1988). Methods for collecting follicular oocytes from mares. *Theriogenology*. 29, 1007–1018.

Westhusin, M.E., Burghardt, R.C., Rugila, J.N., et al. (2001). Potential for cloning dogs. *J. Reprod. Fertil.* Suppl. 57, 287–293.

Westhusin, M., Liu, L., Rugila, J., et al. (2002). Cloning the first dog: How close are we? *Proc. Soc. Therio.* 351–356.

Woods, G.L., White, K.L., Vanderwall, D.K., et al. (2002) Cloned mule pregnancies produced using nuclear transfer. *Theriogenology*. 58, 779–782 (abstract).

Woods, G.L., White, K.L., Vanderwall, D.K., et al. (2003). A mule cloned from fetal cells by nuclear transfer. *Science*. 29 May 2003.

Vajta, G., Lewis, I.M., Hyttel, P., et al. (2001). Somatic cell cloning without micromanipulators. *Cloning*. 3, 89–95.232

Vajta, G. (2000). Vitrification of the oocytes and embryos of domestic animals. *Anim. Reprod. Sci.* 60–61, 357–364.

Vignon, X., Chesne, P., Le Bourhis, D., et al. (1998). Developmental potential of bovine embryos reconstructed from enucleated matured oocytes fused with cultured somatic cells. *C. R. Acad. Sci. III.* 321, 735–745.

Wakayama, T., Perry, A.C., Zuccotti, M., et al. (1998). Full term development of mice from enucleated oocytes injected with cumulus cell nuclei. *Nature*. 394, 369–374.

Wakayama, T., Rodriguez, I., Perry, A.C., et al. (1999). Mice cloned from embryonic stem cells. *Proc Natl. Acad. Sci. USA.* 96, 14984–14989.

Wakayama, T., and Yanagimachi, R. (2001). Mouse cloning with nucleus donor cells of different age and type. *Mol. Reprod. Dev.* 58, 376–383.

Wang, W.H., and Keefe, D.L. (2002). Spindle observation in living mammalian oocytes with the polarization microscope and its practical use. *Cloning Stem Cells.* 4, 269–276.

Wells, D.N., Misica, P.M., and Tervit, H.R. (1999). Production of cloned calves following nuclear transfer with cultured adult mural granulosa cells. *Biol. Reprod.* 60, 996–1005.

Wells, D.N., Laible, G., Tucker, F.C., et al. (2003). Coordination between donor cell type and cell cycle stage improves nuclear cloning efficiency in cattle. *Theriogenology*. 59, 45–59.

Westhusin, M., Hinrichs, K., Chio, Y.H., Shin, T., Kreamer, D. (2003). Cloning companion animals (horses, cats, and dogs). *Cloning Stem Cells.* 301–17.

Whittingham, D.G., and Siracusa, G. (1978). The involvement of calcium in the activation of mammalian oocytes. *Exp. Cell. Res.* 113, 311–317.

Willadsen, S.M. (1986). Nuclear transplantation in sheep embryos. *Nature*. 320, 63–65.

Wilmut, I., Schnieke, A.E., McWhir, J., et al. (1997). Viable offspring derived from fetal and adult mammalian cells. *Nature*. 385, 810–813.

Woods, G.L., White, K.L., Vanderwall, D.K., et al. (2003). A mule cloned from fetal cells by nuclear transfer. *Science*. 301, 1063.

Wrenzycki, C., Wells, D., Herrmann, D., et al. (2001). Nuclear transfer protocol affects messenger RNA expression patterns in cloned bovine blastocysts. *Biol. Reprod.* 65, 309–317.

Yamazaki, Y., Makino, H., Hamaguchi-Hamada, K., et al. (2001). Assessment of the developmental totipotency of neural cells in the cerebral cortex of mouse embryo by nuclear transfer. *Proc. Natl. Acad. Sci. USA.* 98, 14022–14026.

Yanagimachi, R. (2002). Cloning: experience from the mouse and other animals. *Mol. Cell. Endocrinol.* 187, 241–248.

Young, L.E., Sinclair, K.D., and Wilmut, I. (1998). Large offspring syndrome in cattle and sheep. *Rev. Reprod.* 3, 155–163.

Zhou, Q., Jouneau, A., Brochard, V., et al. (2001). Developmental potential of mouse embryos reconstructed from metaphase embryonic stem cell nuclei. *Biol. Reprod.* 65, 412–419.

Chapter 11

Introduction to Comparative Placentation

Cheryl S. Rosenfeld

Evolution of the Placenta

Leonardo da Vinci's drawing of the human fetus in a ruminant placenta underscores the ancient misconception that all mammals had one form of placentation. We now realize that the placenta is the most species-diverse organ and that, while it is an ephemeral, it is essential for conceptus development. No inter-relationships exist between placental classification, taxonomy, and evolution hierarchy (Leiser and Kaufmann, 1994). While some orders, such as carnivore, lagomorpha, and rodentia, are rather homogenous in placental structure, other orders, such as insectivores and primates, display striking variability. Primates and rodents have similar placental structure, which highlights the fact that no single form of placentation is more evolved than another.

Despite its morphological variability, the placenta always serves similar functions. It permits the developing fetus to acquire nutrients from the mother and to dispose of its waste products via the maternal vasculature. The fetus communicates with the mother via hormones, cytokines, etc. (as further discussed later and in chapter 12). The placenta provides structural support for the conceptus and a barrier to blunt an immune attack against the conceptus.

General Features of the Placenta

In ancient times, the placenta was considered to resemble a funnel (flattened) cake. Hence, in Latin *placenta* means cake. In all species, the placenta is comprised of both fetal and maternal portions. Depending on the species, the union of these two tissues (implantation) may occur via superficial attachment or invasion of the fetal tissue into the maternal tissue (King et al., 1982). As mentioned above, the placenta facilitates the exchange of gases and nutrients between the fetus and mother. Nonetheless, it prevents mixing of fetal and maternal blood. The placenta is classified as an endocrine organ due to its productions of hormones. However, the specific hormones the placenta produces vary across species. In this chapter, we explore the development, morphology, and functions of the various domestic animal placentae.

Implantation/Placentation

As the preimplantation embryo develops, it advances from the morula to the blastocyst stage (Perry, 1981). The outer ectodermal cells of the blastocyst that are destined to become the placenta are termed *trophectodermal* or *trophoblast* cells and the inner cell mass will become the embryo proper. The embryo journeys from the oviduct to the uterus during this developmental period. In the uterus, it initially acquires nutrients via secretions from the uterine glands, which are termed *histiotrophe*. Eventually, however, the developing embryo must attach to the uterus to obtain nutrients via the maternal blood vessels (hemotrophe). Placentation is defined as the formation and attachment of the placenta to the uterus.

The extraembryonic membranes develop from all three germ cell layers (*ectoderm, mesoderm,* and *endoderm*). These membranes include the yolk sac, amnion, chorion, and allantois. The yolk sac is derived from the foregut, and thus, it is considered to be composed of *splanchnopleure* (endoderm and splanchnic mesoderm). The allantois is also derived from splanchnopleure, but it originates as an outbranching of the hindgut. Both the yolk sac and allantois are considered to be vascular because of the blood vessels within the splanchnic mesoderm.

The other two extraembryonic membranes, chorion and amnion, are derived from *somatopleure*, which includes ectoderm and somatic mesoderm. Somatic mesoderm is devoid of blood vessels, and thus, these two membranes are avascular.

Types of Placentae

Most animal species have two main types of placentae: yolk sac and chorioallantoic. Other terms employed for the yolk sac placenta include *choriovitelline* or *omphaloid* placenta. The yolk sac placenta represents a fusion of yolk sac and chorion, and is transient in most domestic animal species.

The chorioallantoic (allantoic) placenta is the major placenta type in most eutherian animals. Several structural differences are present among the species and are the subject of the next section.

Classification of Chorioallantoic Placentae

Several placental classification schemes have been developed based on the gross and histological appearances.

The first classification scheme is based on the amount of maternal tissue lost at birth. Gross anatomy of the contact areas between maternal and fetal tissue is the second method used to characterize the varying placentae. The third and fourth placental classification schemes are based on the number of layers separating maternal blood from fetal blood and the appearance of the chorioallantoic projections, respectively.

Amount of Maternal Tissue Lost at Birth

This classification scheme includes two types: *non-deciduate* and *deciduate*. In the non-deciduate placenta, minimal to no loss of endometrium occurs at birth, and correspondingly there is little blood loss. This form of placentation is typical of ungulates and generally occurs in species with non-invasive placentae, in which the chorioallantois can easily be peeled away from the underlying endometrium. However, retained placentae can still occur in species in which the fetal placental tissue can be separated away from the maternal tissues. The deciduate form of placentation entails portions of the endometrium (deciduas) being shed at parturition (birth) and associated hemorrhage. Carnivores, such as canines and felines, are the primary species that have deciduate placentation.

Gross Anatomy of Contact Areas

The chorion is the principal layer that contacts the maternal endometrium, and this layer can be subsequently divided into two main types: *chorion laeve* and *chorion frondosum*. The chorion laeve portion is smooth and not modified for exchange with maternal blood vessels. In contrast, the chorion frondosum is highly branching, forming either folds or villi, and these modifications increase the surface area for exchange of gases, nutrients, and waste. Four principle chorion frondosum sub-types are present among the various species: diffuse, cotyledonary, zonary, and discoid.

Diffuse Placenta

This form of placentation is present in the mare and sow, and it is characterized by the fact that the entire chorion is solely comprised of chorionic frondosum, and thus the entire surface area is modified for exchange with maternal blood vessels.

Cotyledonary (Multiplex) Placenta

Ruminants are the main species that have this form of placentation. The chorion frondosum is localized to areas of the placenta termed cotyledons (Benirschke, 1983; Leiser and Kaufmann, 1994). The fetal cotyledons attach to the maternal caruncles of the endometrium to form *placentomes*.

Zonary Placenta

In carnivores and mustelids, the chorion frondosum forms a band (zone) that is modified for exchange and attachment to the maternal placenta. Depending on the species, one or two bands may be present.

Discoid Placenta

In rodents and humans, the chorion frondosum is shaped like a disc, which results in the term discoid placenta. It might seem surprising that these two dissimilar species would have discoid placentae, but in fact there are several similarities between rodent and human placentae. For comparison of these four types of chorion frondosum placentae and their associated species please see Chapter 12, "Comparative Placentation."

Number of Layers Separating Fetal and Maternal Blood

Another chief classification scheme for the various placentae is the number of cellular layers that separate maternal blood from fetal blood. The fetal layers are the same for all species, but the number of maternal layers differ between species. Six possible layers separate fetal and maternal blood: uterine endothelium, uterine connective tissue (lamina propria), uterine epithelial (endometrial) lining, chorionic epithelium (trophoblast or cytotrophoblast cells), fetal connective tissue, and fetal endothelium of allantoic blood vessels. Based on this classification scheme, there are four main types: epitheliochorial, synepitheliochorial (syndesmochorial), endotheliochorial, and hemochorial.

Epitheliochorial

In this form of placentation, all three maternal layers are intact, which results in the complete six layers (maternal endothelium, maternal connective tissue, maternal epithelium, fetal epithelium, fetal connective tissue, and fetal endothelium) separating maternal blood from fetal blood. The main species in which this form of placentation is present include the mare, sow, and some ruminants (see below).

Synepitheliochorial (Syndesmochorial)

In several ruminant species, e.g. cattle and sheep, some chorionic epithelial cells are binucleated and migrate and fuse with the maternal epithelium (Wooding, 1992). Multinucleated giant cells present on the fetal side are termed trophoblastic giant cells, and those on the maternal side are cryptal giant cells. As discussed below, these multinucleated cells produce various hormones and proteins.

This fusion of maternal and fetal epithelial cells results in areas where the chorion directly contacts the lamina propria of the endometrium. These regions have five layers (maternal endothelium, maternal connective tissue, fetal epithelium, fetal connective tissue, and fetal endothelium) separating maternal from fetal blood.

Endotheliochorial

This type of placentation is characterized by the loss of uterine epithelial lining and underlying connective tissue layer, which results in the chorion contacting the endothelium of the maternal capillaries. Only four layers (maternal endothelium, fetal epithelium, fetal connective tissue, and fetal endothelium) separate maternal blood from fetal blood in this case. Carnivores, felines, and canines are the classic species example for endotheliochorial placentation.

Hemochorial

In this case, maternal blood directly bathes the trophoblast cells. With only three layers separating maternal blood from fetal blood, nutrient and gas exchange readily occurs in these species. Primates and rodents are the main species that have this form of placentation. Interestingly, armadillos and bats also have the hemochorial form of placentation (Anderson, 1969).

Appearance of Chorioallantoic Projections

The chorioallantoic membrane forms diverse projections to further increase the surface area for exchange between mother and conceptus. These projections can be classified as one of three types: folded, villous, or labyrinthine. The sow has the folded chorioallantoic membranes, which can be further sub-divided into macroscopic, or gross, folds (plicae) and microscopic folds (rugae). In the villous form, fetal villi fit into maternal crypts; this type is present in mares and ruminant animals. In placentae in which the chorioallantois forms a complex maze-like network, this is termed labyrinthine; it is present in dogs, cats, rodents, and humans.

Porcine Placenta

Preimplantational porcine embryos can have a variety of morphologies ranging from spherical (day 10.5 to day 11) to tubular (day 11.5) to filamentous (day 12). The embryos attach twelve to thirteen days after ovulation, and gestation lasts approximately 114 to 115 days. Conceptuses must be present in both uterine horns to prevent luteolysis and subsequent abortion (Dhindsa and Dziuk, 1968).

Maternal recognition of pregnancy in pigs is presumed to be due to the production of estrogen by the conceptus, which is thought to redirect $PGF_{2\alpha}$ into the uterine lumen. This re-direction of $PGF_{2\alpha}$ away from the ovary thus confers protection for the CL and the pregnancy is maintained (Bazer and Thatcher, 1977; reviewed in Roberts et al., 1996). The chorioallantoic porcine placenta is fully established at day 24 of gestation (Dempsey et al., 1955).

Because the chorion layer does not erode into the uterus, the porcine placenta is considered non-deciduate with no loss of uterine tissues at birth, and epitheliochorial, with the entire six layers separating maternal blood from fetal blood. The entire chorionic layer is modified for exchange, and thus sows have diffuse placentation. The chorioallantoic membrane is folded with both plicae (macroscopic) and rugae (microscopic) folds.

While the fetuses are able to obtain some nutrients via the maternal blood supply (hemotrophe), the uterine gland secretions (histiotrophe) provide the bulk of the nutrient supply to developing fetuses. The uterine gland secretions collect in certain areas of the placenta called *areolae*, which are directly above uterine glands and first appear at day 17 of gestation (reviewed in King et al., 1982). The trophoblast cells in this region are extremely tall columnar with bulbous microvilli that aid in absorption of the maternal nutrients and have large endocytotic vesicles containing histiotrophe (Raub et al., 1985; Roberts, 1986). In response to progesterone, the porcine endometrial glands produce a unique iron-transport protein termed *uteroferrin* that is taken up by the chorionic epithelial cells overlying the areolae (Roberts et al., 1986). As in most species, the fetal connective tissue appears mesenchymal or mucus-like, and thus, appears pale-staining.

Equine Placenta

In most species, fetal hormones or cytokines increase the CL lifespan, and thereby are considered the signal for maternal recognition of pregnancy. However, no such maternal recognition of pregnancy hormones or cytokines has been identified in equids. Instead, a preimplantational equid embryo traverses both uterine horns, which in some uncertain manner signals to the mother that she is pregnant.

Attachment of the embryos commences 35 to 40 days after ovulation, and gestation lasts approximately 340 days. Similar to the porcine placenta, the equine placenta is non-deciduate, diffuses, and epitheliochorial. However, the equine chorioallantoic membrane is comprised of villi that associate with maternal crypts. While the entire chorion is modified for exchange, fetal and uterine tissues interact in certain discrete areas termed *microcotyledons* (*microplacentomes* or *microcaruncles*). Placentomes of ruminant placentae can be visualized grossly whereas microcotyledons of the equine placenta can only be identified microscopically. Each microcotyledon is invested with one areola, where the uterine gland secretions collect to nourish the fetus.

Endometrial cups are a specialized feature of equine placentae. This term is a misnomer because these cells are of fetal (chorionic) rather than maternal origin. Portions of the chorionic epithelium detach from the chorion at about day 30 to day 35 of gestation. These chorionic cells then colonize and embed within the endometrium. The resulting endometrial cups elaborate equine chorionic gonadotropin (eCG), which is also called pregnant mare serum gonadotropin (PMSG).

Equine chorionic gonadotropin is identical in amino acid sequence to pituitary LH, and thus, stimulates additional ovarian follicular development. The resulting follicles produce high concentrations of estrogen (*equillin*). An interesting side note: estrogen-like compounds have been touted for various uses in humans, and therefore brood mare farms have been created to collect this estrogen-enriched urine from pregnant mares and purify it for use in humans.

The additional ovarian follicles eventually undergo luteinization and become secondary (accessory) corpora lutea. It is not certain whether these follicles undergo a "silent" ovulation or merely luteinize without releasing an egg in the process of luteinization. These additional CL result in a further increase of serum progesterone concentrations to maintain the pregnancy. As eCG ultimately increases progesterone concentrations, it is possibly required for boosting progesterone production by the ovary during the first half of pregnancy. It does not have the same early function as hCG in the human, which serves to rescue the CL of pregnancy around the time of implantation. Because endometrial cup cells are a hemi-allograft and genetically foreign to the mother, she eventually amounts an immune attack against them, which renders the endometrial cups non-functional at about day 120 of gestation. At this point, the placenta assumes the progesterone-producing role.

Hippomanes, which represent free-floating allantoic calculi, are another peculiarity of the equine placenta. Furthermore, the equine placenta, unlike that of other species placenta that have loose areolar connective tissue, is comprised of dense irregular connective tissue.

Ruminant Placenta

The cow, ewe, and doe are the main focus of this section on ruminant animals. A critical window for maternal recognition of pregnancy exists in cattle and sheep (Betteridge et al., 1980; Moor and Rowson, 1966). In cattle, a viable conceptus must be present in the uterus at day 16 for the CL to be maintained. Between days 15–17 of gestation (Northey and French, 1980), bovine conceptuses produce a luteotrophic factor that is now known to be IFN-τ (further discussed below). In sheep, this critical window for maternal recognition of pregnancy occurs at approximately day 12 of gestation (Rowson and Moor, 1967). Adhesion of the bovine conceptus to the underlying maternal endometrium occurs at about day 19 of gestation, but fetal villi and maternal crypts in the placentomes are not fully well-developed until about day 32 of gestation (Wathes and Wooding, 1980). In sheep, adhesion of the fetal to the maternal tissue develops between days 16 to 18 of gestation (Guillomot et al., 1981). Pregnancy in cows and small ruminants lasts 280 and 150 days, respectively.

The ruminant placenta is partially to non-deciduate, epitheliochorial to synepitheliochorial, and cotyledonary (placentomatous), and includes fetal villi inserting into maternal crypts (Mossman, 1987; Wooding, 1992; Leiser and Kaufmann, 1994; Wooding and Flint, 1994). The most well-developed and vascularized placentomes are situated near the conceptus in the middle of the pregnant horn (Leiser et al., 1997). Uterine endometrial glands are present in the inter-caruncular areas. Chorionic ridges and areolae have been identified in the inter-caruncular areas (Björkman, 1954).

Unique cells of the ruminant placenta include binucleate and trinucleate cells. Around day 17 of gestation, some of the chorionic cells develop into binucleate cells (trophoblastic giant cells), and by day 21, the chorionic epithelium is comprised of approximately 20 percent binucleate cells. These cells may migrate across the uterine epithelium and subsequently fuse with maternal cells, resulting in trinucleate cells (cryptal giant cells) and later synctial plaques (Wathes and Wooding, 1980; King et al., 1982; Wooding et al., 1997). Binucleate cells in sheep and cattle produce placental lactogen and a variety of other hormones and factors that presumably regulate fetal-maternal interactions (Flint et al., 1979; Wooding, 1981; Beckers et al., 1998).

This fusion of fetal and maternal cells leads to contact of fetal epithelium and maternal connective tissue (synepitheliochorial), and thus, only five layers separate maternal from fetal blood in these regions. In contrast, in those areas where there is no fusion of maternal and fetal epithelial cells, six layers separate maternal from fetal blood, and consequently, these areas are considered to be an epitheliochorial form of placentation.

While the general features of ruminant placenta extend across several taxa, there are individual species differences that are noteworthy. The placentome that results from the union of maternal caruncle with fetal cotyledon can either be convex (cow) or concave (ewe and doe). In black-faced ewes in particular, these areas might appear black in color because of accumulation of ectopic melanin in these regions. The number of cotyledons can also vary with each species. For instance, cows can have 75 to 120 and ewes and does can have 80 to 100 (Noden and DeLahunta, 1985). Amazingly, several deer species only have a few large cotyledons (oligocotyledonary placentation) that correspond to the few uterine caruncles, which hunters often refer to incorrectly as birth scars (McMahon et al., 1997; Wooding et al., 1997; McMahon et al., 1997). Nonetheless, all ruminant species have evolved sufficient capacity for transfer of nutrients and gases in these regions to sustain the fetus.

Carnivore Placenta

The principle carnivore species considered here are the dog and cat. Canine and feline embryos have delayed implantation, which is initiated at 11 to 12 and 14 to 17 days postovulation, respectively. The gestation periods of dogs and cats last for approximately 63 days.

The carnivore placenta is deciduate, endotheliochorial, and zonary, and the chorioallantoic membrane is the labyrinthine form (Anderson, 1969; Leiser and Koob, 1993). The labyrinth portion can be subdivided into several regions. The first is the lamellar region, where the chorionic villi branch and fuse extensively. The canine lamellae tend to branch more than the feline form. In the canine, the lamellae thus appear irregular and it is difficult to discern the individual layers. In contrast, the sheets of the feline lamellae are readily distinguished. The lamellae are comprised of fetal blood vessels lined by fetal endothelium, a core of fetal connective tissue, and two fetal epithelial layers—*cytotrophoblasts* and *synctiotrophoblasts* (*syntrophoblasts*). The latter cells represent a multinucleated mass of fused cytotrophoblast (Leiser and Koob, 1993). These cells erode the uterine epithelium and lamina propria, resulting in chorionic cells residing next to the maternal endothelial cells.

Decidual cells reside at the bases of the lamellae, particularly in the feline placenta. These cells are identified by their location, large size, and euchromatic nuclei, as well as prominent nucleoli in some of the cells. The origin and function of decidual cells is uncertain, but they might originate from either the bone marrow or endometrial fibroblasts. It is speculated that one role for these cells is to prevent an immune attack against the placenta. However, no definitive evidence exists to support this claim.

The spongy layer deep to the lamellae is comprised of dilated (ectatic) uterine glands. As the labyrinth region erodes the luminal epithelium and occludes the ducts of the endometrial glands, the presumption is that the uterine gland secretions accumulate in the underlying uterine glands. These uterine glands are lost at birth. In the canine placenta, the supraglandular layer is deep to the spongy layer and consists of dense irregular connective tissue. The deep glandular layer is deep to the supraglandular layer and resides above the myometrium. This layer includes uterine glands, which after parturition regenerate the endometrial lining and uterine glands whose predecessors were shed at birth. This layer is more prominent in the dog than in the cat.

Marginal hematomas are commonly present in most carnivore placentae. The placenta at the periphery of the attachment zone appears black to green because of marginal hematomas, which potentially represent a source of iron for the developing conceptus.

Placental Hormones and Proteins

The placenta of all various species produce a wide array of hormones and other factors, whose main function is to aid in the survival of the conceptus during pregnancy and after birth (mammary development). Some of these hormones may achieve this goal by signaling to the mother that she is pregnant and preventing a new ovarian cycle from initiating. These hormones or factors are often said to be required for maternal recognition of pregnancy. Others aid in nutrient acquisition or prolongation of the corpus luteum, which elaborates progesterone. In many species, the placenta itself may produce progesterone and other steroid hormones that suppress another estrous cycle. The diverse placental hormones are discussed in Chapter 12, "Comparative Placentation." Samplings of placental hormones relevant to the domestic animals are discussed below.

Human Chorionic Gonadotropin

The placentae of humans and non-human primates produce a chorionic gonadotropin (CG), which has a wide-range of effects (Licht et al., 2001; Cameo et al., 2004; Keay et al., 2004). The best characterized of these is the ability of CG to extend the CL lifespan, i.e. luteotropic effect. In response to CG, the CL continues to elaborate progesterone and relaxin. CG is thus considered to be the maternal recognition of pregnancy signal in primates. CG may also promote a favorable uterine environment for the conceptus by facilitating blastocyst implantation into the endometrium, inducing vasodilation of myometrial blood vessels, and myometrial smooth muscle relaxation (Licht et al., 2001; Cameo et al., 2004; Keay et al., 2004). CG may stimulate progesterone synthesis in the conceptus (Keay et al., 2004).

Human CG may be detected seven to eight days after gestation in maternal serum and a few days later in the urine. CG is composed of a non-covalently bound α- and β-subunit with the β-subunit conferring specificity of this hormone. Peak level of hCG is detected in the maternal serum at seven to nine weeks gestation, whereupon this hormone begins to decline (Kletzy et al., 1985). Interestingly, in late pregnancy, female conceptuses produce higher concentrations of hCG than males (Obiekwe et al., 1983; Steier et al., 2004; Gol et al., 2004). CG has been clinically useful in pregnancy diagnosis and monitoring and prenatal screening, and the purified or recombinant form of CG can be used to induce ovulation as part of a superovulatory regimen in humans and several other species, including domestic animals (Keay et al., 2004).

Interferon-τ (IFN-τ)

IFN-τ is produced exclusively by the ruminant placenta and is the maternal recognition of pregnancy signal in these species (Roberts et al., 2003). IFN-τ is produced by small and large ruminant placentae between days 10 and 25 of gestation with peak activity on days 14 to 16 (Roberts et al., 1999; Spencer and Bazer, 2004). The net effect of IFN-τ is to prolong the CL lifespan by suppressing the production of the luteolytic factor $PGF_{2\alpha}$ by the endometrium (Roberts et al., 1999; Spencer and Bazer, 2004). It is believe that IFN-τ abates the luteolytic cascade by entailing inhibition of uterine estrogen receptor expression, which in turn causes the loss of uterine oxytocin receptor from the uterine cells. Binding of oxytocin to its uterine cognate receptor induces the release of $PGF_{2\alpha}$ by the endometrium. In the absence of uterine oxytocin receptor (OTR), oxytocin is incapable of stimulating the release of $PGF_{2\alpha}$. Similar to hCG, bovine female conceptuses initially produce higher concentrations of IFN-τ than their male counterparts (Larson et al., 2001; Kimura et al., 2004).

Pregnancy-associated Glycoproteins

Pregnancy-associated glycoproteins (PAG) are classified as inactive members of the aspartic proteinase family, and thus, these proteins are related to pepsin and chymosin as well as cathepsins (Xie et al., 1991). The ruminant placenta produces several isoforms of the PAG. The porcine, equine, and feline placentae express PAG or PAG-like molecules (Hughes et al., 2003). While these ruminant proteins are produced in large amounts, particularly by ruminant placentae binucleate cells, their function is uncertain. Even though the function of these proteins remains elusive, PAG are clinically useful in pregnancy determination in cattle and small ruminants because these proteins can be detected in pregnant maternal plasma or serum (Perenyi et al., 2002; Karen et al., 2003; Gonzalez et al., 2004). Please see Chapter 12, "Comparative Placentation," for more details.

Placental Lactogens and Prolactin

The placentae of ruminant artiodactyls, rodents, and humans produce a variety of compounds that are related to pituitary prolactin and growth hormone (Byatt et al., 1992; Forsyth, 1994; Anthony et al., 1995). These placental compounds are classified as either placental lactogens (PL) or prolactin-related proteins. Their precise functions are uncertain, but these molecules presumably regulate maternal and fetal metabolism and possibly increase insulin-like growth factor (IGF) in the conceptus, which may increase fetal growth. Ruminant PL has both lactogenic and somatogenic effects and therefore may stimulate mammogenesis in preparation for lactation. In late gestation, the concentration of PL increases in the maternal circulation but decreases in the fetal circulation, which further suggests a role for PL in the dam (Byatt et al., 1992).

Equine Chorionic Gonadotropin (Pregnant Mare Serum Gonadotropin)

As mentioned in the section on the equine placenta, eCG is produced by endometrial cup cells (Murphy and Martine, 1991; Hoppen, 1994; Allen, 2001). At days 35 to 37 of pregnancy, these fetal cells migrate from the chorionic girdle region and infiltrate into the underlying endometrium. These cells begin to produce eCG (or PMSG), which is similar to other gonadotropins and comprised of α- and β-subunits. Within each equid species, the α-subunit is identical among all of the gonadotropins. The β-subunit of eCG confers specificity of this hormone and is identical to its equine luteinizing hormone counterpart.

Because eCG is produced after implantation has occurred, this hormone is not considered the equine maternal recognition of pregnancy signal. Instead, eCG stimulates additional follicular development culminating in accessory or secondary CL that helps to maintain the elevated progesterone concentrations during mid-gestation. Peak eCG secretion occurs during 60 to 80 days of gestation followed by a gradual decline until 130 days of gestation. At this time, the maternal immune system mounts an immune attack against the fetal endometrial cup cells, which produce eCG. After 130 days of gestation, the equine placenta, as discussed below, assumes the progesterone-producing role.

Steroid Hormones

In several domestic animal species, including ruminants, equids, and possibly swine, the placenta synthesizes progesterone during the latter half of gestation (Knight, 1994; Hoffman and Schuler, 2002; Ousey et al., 2003). The CL is the primary structure responsible for elaborating progesterone. However, in late gestation, particularly in the horse and other species, the placenta assumes the role of producing progesterone that is necessary for the pregnancy to continue (Silver, 1994). In sheep, placental progesterone may suppress the uterine immune attack on the developing conceptus (Hansen, 1998).

Estrogen is another steroid hormone that is produced by the placentae of several domestic animals (Choi et al., 1997). In the pig, estrogen production by the conceptus is essential for maternal recognition of pregnancy (Knight, 1994; Choi et al., 1997). Estrogen from the porcine conceptus redirects endometrial PGF_2 into the uterine lumen and consequently, away from the utero-ovarian vasculature and CL. By shifting PGF_2 away from the CL, estrogen prevents luteolysis, and thus the CL is maintained.

Conclusions

There is striking diversity in the placental architecture of the various domestic animal species. Yet, in all eutherian species, the placenta is essential for nutrient, gas, and waste exchange and maternal-fetal communication. The placenta includes both fetal and maternal tissues and the juxtaposition of these tissues permits the conceptus to be nourished either by the endometrial glands (histiotrophe) or maternal blood vessels (hemotrophe). Placental hormones moderate the dialogue between mother and conceptus, and, depending on the species, the placenta can produce a wide array of hormones. The common feature of most placental hormones is that they create a maternal environment that is conducive for conceptus survival and development.

Acknowledgements

The author wishes to thank Dr. R. Michael Roberts for his critical review of this chapter and Jennifer L. Kent for her clerical assistance.

Bibliography

Allen, W.R., and Stewart, F. (2001). Equine placentation. *Reprod. Fertil. Dev.* 13:623–34.

Anderson, J.W. (1969). Ultrastructure of the placenta and fetal membranes of the dog. I. The placental labyrinth. *Anat. Rec.* 165:15–35.

Anthony, R.V., Pratt, S.L., Liang, R., and Holland, M.D. (1995). Placental-fetal hormonal interactions: impact on fetal growth. *J. Anim. Sci.* 73:1861–71.

Bazer, F.W., and Thatcher, W.W. (1977). Theory of maternal recognition of pregnancy in swine based on estrogen controlled endocrine versus exocrine secretion of prostaglandin F2alpha by the uterine endometrium. *Prostaglandins.* 14:397–400.

Beckers, J.F., Zarrouk, A., Batalha, E.S., Garbayo, J.M., Mester, L., and Szenci, O. (1998). Endocrinology of pregnancy: chorionic somatomammotropins and pregnancy-associated glycoproteins: review. *Acta. Vet. Hung.* 46:175–89.

Benirschke, K. (1983). Placentation. *J. Exp. Zool.* 228:385–9.

Betteridge, K.J., Eaglesome, M.D., Randall, G.C., and Mitchell, D. (1980). Collection, description and transfer of embryos from cattle 10–16 days after oestrus. *J. Reprod. Fertil.* 59:205–16.

Björkman, N. (1954). Morphological and histochemical studies on the bovine placenta. *Acta. Anat. (Basel).* 22:1–91.

Byatt, J.C., Warren, W.C., Eppard, P.J., Staten, N.R., Krivi, G.G., and Collier, R.J. (1992). Ruminant placental lactogens: structure and biology. *J. Anim. Sci.* 70:2911–23.

Cameo, P., Srisuparp, S., Strakova, Z., and Fazleabas, A.T. (2004). Chorionic gonadotropin and uterine dialogue in the primate. *Reprod. Biol. Endocrinol.* 2:50.

Choi, I., Collante, W.R., Simmen, R.C., and Simmen, F.A. (1997). A developmental switch in expression from blastocyst to endometrial/placental-type cytochrome P450 aromatase genes in the pig and horse. *Biol. Reprod.* 56:688–96.

Dempsey, E.W., Wislocki, G.B., and Amoroso, E.C. (1955). Electron microscopy of the pig's placenta, with special reference to the cell membranes of the endometrium and chorion. *Am. J. Anat.* 96:65–101.

Dhindsa, D.S., and Dziuk, P.J. (1968). Effect on pregnancy in the pig after killing embryos or fetuses in one uterine horn in early gestation. *J. Anim. Sci.* 27:122–6.

Flint, A.P., Henville, A., and Christie, W.B. (1979). Presence of placental lactogen in bovine conceptuses before attachment. *J. Reprod. Fertil.* 56:305–8.

Forsyth, I.A. (1994). Comparative aspects of placental lactogens: structure and function. *Exp. Clin. Endocrinol.* 102:244–51.

Gol, M., Altunyurt, S., Cimrin, D., Guclu, S., Bagci, M., and Demir, N. (2004). Different maternal serum hCG levels in pregnant women with female and male fetuses: does fetal hypophyseal-adrenal-gonadal axis play a role? *J. Perinat. Med.* 32:342–5.

Gonzalez, F., Cabrera, F., Batista, M., Rodriguez, N., Alamo, D., Sulon, J., Beckers, J.F., and Gracia, A. (2004). A comparison of diagnosis of pregnancy in the goat via transrectal ultrasound scanning, progesterone, and pregnancy-associated glycoprotein assays. *Theriogenology.* 62:1108–15.

Guillomot, M., Flechon, J.E., and Wintenberger-Torres, S. (1981). Conceptus attachment in the ewe: an ultrastructural study. *Placenta.* 2:169–82.

Hansen, P.J. (1998). Regulation of uterine immune function by progesterone—lessons from the sheep. *J. Reprod. Immunol.* 40:63–79.

Hoffmann, B., and Schuler, G. (2002). The bovine placenta; a source and target of steroid hormones: observations during the second half of gestation. *Domest. Anim. Endocrinol.* 23:309–20.

Hoppen, H.O. (1994). The equine placenta and equine chorionic gonadotrophin—an overview. *Exp. Clin. Endocrinol.* 102: 235–43.

Hughes, A.L., Green, J.A., Piontkivska, H., and Roberts, R.M. (2003). Aspartic proteinase phylogeny and the origin of pregnancy-associated glycoproteins. *Mol. Biol. Evol.* 20:1940–5.

Karen, A., Beckers, J.F., Sulon, J., el Amiri, B., Szabados, K., Ismail, S., Reiczigel, J., and Szenci, O. (2003). Evaluation of false transrectal ultrasonographic pregnancy diagnoses in sheep by measuring the plasma level of pregnancy-associated glycoproteins. *Reprod. Nutr. Dev.* 43:577–86.

Keay, S.D., Vatish, M., Karteris, E., Hillhouse, E.W., and Randeva, H.S. (2004). The role of hCG in reproductive medicine. *Bjog.* 111:1218–28.

Kimura, K., Spate, L.D., Green, M.P., Murphy, C.N., Seidel Jr., G.E., and Roberts, R.M. (2004). Sexual dimorphism in interferon-tau production by in vivo-derived bovine embryos. *Mol. Reprod. Dev.* 67:193–9.

King, G.J., Atkinson, B.A., and Robertson, H.A. (1982). Implantation and early placentation in domestic ungulates. *J. Reprod. Fertil.* Suppl. 31:17–30.

Kletzky, O.A., Rossman, F., Bertolli, S.I., Platt, L.D., and Mishell Jr., D.R. (1985). Dynamics of human chorionic gonadotropin, prolactin, and growth hormone in serum and amniotic fluid throughout normal human pregnancy. *Am. J. Obstet. Gynecol.* 151:878–84.

Knight, J.W. (1994). Aspects of placental estrogen synthesis in the pig. *Exp. Clin. Endocrinol.* 102:175–84.

Larson, M.A., Kimura, K., Kubisch, H.M., and Roberts, R.M. (2001). Sexual dimorphism among bovine embryos in their ability to make the transition to expanded blastocyst and in the expression of the signaling molecule IFN-tau. *Proc. Natl. Acad. Sci. USA.* 98:9677–82.

Leiser, R., and Koob, B. (1993). Development and characteristics of placentation in a carnivore, the domestic cat. *J. Exp. Zool.* 266:642–56.

Leiser, R., Krebs, C., Klisch, K., Ebert, B., Dantzer, V., Schuler, G., and Hoffmann, B. (1997). Fetal villosity and microvasculature of the bovine placentome in the second half of gestation. *J. Anat.* 191 (Pt 4):517–27.

Licht, P., Russu, V., and Wildt, L. (2001). On the role of human chorionic gonadotropin (hCG) in the embryo-endometrial microenvironment: implications for differentiation and implantation. *Semin. Reprod. Med.* 19:37–47.

McMahon, C.D., Fisher, M.W., Mockett, B.G., and Littlejohn, R. P. (1997). Embryo development and placentome formation during early pregnancy in red deer. *Reprod. Fertil. Dev.* 9:723–30.

Moor, R.M., and Rowson, L.E. (1966). The corpus luteum of the sheep: functional relationship between the embryo and the corpus luteum. *J. Endocrinol.* 34:233–9.

Murphy, B.D., and Martinuk, S.D.. (1991). Equine chorionic gonadotropin. *Endocr. Rev.* 12:27–44.

Noden, D.M., and de Lahunta, A. (1985). *The Embryology of Domestic Animals: Developmental Mechanisms and Malformations.* Baltimore: William and Wilkins.

Northey, D.L., and French, L.R. (1980). Effect of embryo removal and intrauterine infusion of embryonic homogenates on the lifespan of the bovine corpus luteum. *J. Anim. Sci.* 50: 298–302.

Obiekwe, B.C., and Chard, T. (1983). A comparative study of the clinical use of four placental proteins in the third trimester. *J. Perinat. Med.* 11:121–6.

Ousey, J.C., Forhead, A.J., Rossdale, P.D., Grainger, L., Houghton, E., and Fowden, A.L. (2003). Ontogeny of uteroplacental progestagen production in pregnant mares during the second half of gestation. *Biol. Reprod.* 69:540–8.

Perenyi, Z.S., Szenci, O., Sulon, J., Drion, P.V., and Beckers, J.F. (2002). Comparison of the ability of three radioimmunoassay to detect pregnancy-associated glycoproteins in bovine plasma. *Reprod. Domest. Anim.* 37:100–4.

Perry, J.S. (1981). The mammalian fetal membranes. *J. Reprod. Fertil.* 62:321–35.

Raub, T.J., Bazer, F.W., and Roberts, R.M. (1985). Localization of the iron transport glycoprotein, uteroferrin, in the porcine endometrium and placenta by using immunocolloidal gold. *Anat. Embryol. (Berl)* 171:253–8.

Roberts, R.M., Ealy, A.D., Alexenko, A.P., Han, C.S., and Ezashi, T. (1999). Trophoblast interferons. *Placenta.* 20:259–64.

Roberts, R.M., Ezashi, T., Rosenfeld, C.S., Ealy, A.D., and Kubisch, H.M. (2003). Evolution of the interferon tau genes and their promoters, and maternal-trophoblast interactions in control of their expression. *Reprod. Suppl.* 61:239–51.

Roberts, R.M., Raub, T.J., and Bazer, F.W. (1986). Role of uteroferrin in transplacental iron transport in the pig. *Fed. Proc.* 45:2513–8.

Roberts, R.M., Xie, S., and Mathialagan, N. (1996). Maternal recognition of pregnancy. *Biol. Reprod.* 54:294–302.

Rowson, L.E., and Moor, R.M. (1967). The influence of embryonic tissue homogenate infused into the uterus, on the lifespan of the corpus luteum in the sheep. *J. Reprod. Fertil.* 13:511–6.

Silver, M. (1994). Placental progestagens in the sheep and horse and the changes leading to parturition. *Exp. Clin. Endocrinol.* 102:203–11.

Spencer, T.E., and Bazer, F.W. (2004). Uterine and placental factors regulating conceptus growth in domestic animals. *J. Anim. Sci.* 82 E-Suppl:E4–13.

Steier, J.A., Bergsjo, P.B., Thorsen, T., and Myking, O.L. (2004). Human chorionic gonadotropin in maternal serum in relation to fetal gender and utero-placental blood flow. *Acta. Obstet. Gynecol. Scand.* 83:170–4.

Wathes, D.C., and Wooding, F.B. (1980). An electron microscopic study of implantation in the cow. *Am. J. Anat.* 159: 285–306.

Wooding, F.B. (1981). Localization of ovine placental lactogen in sheep placentomes by electron microscope immunocytochemistry. *J. Reprod. Fertil.* 62:15–9.

Wooding, F.B. (1992). Current topic: the synepitheliochorial placenta of ruminants: binucleate cell fusions and hormone production. *Placenta.* 13:101–13.

Wooding, F.B., Morgan, G., and Adam, C.L. (1997). Structure and function in the ruminant synepitheliochorial placenta: central role of the trophoblast binucleate cell in deer. *Microsc. Res. Tech.* 38:88–99.

Xie, S.C., Low B.G., Nagel, R.J., Kramer, K.K., Anthony, R.V., Zoli, A.P., Beckers, J.F., and Roberts, R.M. (1991). Identification of the major pregnancy-specific antigens of cattle and sheep as inactive members of the aspartic proteinase family. *Proc. Natl. Acad. Sci. USA.* 88:10247–51.

Chapter 12

Comparative Placentation

Bhanu Prakash Telugu and Jonathan A. Green

Introduction

For more than 500 million years, the extraembryonic membranes of vertebrates have been serving the growing fetus' needs for gas exchange, nutrient acquisition, waste excretion, and protection from temperature fluctuations and jostling from physical movement of the egg or mother. The establishment of the earliest membrane, the yolk sac, was coincident with the evolution of egg-laying vertebrates. Subsequent development of the amnion and chorioallantoic membranes further permitted egg laying on land. While in viviparous species, the extraembryonic membranes have become even further specialized to permit nutritional, respiratory, and other roles to be performed inside the maternal reproductive tract.

The extraembryonic membranes of vertebrates are structurally diverse and play many distinct roles, depending on the species. Consequently, the study of these membranes is a rather fascinating area of research. Due to the considerable complexity and wealth of information available, this chapter will focus exclusively on the extraembryonic membranes of mammals, specifically those of eutherians. Interested readers can consult numerous other sources for information on the extraembryonic membranes of mammals in other taxa such as the metatherians (marsupials) or monotremata (platypus) (Roberts and Breed, 1994; Hughes and Hall, 1998; Freyer, 2002; Claudia Freyer, 2003).

The placenta has been defined by Mossman as "an apposition of parental (usually maternal) and fetal tissue for the purpose of physiological exchange" (Mossman, 1937). Steven described the eutherian placenta as "an arrangement of one or more transporting epithelia between fetal and maternal circulations" (Steven and Morris, 1975). Along with providing nourishment to their young via mammary secretions, the placenta is a distinguishing feature of eutherian mammals.

In these species, it is the organ that creates the interface for nutrient and waste exchange between the dam and the fetus growing in her womb. The placenta is also an important source of signaling molecules capable of manipulating maternal physiology to maintain an environment conducive to a successful pregnancy. In light of the conserved and important roles played by the placenta, some have suggested that similarities in placenta structure can be used to estab-

lish phylogenetic relationships (Luckett, 1993; Pijnenborg and Vercruysse, 2004). In some cases, such efforts have shown utility (e.g. H.W. Mossman's grouping of rodents with lagomorphs and tenrecs with elephant shrews) (Mossman, 1937). However, such efforts have also led some to assume phylogenetic relationships between species that are not consistent with either morphological or molecular data (Mossman, 1987).

Despite the fact that it has common functions across species, the placenta (specifically, the vascularized chorioallantoic membrane) is arguably the most diverse organ within the eutherians. Placentas vary dramatically in their gross shape as well as in the depth of implantation into maternal tissues (Leiser and Kaufmann, 1994). For example, in rodents and great apes, the trophoblasts (outer cell type of the placenta) invade extensively into the uterine lining, breaching maternal vessels to become bathed in maternal blood (Cross, 1994). At the other extreme is the noninvasive placenta of swine. In these animals, no erosion of the uterine lining occurs (Leiser and Kaufmann, 1994). Carnivores exhibit an invasiveness that is intermediate between these examples (Leiser and Kaufmann, 1994). Such diversity among placentas clearly leads to rather striking differences in the endocrinological, immunological, and metabolic "dialogue" that takes place between the fetus and mother.

Several approaches have been used to define and categorize placenta types. This chapter includes a brief overview of these categories. In addition, several examples of the placenta forms used by individual species are presented to give the reader an appreciation for the striking differences in placentation among species. How these placenta types may be associated with eutherian phylogeny is also presented, as is discussion of why different placenta types might have evolved.

Embryonic and Conceptus Development

Upon fertilization of the oocyte, a series of cell divisions occur that result in the formation of a mass of cells (the morula) encased within a glycoprotein coat, the zona pellucida. The morula is soon transformed into a hollow ball of cells, the blastocyst, which represents the first morphologically obvious cell differentiation event in early mammalian development. At this stage, the embryo consists of an inner cell mass (ICM), and an outer sphere of cells, the trophoblast, surrounding a fluid-filled cavity (blastocoelic cavity) (see Figure 12.1).

In some species (e.g. mouse, human) the ICM is appropriately named because it is literally internal—it is covered by polar trophoblast on one side, while the other side is exposed to the blastocoele fluid. However in other species (e.g. swine and ruminant ungulates), the term inner cell mass is somewhat of a misnomer because these cells are actually contiguous with the trophoblast. In these species, the ICM becomes exposed to the extraembryonic environment because the overlying trophoblasts quickly degenerate once the blastocyst escapes from the zona pelucida (Fléchon, 2004).

In regard to cell lineage specification, the trophoblast cells of the blastocyst contribute exclusively to the extraembryonic membranes, while the ICM develops into the embryo/fetus, but also contributes to the components of the yolk sac, amnion, and allantois.

Immediately after blastocyst formation, endoderm cells (arising from the ICM adjacent to the blastocoele) begin to spread along the inner surface of the trophoblast until they eventually line the blastocoelic cavity (see Figure 12.1). This two-layered structure (the bilaminar omphalopleure) creates the yolk sac cavity bound by extraembryonic endoderm and trophoblast (except in the region of the embryonic disc). Later in development, mesoderm in most species—arising from ingression of embryonic ectoderm through the primitive streak of the embryonic disc—begins to spread between the embryonic ectoderm and embryonic endoderm and between the trophectoderm and the extraembryonic endoderm (see Figure 12.1). Outside the embryonic disc, the mesoderm/trophoblast combination comprises the *chorion* or *somatopleure*. The mesoderm plus extraembryonic endoderm combination comprises the yolk sac *splanchnopleure*. As these different tissues are formed, a space is created between them; this is the *exocoelom*.

The mesodermal tissue associated with the yolk sac endoderm soon develops a blood supply, thus establishing the first efficient maternal fetal exchange system—the yolk sac placenta. When the yolk sac is in contact with trophoblast, the structure is referred to as the *trilaminar omphalopleure* or *choriovitelline membrane* (see Figure 12.1). Later in development, the *allantois*, arising initially as splanchnopleure (in most species), grows as a projection into the exocoelom until it comes into contact with the chorion. Vascularization of the allantois to create the umbilical vessels results in the establishment of the chorioallantoic placenta (see Figure 12.1).

In many eutherian mammals, the expanding allantois displaces the yolk sac from the trophoblast. Therefore, the yolk sac placenta formed early in pregnancy is soon superseded by the establishment of a chorioallantoic placenta. In some mammals (e.g. humans), a true yolk sac placenta is never formed. In others (e.g. rodents and lagomorphs), the yolk sac placenta persists until term. In these species, there is either a partial or complete inversion of cell layers such

that the yolk sac endoderm actually forms an absorptive epithelium that faces the maternal tissues (described later in the chapter). This arrangement is often referred to as an "inverted yolk sac placenta."

Fetal Membranes

There are four extraembryonic membranes in the eutherian embryos.

Chorion (Ectoderm and Mesoderm)

The chorion is the outermost tissue covering the fetal membranes; it consists of trophoblasts with their underlying mesenchyme. It is in direct apposition with maternal tissues. The chorion associates with other extraembryonic membranes and contributes to the development of the chorioallantoic or choriovitelline placenta. Regardless of the depth of invasion into the maternal endometrium, the chorion represents the principal membrane involved in the exchange of nutrients, gases, waste material, etc. It also plays a key role in protecting the embryo from maternal immunosurveillance and is actively involved in the synthesis and secretion of compounds (such as protein and steroid hormones, chemokines, etc.) that influence both maternal and fetal physiology to establish and maintain a successful pregnancy.

Amnion

The presence or absence of an amnion forms the basis for classification of vertebrates into two broad categories. Birds, reptiles, and mammals that possess an amnion are collectively referred to as amniotes; whereas, fishes and amphibians that lack an amnion are classified as anamniotes. In most species, the amnion is derived by the folding of chorion, thereby forming a sac (amniotic sac) around the fetus (see Figure 12.1). In some animals (e.g. rodents) it forms by cavitation. The amniotic sac is filled with fluid (*liquor amnii*) that bathes the fetus. The amniotic fluid was initially considered solely nutritional. In 1651, Sir William Harvey wrote that the amniotic fluid is "like the colliquament in the hen's egg, it is a fluid destined by nature for the nourishment of the fetus" (Harvey, 1651).

It is now known that the amniotic fluid is not merely nutritional but plays a crucial role in cushioning the embryo from sudden blows/movements and allowing the developing fetus room to grow free of uterine restrictions. It also helps in maintaining constant temperature and plays a vital role in the development of the lungs and other organs. The amniotic membrane itself participates in the homeostatic maintenance of the amniotic fluid.

Yolk Sac (Vitelline Sac, Umbilical Vesicle, Vesicular Umbilicus)

"The yolk sac is the most primitive vertebrate fetal membrane" (Mossman, 1987). It is a derivative of endoderm. In macrolecithal embryos of reptiles and birds, where a large amount of yolk is preserved in the yolk sac, it provides the

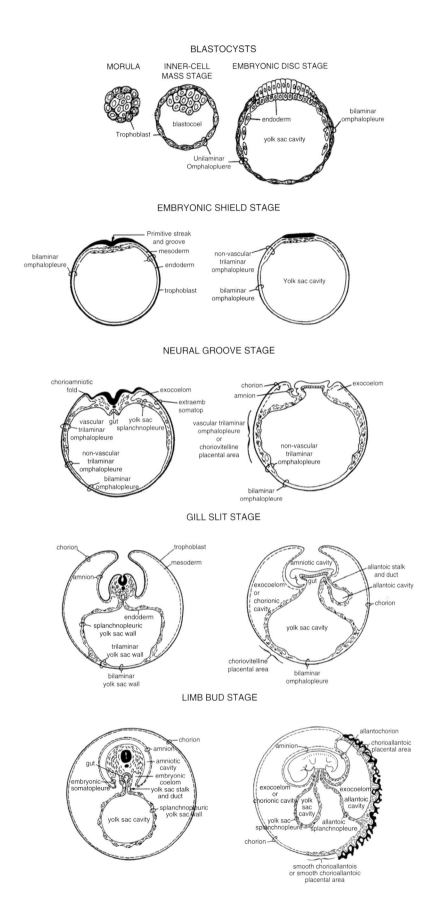

BLASTOCYSTS

MORULA   INNER-CELL   EMBRYONIC DISC STAGE
            MASS STAGE

blastocoel

Trophoblast

Unilaminar
Omphalopluere

endoderm

yolk sac cavity

bilaminar
omphalopleure

EMBRYONIC SHIELD STAGE

Primitive streak
and groove

bilaminar
omphalopleure

mesoderm

endoderm

trophoblast

non-vascular
trilaminar
omphalopleure

bilaminar
omphalopleure

Yolk sac cavity

NEURAL GROOVE STAGE

chorioamniotic
fold

exocoelom

extraemb
somatop

vascular   gut   yolk sac
trilaminar   splanchnopleure
omphalopleure

non-vascular
trilaminar
omphalopleure

bilaminar
omphalopleure

chorion

amnion

exocoelom

vascular trilaminar
omphalopleure
or
choriovitelline
placental area

non-vascular
trilaminar
omphalopleure

bilaminar
omphalopleure

GILL SLIT STAGE

chorion

amnion

endoderm

splanchnopleuric
yolk sac wall

trilaminar
yolk sac wall

bilaminar
yolk sac wall

trophoblast

mesoderm

amniotic cavity

exocoelom
or
chorionic
cavity

gut

yolk sac cavity

choriovitelline
placental area

allantoic stalk
and duct

allantoic cavity

chorion

bilaminar
omphalopleure

LIMB BUD STAGE

chorion

amnion

amniotic
cavity

embryonic
coelom

yolk sac stalk
and duct

splanchnopleuric
yolk sac wall

yolk sac cavity

gut

embryonic
somatopleure

allantochorion

chorioallantoic
placental area

aminion

exocoelom
or
chorionic cavity

yolk sac
splanchnopleure

yolk
sac
cavity

allantoic
splanchnopleure

exocoelom

allantoic
cavity

chorion

smooth chorioallantois
or smooth chorioallantoic
placental area

Figure 12.1. Stylized diagrams of transverse (left side) and sagittal (right side) sections of eutherian embryos depicting fetal membranes in developmental transition. These diagrams illustrate many of the tissues and structures described throughout the chapter. Modified from Mossman, 1987.

bulk of the nutritional support for the embryo. In mammals with microlecithal embryos, the importance and utility of the yolk sac has been challenged.

In most species (except anthrapoids), an initial yolk sac placentation (choriovitelline) is usually transitory and is later usurped by a definitive chorioallantoic membrane. However, rodents possess a yolk sac placenta alongside a chorioallantoic placenta. In these species, along with lagomorphs and insectivores, an *inverted yolk sac* is present. It is referred to as "inverted" because the fetal endoderm and underlying mesoderm are exposed to the maternal tissues due to the loss of the non-vascularized bilaminar yolk sac layers abutting the endometrium (described later in the chapter). Despite its transient nature in most mammals, the yolk sac is still a vital organ. It acts as a source of germ cells that later colonize the gonads. It is also the site at which hematopoietic cells first begin to form.

Allantois

In most vertebrates, the allantois is an endodermally derived vascular evagination that originates from the ventral surface of the hindgut. It is primarily involved in the storage (birds, reptiles) or removal of wastes generated by the embryo and in gaseous exchange. In eutherians, the allantois contributes to the vascular mesenchyme of the chorioallantoic placenta and hence is involved in fetal-maternal exchange. The extent of allantoic development varies in different species of mammals. In the pig, for example, the allantois is extensive and fills the entire exocoelom. In rodents and humans, it is a mere evagination contributing to the vascular mesenchyme of the placenta.

Types of Feto-maternal Interdigitation

Folded, lamellar, trabecular, villous, and labyrinthine are different terms used to describe the conformations of interacting tissues at the feto-maternal interface (see Figure 12.2). The simplest form of association is the folded type and perhaps the most extreme is the labyrinthine form. A folded type of arrangement is seen in the placentation of swine, where the chorionic surface closely apposes the primary and secondary folds (later in pregnancy) of the uterus.

When the folds of interacting surface are further drawn out, the result is a lamellate organization, which is observed in carnivores such as the domestic cat. In this model, the maternal and fetal tissues form a series of tall, closely packed sheets.

In the trabeculate design, which is observed in some primates, the folds are incomplete and engage in secondary branching.

In line of growing complexity, a villous configuration is observed in placenta of humans. In this type, the fetal tissue initiates a complex branching process that culminates in a three-dimensional tree-like structure with numerous slender villi.

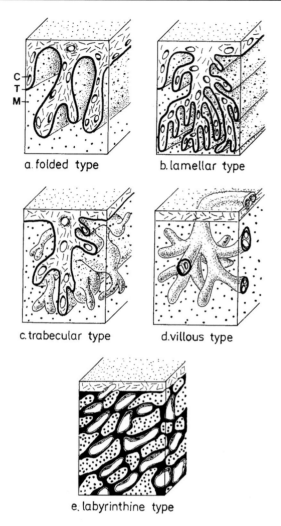

Figure 12.2. Illustrations of the different types of interdigitation of fetal chorion and maternal tissues. **M:** maternal tissues; **T:** trophoblast (black); **C:** fetal capillaries and connective tissue. From Kaufmann and Burton, 1994.

Finally, the labyrinthine pattern is observed in the placenta of rodents. It consists of a complex three-dimensional meshwork of vascularized fetal trophoblast creating cavities through which maternal blood flows. This arrangement has been described as being analogous to the "substance and pores of a sponge" (Kaufmann and Burton, 1994).

Classification of Placental Membranes

Placentas have been categorized in a number of ways. Most of the classification systems are based on morphological characteristics such as the appearance of the extraembryonic tissues and associated organs, placental shape, or the type and number of cell layers between the maternal and fetal circulations (Steven and Morris, 1975; Leiser and Kaufmann, 1994; Carter and Enders, 2004). The two principal means of classification are based on:

- The gross shape and distribution of the chorionic tissues most intimately interacting with the uterine tissues.

- The number of cell types separating the maternal and fetal circulations.

Classification Based on Placental Shape

Four general placental types have been established based on the shape of the placenta. These will be summarized briefly here, with expanded descriptions later in this chapter.

Diffuse Placenta

Examples of the diffuse placenta can be observed in the pig and horse (King, 1993b). In swine, the placenta is completely non-invasive. The chorionic villi are not localized to a particular region but are instead distributed nearly over the entire surface of the uterine lumenal epithelium (see Figure 12.3). The closely packed and convoluted chorionic villi yield an extensive surface area to facilitate movement of diffusible molecules between the maternal and fetal circulations and participate in the uptake of nutritional secretions from uterine glands. The equine placenta, while still considered diffuse, is distinct from the sow placenta in that it possesses localized regions of contact known as *microcotyledons* and an invasive trophoblast population known as chorionic girdle cells that, upon migration into the uterine endometrium, can form transitory structures known as *endometrial cups* (described later).

Cotyledonary Placenta

Ruminant ungulates possess a cotyledonary placenta (Steven and Morris, 1975). The cotyledons are vascularized villous trophoblasts that intercalate into aglandular structures in the uterine endometrium known as caruncles (see Figure 12.3). The fetal cotyledons begin to associate with maternal caruncles early in gestation and interdigitation of these tissues is well underway by day 35 in ewes and day 45 in cattle. Together, the combined unit of cotyledons and caruncles is referred to as a *placentome*.

Zonary Placenta

Numerous species, including carnivores, possess a zonary placenta. This type consists of a band of chorion surrounding the middle of the fetus (see Figure 12.3). This zone of chorion forming the most intimate contact with the maternal uterus is the basis for the name of this placenta type.

Discoid Placenta

Higher primates and rodents possess a placenta that is characterized by one or more distinct discs comprised of localized regions of fetal chorion that interface with uterine tissues, thus the descriptive name "discoid" (see Figure 12.3).

Placental Classification Based on the Number of Intact Cell Layers at the Fetal-maternal Interface

This system was first proposed by O. Grosser in 1909 and 1927 and is described and referred to by Mossman (1987), Steven and Morris (1975), and Amoroso (1952). It is generally considered one of the most useful and instructive methods for functionally describing placental types. In this system, the extraembryonic membranes are classified within one of four broadly descriptive headings: hemochorial, endotheliochorial, syndesmochorial, and epitheliochorial (see Figure 12.4). Grosser's system has since been amended by the replacement of syndesmochorial with the more descriptive heading "synepitheliochorial," which more accurately describes the type of placenta present in ruminant ungulates (Wooding, 1992).

Hemochorial Placenta

The hemochorial placenta of rodents, lagomorphs (rabbits and hares), higher primates, and several other groupings is a highly invasive entity in which the trophoblasts of the chorion penetrate the maternal uterine epithelium, the underlying connective tissue (stroma), and the endothelium of the maternal vasculature to establish direct contact with

Diffuse   **Cotyledonary**

Zonary   **Discoid**

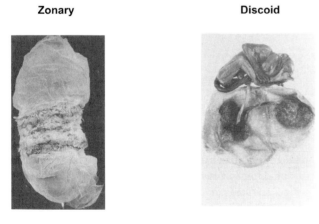

Figure 12.3. Illustrations of four main placenta classifications based on the gross shape of the vascularized fetal membranes in contact with maternal tissues. The four categories are diffuse (pig placenta), cotyledonary (bovine placenta), zonary (dog placenta), and discoid (monkey placenta). From Kaufmann and Burton, 1994.

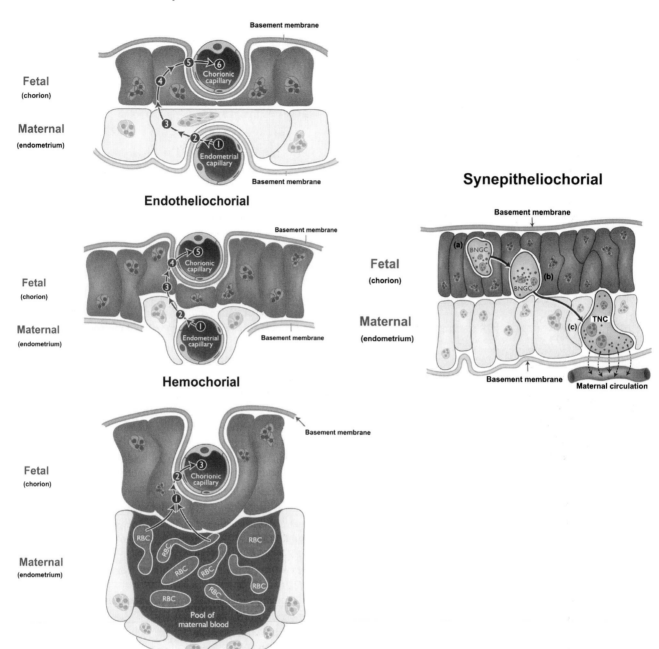

Figure 12.4. Stylized illustrations of the tissue layers separating the fetal and maternal vasculatures based on a modification of Grosser's placental classification system. The three main categories are epitheliochorial (six tissue types separating fetal and maternal blood), endotheliochorial (four tissues) and hemochorial (three tissues); the internal layers are depicted by numbers 1–6, depending on the type. A derivation from the epitheliochorial form is the synepitheliochorial form of the ruminant ungulates. This placenta form has a specialized trophoblast population of Binucleate giant cells (BNGC) or Binucleate cells (BNC) capable of migrating (route a, b, and c) and fusing with uterine epithelial cells to form a syncytial cell type (TNC, or trinucleated cell) or a syncytial cell layer, depending on the species. Modified from Senger, 2003.

maternal blood. There are only three cell types between the fetal and maternal blood: fetal trophoblast, fetal connective tissue or interstitium, and the fetal endothelial cells comprising the fetal capillaries. A further distinguishing characteristic within this grouping is in the number of trophoblast cell layers present. The hemochorial placenta can be further designated hemomonochorial, hemodichorial, or hemotrichorial depending on whether there are one, two, or three layers of trophoblast present, respectively (Enders, 1965; Enders and Welsh, 1993; Enders and Blankenship, 1999).

Endotheliochorial Placenta

The endotheliochorial placenta is a widespread type and is represented in most carnivores, insectivores, some bats, and numerous other phylogenetic orders (Carter and Enders, 2004; Mess and Carter, 2006). It is similar to the hemochorial placenta in that its invading trophoblasts breach the uterine epithelium and stroma. However, the trophoblasts do not directly contact circulating maternal blood. Rather, they become associated with the endothelium of the maternal capillary network. Therefore, species with an endotheliochorial placenta have four cell layers between the fetal and maternal circulations.

Epitheliochorial Placenta

The epitheliochorial placenta is the least invasive type of placenta wherein both the luminal epithelium (LE) of the uterine endometrium and the epithelium of the chorionic villi remain intact. In the sow there is no erosion of the LE. In horses, there is only moderate and transient invasion of the LE and uterine stroma by a subset of trophoblasts (chorionic girdle trophoblasts). In these species, the uterine epithelium remains intact and there are six cell layers separating the maternal and fetal circulations.

Synepitheliochorial Placenta

The synepitheliochorial placenta of ruminant ungulates is derived from the epitheliochorial type. These animals possess specialized binucleated trophoblast cells that fuse with the uterine epithelium (described later). In some animals in the Ruminantia suborder (e.g. domestic cattle), this fusion event results in the production of short-lived trinucleated cells. In others (e.g. sheep and goats), continued migration and fusion of the binucleated trophoblasts can form an extensive fetal-maternal syncytial cell layer. These animals have five to six cell types between the fetal and maternal circulatory systems, depending on whether or not a syncytium is present.

Phylogeny and Placenta Evolution

One recurring suggestion regarding the evolution of the eutherian placenta is that the epitheliochorial placenta is the most primitive form and that the hemochorial type represents a derived form that is a culmination of evolutionary steps from the epitheliochorial form progressing through the synepitheliochorial (or syndesmochorial) and endotheliochorial types (Pijnenborg, 1981; Pijnenborg, 1985; Mossman, 1987, 1991; Haig, 1993; Luckett, 1993). Perhaps the reason the epitheliochorial placenta has often been considered a primitive form arose from the observation that some marsupials, with their poorly developed neonates, possess an epitheliochorial type. There may also have been a certain logic to the underlying assumption that the decreased numbers of cell layers present in endotheliochorial and hemochorial placentas were somehow inherently

more efficient due to a more ready access to maternal blood.

In fact, recent advances in molecular phylogenetics have increased our confidence in assigning eutherian orders to different clades (see Figure 12.5) (Murphy, 2001). With such information in hand, it has become clearer that the primordial form of chorioallantoic placentation in eutherians was most likely of an invasive endotheliochorial or hemochorial type (Mess and Carter, 2006; Wildman, 2006). Some have argued that the hemochorial placenta is actually a derived state, with transformations having occurred in all major clades (Carter and Enders, 2004).

While this point is still debatable, more confidence exists that the epitheliochorial placenta is an adaptive form that arose independently in two of the clades (Laurasiatheria and Euarchontoglires) (see Figure 12.5). More specifically, epitheliochorial placentas are found in species in the Cetartiodactyla, Perissodactyla, and Pholidota orders of Laurasiatheria and the Strepsirhina suborder of Euarchontoglires (see Figure 12.5) (Carter, 2001; Carter and Enders, 2004; Mess and Carter, 2006).

Indeed, the decrease in invasiveness of the trophoblasts of these species appears to be an evolutionary adaptation occurring in the maternal uterus, possibly in an attempt to thwart excessive manipulation of the mother's physiology by the embryo (Haig, 1993, 1996; Crespi and Semeniuk, 2004; Vogel, 2005). Evidence supporting this point can be found in the pig, a species with an epitheliochorial diffuse type of placenta. Porcine cytotrophoblasts possess an inherently invasive character. When they are transferred to ectopic sites, they migrate through and degrade the surrounding tissue (Samuel, 1971; Samuel and Perry, 1972).

These observations are quite intriguing and they return to the point raised at the beginning of this chapter. Specifically, once a functional placenta was developed in the eutherian lineages, why have placentas continued to diverge so drastically and rapidly even within the same phylogenetic order? David Haig and others have argued that one explanation for such changes is that there is a good deal of fetal-maternal conflict taking place between the embryo and the mother (Haig, 1993, 1996; Crespi and Semeniuk, 2004). One such example regards nutrient partitioning, in which the interests of the fetus and those of the mother are not necessarily identical. The fetus would prefer essentially unlimited resources from the mother, while the mother must partition resources to not preclude care of current and future offspring. Selective imprinting of genes appears to be a means by which fetal-maternal conflict is manifested (Haig, 1993, 1996; Iwasa, 1998).

Theoretically, it should be possible to gain a more mechanistic understanding of placental evolution and function by using modern molecular and proteomic tools. One would predict that the diversity among placentas would be reflected in differences in gene expression either from novel expression patterns of conserved genes, from the acquisition of novel placentally expressed genes, or from a combination

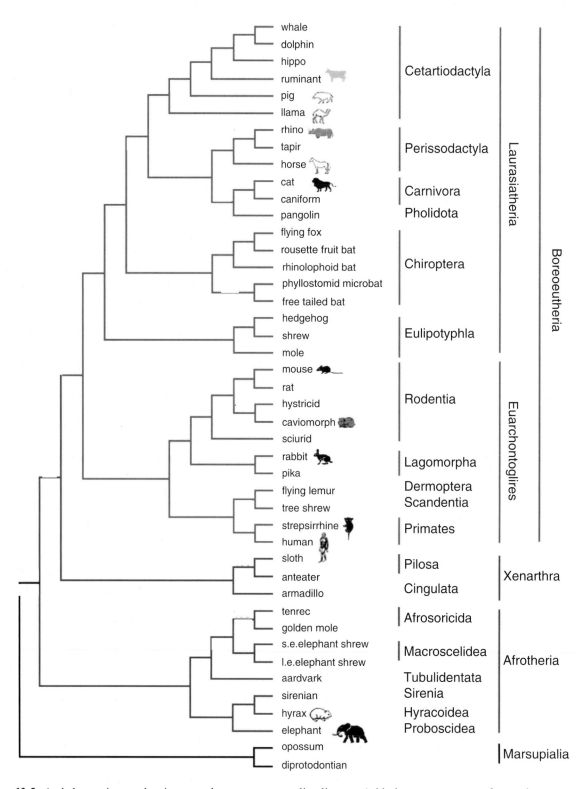

Figure 12.5. A phylogenetic tree showing several common mammalian lineages (with the common name of a species representative), along with the names of the 19 eutherian orders and their grouping within superordinal clades. The more ancient groupings are represented by the Xenarthra and Afrotheria clades. The more recently evolved groups are the Laurasiatheria and Euarchontoglires clades. Illustrations are presented for those species whose placentas are described in this chapter. Modified from Murphy, 2001.

of these two mechanisms. In fact, both phenomena appear to be involved in placental evolution.

Due to its important role as a genetic model, most of our knowledge regarding genes and gene products important for placental development has been identified in the laboratory mouse. Several genes known to be important for placenta development in rodents (e.g. Gcm1, Hand1, Mash2, Dl×3) have also been shown to be important for placenta development in humans and other species (Riley, 1998; Morasso, 1999; Anson-Cartwright, 2000; Cross, 2003a; Degrelle, 2005). These observations suggest that, despite the overt differences between placentas, the basic mechanisms underlying placenta development are conserved.

Even so, dramatic differences between placentas do exist, which should be reflected in either the existence of placenta-specific transcripts or possibly even in the birth of novel genes generated by gene duplication followed subsequently by acquisition of novel functions. This assumption indeed seems to be the case. Several gene families that are restricted to a single phylogenetic order and are unique to each placental type have been identified (Green, 1998; Roberts, 1999; Green, 2000; Sol-Church, 2002; Hughes, 2003b; MacLean, 2003; Soares, 2004).

One of the more extreme examples of the complexity and diversity that can arise in gene families is found in the rodent PRL/growth hormone gene family. More than two dozen of these genes are known to be transcribed by different trophoblast and decidual cell types at the placental uterine interface (Soares, 2004). Other examples of lineage-specific expansion of placenta-expressed genes are illustrated by the growth hormone locus in the great apes (Lacroix, 2002; Soares, 2004), the pregnancy-associated glycoproteins (Green, 1998; Hughes, 2003a) of ungulates in the Cetartiodactyla order, the interferon-tau genes (Leaman, 1992; Roberts, 1997; Roberts, 1999) and the trophoblast Kunitz domain proteins (MacLean, 2003) of the Ruminantia suborder of Cetartiodactyla, and the placentally expressed cathepsins (Sol-Church, 2002) of Rodentia.

The role for some of these gene products has been determined (e.g. interferon tau and some of the rodent prolactin-related proteins). However, the role of others (e.g. the pregnancy-associated glycoproteins) remains a mystery. What is clear is that the diversity of placenta types among the eutherians is matched by a tremendous complexity in placenta-specific gene transcription that will likely be the focus of considerable research for years to come.

The rest of this chapter is designed to give the reader an appreciation for the extensive structural and morphological differences in eutherian chorioallantoic membranes. There is a tremendous source of variation between species in basic placental organization and shape, and in the depth of trophoblast invasiveness in the uterine endometrium. Much of the following information provides a comparative overview of placentas. Each of the major placenta types (based on Grosser's definitions) will be presented in some detail, with an emphasis placed on one or a few model species representing that placenta type. In addition, other species represented within each placenta type will also be presented, but in a more condensed form, to illustrate unusual or interesting deviations.

As was indicated earlier, the endotheliochorial type of placenta may well be the ancestral form for eutheria (Mess and Carter, 2006). Two species possessing endotheliochorial placentas will be described in this chapter (domestic cat and elephant).

Most of the other examples provided will be for species possessing epitheliochorial or hem1ochorial placentas. There are a couple of reasons for this: The first is because there is a vast literature devoted to these placenta types. Rodent and human placentas (hemochorial type) have been studied extensively because the former represents such an important research model and the latter due to the need to promote and enhance human health and quality of life. Many examples of epitheliochorial placentas are found in the Artiodactyla order, which includes the ruminant ungulates, swine, horses, and camels, all of which have been used extensively for food and clothing or as work animals. Not surprisingly, there is considerable interest in increasing reproductive efficiency in these agriculturally important animals. Therefore, a good deal of information has been published describing their reproductive characteristics.

The second reason for emphasizing epitheliochorial and hemochorial placentas in the following descriptions is because it nicely illustrates the point that placentas, even those within the same categories defined by Grosser, are evolving rapidly and are remarkably divergent organs.

Endotheliochorial Placentation

The endotheliochorial type of placenta is found throughout eutheria and likely represents one of the more ancestral forms. Distinct forms of the endotheliochorial placenta are represented by the domestic cat and the elephant. Descriptions for placentas from both these species are described below.

Endotheliochorial Placentation in the Domestic Cat (*Felis domestica*)

Site of first attachment	antimesometrial
Depth of attachment	subepithelial
Yolk sac orientation	mesometrial
Choriovitelline placenta	temporary
Splanchnopleuric yolk sac	large, free, permanent

Chorioallantoic placenta

Shape	zonary
Pattern	lamellar
Interhemal membrane	endotheliochorial
Nonvillous chorioallantois	large
Allantoic sac	large
Distinguishing features	implantation girdle, hemophagous zones

The placenta of the cat has all the hallmarks of a typical endotheliochorial placenta (Leiser and Enders, 1980a, 1980b; Leiser and Kobb, 1993); hence, it will serve as a model to illustrate the salient features of this class of placenta.

The mature placenta of the domestic cat has a zonary shape and the trophoblasts exhibit a lamellar structure. Though the definitive chorioallantoic placenta is categorized as endotheliochorial, overall it exhibits a range of transitional stages of invasion into the maternal endometrium, from a superficial epitheliochorial to a deeper hemochorial type within the same placenta. For example, in the central region of the embryo, which is surrounded by a girdle-like formation of chorioallantoic villi, the extent of invasion in the uterus is subepithelial.

The chorion bypasses the luminal epithelium and reaches up to and surrounds the endothelia of the maternal blood vessels. The endothelial cells remain intact; hence the cat placenta is an endotheliochorial type according to Grosser's nomenclature (Grosser, 1909, 1927). In the region bordering the girdle, called the *hemophagous zones*, the endometrial vessels are transiently ruptured, exposing the fetal trophoblast to maternal blood; hence the pattern in these regions corresponds to a hemochorial type (Creed and Biggers, 1963; Leiser and Enders, 1980b; Leiser, 1982). Finally, in the paraplacental polar zones, which make up the rest of the embryonic surface, the chorioallantois is smooth and is simply apposed to the endometrial luminal epithelium with no invasion at all, thus constituting an epitheliochorial arrangement (Leiser and Enders, 1980a).

Implantation and Placentation in the Cat

The blastocysts of the cat enter the uterus by five days post-conception (dpc) and are spaced evenly by eight dpc (Denker, 1978b; Leiser, 1982). The blastocysts expand gradually within the implantation chamber formed by the uterus, and are visible as reddish swellings from the exterior. The trophoblast of the embryo does not establish extensive contact with maternal endometrium until about day 12.5, the period when implantation is initiated (Leiser and Kobb, 1993). At this time, the trophectoderm appears as a simple cuboidal or columnar epithelium (Dickmann, 1979). The luminal epithelium of the endometrium possesses microvilli on their apical surface, the uterine glands are enlarged, and the interglandular mesenchyme is edematous (Leiser and Kobb, 1993).

Implantation of the embryo begins with the close apposition of columnar trophoblast cells with the uterine epithelium in the antimesometrial side of the uterus. The trophoblast shows signs of significant endocytic activity, actively taking up uterine glandular secretions, the *histotroph* (Leiser and Kobb, 1993). In the ensuing adhesion phase, the initial contacts between the trophoblast and uterine epithelium are reinforced by microvillar interdigitation and establishment of junctional complexes (Leiser and Kobb, 1993). However, this phase is brief and is soon followed by the invasive phase.

The transient junctional complexes that are established in the adhesion phase are disrupted as the trophoblast invades the degenerating uterine epithelium. Some of the cytotrophoblasts at this stage undergo numerous nuclear divisions forming a syncytiotrophoblast, which constitutes the invasive front for the progressing trophoblast layer (Leiser, 1979). The uterine epithelium shows signs of lateral cell fusions and significant cell death. The invading syncytiotrophoblast is extremely phagocytic, engulfing the degenerating and necrosed uterine epithelia (Leiser, 1979). The invading syncytiotrophoblast progresses further within the partially degenerating stromal mesenchyme, reaching the maternal capillaries. The endothelial cells of maternal blood vessels in cats are enlarged and the invading syncytiotrophoblasts do not rupture these enlarged endothelia.

The maternal mesenchyme frequently persists as a sandwiched layer between the syncytiotrophoblast and capillary endothelium, forming the *interstitial membrane* (Wilmsatt, 1962; Wynn, 1971; Bjorkman, 1973). This membrane has been suggested to play an important role in regulating trophoblast growth and differentiation (Rasweiler, 1991, 1993). Therefore, by 14 dpc the endotheliochorial pattern of interhemal membrane is established (see Figure 12.6).

The syncytiotrophoblast continues to expand due to continued proliferation of cytotrophoblast. It becomes filled and expanded by fetal mesenchyme, forming the primitive villi of, by now, the trilaminar choriovitelline placenta (Amoroso, 1952). The villi are distributed all over the embryo, except at the antimesometrial end, where the amniotic folds meet to form an amniotic cavity around the conceptus.

Soon after amniogenesis, the allantois appears as an evagination from the hindgut. It soon expands and fills the exocoelomic cavity, displacing most of the vascularized yolk sac from the chorion (Amoroso, 1952). Blood vessel formation quickly begins within the mesoderm of the allantois that protrudes into the fetal chorionic villi. The allantois also vascularizes the amnion. Therefore, the placenta of cats, among a few other species, is a deviation from the general rule that the amnion is avascular.

The chorioallantoic villi extend into the maternal endometrium forming continuous lamellae alternating with maternal lamellar folds (see Figure 12.6). The core of the lamellae on the fetal side is made up of mesenchyme and fetal capillaries covered by a layer of cytotrophoblast, and overlaid by a single layer of syncytiotrophoblast. The syncytiotrophoblast interfaces with maternal decidual cells and enlarged endothelial cells of the maternal blood vessels (Wynn and Byorkman, 1968; Malasinne 1974).

Grossly, the events of implantation and uterine invasion are first initiated in the antimesometrial end in the abembryonic region, which progresses as a ring in the mesometrial direction, forming an implantation girdle by 15 dpc

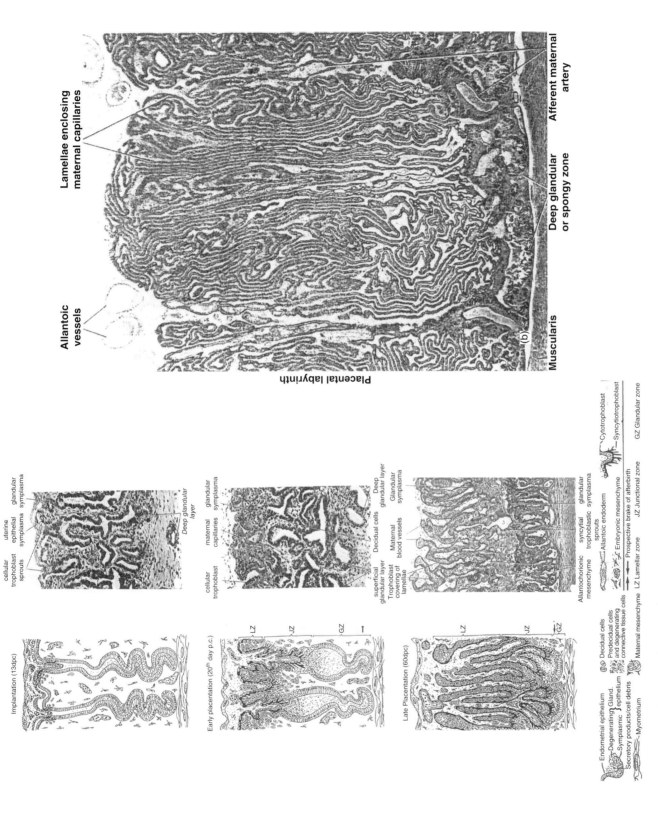

Figure 12.6. Illustrations and histological sections showing the events of placentation taking place during the establishment of the endotheliochorial placenta of the domestic cat. The panels on the left are illustrations of trophoblast-maternal interactions taking place during implantation and early and late placentation; these are presented to help clarify the histological sections in the center and on the right. The sections are from Wooding and Flint, 1994, and the illustrations are from Leiser and Kobb, 1993.

(Leiser and Kobb, 1993). The embryo at this stage therefore consists of an equatorial implantation girdle and two smooth paraplacental tips, one on either side of the girdle. The lamellated villi of the chorioallantois populate this girdle zone; hence the name zonary placenta (Amoroso, 1952; Malasinne, 1974).

Above this lamellar zone is a specialized region called the *junctional zone* (see Figure 12.6). In this region the maternal and fetal cell populations freely intermingle with one another. Beyond the junctional zone is a region of high gland density called the *glandular zone*. With the expansion of the fetal lamellae toward the maternal side, the junctional zone is progressively pushed towards the glandular zone, compressing the latter in the process. These compressive forces, in addition to the continued accumulation of glandular secretions (due to the blockade of the glandular ducts by the enlarging lamellae and degenerating maternal tissue), results in a swollen and spongy appearance of the glands in this zone near the conceptus (Rau, 1925).

In late pregnancy, due to dense materno-fetal lamellation, the lamellar zone of the placental girdle becomes 4 to 6 mm in thickness. This makes up to one-third of the chorioallantoic sac and represents a principal region for placental transfer. This is because the thickness of the endothelia of fetal and maternal blood vessels becomes reduced, which is further aided by the loss of cytotrophoblast cells and thinning of syncytiotrophoblast cell layers. These changes result in an effective diffusion distance of as little as 1.5 μm in this zone (Leiser and Kobb, 1993).

Hemophagous Organ of the Paraplacenta (Paraplacental Extravasate Zone)

In the margin between the placental girdle and the free paraplacental polar zone on either side, is a macroscopically visible extravasated region called the *hemophagous zone* or *paraplacental extravasate zone* (Creed and Biggers, 1963). At the time of parturition in the cat, due to the accumulation of blood pigment residues such as bilivirdin, this region appears as a green or brown border to the placental girdle (Janssen, 1933; Burton, 1987b). Histologically, this region consists of hematomas formed as a result of the rupture of blood vessels by the penetrating cytotrophoblast and the syncytiotrophoblast. The ruptured blood vessels are quickly repaired, and the overlying epithelium reformed; therefore, the hematoma is a stagnant pool of blood as opposed to circulating blood as is observed in the placenta of the hyena (Dempsey, 1969; Oduor-Okelo and Neaves, 1982; Wynn, 1990).

The fetal side of the hematomas is lined by columnar cytotrophoblast cells which engage in active phagocytosis of the maternal blood (Leiser and Enders, 1980b). It is reported that these cells later slip into a digestive or resting phase in which they accumulate inclusions within the cytoplasm. This process provides iron and other essential nutrients to the fetal cat (Baker and Morgan, 1973; Malasinne,

1977; Kehrer, 1978; Leiser and Enders, 1980b). The maternal side of the hematoma is either lined by an intact epithelium or a syncytium of laterally fused epithelial cells.

Paraplacental Free Polar Zone

The paraplacental free polar zone represents the remainder of the embryonic surface until about 50 dpc, when it associates with the analogous regions on adjoining fetuses, forming the paraplacental interfetal polar zone (Leiser and Enders, 1980a, 1980b; Leiser and Kohler, 1984). Contact between these zones is frequently accomplished by the interdigitation of trophoblast microvilli or just a plain apposition. They are frequently interspersed by degenerating interplacental material, which is phagocytosed by the trophoblasts in these zones (Leiser and Kobb, 1993).

The free polar zone is a thin layered sac of chorioallantoic vesicle, loosely apposed to the uterine luminal epithelium. The trophoblast layer is monolayered with no signs of syncytial formation or invasion. Similarly, the uterine luminal epithelium is largely intact and shows no signs of degeneration. This region is reminiscent of the precontact phase or preadhesion phase of the embryo. The cytotrophoblasts have a microvillous brush border on their apical surface and are actively involved in pinocytosis. They also appear to form areolae-like structures over the mouths of the uterine glands, which continue to secrete throughout the pregnancy. At term, though the free polar zone represents more than 50 percent of the placenta itself, it constitutes less than 5 percent of the total surface area represented in the interhemal area (Leiser and Kohler, 1983, 1984).

Endotheliochorial Placentation in the African Elephant (*Loxodonta africana*)

Site of first attachment	antimesometrial
Depth of attachment	superficial
Yolk sac orientation	mesometrial
Choriovitelline placenta	temporary, large
Splanchnopleuric yolk sac	temporary? (see text below), small, free

Chorioallantoic placenta

Shape	complete zonary? (see discussion below)
Pattern	labyrinthine
Interhemal membrane	endotheliochorial
Nonvillous chorioallantois	present
Allantoic sac	permanent, four-lobed, large
Distinguishing features	narrow placental hilus, fan-shaped evaginating maternal stromal folds in girdle zone, verrucae or pustules or buttons on chorioallantois.

Our current understanding on the placentation of African elephants comes from the early efforts of Perry and Amoroso (Perry 1953; Amoroso and Perry, 1964; Perry, 1974) and much more recently from Allen et al. (2003). The salient features of their observations are presented here. However, for a more detailed account on elephant placentation, the readers are directed to the above references. Though the placenta of the African elephant is the principal focus of discussion here, it has been noted from afterbirths of *Elephas indicus* that the placenta of Indian (Asiatic) elephants is similar to that of their African counterparts (Cooper, 1964).

The early conceptus of the elephant becomes lodged within one of the three to four star-shaped grooves of the uterus (Amoroso and Perry, 1964). The shape of the uterine lumen is believed to be due to high toncity experienced within the uterine horns at this stage. The pregnancy in the elephant is typically confined to one uterine horn and the growing fetus does not seem to encroach into the uterine body or the non-gravid uterine horn. As pregnancy advances, the allantoic sac transforms into an enormous four-lobed sac that vascularizes the entire chorion as well as the amnion (Amoroso and Perry, 1964). The umbilical cord attaches mesometrially.

Implantation of the conceptus begins with the development of a ribbon-like girdle zone in the equatorial region of the fetus, similar to carnivores. There are conflicting reports about the extent of girdle formation. Mossman reported that the annular ring of the girdle zone is incomplete in the embryonic disc zone (Mossman, 1987). However, the more recent observations by Allen et al. (2003) contradicts this. According to their observations, the lamellate zone in the girdle is ring-shaped and is complete. It appears pale initially, but with advancing pregnancy it becomes reddish brown in color. The marginal hemophagous zones that form later appear brown in color.

Due to the development of a zonary placenta along with marginal hematomas, the placental membranes of the African elephant have been likened to the zonary placenta of carnivores. Mossman, however, contends that the fetal membranes of the elephant (African or Asiatic) are not as close to those of carnivores as they might appear grossly. The first underlying reasons for his argument is that the source of maternal blood for the hemophagous organ is different from the carnivore placenta. The source of blood in the elephant is the ruptured blood vessels of the endotheliochorial labyrinth (Amoroso and Perry, 1964). This is different from the endometrial origins in the carnivore placenta (Leiser and Kobb, 1993). Second, the yolk sac is absent at term in elephants, as opposed to the free and permanent yolk sac in carnivores (Amoroso and Perry, 1964; Leiser and Kobb, 1993). The yolk sac in elephants is oriented mesometrially and disappears early in development, when the fetus weighs about 10 gm (Mossman, 1987). Other major differences are presented below.

One of the characteristic features of the lamellate zone of the elephant fetus is that there is no invasion of trophectoderm much beyond the line of maternal endometrial epithelia (see Figure 12.7a). Instead, as Allen et al. (2003) describe, there is an induction of an upward growth of the maternal endometrium and its associated vasculature into the invested trophectoderm. Additionally, the trophectoderm in the girdle zone remains cellular at all stages of gestation observed.

There is no syncytia formation as seen in the carnivore placenta (Leiser, 1982). The trophectoderm in the initial stages of lamellogenesis is seen apposed, but not attached to the luminal epithelium. It later develops finger-like projections which penetrate the luminal epithelium and uproot it in the form of sheets from the underlying basement membrane. This uprooted luminal epithelium is later engulfed by the expanding trophoblast. It also needs to be noted here that the uterine epithelium does not fuse laterally with other epithelial cells and form *symplasma*, as has been noticed in cats (Leiser, 1982) and other carnivores. The basement membrane of the endometrial epithelium persists and is analogous to the *interhemal membrane* of the carnivores.

As the trophoblast is advancing, there seem to be a simultaneous "frond-like" protrusion of the maternal stroma growing vertically from the endometrium, as a result of blood vessels and capillaries projecting into them (see Figure 12.7a). These stromal folds elongate and become plate-like and branch out extensively, resulting in an increase in the area of contact with the trophectoderm. Allen et al. (2003) compared these formations to a "fan shape of displaying peacock tail".

With the advancement of pregnancy, the gross thickness and complexity of the lamellate zone increases. This expansion seems to stem from the elongation and branching of the stromal folds that have formed initially, rather than from the development of new stromal outgrowths. With the elongation of the maternal stromal folds, the extracellular matrix stretches out and becomes thin, reducing the interhemal distance to less than 3 µm (see Figure 12.7b) (Allen et al., 2003). These changes, therefore, bring the trophectoderm along with its capillary network in close apposition with the endothelia of maternal blood vessels (Allen et al., 2003).

At the edges of the enlarging placental band, the elongating placental lamellae fold sideways on to the endometrial surface forming channels which are later filled with the maternal blood extravasated from the blood vessels within the lamellate zone (see Figure 12.7a). The trophoblast cells exposed to the maternal blood in the extravasate zone are involved in active phagocytosis of blood cells, becoming engorged in the process. They appear "flocculent" due to the digestion of these blood cells and therefore constitute a major route for transfer of iron to the growing fetus. These lateral hemophagous zones continue to grow as the pregnancy advances in the fetus (Allen et al., 2003).

A more surprising aspect of elephant placentation as Allen et al. (2003) have noted, is the narrowness of the placental hilus that initially forms during the sprouting of the stromal folds. Though the lamellate girdle zone increases in width to more than 12 cm and attains a thickness up to 4 cm, the original hilus, which is about 2 to 4 cm in width,

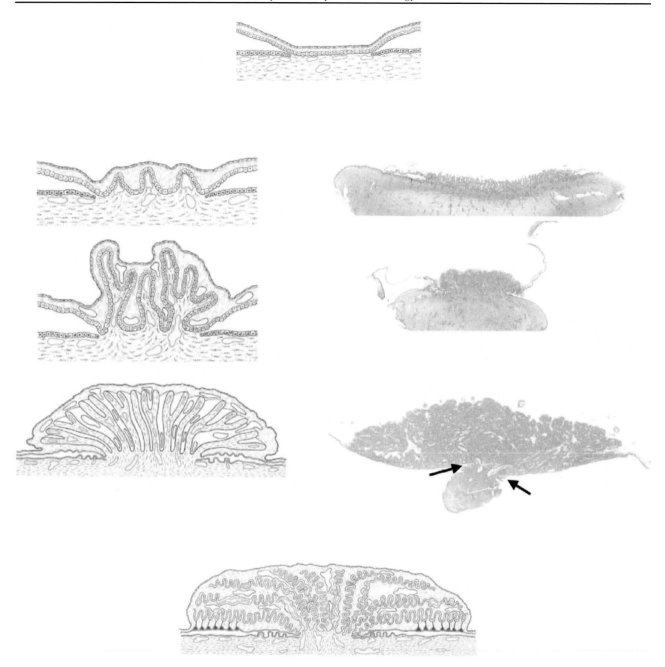

Figure 12.7a. Illustrations and histological sections representing different stages of endotheliochorial placentation in the elephant. Top panel: replacement of the uterine lumenal epithelium by trophoblasts in the equatorial region. Left side panels: illustrations demonstrating the upgrowth, elongation, and subsequent branching of uterine stromal villi above the endometrial surface. Right side panels: histological sections for the developmental stages shown on the left. Moving from top to bottom, they were collected from 1.6 g, 5.15 g, and 120 g fetuses, respectively. The **arrows** indicate the narrow hilus that connects the placenta and the endometrium. Bottom panel: illustration of a mature placenta; leaking of maternal blood into the lateral clefts (arising from the extensive elongation of the stromal lamellae) creates the hemophagus zones. Illustrations and histological sections from Allen et al., 2003.

does not seem to increase proportionately. More significantly, this original hilus zone carries all the maternal blood vessels that form an intensive network within the lamellate zone (see Figure 12.7a).

Therefore, it is not surprising that there is intense bleeding during parturition when the fetus, along with the after-birth, is ripped off in one instance from the zone of attachment, the hilus of the uterus. Parturition in the elephant appears to be effortless, as the mother assumes a standing posture. The sheer weight of the fetus forces the breakage of afterbirth from the uterus to pass through the vaginal canal (Allen et al., 2003).

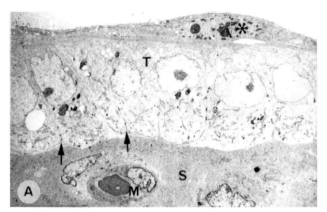
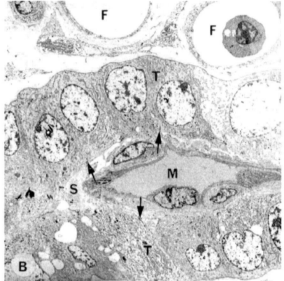
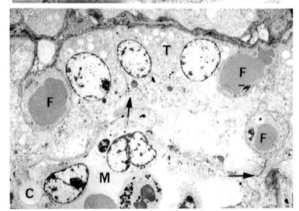

Figure 12.7b. Electron micrographs of the elephant fetal-maternal interface. **A:** embryonic day 17 showing trophoblast (**T**) with endoderm (*) in direct apposition to maternal uterine stroma (**S**). **Arrows** indicate apical junctional complexes between the trophoblasts. The maternal capillaries (**M**) are indicated. **B:** placenta image from a conceptus with a 5.15 g fetus. The trophoblasts surround some of the maternal capillaries; a thin layer of maternal stroma is present. Fetal capillaries (**F**) are visible. **C:** placenta image from a conceptus with a 44 kg fetus. In a mature placenta, the fetal capillaries indent the trophoblast layer, which still contains apical junctional complexes and completely encompasses the endothelium of the maternal capillaries. Images from Allen, 2003.

The placenta of elephants also has unusual structures called *verrucae* or pustules or buttons on the inner side of the chorioallantoic surface. These are made of numerous blood vessels enmeshed within loose mesenchyme. Besides verrucae, the placenta also possesses polypoid-like structures that might have arisen from these pustules (Amoroso and Perry, 1964; Allen et al., 2003).

Epitheliochorial Placentation

The epitheliochorial type of placenta is only found in a couple of phylogenetic orders and likely represents a more recently evolved placenta type. Even so, striking differences exist between species with epitheliochorial placentas, for example, the placentas of swine and equids. Descriptions for placentas from several species that possess epitheliochorial placentas are described below.

Epitheliochorial Placentation of Swine (*Sus scrofa*)

Site of first attachment	mesometrial
Depth of attachment	superficial
Yolk sac orientation	mesometrial
Choriovitelline placenta	temporary
Splanchnopleuric yolk sac	temporary, small and free
Chorioallantoic placenta	
Shape	diffuse
Pattern	villous
Interhemal membrane	epitheliochorial
Nonvillous chorioallantois	small, irregular at the tips of the extraembryonic membranes
Allantoic sac	permanent, large
Distinguishing features	areolae and arcades

Perhaps the most basic and simple chorioallantoic placentation of eutherian mammals exists in swine. Therefore, it often serves as a model for comparison when studying placentation in other eutherian mammals. Porcine blastocysts escape their zonas early in the second week of pregnancy and begin to enlarge. By 10 dpc they form spherical vesicles of 8 to 10 mm in diameter (see Figure 12.8a) (Perry, 1981; King, 1993b). During this stage, the conceptuses are distributed evenly within the uterine lumen by active peristaltic movements of the myometrium, which fade gradually as the blastocyst becomes fixed in position (Keye, 1923).

The conceptuses begin to elongate from day 12 of the approximately 114-day gestation period. This results in elongated, slender blastocysts that can reach a length of 1 m or longer (see Figure 12.8a) (Heuser and Streeter, 1929; Patten, 1948; Anderson, 1978; Perry, 1981). They form highly convoluted structures that occupy a relatively small portion within the uterine horn. The elongated blastocysts now make contact with neighboring conceptuses. This distribution seems to be a function of contact with neighboring conceptuses, since the length of the conceptus tends to be larger in pregnancies with fewer conceptuses (Perry, 1981). On average there must be at least four viable conceptuses

present for the pregnancy to proceed much beyond the third week.

In swine, conceptus-derived estrogen is essential to change the course of secretion of the antiluteolytic compound, prostaglandin ($PGF_{2\alpha}$), from an endocrine pattern (into the maternal circulation) to an exocrine secretory pattern (into the uterine lumen). The result is that this luteolysin fails to gain access to the corpora lutea to cause their demise (Dhindsa and Dziuk, 1968; Perry, 1973; Perry, 1976; Bazer and Thatcher, 1977; Bazer, 1982; Geisert, 1982b; Bazer, 1984).

The rapid increase in the length of the pig conceptus to form a convoluted thread by day 12 is accompanied by only a minor concomitant increase in DNA or RNA synthesis or cell division, which suggests that the initial extensive elongation is mainly due to cellular rearrangements (Geisert,

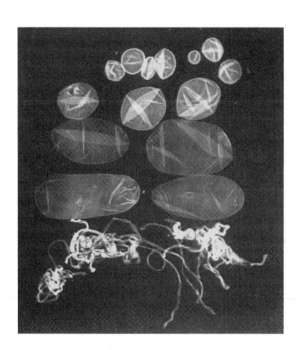

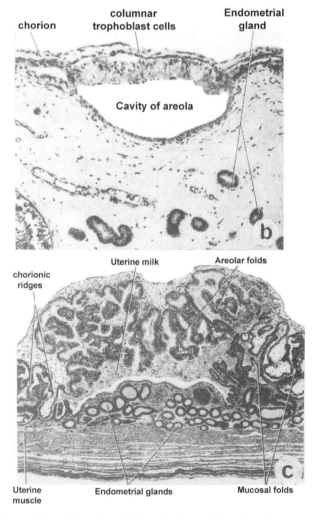

Figure 12.8a. Early conceptus development in swine and the establishment of specialized trophoblasts for the uptake of uterine gland secretions. Left panel: picture illustrating the transition of porcine conceptuses from small spherical to long filamentous structures. From Roberts and Bazer, 1988. Right panels: the development of specialized absorptive trophoblasts over the openings of uterine glands and the development of areola. The top panel was taken from a 23 dpc conceptus and the bottom panel was taken from a mature placenta at 111 dpc. From Wooding and Flint, 1994.

1982a; Mattson, 1990). The attachment of conceptuses to the endometrium is initiated at this stage and is usually accompanied by hyperemia of the uterus (Perry and Rowlands, 1962). The attachment is underway by day 18 with a transient loss of microvilli on the trophectoderm, presumably to facilitate closer association between the maternal and fetal layers (Keys and King, 1990). Once the union between the chorion and the uterine epithelial cells is achieved, the chorionic microvilli quickly reform and interdigitate with microvilli on uterine epithelial cells (Dantzer, 1985; Hasselager, 1985).

These noticeable external developments correspond with marked internal reorganization. For a more detailed perusal of these events, the readers are referred to an excellent review by Perry (1981). The mesodermal primordium originates as ectoderm erupting from the primitive streak that spreads between the endoderm and ectoderm separating them. This mesoderm contributes to both embryonic and extraembryonic mesenchyme.

Immediately following the generation of the extraembryonic mesoderm, a cavity forms as mesoderm begins lining both the extraembryonic endoderm and ectoderm, respectively. This cavity is referred to as *extraembryonic coelom* or *exocoele* (see Figure 12.8b). The mesoderm associated with the overlying trophoblast forms the *somatopluere* or chorion. The chorion adjacent to the embryonic disc develops evaginations known as amniotic folds that grow and subsequently converge over the embryonic disc, forming the amniotic sac around the fetus. It eventually loses contact with the chorion (see Figure 12.8b).

The embryonic disc at this stage transforms from a saucer-shaped structure into a tubular form and is contiguous with the developing yolk sac on the ventral side. The endoderm of the yolk sac together with the mesoderm overlying it constitute the bilaminar splanchnopluere which eventually reaches the chorion and establishes contact with it. The mesoderm of the yolk sac becomes vascularized, forming a choriovitelline placenta that is transient. The expanding exocoelom separates the yolk sac from chorion and by day 20 the yolk sac becomes inconspicuous (see Figure 12.8b).

An evagination from the posterior of the hindgut, which is called the allantois, develops. It is an endodermal derivative and is lined by mesoderm. The initial cylindrical allantois following the segregation of yolk sac from chorion fills the entire exocoelom and subsequently associates with chorion, forming the chorioallantois (see Figure 12.8b). The mesoderm of the allantois eventually becomes vascularized, establishing the definitive pig placenta.

The chorion of the porcine placenta forms neither a syncytium with the maternal epithelium (as for ruminant ungulates, see below) nor is there any compelling evidence of trophoblasts migrating or invading into the endometrium (Dantzer, 1985). An intact uterine epithelium persists throughout gestation, and therefore the porcine placenta is an epitheliochorial type (see Figure 12.8c).

The area of contact between the placenta and the endometrium reaches a maximum at midgestation, at which point it declines until term (Dantzer and Nielsen, 1984). Initial associations with the uterine epithelium begin adjacent to the embryo and spreads, toward the extreme ends of the conceptus. During the fourth week, the chorion evolves villi that penetrate into troughs within the endometrium to increase the intimacy and complexity of association (Michael, 1985; Wigmore and Strickland, 1985). The fetal and maternal villi become narrower on the sides and tips as development proceeds (Steven, 1983). The villi are lined by extensive vascular networks that progressively indent them, resulting in an effective decline of interhemal distance to as little as $2\,\mu m$ as opposed to 20 to $100\,\mu m$ at the base of the villi (see Figure 12.8c) (Steven, 1983; Wooding and Flint, 1994). The net result is a considerable increase in the surface area and a minimal barrier for diffusion.

The chorionic membranes adjacent to the mouths of the uterine glands become corrugated, forming specialized regions for nutrient uptake called areolae (see Figure 12.8a) (Amoroso, 1952). These areolae serve to locally enhance the surface area for absorption of glandular secretions (King, 1982). They are lined by specialized trophectodermal cells that actively uptake secretions of the glands which are important for fetal growth. Although the placenta is fully formed by day 30, the areolae continue to increase in number and size throughout gestation (see Figure 12.8a) (Dantzer, 1981; Friess, 1981). By term, around 7,000 evenly spaced areolae are observed per fetus. These areolae constitute about 10 percent of the total absorptive surface by mid-gestation, almost tripling in area until term (Brambel, 1933). The areolae represent an important structural modification for nutrient acquisition in swine and other species, such as the horse, with epitheliochorial placentas.

These species rely heavily on histotrophic nutrition, especially for macromolecules and metals, such as iron, that cannot easily traverse the interhemal membrane (Gitlin, 1964; Baker and Morgan, 1970). The secretions of the uterine glands are rich in these macromolecules and are comparable to an "enriched embryo culture medium" (Roberts and Bazer, 1988). In species such as lagomorphs and humans with hemochorial placentas, the chorion comes in direct contact with maternal blood and actively takes up macromolecules by means of receptors and coated pits present on their cell surface (Whyte, 1980; Malassine, 1987; Bright, 1994). For example, they have receptors for transferrin on their apical surface which conjugates with circulating transferrin- iron complexes, subsequently internalizing it and releasing iron inside the cells (Faulk and Galbraith, 1979; Wada, 1979; Turkewitz and Harrison, 1989).

In swine, the lack of direct access to maternal blood is circumvented by copious secretion of nutrients by the uterine glands throughout pregnancy. For instance, the iron complexed in a specialized acid phosphatase glycoprotein

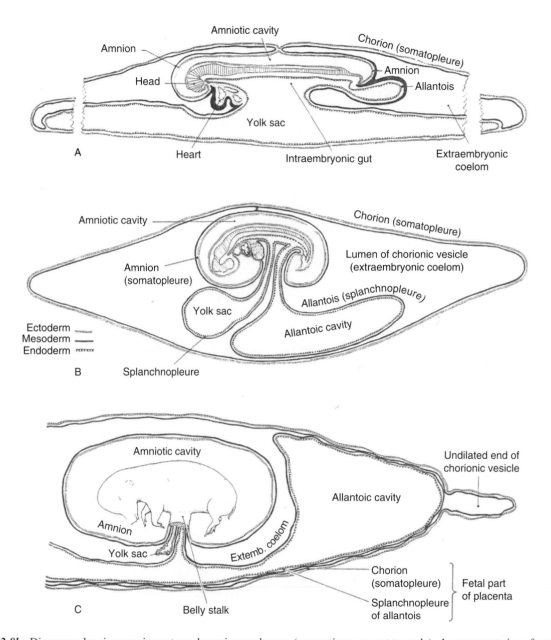

Figure 12.8b. Diagrams showing porcine extraembryonic membranes (proportions are not to scale). **A:** representative of embryos with 15 to 20 somites. **B:** representative of embryos 4 to 6 mm in length. **C:** representative of embryos approximately 30 mm in crown-rump length. From Carlson, 1981.

called uteroferrin is secreted in large quantities (up to 1 gm can be recovered on day 60) via uterine glands from day 35 until day 105 of gestation (Palludan, 1969; Murray, 1972; Chen, 1973; Chen, 1975; Basha, 1979; Roberts and Bazer, 1980; Buhi, 1982). According to the accepted model, secreted uteroferrin is subsequently picked up by the chorioallantois. The uteroferrin in the allantoic sac (Bazer, 1975) then transfers the iron to fetal transferrin via a low-

molecular-weight intermediary. This fetal transferrin then distributes iron to the developing fetus (Buhi, 1982).

Epitheliochorial Placenta of the Domestic Horse (*Equus caballus*)

Site of first attachment	mesometrial
Depth of attachment	superficial
Yolk sac orientation	mesometrial

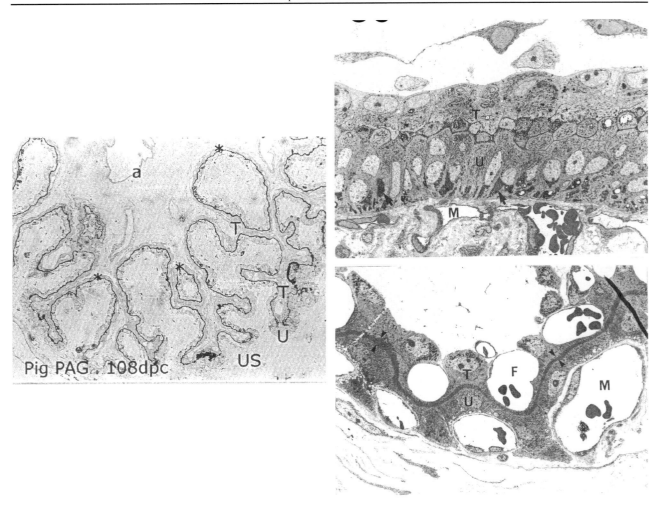

Figure 12.8c. Histological sections of the fetal-maternal interface in domestic pigs. Left panel: immunocytochemistry of a 108 dpc pig placenta with an antibody to the trophoblast product, porcine pregnancy-associated glycoprotein 2. The intense staining highlights the microvillar junction between cellular trophoblasts (**T**) and the intact uterine epithelial cells (**U**). From Wooding, 2005. Right panels: electron micrographs of the fetal-maternal interface at 16 dpc (top) and 109 dpc (bottom). Of particular interest is the narrow diffusion distance between the fetal (**F**) and maternal (**M**) capillaries in the mature placenta. From Wooding and Flint, 1994.

Choriovitelline placenta	temporary, large
Splanchnopleuric yolk sac	temporary
Chorioallantoic placenta	
Shape	diffuse
Pattern	villous
Interhemal membrane	epitheliochorial
Nonvillous chorioallantois	small areas at uterotubal junctions and cervix
Allantoic sac	permanent, very large
Unique cell types	chorionic girdle cells
Distinguishing features	microcotyledons, endometrial cups

The equine conceptus sheds its zona pellucida by day 9 (the equine pregnancy lasts 315 to 360 days) but it remains enclosed in a noncellular capsule, which does not dissolve until about day 22 (Betteridge, 1982; Steven, 1982; Ginther, 1992). Consequently, the equine conceptus never achieves the long filamentous structure developed in ruminants and swine, but rather, it persists as a spherical structure for a much longer time relative to other livestock species (King, 1993b).

Furthermore, the equine conceptus is quite mobile, traversing both horns several times daily, prior to becoming fixed in position by day 16 of pregnancy (van Niekerk and Allen, 1975; Ginther, 1983a, 1983b). In fact, this mobility during the first two weeks of gestation is required for the maintenance of the pregnancy. The pregnancy generally fails if the mobility of the conceptus is restricted (Ginther, 1983a; McDowell, 1988). The mobility of the conceptus permits access to most of the uterine lumen and is probably functionally analogous to the extensive conceptus elongation observed in ruminant ungulates (described below) and swine (described above).

By day 20, erythropoesis and angiogenesis is noticeable within the yolk sac and by day 22 a fetal circulation is becoming established (Enders and Liu, 1991a). Many significant events such as amniogenesis, establishment of a choriovitelline circulation, and the rupture of the capsule coincide on day 22 (Enders and Liu, 1991a). This does not seem to be a mere coincidence, but rather appear to be scrupulously orchestrated events that initiate feto-maternal exchange. The allantois is visible at this stage as a small diverticulum and does not dislocate the yolk sac, but by day 32 it begins to do so. The embryo, though initially aligned antimesometrially, will now be displaced mesometrially by the expanding allantois. By day 38 the allantois vascularizes approximately 90 percent of the chorion and fuses with it to form the chorioallantois (Steven, 1982).

In the horse, the association between the chorion and the luminal epithelia becomes quite convoluted and complex as pregnancy progresses. Microvilli from the chorionic surface penetrate into endometrial invaginations. However, unlike the pig, the microvilli undergo extensive secondary and tertiary branching which is complemented by corresponding invaginations of the uterine epithelium (Baur, 1977). The result is the formation of microcotyledons that serve to dramatically increase the surface area between the fetal and maternal tissues to promote the exchange of nutrients and metabolites (see Figure 12.9a) (Samuel, 1974; Steven, 1982).

By day 150, the placenta consists of thousands of small globular microcotyledons, each 1 to 2 mm in diameter and packed closely together in the endometrium. It should be noted, however, that these structures are distinct from the cotyledons of ruminants (see below). They are much more extensive in number and considerably smaller than ruminant cotyledons (see Figure 12.9a). Furthermore, there is

no erosion of the luminal epithelium. Therefore, like the pig, equids have an epitheliochorial placenta (Mossman, 1987).

Chorionic Girdle Cells and Endometrial Cups of Equine Placenta

One of the distinguishing characteristics of the equine placenta is the existence of an invasive population of cells within the chorion known as chorionic girdle cells. They are a strip of specialized trophoblast cells that appear at the margin between the yolk sac and the chorioallantois and extend around the spherical conceptus (see Figure 12.9b) (Allen, 1982; Enders and Liu, 1991a). The chorionic girdle, which is visible by day 25, attains its maximum width by day 35 and develops extensive folds and ridges that project into folds within the uterine lining. The cells are initially tall and columnar and by day 32 become stratified (Enders and Liu, 1991a).

By day 34 the binucleate cells within the girdle begin to migrate across the maternal-fetal interface to penetrate the uterine epithelium and enter the underlying stroma (Allen, 1973; Enders and Liu, 1991b). As the superficial layer of cells make their way into the maternal stroma through the luminal epithelium they become separated from the basal layers. By day 37 to day 38, many of the cells that were not able to make contact with the uterine epithelium to pass through the luminal barrier begin to degenerate. Once within the maternal stroma, the girdle cells do not proliferate but instead enlarge and coalesce to form the endometrial cups (see Figure 12.9b). Those regions of uterine epithelium destroyed by the girdle cell invasion are quickly regenerated to cover the endometrial cups (Enders and Liu, 1991b). Consequently, the endometrial cups are not attached to the placenta; instead, they are differentiated cell bodies buried within the uterine stroma.

The endometrial cups are endocrine cells that synthesize a powerful gonadotropin, equine chorionic gonadotropin (eCG). The amount of eCG produced seems to be positively correlated with the number of chorionic girdle cells and the latter is a function of genotype. For example, fetuses generated by stallion-mare matings produce much larger cups than either jack-jenny or stallion-jenny matings (Allen, 1982).

Equine CG is a placental form of luteinizing hormone (LH) and is produced from about day 40 to day 100 of pregnancy (Ginther, 1983a; Sherman, 1992). Equine CG is believed to stimulate the ovulation or luteinization of follicles to promote the development of secondary or accessory corpora lutea (Urwin and Allen, 1982). The level of eCG within the maternal circulation peaks around day 70, then declines steadily until it is no longer detectable after day 150 (Ginther, 1992). By the end of the first trimester, maternal leukocytes begin to attack the endometrial cups causing them to become necrotic and to slough into the uterine lumen (Allen, 1973; Allen, 1982).

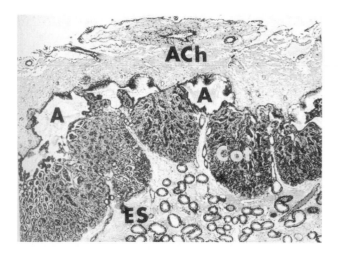

Figure 12.9a. Histological section of a mature equine placenta showing the microcotyledons (**Cot**) and areolae (**A**) over the mouths of the uterine glands in the endometrial stroma (**ES**). **ACh:** allantochorion. From Bjorkman, 1970.

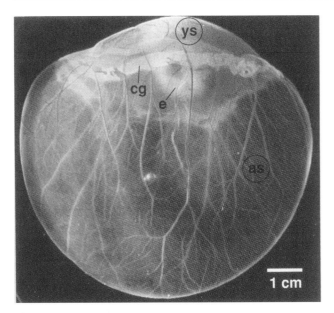 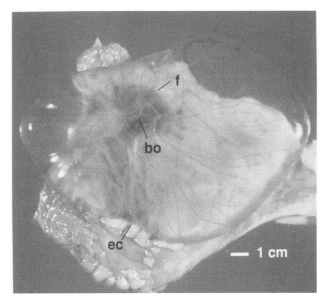

Figure 12.9b. Placentation in the horse. Left panel: a 36 dpc horse conceptus possessing a strip of specialized chorionic girdle (**cg**) trophoblasts; (**e**) embryo; (**ys**) yolk sac. Right panel: a 60 dpc conceptus that has been partially separated from the endometrium; (**ec**) endometrial cups; (**f**) fetus; (**bo**) bilaminar omphlampleur. From Ginther, 1992.

Following the demise of the endometrial cups, and the accessory corpora lutea, the placenta takes over the production of progesterone for the remainder of the pregnancy. Beyond progesterone, the placenta of horses also produce unique unsaturated estrogens referred to as *equilin* and *equilenin* (Allen, 1975; Pashen, 1983; Haluska and Currie, 1988).

Placentation in Rhinocerotidae (*Rhinoceros unicornis, Diceros bicornis*)

Depth of attachment	superficial
Splanchnopleuric yolk sac	permanent, small
Chorioallantoic placenta	
Pattern	villous (complex villi)
Interhemal membrane	epitheliochorial
Allantoic sac	permanent, large

A comprehensive description of placenta in rhinocerotidae has been provided by Benirshke and Lowenstein (1995). Some of the important observations of their discussion are presented here. The placenta of the rhinoceros is diffuse and epitheliochorial. Of the five different species of rhinoceros, the placenta of the Indian rhinoceros (Lang, 1957; Ludwig and Muller, 1965) and the African rhinoceros (Ludwig, 1962) have been studied in some detail. However, almost all studies have been performed on the "afterbirth" or delivered placenta and there have been no reported *in utero* studies. Therefore, the timing of implantation and earliest embryonic events remain largely unknown.

The placenta of rhinos extends into both horns of the uterus, whereas the fetus is confined to one. The allantois fills the entire exoceoleom and vascularizes both the amnion and chorion. The umbilical cord is attached in the region of the junction of the two horns and ruptures before birth.

The most comprehensive work on Indian rhinoceros placenta has been performed by Ludwig et al. (Ludwig and Muller, 1965). These authors identified areas of denuded villus formation called "streets" and hence described the placenta as *placenta villosa diffusa incompleta*. These villus-free streets are the regions where the allantois and chorion are supposedly anchored by thin fibers. They also seem to attach large vessels that traverse this space (Dolinar, 1965).

Two types of villi, the leaf-like villi and the folded villi, have been reported in the rhino placenta. The epithelium lining the former is cuboidal and that lining the latter is columnar. The leaf-like villi are likened to the villi of equids (Amoroso, 1952; Dolinar, 1965; Ludwig and Villiger, 1965). Occasional binucleate trophoblastic cells, possibly analogous to those of bovine and equine placentas, have been reported but there are no indications that they invade the maternal endometrium (Ludwig and Muller, 1965). Based on these observations it was claimed that the rhino placenta is intermediate between cattle and horse placentas. However, such a position cannot be justified until more detailed histological evidence is collected.

The gross thickness of the rhinoceros placenta is never greater than 3 μm and is even thinner in the regions of the streets (Dolinar, 1965). In some species, the amnion and or allantois contain pustules which accumulate urinary wastes within the allantoic sac and develop into olive green or brown crystal-laden *hippomanes*. These structures either remain attached to the allantois or remain free.

Epitheliochorial Placentation in Camelidae (*Camelus bactrianus, C. dromedarius, Lama guanicoe, L. glama, L. pacos, Vicugna vicugna*)

Depth of attachment	superficial
Choriovitelline placenta	temporary
Splanchnopleuric yolk sac	temporary, small and free

Chorioallantoic placenta

Shape	diffuse
Pattern	villous, short branched villi
Interhemal membrane	epitheliochorial
Allantoic sac	permanent, large
Unique cell types	unique multinucleated giant cells

Camelids have a diffuse epitheliochorial placenta. The blastocyst is spherical in shape in the earlier stages of development, and it elongates in due course (Tibary, 1997). By 14 dpc, the trophoblast appears as a single layer of epithelial cells with free microvilli on the apical border. The luminal epithelial cells also possess microvilli on their interactive surface.

During the apposition phase, the surface microvilli are lost on both the luminal epithelium and trophoblast and are drawn even closer to one another by the loss of glycocalyx. Soon after, the microvilli reappear in the apposing epithelia, becoming interdigitated to reinforce the attachment (Abd-Elnaeim, 1999). The trophoblast cells do not seem to form apical junctional complexes with the luminal epithelium nor do they invade it. These events are similar to placentation in the pig. However, the penetration of the villi into the glands as seen in pig placentation is absent in camels.

At 25 dpc, the enlarging allantoic sac displaces the yolk sac from the trophoblast surface. The yolk sac subsequently shrinks and remains vestigial (Skidmore, 1996). By 30 dpc,

implantation is complete in camels (in the alpaca and llama it is complete by day 22) (Tibary, 1997).

Vasculogenesis in the allantois quickly follows, establishing a functional chorioallantoic placenta. In later stages of gestation numerous folds appear in the chorioallantoic and endometrial surface, which significantly increase the interacting surface for exchange and also strengthen the attachment.

Pregnancies are typically established in the left uterine horn in camels. There are reports demonstrating that embryos placed in the right horn migrate and subsequently inhabit the left uterine horn (Ghazi, 1994; Tibary, 1997; Sumar, 1999). However, by 56 dpc the placenta expands to fill the right uterine horn as well.

The placenta of camelids is highly vascularized. As the pregnancy advances, the capillaries of the blood vessels indent the epithelia of both the chorioallantois and endometrium. The endothelia of the fetal blood vessels and epithelia become progressively thin and as a result, the interhemal distance can become reduced to as little as 2 μm.

Camelids possess a unique population of multinucleate giant cells that are apparent by day 35 (van Lennep, 1963; Skidmore, 1996). Skidmore et al. provided histological evidence to suggest that the multinucleate cells originated by the fusion of mononucleate trophectoderm cells. These giant cells are found in isolated areas of trophectoderm and a significant percentage tend to predominate in the areolae-like structures found over glandular orifices by day 35 (see Figure 12.10). Though the abundance of giant cells drops markedly in the second half of pregnancy, a significant percentage still persists until term.

The origin of the giant cells of camels and their purported function is the subject of some debate. Skidmore

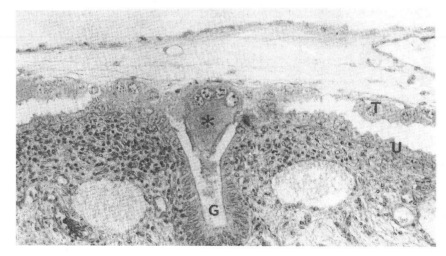

Figure 12.10. Histological section of the placenta-uterine interface of camels. Multinucleated giant trophoblast cells (*) have been described; these are often spotted over the mouths of endometrial glands (**G**). **T**: trophoblast. **U**: uterine epithelium. From Skidmore, 1996.

et al. have argued that the giant cells of camels are different from the binucleate cells of ruminants and horses because they are neither migratory nor invasive (Skidmore, 1996). Based on the current available evidence, they also seem to possess an extensive secretory capacity (Allen and Moor, 1972; Allen, 1973; Wooding, 1982a, 1983; Wooding, 1992; Skidmore, 1996). Furthermore, they seem to differ from rodent giant cells in that they are generated by the fusion of trophoblast cells rather than by endoreduplication (Deane, 1962).

The distribution of these cells suggests an absorptive role. This is because the giant cells tend to predominantly populate the blood vessels of the chorioallantois or the areolae, along with the absorptive columnar trophoblast cells (Skidmore, 1996). However, it is important to note that this claim is circumstantial, because there is no direct evidence to support it. Another interesting hypothesis regarding their function involves constitutive secretion of protein or steroid compounds. However, regulated secretion of proteins by these cells is ruled out because there are no requisite secretory granules or enlarged golgi bodies within their cytoplasm (Skidmore, 1996). There are also some reports of binucleate cells in the camelid placenta (Gorokhovskii, 1975). Whether these cells represent intermediates in the generation of multinucleate giant cells or constitute a unique subpopulation of trophoblasts remains to be determined.

Hippomanes seem to be a common occurrence in the allantoic sac of camelids. A more interesting feature of camelid placentation, however, is the occurrence of a so called "fourth" placental membrane or *epidermal membrane*. It is supposedly a derivative of the squamous surface of the embryo that adheres to its mucocutaneous junctions. Histologically, it is made of squamous cells and has no connective tissue; therefore it is likely a pseudomembrane (Fowler and Olander, 1990; Fowler, 1998).

Diffuse Epitheliochorial Placentation in Bush Babies (*Galago crassicaudata*)

Site of first attachment	mesometrial
Depth of attachment	superficial
Yolk sac orientation	mesometrial
Choriovitelline placenta	large, temporary
Splanchnopleuric yolk sac	temporary
Chorioallantoic placenta	
Shape	diffuse
Pattern	villous
Interhemal membrane	epitheliochorial
Nonvillous chorioallantois	at cervix
Allantoic sac	very large, lobed
Distinguishing features	chorionic vesicles

Bush babies, along with lorises, lemurs, aye-ayes, and related animals, are referred to as *prosimians*. They are the inhabitants of Madagascar and Southeast Asia and, with the exception of tarsiers, are placed in the same suborder (Strepsirrhini). Mossman (1987) described the placenta of

bush babies as an equid type because it is diffuse and epitheliochorial, similar to that of horses (and pigs) (Enders, 1965). Their placentas also possess additional characteristics such as the presence of a temporary and free yolk sac orientated mesometrially and a large allantoic sac (Mossman, 1987).

The similarity of prosimian placentas with those of horses and swine is a very interesting observation. Bush babies belong to the same phylogenetic order (Anthropoidea) as humans and other great apes; these species possess invasive hemochorial placentas (Enders, 1965). Therefore, this situation constitutes one of the common paradoxes of placentation in eutherian evolution, in which related species, often within the same order, can have drastically different placental (chorioallantoic) organization.

The fine structure of the *Galago crassicaudata* placenta has been described in detail by King (1984). The epitheliochorial placenta is diffuse, with the chorionic villi evenly distributed over the entire placenta. Microvilli are observed on the surface of trophoblast cells which closely interdigitate with the microvilli on the uterine epithelium. The chorionic villi also closely align with maternal crypts or folds, as seen in the pig. The chorionic epithelium is supplied with an abundant supply of fetal blood vessels that can indent the epithelium in the advanced stages of pregnancy (105 dpc of 132-day gestation period).

The trophoblast cells over the capillaries in these regions become attenuated with fewer organelles. However, the endothelial cells of the fetal blood vessels remain continuous at all stages of pregnancy. In contrast, the maternal capillaries indenting the uterine luminal epithelium appear collapsed with occasional fenestrae on their surface. In addition to these, prominent pits are identified at the tip and the base of the villi. These pits are lined by trophoblast cells which are columnar, as opposed to the cuboidal cells over the remainder of the chorionic epithelium. These structural changes in the interacting sides in late gestation serve to improve the diffusion of material across the interhemal barrier.

Chorionic Vesicles of Bush Baby Placenta

In the regions opposite the uterine glands, specialized invaginations appear on the chorion, which are referred to as *chorionic vesicles* (see Figure 12.11). These structures are functionally analogous to the areolae of pig and horse placentas. The chorionic vesicles are overlaid by a single layer of columnar epithelial cells which have numerous microvilli on their surface along with coated pits and vesicles, suggesting an absorptive function (see Figure 12.11). The mesoderm of these vesicles possess a rich vasculature; however, the capillaries do not indent the epithelia in these zones. Another interesting feature is the presence of smooth muscle cells in the underlying mesoderm. The importance of these structures remains a mystery. The many characteristics of the chorionic vesicles point toward a role in histotrophic nutrition, actively taking up macromolecules in the

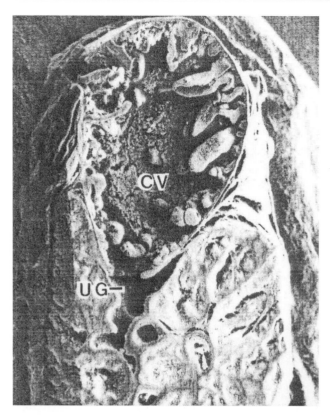

Figure 12.11. Electron micrograph of bush baby chorionic vesicle (**CV**) over the opening of a uterine gland (**UG**). Note the extensive trophoblastic villi along the wall of the vesicle. From King, 1984.

milieu secreted by the uterine glands (Amoroso, 1952; King, 1982).

Synepitheliochorial Placentation (Grosser's "Syndesmochorial" Placenta, Revised)

The synepitheliochorial placenta is found only in ruminant ungulates and appears to be an adaptive modification of the epitheliochorial type. In the following sections, particular attention is placed on those placenta features and cell types that distinguish the synepitheliochorial placenta from the epitheliochorial placenta.

Synepitheliochorial Placenta of Ruminant Ungulates
(***Bos taurus, Ovis aries, Capra hircus, Cervus elaphus barbarus, Tragulus javanicus***)

Site of first attachment	mesometrial
Depth of attachment	superficial
Yolk sac orientation	mesometrial
Choriovitelline placenta	temporary
Splanchnopleuric yolk sac	small, free, temporary

Chorioallantoic placenta

Shape	diffuse cotyledonary
Pattern	villous
Interhemal membrane	synepitheliochorial
Nonvillous chorioallantois	large
Allantoic sac	large
Unique cell types	moderately invasive binucleate cells
Distinguishing features	placentomes (fetal cotyledons plus uterine caruncles)

Grosser described the ruminant placenta as syndesmochorial with the assumption that the uterine epithelium was lost, leading to a direct apposition of trophoblast with maternal connective tissue (Grosser, 1909, 1927). Recently, as a result of detailed histological evidence accumulated by Wooding and others, it is now understood that the uterine epithelium can be altered but remains intact for the most part. Instead of an erosion of uterine epithelium, specialized trophoblasts (binucleate trophoblast cells) can fuse with uterine epithelial cells to form a feto-maternal syncytial cell layer (Wooding 1982a, 1982b, 1984). Hence, the term syndesmochorial placenta has been revised to the more accurate synepitheliochorial placentation, wherein "syn" stands for the feto-maternal syncytium and "epitheliochorial" signifies the persistence of a maternal epithelium at the fetal-maternal interface (Wooding, 1992).

In ruminant ungulates, the morula enters the uterus about day 4 to day 5 (Rowson and Moor, 1966). The blastocyst sheds the zona pelucida around day 8 or day 9 (Rowson and Moor, 1966), and becomes positioned in the center of the uterine horn ipsilateral to the ovulated ovary (Lee, 1977). Transuterine migration of blastocysts is rarely reported in cows, but is seen in 8 percent of the ewes with single ovulations (Scanlon, 1972). The positioning is predominantly due to myometrial contractions of the uterus.

Once positioned, the embryo does not implant immediately but instead, starting around day 10 (sheep) to day 12 (cattle) begins to elongate from a spherical form to a tubular form and eventually transforms into a filamentous structure (Wintenberger-Torres and Flechon, 1974; Betteridge, 1980; Spencer, 2004). The elongating embryo, by day 13 in sheep and day 15 in cattle, establishes firm apposition with the maternal epithelium by developing small chorionic villus projections or papillae that penetrate into the openings of the uterine glands (Wooding and Staples, 1981; Guillomot and Guay, 1982; Wooding, 1982). Interestingly, goats lack these papillae.

The conceptus then expands progressively and fills the entire uterus by day 16 in sheep and days 19 to 20 in cattle (Wintenberger-Torres and Flechon, 1974; Wales and Cuneo, 1989; King, 1993b). The pre-attachment phase is much longer than in the human and mouse, allowing for greater development prior to implantation. Not surprisingly then, ungulate embryos have a much greater reliance on uterine glandular secretions than do those species that implant immediately. Furthermore, once implantation does occur, it is not a blastocyst that implants but a much more differentiated conceptus.

Attachment and implantation begin near the embryonic disc and spread to the ends of the conceptus (King, 1982). The events of implantation are similar between sheep and cattle, although the events are delayed by two to three days in cattle. In sheep, the process is initiated with a transient loss of microvilli on the tropectodermal cells between 13 and 15 dpc; however, the microvilli remain intact on the luminal epithelium (Guillomot, 1981, 1982, 1993). This loss of microvilli in the chorion (trophectoderm) permits a close apposition of trophoblast with the luminal epithelium. By 16 dpc, the maternal microvilli begin to penetrate the folds of the chorionic cells. The microvilli on the trophoblast soon reappear and interdigitation begins by day 18 and is completed by day 22. In cattle it is completed by day 27 and in goats between days 25 and 28 (King, 1982).

In the regions of the maternal uterine caruncles (focally dense connective tissue formations covered by columnar epithelium), the initial attachments are reinforced and the surface area is increased due to the penetration of chorionic villi (cotyledons) into crypts within the caruncular endometrium. Lengthening and branching of the villi, along with coincident development of a blood supply in the expanding villi, results in the production of mature placentomes (see Figure 12.12a) (King, 1993a). Because the cotyledons are the most prominent feature of the mature ruminant placenta, it is often referred to as a cotyledonary placenta.

The *Tragulidae* family, which includes species such as the mouse deer, is an exception to this generalization. The mouse deer has a diffuse placenta with no caruncles or placentomes. To date, this is the only animal classified in the *Ruminantia* suborder that does not possess a cotyledonary placenta. However, these animals do possess binucleate trophoblast cells (described below) dispersed within the trophoblastic villi (Kimura, 2004). These observations suggest that the placenta of mouse deer represents an intermediate stage between the epitheliochorial placenta of swine and the derived cotyledonary synepitheliochorial placenta of most other ruminant ungulates.

The number of caruncles that are present within the uterus determines the maximum possible number of placentomes that can be established. This number is species-specific and is fixed at birth. It ranges from three to eight in deer to 20 to 150 in sheep, goats, and cattle (Mossman, 1987; Wooding and Flint, 1994). The decrease in the number of placentomes within deer is presumably offset by a corresponding increase in the size of individual placentomes. This also holds true for twin pregnancies in sheep and goats. Although in theory the twins have only about half the total number of available caruncles compared to singletons (though singletons do not use all the available caruncles), the individual size and total mass of placentomes is larger than that observed in singleton pregnancies. In fact, there is a positive correlation between placentomal mass and the size of the fetus (Bell, 1984, 1991; Wooding

and Flint, 1994). Across species, the placentomes also differ in gross morphology; they are convex in cattle, concave in sheep and goats, and flat in antelopes (Figure 12.12a).

The mature placentome develops an extensive blood supply and is the main site of exchange for easily diffusible nutrients. The caruncular regions are separated by glandular endometrium that is responsible for the secretion of large macromolecules into the uterine lumen. By the fourth week of pregnancy, absorptive areas form within the chorionic membrane over the uterine glands, providing further indication that the glandular regions are involved in the transport of larger, less soluble nutrients (Wilmsatt, 1950).

There are also reports of hemophagous zones within the placentomes of some species (see Figure 12.12a). They are presumably formed by the leakage of blood from the blood vessels at the base of the chorionic villi, subsequently undergoing hemolysis and forming colored deposits. These zones are thought to be an important source of iron for the growing fetus. However, these observations are somewhat inconsistent and there are no such zones in the placenta of the cow (Byorkman, 1969; Myagkaya and Vreeling-Sindelarova, 1976).

Binucleate Cells of Ruminants

A unique feature of the ruminant placenta is the population of fetal chorionic binucleate cells (BNC). The BNCs first become apparent around day 16 in sheep (Boshier, 1969), day 18 in goats (Wango, 1990b), and day 17 in cattle (Greenstein, 1958). These time points correspond roughly to the period of trophoblast attachment to the uterine epithelium. The BNC eventually constitute 15 percent to 20 percent of the chorionic epithelium within the mature placenta (see Figure 12.12a) (Wooding, 1992). Their numbers remain fairly constant throughout gestation, until one or two days prior to parturition, when they suddenly dwindle in sheep and goats (Wooding, 1986; Wooding and Flint, 1994).

There are no known stem cells or reserves for the genesis of binucleate cells and they are believed to originate from mononuclear trophoblast cells (MNC) (Wooding and Flint, 1994; Wooding, 1997). In addition, there are no known developing cues or signals that underpin the progenitors of BNC; apparently any MNC can give rise to a BNC. At first, the MNC undergoes a horizontal division to give rise to two MNC. One of the MNC is included within the tight junctions of trophectoderm and the other is free (Lawn, 1969; Boshier and Holloway, 1977). The latter undergoes a nuclear division without subsequent cytokinesis to give rise to a cell with two nuclei (Wooding, 1997). This BNC is a terminally differentiated cell that has lost its ability to divide, but it does undergo further development and matures. At maturity, it possesses two nuclei and an extensive network of rough endoplasmic reticulum and large golgi bodies. The golgi bodies produce a substantial number of cytoplasmic granules that make up to 50 percent of the total cell volume.

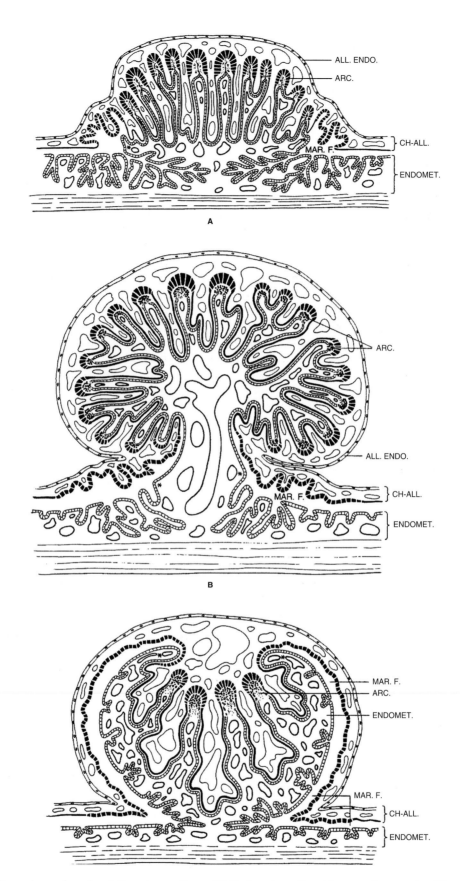

Figure 12.12a. Gross shape of ruminant placentomes. Top: a "flat" placentome found in some deer species. The cotyledons are straight and relatively unbranched. Middle: a "convex" placentome typically found in Bovinae, giraffes, and some deer. Bottom: a "concave" placentome characteristic of Caprinae (sheep and goats). All illustrations: **ENDO.:** endoderm of the allantois; **ARC:** arcade; **CH-ALL:** chorioallantois; **ENDOMET:** endometrium; **MAR. F.:** marginal folds of the allantochrorion; *: approximate border between the glandular endometrium and the aglandular caruncular endometrium. From Mossman, 1987.

Although, endoreduplication has been opined as the basis for BNC production, there is no conclusive evidence to rule out the possibility that a fusion event between two MNC could occur as a means for generating BNC.

Nevertheless, the BNC, once matured, sets its migration toward the uterine epithelium. It forms a cytoplasmic vesicle as it squeezes its contents through the microvillar junctions of the trophoblast and luminal epithelia. It fuses with an apposing uterine epithelial cell forming a hybrid feto-maternal trinucleate cell (TNC) (see Figure 12.12b) (Wooding, 1997). During the fusion event, the cytoplasm and nuclei of the two cells mix thoroughly and the secretory granules of the BNC that were originally in the basolateral region make their way toward the maternal side of the nascent TNC (Wooding, 1987). Soon after, the granular contents are expelled toward the maternal stroma (see Figures 12.12b and 12.12c). Following fusion, the microvillar junctions reappear in the TNC; it reforms part of the apical tight junctions with the adjacent trophoblast cells, thus retaining a protective seal between the two interfacing epithelia (Wooding, 1997).

The newly formed trinucleate cells can undergo expansion as a result of continued binucleate cell migration and fusion to form syncytial plaques (Wooding, 1984). The extent of syncytium formation depends on the species. In the placentomes of sheep, the syncytium is quite extensive. These syncytial plaques contain up to 20 to 24 nuclei; they are bordered by tight junctions and they persist throughout pregnancy (Morgan and Wooding, 1983). The syncytium is presumably maintained by the continued migration of binucleate cells, because nuclear divisions are not observed within the syncytium (Wooding, 1981; Wooding, 1993).

In cattle, no extensive syncytium is present beyond about day 40 of gestation (King, 1979; Wathes and Wooding, 1980; King, 1982). After that time, the migration and fusion of binucleate cells is limited to the generation of short-lived trinucleated cells that are soon replaced by epithelial cells (see Figure 12.12b) (Wooding and Wathes, 1980).

In the intercotyledonary regions of sheep and goats, syncytial plaques are found initially, but they are soon replaced by proliferating cells of the glandular epithelium (King, 1981; King and Atkinson, 1987; Wooding and Flint, 1994). Thereafter, occasional migrations of BNC result in the formation of TNC, but not a syncytium.

An endogenous Jaagsiekte sheep retrovirus (enJSRV) envelope (*env*) protein mRNA and its endogenous receptor hyaluronidase 2 (HYAL2) message has been found to be localized exclusively to BNC and syncytial plaques within the placentomes of sheep throughout gestation (Dunlap, 2005). This is a notable observation because a similar retroviral envelope protein, *syncytin*, produced by a human endogenous retrovirus-W, has been found in the syncytial trophoblast of humans. Syncytin is a fusogenic membrane protein that is involved in the fusion of cytotrophoblast cells

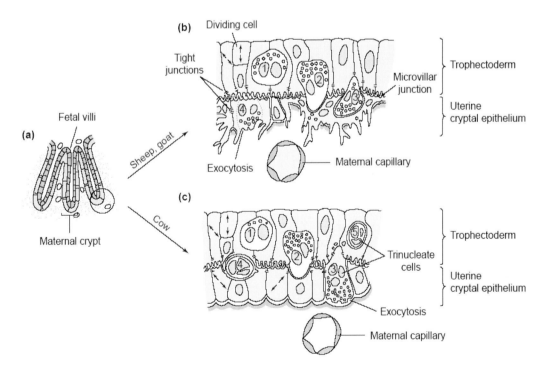

Figure 12.12b. Diagram illustrating the characteristics of trophoblast binucleate cells in the ruminant placentome. **A:** cotyledonary villi penetrating crypts of the uterine caruncles. **B:** in some ruminant species, extensive migration and fusion of trophoblast binucleate cells with uterine epithelia produce a fetal-maternal syncytial cell layer. **C:** in cattle, binucleate cell fusion with uterine epithelial cells produces short-lived trinucleate cells that are resorbed upon release of secretory granule products into the maternal stroma. From Green, 1998.

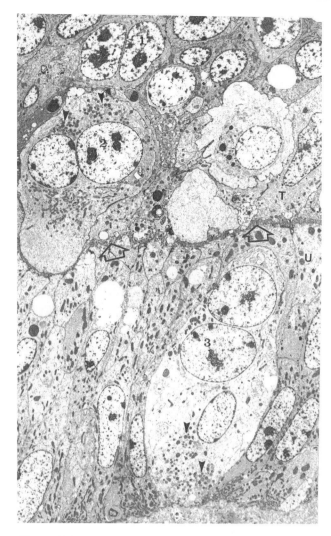

Figure 12.12c. Electron micrograph of the bovine placenta-uterine interface at 20 dpc. Trophoblast binucleate cells (1 and 2) with secretory granules **(arrowheads)** are shown migrating through the microvillar junction **(open arrows)**. Also shown is a fetal-maternal trinucleate cell (3) within the uterine epithelium **(U)**. **T:** trophectoderm. From Wooding and Flint, 1994.

to form syncytia (Mi, 2000). With the identification of an additional retroviral envelope protein in sheep, the argument about a critical role of retroviruses in the evolution of placenta and viviparity in mammals gains further momentum (Villarreal, 1997; Harris, 1998; Stoye and Coffin, 2000; Muir, 2004).

Binucleate cells are endocrine cells that produce steroid (progesterone), prostaglandin (PGI_2, PGE_2), and protein hormones (placental lactogens), as well as protein products with no known function (pregnancy-associated glycoproteins) (Reimers, 1985; Duello, 1986; Xie, 1991; Green, 2000; Wooding, 2005). These proteins, which are packaged in the BNC secretory granules, are released toward the

maternal tissues subsequent to BNC fusion. They can then diffuse into the maternal capillary network to be distributed throughout the maternal circulation (Wooding, 1992; Green, 2005). Therefore, binucleate cells have two principle functions during pregnancy: to form the fetomaternal syncytium required for successful implantation and placentomal growth, and to produce and deliver steroid and protein hormones.

The fusion of binucleate cells with uterine epithelial cells is the extent of invasive implantation in ruminant ungulates. However, it almost certainly allows the conceptus to establish a more intimate endocrinological and immunological dialogue with the mother than is observed in species such as the pig, in which no erosion of the uterine epithelium occurs.

Hemochorial Placentation

The hemochorial type of placenta, like the endotheliochorial type, represents an "invasive" form in which the trophoblasts breach the epithelial barrier of the uterus. Like the endotheliochorial form, it is also found in many eutherian orders. This section contains descriptions of hemochorial placentas from several species that possess this placental type.

Hemotrichorial Placenta of Laboratory Mice (*Mus musculus*)

Site of first attachment	antimesometrial
Depth of attachment	deep
Yolk sac orientation	antimesometrial
Splanchnopleuric yolk sac	complete inversion, permanent, large, mesometrial half usually villous
Chorioallantoic placenta	
Shape	discoid
Pattern	labyrinthine
Interhemal membrane	hemotrichorial
Nonvillous chorioallantois	none
Allantoic sac	none
Unique cell types	trophoblast giant cells, intravascular trophoblasts, syncytial trophoblasts, interstitial glycogen trophoblast cells
Distinguishing features	spongiotrophoblast, completely inverted yolk sac

In many ways the placenta of the mouse represents a striking departure from the type of placentas we have examined so far. In species such as ruminants, swine, and horses, in which the depth of invasion is limited to the superficial layers of the endometrium (at most), the embryo develops extraembryonic membranes before it implants. Paradoxically in rodents and other species with hemochorial placentas, where the depth of invasion is much deeper, implantation precedes the development of fetal membranes. In these species, the blastocyst invades maternal endometrium at a time prior to gastrulation and when only a few cell lineages can be defined. Another distinguishing characteristic of the rodent placenta is that it develops both a yolk sac and a chorioallantoic placenta that function simultaneously.

By day 3.5, the embryo of the mouse is still enclosed within the zona pellucida and contains two distinct cell lineages—the outer trophectoderm and the inner cell mass. The trophectoderm, which gives rise to various trophoblast cell populations, is the first cell lineage to differentiate. The

blastocyst hatches from the zona pellucida by day 4.5 and begins to implant (see Figure 12.13a). At this stage it possesses three clearly defined cell layers—the outer trophectoderm, ICM, and primitive endoderm. The primitive endoderm cells are a group of 20 to 25 cells originating from the ectodermal cells of the ICM lining the blastocoelic cavity (Nadijcka and Hillman, 1974). These cells proliferate, migrate, and subsequently line the inside of the trophectoderm, forming the primitive yolk sac (see Figure 12.13a) (Wartiovaara, 1979; Leivo, 1980).

When the blastocyst begins to implant by day 4.5, the otherwise hostile uterine environment becomes receptive to

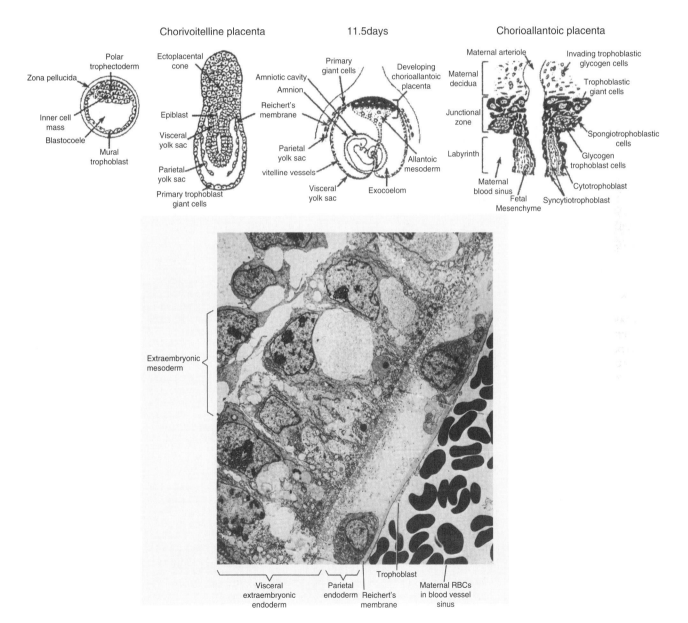

Figure 12.13a. Top: illustrations showing mouse placenta development and defining several tissue types and membrane structures. From Malassine, 2003. Bottom: electron micrograph of the rodent yolk sac cavity created by the close apposition of the villous visceral endoderm and parietal endoderm (along with its thick Reichert's membrane). From Nagy, 2003.

the embryo. This results from a sequence of events that immediately precede implantation. These events include a transient pulse of estradiol production from the ovary on day 4, loss of MUC-1 glycoprotein lining the luminal epithelia (Kimber and Lindenberg, 1990; Kramer, 1990), localized expression of heparin-binding-EGF at the site of implantation (Raab, 1996), as well as other changes (Dey, 2004). These events correspond with concurrent changes in the blastocyst as well, such as an increase in cell number and changes in adhesive properties due to alteration of the integrin profile on the surface trophectoderm cells (Armant, 2000; Wang, 2000; Armant, 2005).

The uterine lumen begins to decrease in size following an even spacing of embryos; as a result, the embryos become confined to 'crypts' within the lumen. This achieves two important objectives: it confines the embryo to the site of attachment and it allows for close apposition and interaction with the uterine wall at the time of apposition (Enders, 1980; Armant, 2005). Next, the blastocyst adheres to the maternal endometrium by its abembryonic pole antimesometrially (Amoroso, 1952; Kaufmann, 1983).

At the site of the attachment, the underlying maternal stroma undergoes the decidual reaction, a process that transforms it into a specialized structure known as a "deciduum," which means "the thing that falls off" (Nagy, 2003). The luminal epithelium adjoining the embryo by now undergoes apoptosis, exposing the embryo to the underlying maternal stroma (Schlafke, 1985; Parr, 1987). This confers an invasive phenotype to the trophectodermal cells, presumably as a result of changes in integrin expression again, and they begin to invade into the maternal endometrium (Blankenship and Given, 1992; Carson, 2000; Armant, 2005).

After implantation has taken place, the trophectoderm begins to differentiate into different cell types. The trophectoderm cells lining the blastocyst cavity farthest from the ICM (mural trophectoderm cells) cease to divide, undergo endoreduplication, and transform into polyploidic *primary trophoblast giant cells* (see Figure 12.13a) (Gardner, 1983a; Varmuza, 1988; Zybina and Zybina, 1996; Gardner, 2000). The giant cells in mice are unique in that the ploidy of these cells can reach up to 1,000 N as opposed to 4 to 16 N in human syncytiotrophoblasts and binucleate cells of ruminants (Berezowsky, 1995; Zybina and Zybina, 1996; Klisch, 1999).

The trophectoderm, in close association with the ICM, remains diploid and is referred to as *polar trophectoderm*. This undifferentiated state is maintained by FGF-4 production by the ICM (Chai, 1998; Tanaka, 1998; Rossant and Cross, 2001). The polar trophectoderm cells soon begin to migrate in all directions within the endometrium. They also migrate onto the sides of the embryo replacing the degenerating mural trophoblast giant cells and transforming into giant cells in the process (Cross, 1994; Hemberger and Cross, 2001; Rossant and Cross, 2001).

This sub-population of polar trophectoderm that become separated from the ICM also undergo a similar fate as was observed for the mural trophoblasts. They too stop dividing, undergo endoreduplication, and become giant cells. These are called *secondary trophoblast giant cells* (Cross, 1994; Rossant and Cross, 2001). These giant cells later invade the maternal spiral arteries and, once there, are referred to as *endovascular trophoblast giant cells* (Pijnenborg, 1981; Redline and Lu, 1989; Adamson, 2002). Their invasion route is strictly limited to the maternal arteries.

In contrast, a group of *glycogen trophoblast cells* are also seen in rodents that are interstitial and do not invade the maternal arteries (see Figure 12.13a) (Adamson, 2002). The origin of these cells is unclear; however, they are thought to arise from spongiotrophoblast that emerges later in development (Adamson, 2002). In stark contrast to the secondary trophoblast giant cells, the polar trophectoderm cells immediately adjacent to the ICM are still maintained in a diploid state; therefore it appears that the proximity and, thereby, access to signals from the ICM, are critical for maintenance of ploidy and a less differentiated state in mouse trophoblasts (Rossant and Cross, 2001).

The polar trophectoderm cells by day 6 undergo rapid proliferation and differentiation into two subpopulations of cells, the *extraembryonic ectoderm* and the *ectoplacental cone* (see Figure 12.13a) (Gardner, 1973; Adamson, 2002). The extraembryonic ectoderm grows and expands toward the blastocyst cavity, pushing the ICM further down into the cavity (see Figure 12.13a). With the growth of the ectoplacental cone the uterine epithelia and capillaries are breached; subsequently the maternal blood vessels develop and become continuous with the uterine lumen, filling it with blood. The maternal blood also communicates with the spaces in the trophoblast, filling it with blood. These spaces are initially irregular but eventually become organized into defined channels.

Between days 5.5 and 6.5 the primitive ectodermal cells of the inner cell mass, the epiblast, multiply rapidly from about 120 cells to 660 cells (Snow, 1977). These proliferating cells of epiblast become organized into an epithelium, enclosing a small pro-amniotic cavity inside. With the growth of extraembryonic ectoderm toward the cavity the epiblast protrudes further into the yolk sac, forming an egg cylinder. This progressive development of the egg cylinder into the yolk sac leads to the delineation of primitive endodermal cells into two epithelia which are both morphologically and physiologically distinct (Gardner, 1983b). The primitive endodermal epithelium lining the egg cylinder and the extraembryonic ectoderm is the visceral yolk sac epithelium and that lining the trophectoderm is the parietal yolk sac epithelium (see Figure 12.13a).

Gastrulation begins on day 6.5 with the origination of the primitive streak on one end of the epiblast in the junction region between the embryonic and extraembryonic ectoderm (Snow, 1977). The primitive streak represents the future posterior end of the developing embryo. The cells of the epiblast at the primitive streak region become discontinuous and give rise to mesoderm. The mesoderm continues to grow in both embryonic and extraembryonic regions, separating the epiblast from both extraembryonic ectoderm and visceral endoderm in the process. As a result, by day 7 the mesoderm is seen developing adjacent to the visceral yolk sac epithelium surrounding the embryo, which eventually becomes vascularized by day 8. Shortly after, by day 9 short villi are seen developing from the visceral endoderm and a vascularized yolk sac placenta is established (Nagy 2003).

In rodents, the yolk sac placenta plays a crucial role alongside the chorioallantoic placenta. Even prior to the development of a vasculature in the mesoderm, the yolk sac placenta is fully functional. This is because the apical surface of the visceral endodermal cells possesses microvilli and coated pits that are actively involved in the uptake of nutrients from the yolk sac cavity (Hogan and Tilly, 1981; Jollie, 1986, 1990a). This is further aided by a narrow yolk sac cavity and a thin interhemal membrane (Jollie, 1986). The yolk sac cavity is narrowed by the expanding egg cylinder into the cavity, bringing the parietal and visceral endodermal cells bordering the yolk sac cavity closer in space (see Figure 12.13a). The interhemal membrane in the yolk sac is also quite narrow, consisting of the avascular omphalopluere (parietal endoderm cells and discontinuous mural trophectoderm cells) (Enders and Blankenship, 1999).

The interhemal membrane also consists of a specialized basement membrane called *Reichert's membrane* (see Figure 12.13a) (Fatemi, 1987; Mazariegos, 1987). This basement membrane is abundant in extracellular matrix components such as laminin, entactin, heparin sulfate proteoglycans, etc; however, fibronectin is not present (Hogan, 1980; Smith and Strickland, 1981; Semoff, 1982; Amenta, 1983). Reichert's membrane is produced by the parietal yolk sac endodermal cells between themselves and mural trophoblast cells. It is thought to act as a sieve, permitting the yolk sac cavity to be filled with filtrate of maternal blood (Parr and Parr, 1989). In addition to the filtrate, the secretions of parietal and visceral yolk sac epithelia contribute to the contents within the yolk sac cavity. As the pregnancy advances, trophoblast cells surrounding Reichert's membrane become discontinuous, making it the principal barrier between the mother and fetus until about 16 dpc when the membrane degenerates as well. At this point, the visceral endodermal cells are directly exposed to the maternal environment (Welsh and Enders, 1983).

The mesoderm in the posterior region of the extraembryonic ectoderm, and to some extent in the anterior and lateral regions, develops cavities which later coalesce to form the exocoelom (see Figure 12.13b). The mesoderm of the exoceolom, along with the distal rim of extraembryonic ectoderm, metamorphose into chorion, similarly, while the

proximal rim of epiblast on the other end of cavity develops into an amnion (Nagy, 2003). Following this, extraembryonic mesoderm in the posterior streak region buds off into the allantois. The allantois grows, traverses the exocoelom, and contacts the chorion to form chorioallantois by day 8.5 (see Figure 12.13b). This heralds the emergence of the chorioallantoic placenta (Welsh and Enders, 1991b; Enders and Welsh, 1993).

Following contact between the allantois and chorion—in a process often called *chorio-allantoic fusion* (there is in fact no fusion of these two layers)—distinct folds begin to appear in the chorion (Cross, 2003b). These are the sites where fetal villi emerge as a result of growth of stromal cells and blood vessels from allantoic mesoderm. Actually, around day 8 prior to chorioallantoic fusion, a transcription factor called *Glial cells missing-1* (GCM-1) is expressed in focal sites of the chorion (Anson-Cartwright, 2000). These restricted areas of GCM-1 expression subsequently concentrate at the tip of the folds and metamorphose into villi. Therefore, the sites for initiating villi formation are predetermined (Anson-Cartwright, 2000).

Once the villi emerge, they undergo extensive branching analogous to other branching organs, such as lungs, leading to the formation of a highly dense labyrinth by day 9 (Rossant and Cross, 2001; Cross, 2003a; Cross, 2003b). The transcription factor GCM-1 is always found localized to the tip of the developing and branching villi and persists for as long as the villi continue to grow (Eugenia Basyuk, 1999).

Coincident with villus formation, the trophoblast cells within the elongating chorionic villi, which are in direct contact with maternal blood, fuse to form syncytia (West, 1995). In mice in which the gene for GCM-1 has been disrupted, syncytiotrophoblast and the labyrinth fail to develop; the chorioallantoic branching is not initiated and the progression of labyrinth is restricted to the smooth chorion stage (Schreiber, 2000). Therefore, GCM-1 is pivotal in the organization of the placental labyrinth in mice. With the organization of the fetal labyrinth and the chorioallantoic placenta, another front for fetomaternal exchange is established in the mouse (the inverted yolk sac is the other). The interhemal membrane in the labyrinth consists of two layers of syncytiotrophoblast covered by a single layer of mononucleate cell type of unknown origin (Rossant and Cross, 2001). Therefore the placenta of mice is classified as hemotrichorial type (see Figure 12.13c) (King and Hastings, 1977).

The labyrinth is supported by a scaffold of diploid nonsyncytial trophoblast cells, the *spongiotrophoblast*, originating from the ectoplacental cone (Lescisin, 1988; He, 1999). The secondary trophoblast giant cells erode the maternal capillaries and replace the endothelium, thereby forming maternal blood sinuses. The blood eventually traverses through the tortuous channels of the spongiotrophoblast to reach the labyrinth where it directly bathes the vascularized trophoblasts (see Figures 12.13a and 12.13c).

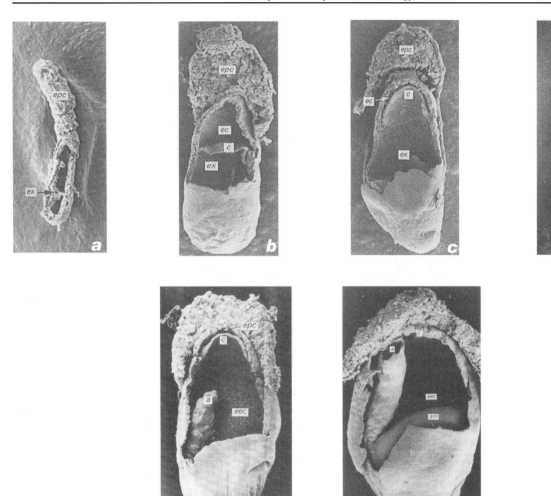

Figure 12.13b. Scanning electron micrographs of rat conceptuses showing the establishment of some extraembryonic structures. Panels A through F represent distinct developmental stages of 8.25, 9.25, 9.5, 9.75, 10, and 10.25 dpc, respectively. **a:** allantois; **am:** amnion; **c:** chorion; **ec:** extraembryonic ectoderm cavity; **epc:** ectoplacental cone; **ex** or **eec:** exocoelom or extra-embryonic coelom. From Ellington, 1985, 1987.

The spongiotrophoblast is not served by a fetal blood supply; therefore, the principal site of maternal fetal exchange is located in the labyrinthine layer. The chorioallantoic vasculature is connected to the growing fetus by the umbilical artery and vein through the allantoic stalk, which later transforms into the umbilical cord. Therefore, the mouse has a functional chorioallantoic placenta only in the second half of pregnancy (Enders and Blankenship, 1999).

Hemodichorial Placenta of Old World Rabbits (*Oryctolagus cuniculus*)

Site of first attachment	antimesometrial and lateral
Depth of attachment	deep
Yolk sac orientation	antimesometrial
Choriovitelline placenta	temporary
Splanchnopleuric yolk sac	large, inverted

Chorioallantoic placenta

Shape	discoid (late in pregnancy)
Pattern	labyrinthine
Interhemal membrane	hemodichorial
Nonvillous chorioallantois	none
Allantoic sac	permanent, very small
Unique cell types	unique decidual cell lamina defining the border of term placenta
Distinguishing features	dicotyledonary placenta

The blastocyst of rabbits undergoes considerable expansion before implantation. It increases from 4 mm in diameter to up to 10 mm by day 8, when definitive contact with the uterus and implantation begins. This increase in the size of the blastocyst is attributed to the abundance of IGF-1 within the secretions of uterine glands by day 7 (Grundker and Kirchner, 1996; Klonisch, 2001). There is also strong evidence that links the EGF/Erb (EGF receptor) system to the enlargement of the blastocyst (Klonisch, 2001). Once

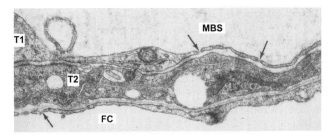

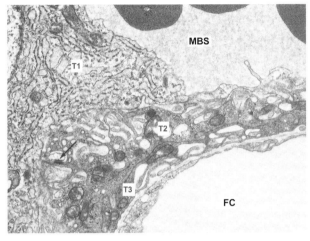

Figure 12.13c. Example of hemotrichorial placenta of myomorph (mouse, rats) rodents. Maternal blood spaces (**MBS**) are bound by (usually) a cellular trophoblast layer (**T1**) that can become thin and discontinuous (**lower panel, arrows**) in places. The second layer (**T2**) is syncytiotrophoblast and is normally the thickest layer. The third layer (**T3**) is in contact with the endothelial cells of the fetal capillaries (**FC**); it is the thinnest and most uniform layer. The top panel represents a *Peromyscus* placenta and the bottom panel represents a *Lemmus* placenta. From King and Hastings, 1977.

the blastocysts are extended and spaced evenly, they initiate establishment of a definitive contact with the endometrium. This attachment or apposition phase is preceded by the loss of MUC-I lining the abembryonic region (Anderson and Hoffman, 1984; Anderson, 1986).

In most species, the period of receptivity is defined by the loss of the apical MUC-1 glycocalyx layer on the luminal epithelium (Johnson, 2001; Brayman, 2004). However, rabbits and primates constitute an exception; in these species, there is an overall increase in the glycocalyx, except for the localized depletion in the abembryonic region (Hey, 1994; Hild-Petito, 1996; Chervenak and Illsley, 2000; Meseguer, 2001). Although it has been attributed to paracrine signaling by the implanting embryo, there are alternative theories that implicate the activity of proteases of trophoblast origin in both rabbits and humans (Olson, 1998; Thathiah and Carson, 2002).

Blastocyst attachment is initially established at the antimesometrial end, which subsequently spreads toward the mesometrial side of the uterus. This is characterized by the apposition and fusion between syncytial trophectoder-

mal knobs and the uterine epithelium (Larsen, 1961; Enders and Schlafke, 1971). This fusion results in the development of syncytial plaques that degenerate into symplasmic masses, which are phagocytosed and replaced by the invading syncytiotrophoblast. A unique population of trophoblast giant cells is also found covering the antimesometrial and lateral aspects of the developing embryo.

Meanwhile, the yolk sac grows antimesometrially and a bilaminar omphalopleure develops by day 7. Vascularization in the yolk sac is poor; therefore, the development of a vascularized trilaminar yolk sac or choriovitelline placenta is temporary in these animals (Enders and Blankenship, 1999). By 16 dpc the avascular bilaminar omphalopleure surrounding the embryo in the antimesometrial end ruptures, thereby exposing the endoderm of the completely inverted yolk sac in a manner similar to the rupturing of Reichert's membrane in rodents (see above). This inverted yolk sac is initially the major site of materno-fetal exchange, until the development of a definitive chorioallantoic placenta in the mesometrial end of the embryo (Enders and Blankenship, 1999).

The syncytiotrophoblasts in the embryonic pole begin their invasion as soon as the amnion is formed by the fusion of amniotic folds (Hoffman, 1990a, 1990b). The syncytiotrophoblasts reach the maternal blood vessels by 9 dpc and rupture the blood vessels by 10 dpc (Pijnenborg, 1981; Hoffman, 1990b). The allantoic vesicle forms by day 9, and it rapidly vascularizes the invading syncytiotrophoblasts, forming the definitive chorioallantoic placenta by 12 dpc. These vascularized chorioallantoic villi increase in complexity and form a placental labyrinth.

The definitive placenta does not develop an ectoplacental cone and subsequently a spongiotrophoblast layer is absent in rabbits. However, similar to rodents, the maternal arteries supplying the developing fetus are invaded by trophectoderm (Hoffman 1990b). The maternal blood flows through the intricate channels of the fetal labyrinth, which is drained by maternal veins (Hafez and Tsutsumi, 1966; Carter, 1971). The interhemal layer in the labyrinth is bilayered, consisting of cellular trophectoderm surrounded by a syncytial layer, which is in contact with maternal blood. Therefore, the definitive placenta of the rabbit is labyrinthine hemodichorial in pattern (see Figure 12.14) (Enders, 1965; Enders and Schlafke, 1971). However, there are occurrences of isolated thick and thin regions within the interhemal membranes. In these regions the cytotrophoblast alone or along with syncytiotrophoblasts becomes exceedingly thin or may even be lost altogether. If the loss of both trophoblast layers does indeed occur, the interhemal region would be of a type best described as hemo-endotheliochorial (Amoroso, 1961; Samuel, 1975).

The placenta of the rabbit, when viewed from the exterior, appears to be discoid. When viewed internally it is bidiscoidal. This bidiscoidal structure is due to the development of two placental folds/cotyledons with a sagittal groove between them. These folds/cotyledons increase in

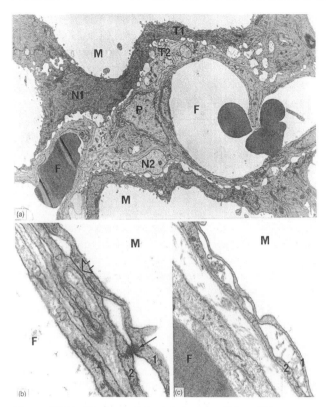

Figure 12.14. The hemodichorial placenta of the rabbit labyrinth region. Maternal blood spaces (**M**) are bound by syncytiotrophoblast (**T1**) and cytotrophoblast (**T2**). Nuclei present in each layer are indicated (**N1 and N2**). The two lower panels demonstrate that there are occasional gap junctions (**open arrow**) and desmosomal junctions (**small arrow**) between T1 and T2. **F:** fetal capillaries. **P:** fetal pericyte. From Wooding and Flint, 1994.

size as the pregnancy advances and the groove narrows; therefore, the placenta of rabbits at term is discoidal (Mossman, 1987).

Probably one of the most interesting and distinguishing features of rabbit placentation is the development of a thin lamina of uninucleate decidual cells adjacent to the myometrium in the decidua basalis at term (Mossman, 1987). These cells are uniform in both size and appearance and mark the plane of separation during parturition. The placenta separates between this layer and the overlying degenerating decidua (Mossman, 1987).

Hemomonochorial Placenta of Guinea Pigs (*Cavia porcellus*)

Site of first attachment	antimesometrial
Depth of attachment	interstitial
Yolk sac orientation	antimesometrial
Choriovitelline placenta	none
Splanchnopleuric yolk sac	complete inversion, permanent, large villous capillary ring

Chorioallantoic placenta	
Shape	discoid
Pattern	labyrinthine
Interhemal membrane	hemomonochorial
Nonvillous chorioallantois	none
Allantoic sac	none

The guinea pig shares many similarities with rodent placentation and interested readers can find several detailed descriptions of guinea pig placentation (Wimsatt, 1975; Kaufmann and Davidoff, 1977; Perry, 1981; Pijnenborg, 1981; Jollie, 1990b). Briefly, following fertilization, the blastocyst enters the uterus and becomes lodged within uterine crypts by day 6. The embryo implants antimesometrially and penetrates the uterine wall completely and is encapsulated within the maternal decidua. The trophoblast, except for the region near the embryonic disc, rapidly invades the maternal decidua and differentiates into trophoblast giant cells. These giant cells are smaller and sparser when compared to the rodent placenta (Perry, 1981). In addition, a continuous layer of trophoblast on the mesometrial half, analogous to the mural trophoblast layer in the mouse, never exists in the guinea pig. Likewise, juxtauterine endoderm cells akin to the parietal endoderm cells in rodents also never appear. Therefore, in guinea pigs, the bilaminar omphalopleure does not form and the inversion of the yolk sac occurs very early in development (Jollie, 1990b).

The epiblast expands into an egg cylinder with a central cavity. The extraembryonic ectoderm above the epiblast gives rise to an invasive *ectoplacenta*. Soon afterwards, a slit appears in the mesoderm in the "waist" region of the egg cylinder. As the slit enlarges, it transforms into exocoelom or exocele. This exocele is bordered by a newly developed amnion on the antimesometrial side and chorion on the mesometrial side (Kaufmann and Davidoff, 1977; Perry, 1981).

As the maternal capillaries are breached by trophoblasts, the maternal blood fills the numerous lacunae that are present within the ectoplacenta. Soon after, a swelling appears on the posterior end of the exocele. This mesodermal evagination transforms into allantois and makes contact with the mesodermal lining of the newly formed chorion under the ectoplacenta, forming the chorioallantois. With the growth of the embryo, the decidua capsularis becomes increasingly thinner and is eventually lost, thereby exposing the mesometrial wall of the uterus. The ectoplacenta and the chorioallantoic placenta now attach themselves to the mesometrial wall to establish a definitive placenta (Kaufmann and Davidoff, 1977).

The definitive chorioallantoic placenta of the guinea pig is discoidal and lobular. Within each lobule is a placental labyrinth. Apart from a few dispersed cytotrophoblast cells, the interhemal membrane in the labyrinth is largely composed of a single layer of syncytial trophoblast. Hence, the placenta of the guinea pig is hemomonochorial labyrinthine in nature (Enders, 1965; Kaufmann and Davidoff, 1977). The apical and basolateral surface of the syncytiotrophoblast that is in contact with maternal blood is microvillous. The syncytia forms specialized pockets which are very close to the basal lamina. These pockets are occasionally interfaced by a thin endothelium lining of the fetal blood vessels. This results in the reduction of interhemal barrier distance in these regions. Because the gestation period of guinea pig is relatively long (68 days), the definitive placenta is functional for a considerable time.

In addition to the chorioallantois, the guinea pig also possesses an inverted yolk sac. So by late gestation, the embryo is seen dangling in the exocele by means of an umbilical cord, the allantoic stalk that connects to the definitive placenta mesometrially, and a secondary umbilical cord which is a group of blood vessels connecting the yolk sac in the antimesometrial pole. Hence, the guinea pig, like rodents, has both chorioallantoic and yolk sac placenta functioning simultaneously until term (Perry, 1981; Jollie, 1990b).

Hemomonochorial Placenta of Humans (*Homo sapiens*)

Site of first attachment	antimesometrial
Depth of attachment	deep
Yolk sac orientation	mesometrial
Choriovitelline placenta	none
Splanchnopleuric yolk sac	free, temporary
Chorioallantoic placenta	
Shape	discoid
Pattern	villous
Interhemal membrane	hemodichorial initially, hemomonochorial later (definitive)
Nonvillous chorioallantois	+, nonvascular
Allantoic sac	rudimentary duct only
Unique cell types	Intravascular cytotroblast giant cells, extravillous cytotrophoblast giant cells
Distinguishing features	amniochorion

Humans possess a hemochorial placenta. It is unique from the mice placenta in that its yolk sac is rudimentary, it possesses a true villous placenta as opposed to a labyrinthine placenta, and it has an amniochorion, to name just a few distinguishing characteristics.

The human blastocyst enters the uterus by day 4 to day 5 and attaches antimesometrially via the side of the embryonic pole on either the dorsal or ventral uterine wall in the midsagittal plane (Enders and Blankenship, 1999; Norwitz, 2001; Paria, 2002). This attachment of the blastocyst to the uterine wall is probably mediated by selectins on the trophoblasts and L-selectin-like ligands on the uterine wall. This phenomenon is reminiscent of leukocyte adhesion to endothelial cells prior to extravasation (Genbacev, 2003; Red-Horse, 2004; Rosen, 2004).

Just prior to implantation, the cytotrophoblast cells surrounding the embryo undergo rapid proliferation and differentiation to form a multinucleated syncytiotrophoblast. This event underpins the beginning of an invasive implantation in the developing embryo. It invades the luminal epithelia and underlying stroma to become completely embedded within the endometrial stroma by 7 to 8 dpc (Enders, 1983). The embryo soon becomes encapsulated within a syncytiotrophoblast, which grows by the fusion of cytotrophoblast cells rather than nuclear division. In humans, a fusogenic intramembrane endogenous retroviral envelope protein called syncytin is implicated in this process (Blond, 2000; Mi, 2000; Frendo, 2003).

By 11 dpc intercellular spaces or lacunae begin to appear within the syncytiotrophoblast layer (lacunar stage) (Boyd and Hamilton, 1970; Enders, 1989, 1993). Due to the invasion and rupture of maternal endothelial cells comprising the endometrial capillaries, the lacunae become filled with maternal blood, which flows sluggishly through the spaces (Knoth and J., 1972; Falck Larsen, 1980; Enders and King, 1991). The syncytial trophoblasts lining the maternal blood have extensive microvilli on their surface, which persists throughout the remainder of pregnancy (King, 1991).

The human blastocyst progresses rapidly through several developmental steps, forming a yolk sac, amnion, and allantoic mesoderm. The amnion is formed by cavitation and later in development fuses with the chorion to form an *amniochorion*. This is one of the distinguishing characteristics of human placenta (Enders and Blankenship, 1999; Sadler, 2000). The yolk sac is larger than the embryo by day 22. It extends in the direction opposite to the embryonic pole by which the embryo implants, i.e., mesometrial. Only the proximal portion of the yolk sac becomes vascularized and eventually the yolk sac becomes a stalked, temporary sac (Enders and King, 1993). The yolk sac, though significant initially, never reaches the chorion, and therefore there is no choriovitelline placenta in the human. The yolk sac eventually becomes rudimentary and is completely gone at term (Enders and King, 1993).

Besides the yolk sac, the allantoic sac in humans does not enlarge; instead it only remains as a stalk. The mesoderm of the allantoic stalk becomes vascularized as it reaches out to the chorion, vascularizing it and converting it into chorioallantois. This early morphogenesis of chorion into chorioallantois is another distinctive characteristic of human, as well as other anthropoid, placentas (Mossman, 1987).

In humans, the villi are formed as a result of proliferation of cytotrophoblast cells through the syncytiotrophoblast. During the early stages of development, distinct

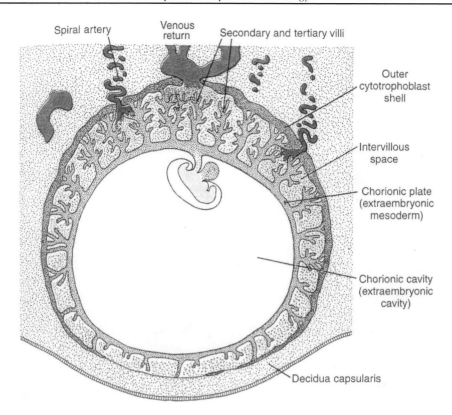

Figure 12.15a. A diagram of human placentation at the second month of development. There are numerous chorionic villi at the embryonic pole. At the abembryonic pole, villi are present but they are fewer in number and poorly developed. From Sadler, 2000.

subpopulations of cytotrophoblasts leave the basement membrane (chorionic plate), penetrate the syncytiotrophoblast, and form columns of cells that eventually make contact with the functional maternal decidua, called the *decidua basalis*, to form anchoring villi (see Figure 12.15a) (Castellucci, 1990).

The cytotrophoblast cells that reach the decidual plate (contribution of the uterine decidua to the placenta) join laterally with adjacent cytotrophoblasts to create the cytotrophoblast shell (see Figure 12.15a). The cytotrophoblast shell attaches the embryo firmly to the maternal deciduum. A portion of the deciduum becomes incorporated into the placenta and together with the cytotrophoblast forms the basal plate. The decidual and trophoblast cells blend together in this junctional zone. These cells are also covered by a fibrinous extracellular material of maternal origin (Pijnenborg, 1981; Aplin, 1991; Blankenship, 1992; Damsky, 1992). In addition to the anchoring villi, there is a subset of villi known as "floating villi" that are freely suspended in the intervillous spaces (see Figure 12.15b) (Boyd and Hamilton, 1970; Burton, 1987a; Kaufmann, 1988; Burton, 1990; Castellucci, 1990). Both the anchoring and floating villi are always covered by a layer of syncytiotrophoblast. In later stages of development the anchoring villi become vascularized, thereby contributing to the absorptive surface.

The invasiveness of cytotrophoblast cells is not limited to the cytotrophoblast shell. A distinct endocrine population called *extravillous cytotrophoblasts* invades the decidua and maternal arterial system. Those extravillous cytotrophoblast cells that stay in the decidua are called *interstitial extravillous trophoblast cells* and those that invade the maternal arteries are *endovascular extravillous trophoblast cells* (Pijnenborg, 1981; Aplin, 1991; Benirschke and Kaufmann, 2000; Cross, 2003a). Though these invasive cytotrophoblast populations are polyploid (4N to 16N), they do not reach the DNA content observed in rodent giant trophoblasts, which can be up to 1,000N (Berezowsky, 1995; Zybina and Zybina, 1996). These cells also express an atypical HLA type-I antigen, HLA-G, which ensures safe trespass into the maternal tissue without falling prey to maternal natural killer- (NK) cells or cytotoxic-T (Tc) cells (Redman, 1984; Bulmer and Johnson, 1985; Loke and Butterworth, 1987; Wells and Bulmer, 1988; Loke and King, 1989; Hunt, 1990; Hunt and His, 1990; Loke and King, 1995; Loke, 1999; Slukvin, 2000).

The expression of HLA-G by trophoblast cells represents a classic case of misguidance put forth by the fetus to elude the immuno-surveillance of the mother (Rouas-Freiss, 1997). The trophoblast cells and fetal cells lack the classical MHC class I; Ia molecules such as HLA-A, B, and C; and MHC class II on their cell surface (Loke and King, 1995).

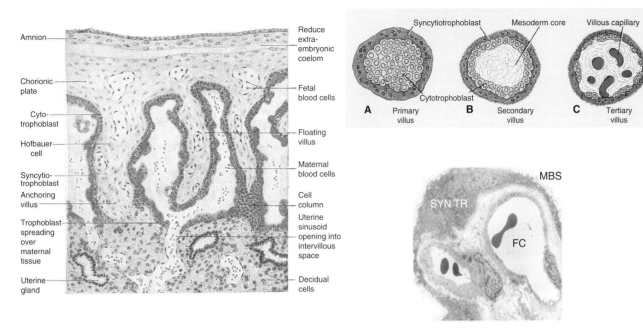

Figure 12.15b. Left panel: illustration showing chorionic villi projecting (downward) into the maternal decidua. Upper right panel: development of primary, secondary, and tertiary placental villi. Left and upper right panels from Sadler, 2000. Lower right panel: electron micrograph of a human hemomonochorial placental villous showing a single layer of syncytiotrophoblast **(SYN TR)** adjacent to the maternal blood sinus **(MBS)**. **FC:** fetal capillaries. Lower right panel from Carter and Enders, 2004; © 2004 Carter and Enders; licensee BioMed Central Ltd.

This renders them incapable of presenting paternal antigens to the Tc cells and thereby avoids the prospect of activating them. However, the lack of MHC molecules would be recorded as "missing self" by the NK-cells prowling the premises, making the trophoblast cells vulnerable to their attack (King, 1997). It is here that the non-classical MHC class-Ib HLA-G molecules come to the rescue of trophoblast. HLA-G is an atypical molecule that resembles MHC-class I molecule in basic organization, but is incapable of presenting paternal antigens (Lee, 1995; Diehl, 1996). It is also shown to be capable of inhibiting NK-cells by interacting with its receptors (Rouas-Freiss, 1997). Therefore, the HLA-G confers protection for the trophoblast cells from both cytotoxic-T cells and NK-cells.

The endovascular extravillous cytotrophoblast cells replace the existing endothelial cells and pericytes of the maternal arteries, producing vascular beds that are non-responsive to vasoactive mediators (Pijnenborg, 1981; Lim, 1997; Kaufmann, 2003). The end result is a permanent widening of the endometrial arterioles, ensuring an unabated supply of maternal blood to the fetus. The maternal blood enters the intervillous spaces and subsequently drains through the basal plate. Following vascularization of the chorioallantoic membranes the fetal blood enters and leaves the villi through the chorionic plate.

The villi in various stages of transitional morphogenesis are seen beginning in the third week. The primary villus

consists of a core of cytotrophoblast surrounded by syncytiotrophoblast (Figure 12.15b). Once mesodermal cells fill the core of the primary villus, it is called secondary villus. This penetration of mesoderm enlarges the secondary villus, which grows toward the decidua. By the end of the third week, angiogenesis and vasculogenesis begins in the core mesodermal cells of the secondary villus, transforming it into tertiary villus (see Figure 12.15b) (Boyd and Hamilton, 1970; Kaufmann, 1981a; Kaufmann, 1985; Burton, 1987a; Mossman, 1987; Burton, 1990; Castellucci, 1990; Sadler, 2000).

Capillaries developed in these tertiary villi become connected to the vessels within the mesoderm of the chorionic plate and connecting stalk, the structure that attaches the developing conceptus to the placenta that later transforms into the umbilical cord. Therefore, by the fourth week of development, when the heart starts to function, a functional vascular system has already become established within the chorionic villi (Sadler, 2000).

In the early weeks of development, the chorionic villi are distributed throughout the entire surface of the chorion. Later, they become confined to the region of greatest blood supply in the embryonic pole or antimesometrial area, thereby forming a discoid placenta. In fact, the word placenta is derived from the Latin word meaning cake, which is an apt description of the disc-shaped placenta of humans. These expanding villi in the embryonic pole are referred to as *chorion frondosum* (bushy chorion) (see Figure 12.15c).

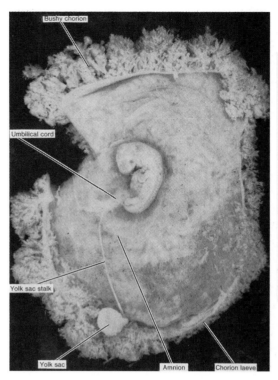

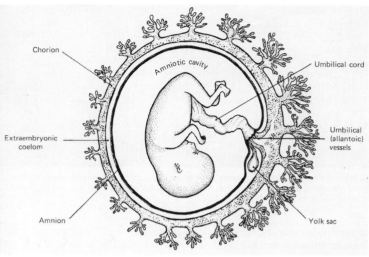

Figure 12.15c. Pictorial (left) and stylized (right) views of the human placenta. From Sadler, 2000.

By the third month, the villi on the rest of the chorionic surface degenerate, forming a smooth chorion or *chorion laeve* (see Figure 12.15c).

These local differences in chorion morphogenesis transcend to changes in the uterine endometrium. While the decidua apposing the chorion frondosum is "decidua basalis," the decidua that surrounds the chorion laeve is called "decidua capsularis." With the growth and expansion of the chorion cavity, the decidua capsularis is stretched and eventually degenerates along with the underlying luminal epithelium that had originally reformed after the interstitial implantation of the embryo. This results in direct apposition of the chorion laeve with the uterine wall on the opposite side of the lumen. Later, the association between the two membranes results in obliteration of the uterine lumen entirely. The decidua of the opposing uterine wall now in contact with the chorionic laeve is called "decidua parietalis" (Sadler, 2000).

From the beginning of the second month, with the completion of development of tertiary villi and establishment of a functional vascular network, the interhemal membrane consists of a continuous layer of syncytiotrophoblast (in contact with maternal blood) and an underlying single layer of cytotrophoblast cells overlying the endothelial cells of fetal blood vessels. Hence, the placenta at this stage can be referred to as hemodichorial type. However, by the beginning of the fourth month, the cytotrophoblast cells become dissociated from one another or are lost, leaving syncytiotrophoblast as the only barrier between the maternal blood and the endothelial cells of the fetal vessels (Figure 15b). Thus, the placenta at this stage is hemomonochorial. Therefore, the placenta of humans transforms from a hemodichorial to a definitive hemomonochorial villous placenta during the course of pregnancy (Kaufmann, 1981b, 1981a; Mossman, 1987; Benirschke and Kaufmann, 2000).

As the pregnancy advances further, the syncytial trophoblast layer becomes progressively thin, thereby reducing the effective distance for diffusion or transcytosis of materials. The syncytiotrophoblast overlying the villi frequently break off, forming multinucleate *syncytial knots*. Though these knots enter the maternal circulation through the intervillous space, they are not associated with any known complications of pregnancy (Ikle, 1964; Billington, 1970; Covone, 1984; Kozma, 1986; Mueller, 1990).

By 4 to 5 months, several septa originate from the decidua basalis that extend into the intervillous space. These growing septa do not reach the chorionic plate and therefore the entire intervillous space is contiguous. As a result of the septal formations, the placenta of humans is divided into approximately 15 to 20 compartments or cotyledons (Sadler, 2000). Each cotyledon consists of tree-like villi, surrounded by maternal blood. The septa of these cotyledons are also lined by fetal-derived syncytium, and therefore a syncytium is always present lining the surfaces exposed to maternal blood.

Hemomonochorial Placenta of the Rock Hyrax
(*Procavia capensis*)

Site of first attachment	central
Yolk sac orientation	mesometrial
Choriovitelline placenta	temporary, large
Splanchnopleuric yolk sac	temporary, large

Chorioallantoic placenta

Shape	complete zonary
Pattern	labyrinthine
Interhemal membrane	hemochorial
Nonvillous chorioallantois	large
Allantoic sac	permanent, large
Distinguishing features	true hemomonochorial placenta (see discussion below)

The rock hyrax or dassie is a unique animal. It is so different from other existing mammals that it has been placed in a separate order (hyracoidean). In fact, the closest relative to the rock hyrax is the elephant, with which it shares a common ancestor. This may come as a surprise because the rock hyrax is a small furry animal about the size of a stocky rabbit or an oversized guinea pig. However, paleontological evidence reveals that hyrax ancestors were once the size of an ox. This is probably why they have a prolonged gestation period of seven to eight months, which is highly atypical for small mammals (Sale, 1965).

The embryonic disc of the rock hyrax is oriented antimesometrially at implantation. The yolk sac is therefore mesometrially aligned; it is free and disappears soon after formation. The allantoic sac is large and surrounds most of the amnion. The allantois vascularizes the amnion in addition to the chorion and, therefore, the rock hyrax represents one of the few species in which the amnion is vascularized (Mossman, 1987).

The definitive placenta of the rock hyrax is classified as a zonary hemochorial labyrinthine placenta (Wislocki and Van der Westhuysen, 1940; Sturgess, 1948). The placenta initially appears as a diffuse placenta, but with the expansion of non-villous chorioallantois (smooth chorioallantois), it becomes zonary.

Histologically, the placenta of the rock hyrax can be divided into three zones (Wislocki and Van der Westhuysen, 1940; Oduor-Okelo, 1983). Zone I consists of trophoblast cells arranged in tall column-like villi which anastomose to form a dense labyrinth. The labyrinth has a number of interconnected spaces that eventually become filled with maternal blood. The trophoblast in this zone is invaded by fetal mesenchyme and is vascularized; therefore, it is the principal site of feto-maternal exchange.

Zone II is the spongiotrophoblast that provides structural support to the labyrinth. The spongiotrophoblast forms tortuous vascular channels for maternal blood to reach the labyrinth. This zone of trophoblast is not invaded by mesoderm and is not vascularized.

Zone III consists of a mixture of columnar and cuboidal basal trophoblast cells. These cells are in direct apposition with the maternal decidua and are highly phagocytic in nature (Oduor-Okelo, 1983). Ultrastructural examination of these cells revealed the remnants of phagocytosed cells. The relative abundance of lysosomes and residual bodies in these cells corroborate their phagocytic behavior (Oduor-Okelo, 1983).

Transient syncytia of 25 to 30 nuclei (giant cells of the decidua) are spotted in the junctional zone between the basal trophoblast cells and maternal decidua. This layer is not continuous and appears sporadically. It has an acidophilic cytoplasm with nuclei arranged haphazardly or along the periphery (Oduor-Okelo, 1983).

The interhemal membrane of rock hyrax in zone I is hemomonochorial. It has a single layer of trophoblast cells on a basement membrane overlying endothelial cells of fetal capillaries (Dempsey, 1969). These trophoblast cells, on their apical surface by which they contact maternal blood, have numerous microvilli and are actively involved in absorption. It must be noted that most of the hemomonochorial placentas that have been described contain syncytial trophoblasts interfacing with maternal blood, and not cytotrophoblasts (Enders, 1965). Therefore, the rock hyrax is one of the few animals that have a cellular hemomonochorial interhemal membrane.

Conclusion

Hopefully the descriptions above have served to illustrate the rich diversity of eutherian placentas. Until recently, our understanding of placental biology has come about through systematic descriptive studies. Such efforts have been invaluable and our knowledge of placenta structure, function, and evolution will only increase in the future. Recent whole genome sequencing efforts coupled with the emergence of relatively low-cost sequencing of genomes and tissue specific cDNA libraries, expression profiling with microarrays, and proteomics tools will enable us to perform comparisons between different species that were undreamed of only a few years ago. These tools hold the potential to disclose hitherto undiscovered genes, regulatory elements, and other biochemical mechanisms involved in placenta biology and will greatly expand our understanding of the fascinating and complex eutherian placenta.

Bibliography

Abd-Elnaeim, M.M., Pfarrer, C., Saber, A.S., Abou-Elmagd, A., Jones, C.J., Leiser, R. (1999). Fetomaternal attachment and anchorage in the early diffuse epitheliochorial placenta of the camel (*Camelus dromedarius*). Light, transmission, and scanning electron microscopic study. *Cells Tissues Organs* 164:141–154.

Adamson, S.L., Lu, Y., Whiteley, K.J., Holmyard, D., Hemberger, M., Pfarrer, C., Cross, J.C. (2002). Interactions between trophoblast cells and the maternal and fetal circulation in the mouse placenta. *Developmental Biology* 250:358–373.

Allen, W.R. (1975). Endocrine functions of the placenta. In: Steven, D.H. (ed) *Comparative Placentation*. London: Academic Press. pp. 214–267.

Allen, W.R. (1982). Immunological aspects of the endometrial cup reaction and the effect of xenogenic pregnancy in horses and donkeys. *J Reprod Fertil* 31:59–94.

Allen, W.R., Hamilton, D.W., Moor, R.M. (1973). The origin of the endometrial cups. II. Invasion of the endometrium by trophoblast. *Anat Rec* 177:485–502.

Allen, W.R., Mathias, S., Wooding, F.B.P., van Aarde, J. (2003). Placentation in the African elephant (*Loxodonta africana*): II Morphological changes in the uterus and placenta throughout gestation. *Placenta* 24:598–617.

Allen, W.R., and Moor, R.M. (1972). The origin of the equine endometrial cups. I. Production of PMSG by fetal trophoblast cells. *J Rep Fert* 29:313–316.

Amenta, P.S., Clark, C.C., Martinez-Hernandez, A. (1983). Deposition of fibronectin and laminin in the basement membrane of the rat parietal yolk sac: Immunohistochemical and biosynthetic studies. *J Cell Biol* 96:104–111.

Amoroso, E.C. (1952). Placentation. In: *Marshall's Physiology of Reproduction*, *Volume 2*, Chapter 15, Parkes, A.S. (ed) London: Longman, Green and Co. pp. 127–311.

Amoroso, E.C. (1961). Placentation. In: Parkes, A.S. (ed) *Marshall's Physiology of Reproduction*. Boston: Little Brown and Co., pp. 127–311.

Amoroso, E.C. and Perry, J.S. (1964). The foetal membranes and placenta of the African elephant (*Loxodonta africana*). *Proc Roy Soc B* 248:1–34.

Anderson, L.L. (1978). Growth, protein content and distribution of early pig embryos. *Anat Rec* 190:143–53.

Anderson, T.L. and Hoffman, L.H. (1984). Alterations in epithelial glycocalyx of rabbit uteri during early pseudopregnancy and pregnancy and following ovariectomy. *Am J Anat* 171:321–334.

Anderson, T.L., Olson, G.E., Hoffman, L.H. (1986). Stage specific alterations in the apical membrane glycoproteins of endometrial epithelialcells related to implantation in rabbits. *Biol Reprod* 34:701–720.

Anson-Cartwright, L., Dawson, K., Holmyard, D., Fisher, S.J., Lazzarini, R.A., Cross, J.C. (2000). The glial cells missing-1 protein is essential for branching morphogenesis in the chorioallantoic placenta. *Nature Genetics* 25:311–314.

Aplin, J.D. (1991). Review: Implantation, trophoblast differentiation and hemochorial placentation, mechanistic evidence in vivo and in vitro. *J Cell Sci* 99:681–692.

Armant, D.R. (2005). Blastocysts don't go it alone. Extrinsic signals fine-tune the intrinsic developmental program of trophoblast cells. *Developmental Biology* 280:260–280.

Armant, D.R., Wang, J., Liu, Z. (2000). Intracellular signaling in the developing blastocyst as a consequence of the maternal-embryonic dialogue. *Seminars In Reproductive Medicine* 18:273–287.

Baker, E. and Morgan, E.H. (1970). Iron transfer across the perfused rabbit placenta. *Life Sci* 9:765–772.

Baker, E. and Morgan, E.H. (1973). Placental iron transfer in the cat. *J Physiol* 232:485–501.

Basha, S.M.M., Bazer, F.W., Roberts, R.M. (1979). The secretion of a uterine specific, purple phosphatase by cultured explants of porcine endometrium dependency upon the state of pregnancy of the donor animal. *Biol Reprod* 20:431–441.

Baur, R. (1977). Morphometry of the placental exchange area. *Advances in Anatomy Embryology and Cell Biology* 53:1–63.

Bazer, F., Marengo, S., Geisert, R., Thatcher, W. (1984). Endocrine vs exocrine secretion of PGF2a in the control of pregnancy in swine. In: Edqvist, L. and Kindahl, H. (eds) *Prostaglandins in Animal Reproduction II* Amsterdam: Elsevier Science Publishers, pp. 115–132.

Bazer, F.W., Chen, T.T., Knight, J.W., Schlosnagle, D.C., Baldwin, N.J., Roberts, R.M. (1975). Presence of a progesterone-induced, uterine specific, acid phosphatase in allantoic fluid of gilts. *J Anim Sci* 41:1112–1119.

Bazer, F.W., Geisert, R.D., Thatcher, W.W., Roberts, R.M. (1982). The establishment and maintenance of pregnancy. In: Cole, D.J.A and Foxcroft, G.R. (eds) *Control of Pig Reproduction*, London: Butterworth Scientific, pp. 227–252.

Bazer, F.W. and Thatcher, W.W. (1977). Theory of maternal recognition of pregnancy in swine based on estrogen controlled endocrine versus exocrine secretion of prostaglandin F2alpha by the uterine endometrium. *Prostaglandins* 14:397–400.

Bell, A.W. (1984). Factors controlling placental and fetal growth and their effects on future production. In: Lindsay, D.H. and Pearce, D.T. (eds) *Reproduction in Sheep*, Cambridge: Cambridge University Press, pp. 144–152.

Bell, A.W. (1991). The whole animal-pregnancy and fetal metabolism. In: Forbes, J.M. and France, J. (eds) *Quantitative Aspects of Ruminant Digestion and Metabolism*, London: Butterworths, pp. 100–145.

Benirschke, K. and Kaufmann, P. (2000). *Pathology of the Human Placenta*, New York: Springer-Verlag.

Benirschke, K. and Lowenstine, L.J. (1995). The placenta of rhinocerotidae. *Verh Ber Erkr Zootiere (Dresden)* 37:15–23.

Berezowsky, J., Zbieranowski, I., Demers, J., Murray, D. (1995). DNA ploidy of hydatiform moles and nonmolar conceptuses: a study using flow and tissue section image cytometry. *Mod Pathol* 8:775–781.

Betteridge, K.J., Eaglesome, M.D., Mitchell, D., Flood, P.F., Beriault, R. (1982). Development of horse embryos up to twenty-two days after ovulation: observations on fresh specimens. *J Anat* 135:191–209.

Betteridge, K.J., Eaglesome, M.D., Randall, G.C.B., Mitchell, D. (1980). Collection, description and transfer of embryos from cattle 10–16 days after oestrus. *J Reprod Fert* 59: 205–216.

Billington, W.D. (1970). Trophoblast extensions from the placenta. *Proc R Soc Med* 63:57–59.

Bjorkman, N. (1973). Fine structure of the fetal-maternal area of exchange in the epitheiochorial and endoteliochorial type of placentation. *Acta Anat* 86:1–22.

Bjorkman, N.H. (1970). *An Atlas of Placental Fine Structure,* Baltimore: Williams and Wilkins.

Blankenship, T.N., Enders, A.C., King, B.F. (1992). Distribution of laminin, type IV collagen, and fibronectin in the cell columns and trophoblastic shell of early macaque placentas. *Cell Tissue Res* 270:241–248.

Blankenship, T.N. and Given, R.L. (1992). Penetration of the epithelial basement membrane during blastocyst implantation in the mouse. *Anat Rec* 233.

Blond, J.L., Lavillette, D., Cheynet, V., Bouton, O., Oriol, G., Chapel-Fernandes, S., Manrand, B., Mallet, F., Cosset, F.L. (2000). An envelope glycoprotein of the human endogenous retrovirus HERV-W is expressed in the human placenta and fuses cells expressing the type D mammalian retrovirus receptor. *J Virol* 74:3321–3329.

Boshier, D.P. (1969). A histological and histochemical examination of implantation and early placentome formation in sheep. *J Reprod Fertil* 19:51–61.

Boshier, D.P. and Holloway, H. (1977). The sheep trophoblast and placental function: an ultrastructural study. *J Anat* 124: 287–298.

Boyd, J.D. and Hamilton, W.J. (1970). *The Human Placenta,* Cambridge: W. Heffer and Sons.

Brambel, C.E. (1933). Allantochorionic differentiations of the pig studied morphologically and histochemically. *Am J Anat* 51:397–459.

Brayman, M., Thathiah, A., Carson, D. (2004). MUC1: A multifunctional cell surface component of reproductive tissue epithelia. *Reproductive Biology and Endocrinology* 2:4.

Bright, N.A., Ockleford, C.D., Anwar, M. (1994). Ontogeny and distribution of Fc gamma receptors in the human placenta. Transport or immune surveillance? *J Anat* 184:297–308.

Buhi, W., Ducsay, C., Bazer, F., Roberts, R. (1982). Iron transfer between the purple phosphatase uteroferrin and transferrin and its possible role in iron metabolism of the fetal pig. *J Biol Chem* 257:1712–1723.

Bulmer, J.N. and Johnson, P.M. (1985). Antigen expression by trophoblast populations in the human placenta and their possible immunobiological relevance. *Placenta* 6:127–140.

Burton, G.J. (1987a). The fine structure of the human placental villus as revealed by scanning electron microscopy. *Scanning Microscopy* 1:1811–1828.

Burton, G.J. (1987b). Review article. Placental uptake of maternal erythrocytes: a comparative study. *Placenta* 3:407–434.

Burton, G.J. (1990). On the varied appearances of the human placenta villous surface visualised by scanning electron microscopy. *Scanning Microscopy* 4:501–507.

Byorkman, N.H. (1969). Light and electron microscopic studies on alterations in the normal bovine placentome. *Anat Rec* 163:17–29.

Carlson, B.M. (1981). *Patten's Foundations of Embryology,* New York: McGraw-Hill.

Carson, D.D., Bagchi, I., Dey, S.K., Enders, A.C., Fazleabas, A.T., Lessey, B.A., Yoshinaga, K. (2000). Embryo Implantation. *Developmental Biology* 223:217–237.

Carter, A.M. (2001). Evolution of the placenta and fetal membranes seen in the light of molecular phylogenetics. *Placenta* 22:800–807.

Carter, A.M. and Enders, A.C. (2004). Comparative aspects of trophoblast development and placentation. *Reprod Biol Endocrine* 2:http://www.rbej.com/content/2/1/46.

Carter, A.M., Gothlin, J., Olin, T. (1971). An angiographic study of the structure and function of uterine and maternal placental vasculature in the rabbit. *J Reprod Fertil* 25:201–210.

Castellucci, M., Scheper, M., Schefen, I., Celora, A., Kaufmann, P. (1990). The development of the human placental villous tree. *Anat Embryol (Berl)* 181:117–128.

Chai, N., Patel, Y., Jacobson, K., McMahon, J., McMahon, A., Rappolee, D.A. (1998). FGF is an essential regulator of the fifth cell division in preimplantation mouse embryos. *Developmental Biology* 198:105–115.

Chen, T.T., Bazer, F.W., Cetorelli, J.J., Pollard, W.E., Roberts, R.M. (1973). Purification and properties of a progesterone-induced basic glycoprotein from the uterine fluids of pigs. *J Biol Chem* 248:8560–8566.

Chen, T.T., Bazer, F.W., Gebhardt, B., Roberts, R.M. (1975). Uterine secretion in mammals: synthesis and placental transport of a purple acid phosphatase in pigs. *Biol Reprod* 13:304–313.

Chervenak, J.L. and Illsley, N.P. (2000). Episialin acts as an antiadhesive factor in an in vitro model of human endometrial-blastocyst attachment. *Biol Reprod* 63:294–300.

Claudia Freyer, U.Z., Renfree, M.B. (2003). The marsupial placenta: A phylogenetic analysis. *Journal of Experimental Zoology Part A: Comparative Experimental Biology* 299A:59–77.

Cooper, R.A., Connell, R.S., Wellings, S.R. (1964). Placenta of the Indian elephant, *Elephas indicas. Science* 146:410–412.

Covone, A.E., Johnson, P.M., Mutton, D., Adinolfi, M. (1984). Trophoblast cells in peripheral blood from pregnant women. *Lancet:* 841–843.

Creed, R.F.S. and Biggers, J.D. (1963). Development of the raccoon placenta. *Am J Anat* 113:417–446.

Crespi, B. and Semeniuk, C. (2004). Parent-offspring conflict in the evolution of vertebrate reproductive mode. *Am Nat* 163:635–653.

Cross, J.C., Baczyk, D., Dobric, N., Hemberger, M., Hughes, M., Simmons, D.G., Yamamoto, H., Kingdom, J.C.P. (2003a). Genes, development and evolution of placenta. *Placenta* 24:123–130.

Cross, J.C., Simmons, D.G., Watson, E.D. (2003b). Chorioallantoic morphogenesis and formation of the placental villous tree. *Ann NY Acad Sci* 995:84–93.

Cross, J.C., Werb, Z., Fisher, S.J. (1994). Implantation and the placenta: key pieces of the development puzzle. *Science* 266:1508–1518.

Damsky, C.H., Fitzgerald, M.L., Fisher, S.J. (1992). Distribution patterns of extracellular matrix components and adhesion receptors are intricately modulated during first trimester cytotrophoblast differentiation along the invasive pathway, in vivo. *J Clin Invest* 89:210–222.

Dantzer, V. (1985). Electron microscopy of the initial stages of placentation in the pig. *Anat Embryol (Berl)* 172:281–293.

Dantzer, V., Bjorkman, N., Hasselager, E. (1981). An electron microscopic study of histiotrophe in the interareolar part of the porcine placenta. *Placenta* 2:19–28.

Dantzer, V. and Nielsen, M.H. (1984). Intracellular pathways of native iron in the maternal part of the porcine placenta. *Eur J Cell Biol* 34:103–9.

Deane, H.W., Rubin, B.L., Driks, E.C., Lobel, B.L., Leipsner, G. (1962). Trophoblast giant cells in placentas of rats and mice and their probable role in steroid hormone production. *Endocrinology* 70:407–419.

Degrelle, S.A., Campion, E., Cabau, C., Piumi, F., Reinaud, P., Richard, C., Renard, J.-P., Hue, I. (2005). Molecular evidence for a critical period in mural trophoblast development in bovine blastocysts. *Developmental Biology* 288:448–460.

Dempsey, E.W. (1969). Comparative aspects of the placentae of certain African mammals. *J Rep Fert* 6:189–192.

Denker, H.W., Eng, L.A., Mootz, U., Hamner, C.E. (1978b). Studies on the early development and implantation in the cat. II. Implantation: proteinases. *Anat Embryol (Berl)* 154:39–54.

Dey, S.K., Lim, H., Das, S.K., Reese, J., Paria, B.C., Daikoku, T., Wang, H. (2004). Molecular cues to implantation. *Endocr Rev* 25:341–373.

Dhindsa, D.S. and Dziuk, P.J. (1968). Effect on pregnancy in the pig after killing embryos or fetuses in one uterine horn in early gestation. *J Anim Sci* 27:122–6.

Dickmann, Z. (1979). Blastocyst estrogen: An essential factor for the control of implantation. *J Steroid Biochem* 11:771–773.

Diehl, M., Munz, C., Keilholz, W., Stevanovic, S., Holmes, N., Loke, Y.W., Rammensee, H.G. (1996). Nonclassical HLA-G molecules are classical peptide presenters. *Current Biology* 6:305–314.

Dolinar, Z.J., Ludwig, K.S., Muller, E. (1965). Ein weiterer Beitrag zur Kenntnis der Placenten der Ordnung Perissodactyla: Zwei Geburtsplacenten des Indischen Panzernashorns. (*Rhinoceros unicornis* L.). *Acta Anat* 61:331–354.

Duello, T.M., Byatt, J.C., Bremel, R.D. (1986). Immunohistochemical localization of placental lactogen in binucleate cells of bovine placentomes. *Endocrinology* 119:1351–1355.

Dunlap, K.A., Palmarini, M., Adelson, D.L., Spencer, T.E. (2005). Sheep endogenous betaretroviruses (enJSRVs) and the hyaluronidase 2 (HYAL2) receptor in the uvine uterus and conceptus. *Biol Reprod* 73:271–279.

Ellington, S.K. (1985). A morphological study of the development of the allantois of rat embryos in vivo. *J Anat* 142:1–11.

Ellington, S.K. (1987). A morphological study of the development of the chorion of rat embryos. *J Anat* 150:247–263.

Enders, A. (1965). A comparative study of the fine structure of the trophoblast in several hemochorial placentas. *American Journal of Anatomy* 116:29–67.

Enders, A. and Blankenship, T. (1999). Comparative placental structure. *Advanced Drug Delivery Review* 38:3–15.

Enders, A.C. (1989). Trophoblast differentiation during the transition from trophoblastic plate to lacunar stage of implantation in the rhesus monkey and human. *Am J Anat* 186:85–98.

Enders, A.C., Hendrickx, A.G., Schlafke, S. (1983). Implantation in the rhesus monkey: initial penetration of endometrium. *Am J Anat* 167:275–298.

Enders, A.C. and King, B.F. (1991). Early stages of trophoblastic invasion of the maternal vascular system during implantation in the macaque and baboon. *Am J Anat* 192:329–346.

Enders, A.C. and King, B.F. (1993). Development of the human yolk sac. In: Nogales, F.F. (ed) *The Human Yolk Sac and Yolk Sac Tumors*, New York: Springer-Verlag.

Enders, A.C. and Liu, I.K.M. (1991a). Lodgement of the equine blastocyst in the uterus from fixation through endometrial cup formation. *J Reprod Fertil* Suppl 44:427–438.

Enders, A.C. and Liu, I.K.M. (1991b). Trophoblast-uterine interactions during equine girdle cell maturation, migration and transformation. *Am J Anat* 192:366–381.

Enders, A.C. and Schlafke, S. (1971). Penetration of the uterine epithelium during implantation in the rabbit. *Am J Anat* 132:219–240.

Enders, A.C., Schlafke, S., Welsh, A.O. (1980). Trophoblastic and uterine luminal epithelial surfaces at the time of blastocyst adhesion in the rat. *Am J Anat* 159:59–72.

Enders, A.C. and Welsh, A.O. (1993). Structural interactions of trophoblast and uterus during hemochorial placenta formation. *J Exp Zool* 266:578–587.

Eugenia Basyuk, J.C.C., Corbin, J., Nakayama, H., Hunter, P., Nait-Oumesmar, B., Lazzarini, R.A. (1999). Murine *Gcm1* gene is expressed in a subset of placental trophoblast cells. *Developmental Dynamics* 214:303–311.

Falck Larsen, J. (1980). Human implantation and clinical aspects. *Prog Reprod Biol* 7:284–296.

Fatemi, S.H. (1987). The role of secretory granules in the transport of basement membrane components: radioautographic studies of rat parietal yolk sac employing 3H-proline as a precursor of type IV collagen. *Connect Tissue Res* 16:1–14.

Faulk, W.P. and Galbraith, G.M.P. (1979). Transferrin and transferrin-receptors of human trophoblast. In: Hemmings, W.A. (ed) *Protein Transmission through Living Membranes*, Amsterdam: Elsevier/North Holland Biomedical Press, pp. 55–61.

Fléchon, J.-E., Degrouard, J., Fléchon, B. (2004). Gastrulation events in the prestreak pig embryo: ultrastructure and cell markers. *Genesis* 38:13–25.

Fowler, M.E. (1998). *Medicine and Surgery of South American Camelids. Llama, Alpaca, Vicuña, Guanaco.* Ames, Iowa: Iowa State University Press.

Fowler, M.E. and Olander, H.J. (1990). Fetal membranes and ancillary structures of llamas (*Lama glama*). *Amer J Vet Res* 51:1495–1500.

Frendo, J.-L., Olivier, D., Cheynet, V., Blond, J.-L., Bouton, O., Vidaud, M., Rabreau, M., Evain-Brion, D., Mallet, F. (2003).

Direct involvement of HERV-W env glycoprotein in human trophoblast cell fusion and differentiation. *Mol Cell Biol* 23:3566–3574.

Freyer, C., Zeller, U., Renfree, M.B. (2002). Ultrastructure of the placenta of the tammar wallaby, *Macropus eugenii*: comparison with the grey short-tailed opossum, *Monodelphis domestica*. *Journal of Anatomy* 201:101–119.

Friess, A.E., Sinowatz, F., Skolek-Winnisch, R., Trautner, W. (1981). The placenta of the pig. II. The ultrastructure of the areolae. *Anat Embryol (Berl)* 163:43–53.

Gardner, R.L. (1983a). Origin and differentiation of extra-embryonic tissues in the mouse. *Int Rev Exp Pathol* 24:63–133.

Gardner, R.L. (1983b). Origin and differentiation of extra-embryonic tissues in the mouse. *Int Rev Exp Path* 24:63–133.

Gardner, R.L. (2000). Flow of cells from polar to mural trophectoderm is polarized in the mouse blastocyst. *Human Reproduction* 15:694–701.

Gardner, R.L., Papaioannou, V.E., Barton, S.C. (1973). Origin of the ectoplacental cone and secondary giant cells in mouse blastocysts reconstituted from isolated trophoblast and inner cell mass. *J Embryol Exp Morphol* 30:561–572.

Geisert, R.D., Brookbank, J.W., Roberts, R.M., Bazer, F.W. (1982a). Establishment of pregnancy in the pig: II. cellular remodelling of the porcine blastocyst during elongation on day 12 of pregnancy. *Biol Reprod* 27:941–955.

Geisert, R.D., Renegar, R.H., Thatcher, W.W., Roberts, R.M., Bazer, F.W. (1982b). establishment of pregnancy in the pig: I. interrelationships between preimplantation development of the pig blastocyst and uterine endometrial secretions. *Biol Reprod* 27:925–939.

Genbacev, O.D., Prakobphol, A., Foulk, R.A., Krtolica, A.R., Ilic, D., Singer, M.S., Yang, Z.-Q., Kiessling, L.L., Rosen, S.D., Fisher, S.J. (2003). Trophoblast L-selectin-mediated adhesion at the maternal-fetal interface. *Science* 299:405–408.

Ghazi, S.R., Oryan, A., Poumiraei, H. (1994). Some aspects of macroscopic studies of the placentation in the camel (*Camelus dromedarius*). *Anat Histol Embryol* 23:337–342.

Ginther, O.J. (1983a). Mobility of the early equine conceptus. *Theriogenol* 19:603–611.

Ginther, O.J. (1983b). Fixation and orientation of the early equine conceptus. *Theriogenol* 19.

Ginther, O.J. (1992). *Reproductive Biology of the Mare: Basic and Applied Aspects.* Cross Plains, WI: Equiservices.

Gitlin, D., Kumate, J., Urrusti, J., Morales, D. (1964). The selectivity of the human placenta in the transfer of plasma proteins from mother to fetus. *J Clin Invest* 43:1938–1951.

Gorokhovskii, N.L., Schmidt, G.A., Shagaeva, V.G., Baptidanova, I.P. (1975). Giant cells in the placenta of the Bactrian camel in the fetal period of development. (In Russian). *Arkh Anat Gistol Embriol* 69:41–46.

Green, J.A., parks, T.E., Avalle, M.P., Telugu, B.P., McLain, A. L., Peterson, A.J., McMillan, W., Mathialagan, N., Xie, S., Hook, R.R., Roberts, R.M. (2005). The establishment of an ELISA for the detection of pregnancy-associated glycoproteins (PAGs) in the serum of pregnant cows and heifers. *Theriogenology* 63:1481–1503.

Green, J.A., Xie, S., Quan, X., Bao, B., Gan, X., Mathialagan, N., Beckers, J.-F., Roberts, R.M. (2000). pregnancy-associated bovine and ovine glycoproteins exhibit spatially and temporally distinct expression patterns during pregnancy. *Biol Reprod* 62:1624–1631.

Green, J.A., Xie, S., Roberts, R.M. (1998). Pepsin-related molecules secreted by trophoblast. *Rev Reprod* 3:62–69.

Greenstein, J.S., Murray, R.W., Foley, R.C. (1958). Observations on the morphogenesis and histochemistry of the bovine pre-attachment placenta between 16–33 days of gestation. *Anat Rec.* 132:321–341.

Grosser, O. (1909). Vergleichende Antomie und Entwicklunsgeschchte der Eihaute und der Placenta. In *Braumuller, Wien und Leipzig*, pp. 1–314.

Grosser, O. (1927). *Fruhentwicklung, Eihautbidung und Placentation des Menschen und der Saugetiere.*

Grundker, C. and Kirchner, C. (1996). Influence of uterine growth factors on blastocyst expansion and trophoblast knob formation in the rabbit. *Early Pregnancy* 2:264–270.

Guillomot, M., Flechon, J., Wintenberger-Torres, S. (1982). Cytological studies of uterine and trophoblastic surface coats during blastocyst attachment in the ewe. *J Reprod Fertil* 65:1–8.

Guillomot, M., Flechon, J.E., Leroy, F. (1993). Blastocyst development and implantation. In: Thibault, C., Levasseur, M.C., and Hunter, R.H.F. (eds) *Reproduction in Mammals and Man*, Paris: Ellipses, pp. 387–411.

Guillomot, M., Flechon, J.E., Wintenberger-Torres, S. (1981). Conceptus attachment in the ewe: an ultrastructural study. *Placenta* 2:169–82.

Guillomot, M. and Guay, P. (1982). Ultrastructural features of the cell surfaces of terine and trophoblastic epithelium during embryonic attachment in the cow. *Anatomical Record* 204:315–322.

Hafez, E.S.E. and Tsutsumi, Y. (1966). Changes in endometrial vascularity during implantation and pregnancy in the rabbit. *Am J Anat* 118:249–282.

Haig, D. (1993). Genetic conflicts in human pregnancy. *Q Rev Biol* 68:495–532.

Haig, D. (1996). Altercation of generations: genetic conflicts of pregnancy. *Am J Reprod Immunol* 35:226–32.

Haluska, G.J. and Currie, W.B. (1988). Variation in plasma concentrations of oestradiol 17β and their relationship to those of progesterone, PGF$_{2\alpha}$ and oxytocin across pregnancy and at parturition in pony mares. *J Reprod Fertil* 84:635–644.

Harris, J.R. (1998). Placental endogenous retrovirus (ERV): structural, functional, and evolutionary significance. *Bioessays* 20:307–316.

Harvey, W. (1651). *De Generatione Animalium.* London: Sydenham Society.

Hasselager, E. (1985). Surface exchange area of the porcine placenta. *Journal of Microscopy* 131:91–100.

He, Y., Smith, S.K., Day, K.A., Clark, D.E., Licence, D.R., Charnock-Jones, D.S. (1999). Alternative splicing of vascular endothelial growth factor (VEGF)-R1 (FLT-1) pre-mRNA is important for the regulation of VEGF activity. *Mol Endocrinol* 13:537–545.

Hemberger, M. and Cross, J.C. (2001). Genes governing placental development. *Trends in Endocrinology and Metabolism* 12:162–168.

Heuser, C.H. and Streeter, G.L. (1929). Early stages in the development of pig embryos, from the period of initial cleavage to the time of the appearance of limb-buds. *Contr Embryol Carnegie Instn* 20:1–29.

Hey, N.A., Graham, R.A., Seif, M.W., Aplin, J.D. (1994). The polymorphic epithelial mucin MUC-1 in human endometrium is normally upregulated with maximal expression in the implantation phase. *J Clin Endocinol Metab* 78:337–342.

Hild-Petito, S., Fazleabas, A.T., Julien, J.A., Carson, D.D. (1996). Mucin (MUC-1) expression is differentially regulated in uterine luminal and glandular epithelium of baboon (*Papio anubis*). *Biol Reprod* 54:939–947.

Hoffman, L.H., Winfrey, V.P., Anderson, T.Z., Olsen, G.E. (1990a). Uterine receptivity to implantation in the rabbit: evidence for a 42kDa glycoprotein as a marker of receptivity. *Troph Res* 4:243–258.

Hoffman, L.H., Winfrey, V.P., Hoos, P.C. (1990b). Sites of endometrial vascular leakage during implantation in the rabbit. *Anat Rec* 227:47–61.

Hogan, B.L.M. (1980). High molecular weight extracellular protens synthesized by endoderm cells derived from mouse teratocarcinoma cells and normal extra-embryonic membranes. *Dev Biol* 76:275–285.

Hogan, B.L.M. and Tilly, R. (1981). Cell interactions and endoderm differentiation in cultured mouse embryos. *J. Embryol Exp Morphol* 62:379–394.

Hughes, A.L., Green, J.A., Piontkivska, H., Roberts, R.M. (2003a). Aspartic proteinase phylogeny and the origin of pregnancy-associated glycoproteins. *Mol Biol Evol* 20:1940–1945.

Hughes, A.L., Green, J.A., Piontkivska, H., Roberts, R.M. (2003b). Aspartic proteinase phylogeny and the origin of pregnancy-associated glycoproteins. *Mol Biol Evol* 20:1940–1945.

Hughes, R.L. and Hall, L.S. (1998). Early development and embryology of the platypus. *Phil Trans R Soc Lond B Biol Sci* 353:1101–1114.

Hunt, J.S., Fishback, J.L., Chumbley, G., Loke, Y.W. (1990). Identification of class I MHC mRNA in human first trimester trophoblast cells by in situ hybridization. *J Immunol* 144:4420–4425.

Hunt, J.S. and Hsi, B.L. (1990). Review: Evasive strategies of trophoblast cells: selective expression of membrane antigens. *Am J Reprod Immunol* 23:57–63.

Ikle, F.A. (1964). Dissemination von Syncytiotrophoblastzellen im mutterlichen Blut wahrend der Graviditat. *Bull Schweiz Akad Med Wiss* 20:62–72.

Iwasa, Y. (1998). The conflict theory of genomic imprinting: how much can be explained? *Curr Top Dev Biol* 40:255–293.

Janssen, A. (1933). Uber die Placenta und Paraplacenta bei der Katze. In *Vet Med Diss*, Hannover.

Johnson, G.A., Bazer, F.W., Jaeger, L.A., Ka, H., Garlow, J.E., Pfarrer, C., Spencer, T.E., Burghardt, R.C. (2001). Muc-1, integrin, and osteopontin expression during the implantation cascade in sheep. *Biol Reprod* 65:820–828.

Jollie, W.P. (1986). Ultrastructural studies of protein transfer across rodent yolk sac. *Placenta* 7:263–281.

Jollie, W.P. (1990a). Development, morphology, and function of the yolk-sac placenta of laboratory rodents. *Teratology* 41:361–381.

Jollie, W.P. (1990b). Development, morphology, and function of the yolk-sac placenta of laboratory rodents. *Teratology* 41:361–381.

Kaufmann, M.H. (1983). Origin, properties and fate of trophoblast in mouse. In: Loke, C. and Whyte, A. (eds) *Biology of tropoblast*, Amsterdam: Elsevier, pp. 23–70.

Kaufmann, M.H. (1985). Basic morphology of the fetal and maternal circuits in the human placenta. *Contributions to Gynecology and Obstetrics* 13:5–17.

Kaufmann, P. (1981a). Entwicklund der plazenta. In: Becker, V., Schiebler, T.H., and Kubli, F. (eds) *Die Plazenta des Menschen*, New York: Thieme.

Kaufmann, P. (1981b). Functional anatomy of the non-primate placenta. *Placenta* (Suppl) 1:13–28.

Kaufmann, P., Black, S., Huppertz, B. (2003). Endovascular trophoblast invasion: implications for the pathogenesis of intra-uterine growth retardation and preeclampsia. *Biol Reprod* 69:1–7.

Kaufmann, P. and Burton, G.J. (1994). Anatomy and genesis of the placenta. In: Knobil, E. and Neill, J.D. (eds) *The Physiology of Reproduction*, New York: Raven Press, pp. 441–484.

Kaufmann, P. and Davidoff, M. (1977). The guinea-pig placenta. *Adv Anat Embryol Cell Biol* 53:5–91.

Kaufmann, P., Luckhard, M., Leiser, R. (1988). Three-dimensional representation of the fetal vessel system in the human placenta. *Troph Res* 3:113–137.

Kehrer, A. (1978). Licht-und elktronenkiskroskroskopische Untersuchungen an der Paraplacenta der Katze. *Z Mikrosk Anat Forsc* 92:119–146.

Keye, J.D. (1923). Periodic variations in spontaneous contractions of uterine muscle in relation to the oestrous cycle and early pregnancy. *Bull, Johns Hopkins Hospital* 34:60–63.

Keys, J.L. and King, G.J. (1990). Microscopic examination of porcine conceptus-maternal interface between days 10 and 19 of pregnancy. *Am J Anat* 188:221–238.

Kimber, S.J. and Lindenberg, S. (1990). Hormonal control of a carbohydrate epitope involved in implantation in mice. *J Reprod Fertil* 89:13–21.

Kimura, J., Sasaki, M., Endo, H., Fukuta, K. (2004). Anatomical and histological characterization of the female reproductive organs of mouse deer (*Tragulidae*). *Placenta* 25:705–711.

King, A., Loke, Y.W., Chaouat, G. (1997). NK cells and reproduction. *Immunology Today* 18:64–66.

King, B.F. (1984). The fine structure of the placenta and chorionic vesicles of the bush baby, *Galago crassicaudata*. *Am J Anat* 169:101–116.

King, B.F. (1991). Absorption of macromolecules by the placenta-some morphological perspectives. *Troph Res* 5:333–347.

King, B.F. (1993a). Development and structure of the placenta and fetal membranes of nonhuman primates. *J Exp Zool* 266:528–540.

King, B.F. and Hastings, R.A. (1977). The comparative fine structure of the interhemal membrane of chorioallantoic placenta from six general of myomorph rodents. *Am J Anat* 149:165–180.

King, G.J. (1993b). Comparative placentation in ungulates. *J Exp Zool* 266:588–602.

King, G.J. and Atkinson, B.A. (1987). The bovine intercaruncular placenta throughout gestation. *Anim Reprod Sci* 12:241–254.

King, G.J., Atkinson, B.A., Robertson, H.A. (1979). Development of the bovine placentome during the second month of gestation. *J Rep Fert* 55:173–180.

King, G.J., Atkinson, B.A., Robertson, H.A. (1981). Development of the intercaruncular area during early gestation and the establishment of the bovine placenta. *J Rep Fert* 61:469–474.

King, G.J., Atkinson, B.A., Robertson, H.A. (1982). Implantation and early placentation in domestic ungulates. *J Reprod Fertil Suppl* 31:17–30.

Klisch, K., Hecht, W., Pfarrer, C., Schuler, G., Hoffmann, B., Leiser, R. (1999). DNA content and ploidy level of bovine placentomal trophoblast giant cells. *Placenta* 20:451–458.

Klonisch, T., Wolf, P., Hombach-Klonisch, S., Vogt, S., Kuechenhoff, A., Tetens, F., Fischer, B. (2001). Epidermal growth factor-like ligands and erbB genes in the peri-implantation rabbit uterus and blastocyst. *Biol Reprod* 64:1835–1844.

Knoth, M. and Larsen, J.F. (1972). Ultrastructure of a human implantation site. *Acta Obstet Gynecol Scand* 51:385–393.

Kozma, R., Spring, J., Johnson, P.M., Adinolfi, M. (1986). Detection of syncytiotrophoblast in maternal peripheral and uterine veins using a monoclonal antibody and flow cytometry. *Hum Reprod* 1:335–336.

Kramer, B., Stein, B.A., Vanderwalt, L.A. (1990). Exogenous gonadotropins serum oestrogen and progesterone and the effect on endomerial morphology in the rat. *J Anat* 173.

Lacroix, M.C., Guibourdenche, J., Frendo, J.L., Pidoux, G., Evain-Brion, D. (2002). Placental growth hormones. *Endocrine* 19:73–79.

Lang, E.M. (1957). Geburt eines Panzernashorns, Rhinoceros unicornis, im Zoologischen Garten Basel. *Säugetierk. Mitt* 5:69–70.

Larsen, J.F. (1961). Electron microscopy of the implantation site in the rabbit. *Am J Anat* 109:319–334.

Lawn, A.M., Chiquoine, A.D., Amoroso, E.C. (1969). The development of the placenta in the sheep and goat: an electron microscopic study. *J Anat* 105:557–578.

Leaman, D.W., Cross, J.C., Roberts, R.M. (1992). Genes for the trophoblast interferons and their distribution among mammals. *Reprod Fertil Dev* 4:349–353.

Lee, N., Malacko, A.R., Ishitani, A., Chen, M.C., Bajorath, J., Marquardt, H., Geraghty, D.E. (1995). The membrane-bound and soluble forms of HLA-G bind identical sets of endogenous peptides but differ with respect to TAP association. *Immunity* 3.

Lee, S.Y., Mossman, H.W., Mossman, A.S., Delpino, G. (1977). Evidence for a specific implantation site in ruminants. *Am J Anat* 150:631–640.

Leiser, R. (1979). Blastocysten implantation bei der Hauskatze. Licht-und elektronenmiskroskopische Untersucung. *Anat Histol Embryol* 8:79–96.

Leiser, R. (1982). Development of the trophoblast in the early carnivore placenta of cat. *Bibl Anat* 22:93–107.

Leiser, R. and Enders, A.C. (1980a). Light and electron microscopic study of the near-term paraplacenta of the domestic cat. I. Polar and paraplacental junctional areas. *Acta Anat.* 106:293–311.

Leiser, R. and Enders, A.C. (1980b). Light and electron microscopic study of the near-term paraplacenta of the near-term paraplacental junctional areas. *Acta Anat.* ••:312–326.

Leiser, R. and Kaufmann, P. (1994). Placental structure: in a comparative aspect. *Exp Clin Endocrinol* 102:122–134.

Leiser, R. and Kobb, B. (1993). Development and characteristics of placentation in a carnivore, the domestic cat. *J Exp Zool* 266:642–656.

Leiser, R. and Kohler, T. (1983). The blood vessels of the cat girdle placenta. Observations on corrosion casts. SEM and histological studies. I. Maternal vasculature. *Anat Embryol (Berl)* 167:85–93.

Leiser, R. and Kohler, T. (1984). The blood vessels of the cat girdle placenta. Observations on corrosion casts,. SEM and histological studies. II. Fetal vasculature. *Anat Embryol (Berl)* 170:209–216.

Leivo, I., Vaheri, A., Timpl, R., Wartiovaara, J.L. (1980). Appearance and distribution of collagens and laminin in the early mouse embryo. *Dev Biol* 76:100–114.

Lescisin, K.R., Varmuza, S., Rossant, J. (1988). Isolation and characterization of a novel trophoblast-specific cDNA in the mouse. *Genes Dev* 2:1639–1646.

Lim, K., Zhou, Y., Jantpour, M., McMaster, M., Bass, K., Chun, S., Fisher, S. (1997). Human cytotrophoblast differentiation/invasion is abnormal in pre-eclampsia. *Am J Pathol* 151:1809–1818.

Loke, Y.W. and Butterworth, B.H. (1987). Heterogeneity of human trophoblast populations. In: Gill, T.J. and Wegmann, T.G. (eds) *Immunoregulation and Fetal Survival*, New York: Oxford University Press, pp. 197–209.

Loke, Y.W., Hiby, S., King, A. (1999). Human leucocyte antigen-G and reproduction. *Journal of Reproductive Immunology* 43:235–242.

Loke, Y.W. and King, A. (1989). Immunology and pregnancy: quo vadis. *Human Reproduction* 4:613–615.

Loke, Y.W. and King, A. (1995). *Human Implantation: Cell Biology and Immunology.* Cambridge: Cambridge University Press.

Luckett, W.P. (1993). Uses and limitations of mammalian fetal membranes and placenta for phylogenetic reconstruction. *J Exp Zool* 266:514–527.

Ludwig, K.S. (1962). Zur Kenntnis der Geburtsplacenten der Ordnung Perissodactyla. *Acta Anat* 49:157–167.

Ludwig, K.S. and Muller, E. (1965). Zur Histochemie der Placenta des Panzernashorns (*Rhinoceros unicornis L.*). *Acta Anat* Suppl 115:155–159.

Ludwig, K.S. and Villiger, W. (1965). Zur Ultrastruktur der Blattzottenepithelien in der Placenta des Indischen Panzernashorns (*Rhinoceros unicornis L.*). *Acta Anat* 62:593–605.

MacLean, J.A., Chakrabarty, A., Xie, S., Bixby, J., Roberts, R.M., Green, J.A. (2003). Family of Kunitz proteins from trophoblast: expression of the trophoblast Kunitz domain proteins (TKDP) in cattle and sheep. *Mol Reprod Dev* 65:30–40.

Malasinne, A. (1974). Evolution ultrastructurle du labyrinthe de placenta de chatte. *Anat Embryol (Berl)* 146:1–20.

Malasinne, A. (1977). Etude ultrastructurale du paaplacenta de chatte: Mechanisme de l'erythrophagocytse par la cellule choriionique. *Anat Embryol (Berl)* 151:267–283.

Malassine, A., Besse, C., Roche, A., Alsat, E., Rebourcet, R., Mondon, F., Cedard, L. (1987). Ultrastructural visualization of the internalization of low density lipoprotein by human placental cells. *Histochemistry* 87:457–464.

Malassine, A., Frendo, J.-L., Evain-Brion, D. (2003). A comparison of placental development and endocrine functions between the human and mouse model. *Hum Reprod Update* 9:531–539.

Mattson, B.A., Overstrom, E.W., Albertini, D.E. (1990). Transitions in trophectodermal cellular shape and cytoskeletal organization in the elongating pig blastocyst. *Biol Reprod* 42:195–205.

Mazariegos, M.R., Leblond, C.P., van der Rest, M. (1987). Radio-autographic tracing of 3H-proline in the endodermal cells of the parietal yolk sac as an indicator of the biogenesis of basement membrane components. *Am J Anat* 179:79–93.

McDowell, K.J., Sharp, D.C., Grumbaugh, W., Thatcher, W.W., Wilcox, C.J. (1988). Restricted conceptus mobility results in failure of pregnancy maintenance in mares. *Biol Reprod* 39:340–348.

Meseguer, M., Aplin, J.D., Caballero-Campo, P., O'Connor, J.E., Martin, J.C., Remohi, J., Pellicer, A., Simon, C. (2001). Human endometrial mucin MUC1 is up-regulated by progesterone and down-regulated in vitro by the human blastocyst. *Biol Reprod* 64:590–601.

Mess, A. and Carter, A.M. (2006). Evolutionary transformations of fetal membrane characters in eutheria with special reference to afrotheria. *J Exp Zool (Mol Dev Evol)* 306B.

Mi, S., Lee, X., Li, X.-P., Veldman, G.M., Finnerty, H., Racie, L., LaVallie, E., Tang, X.-Y., Edouard, P., Howes, S., Keith, J.C., McCoy, J.M. (2000). Syncytin is a captive retroviral envelope protein involved in human placental morphogenesis. 403:785–789.

Michael, K., Ward, B.S., Moore, W.M.O. (1985). In vitro permeability of the pig placenta in the last third of gestation. *Biology of the Neonate* 47:170–178.

Morasso, M.I., Grinberg, A., Robinson, G., Sargent, T.D., Mahon, K.A. (1999). Placental failure in mice lacking the homeobox gene Dlx3. *PNAS* 96:162–167.

Morgan, G. and Wooding, F.B.P. (1983). Cell migration in the ruminant placenta, a freeze fracture study. *Journal of Ultrastructural Research* 83:148–160.

Mossman, H.W. (1937). Comparative morphogenesis of the fetal membranes and accessory uterine structures. *Carnegie Instit Contrib Embryol* 26.

Mossman, H.W. (1987). *Vertebrate Fetal Membranes.* New Brunswick, N.J.: Rutgers University Press.

Mossman, H.W. (1991). Classics revisited: comparative morphogenesis of the fetal membranes and accessory uterine structures. *Placenta* 12:1–5.

Mueller, U.W., Hawes, C.S., Wright, A.E. (1990). Isolation of fetal trophoblast cells from peripheral blood of pregnant women. *Lancet* 336:197–200.

Muir, A., Lever, A., Moffett, A. (2004). Expression and functions of human endogenous retroviruses in the placenta: an update. *Placenta* 25:suppl_AS16–25.

Murphy, W.J., Eizirik, E., O'Brien, S.J., Madsen, O., Scally, M., Douady, C.J., Teeling, E., Ryder, O.A., Stanhope, M.N., de Jong, W.W., Springer, M.S. (2001). Resolution of the early placental mammalian vadiation using Bayesian phylogenetics. *Science* 294:2348–2351.

Murray, F.A., Jr., Bazer, F.W., Wallace, H.D., Warnick, A.C. (1972). Quantitative and qualitative variation in the secretion of protein by the porcine uterus during the estrous cycle. *Biol Reprod* 7:314–320.

Myagkaya, G. and Vreeling-Sindelarova, H. (1976). Erythrophagocytosis by cells of the trophoblastic epithelium in the sheep placenta in different stages in gestation. *Acta Anat* 95:234–248.

Nadijcka, M. and Hillman, N. (1974). Ultrastructural studies of the mouse blastocyst sub-stages. *J. Embryol Exp Morphol* 32:675–695.

Nagy, A., Gertsenstein, M., Vintersten, K., Behringer, R. (2003). *Manipulating the mouse embryo. A laboratory manual.* Cold Spring Harbor, N.Y.: Cold Spring Harbor Laboratory Press.

Norwitz, E.R., Schust, D.J., Fisher, S.J. (2001). Implantation and the survival of early pregnancy. *N Engl J Med* 345:1400–1408.

Oduor-Okelo, D., Musewe, V.O., Gombe, S. (1983). Electron microscopic study of the chorioallantoic placenta of the rock hyrax (*Heterohyrax brucei*). *J Rep Fert* 68:311–316.

Oduor-Okelo, D. and Neaves, W.B. (1982). The chorioallantoic placenta of the spotted hyena (*Crouta, crocuta Erxleben*): an electron microscopy study. *Anatomical Record* 204:215–222.

Olson, G.E., Winfrey, V.P., Matrisian, P.E., NagDas, S.K., Hoffman, L.H. (1998). Blastocyst-dependent upregulation of metalloproteinase/disintegrin MDC9 expression in rabbit endometrium. *Cell and Tissue Research* 293:489–498.

Palludan, B.I., Wegger, I., Moustgaard, J. (1969). Placental transfer of iron. *Royal Veterinary and Agricultural University Yearbook*, Copenhagen: Royal Veterinary and Agricultural University, pp. 62–91.

Paria, B.C., Reese, J., Das, S.K., Dey, S.K. (2002). Deciphering the cross-talk of implantation: advances and challenges. *Science* 296:2185–2188.

Parr, E.L., Tung, H.N., Parr, M.B. (1987). Apoptosis as the mode of uterine epithelial cell death during embryo implantation in mice and rats. *Biology Of Reproduction* 36:211–225.

Parr, M.B. and Parr, E.L. (1989). The barrier role of the primary decidual zone. In: Yoshinaga, K. (ed) *Blastocyst Implantation*, Boston: Adams Pub., pp. 163–169.

Pashen, R.L., Sheldrick, E.L., Allen, W.R., Flint, A.P.F. (1983). Dehydroepiandrosterone synthesis by the foetal foal and its importance as an oestrogen precursor. *J Reprod Fertil* Suppl 32:389–397.

Patten, B.M. (1948). *Embryology of the Pig*. Toronto: Blakiston.

Perry, J.S. (1953). The reproduction of the African elephant, *Loxodonta africana*. *Proc Roy Soc B* 237:93–153.

Perry, J.S. (1974). Implantation, foetal membranes and early placentation of the African elephant, *Loxodonta africana*. *Proc Roy Soc B* 269:109–135.

Perry, J.S. (1981). The mammalian fetal membranes. *J Reprod Fertil* 62:321–335.

Perry, J.S., Heap, R.B., Amoroso, E.C. (1973). Steroid hormone production by pig blastocysts. *Nature* 245:45–47.

Perry, J.S., Heap, R.B., Burton, R.D., Gadsby, J.E. (1976). Endocrinology of the blastocyst and its role in the establishment of pregnancy. *J Reprod Fertil* Suppl 25:85–104.

Perry, J.S. and Rowlands, I.W. (1962). Early pregnancy in the pig. *J Reprod Fertil* 4:175–188.

Pijnenborg, R., Robertson, W.B., Brossens, I. (1985). Morphological aspects of placental ontogeny and phylogeny. *Placenta* 6:155–162.

Pijnenborg, R., Robertson, W.B., Brossens, I., Dixon, G. (1981). Review article: trophoblast invasion and the establishment of haemochorial placentation in man and laboratory animals. *Placenta* 2:71–91.

Pijnenborg, R. and Vercruysse, L. (2004). Thomas Huxley and the rat placenta in the early debates on evolution. *Placenta* 25:233–237.

Raab, G., Kover, K., Paria, B.C., Dey, S.K., Ezzell, R.M., Klagsbrun, M. (1996). Mouse preimplantation blastocysts adhere to cells expressing the transmembrane form of heparin-binding EGF-like growth factor. *Development* 122:637–645.

Rasweiler, J.J.T. (1991). Development of the discoidal hemochorial placenta in the black mastiff bat, *Molassus ater*: Evidence for a role of maternal endothelial cells in the control of trophoblastic growth. *Am J Anat* 191:185–207.

Rasweiler, J.J.T. (1993). Pregnancy in chiroptera. *J Exp Zool* 266:495–513.

Rau, A.S. (1925). Contribution to our knowledge of the structure of the placenta of mustelidae, Ursidae and scuiridae. *Proc Zool Soc* 50:1027–1069.

Red-Horse, K., Zhou, Y., Genbacev, O., Prakobphol, A., Foulk, R., McMaster, M., Fisher, S.J. (2004). Trophoblast differentiation during embryo implantation and formation of the maternal-fetal interface. *J Clin Invest* 114:744–754.

Redline, R.W. and Lu, C.Y. (1989). Localization of fetal major histocompatibility complex antigens and maternal leukocytes in murine placenta. Implications for maternal-fetal immunological relationship. *Lab Invest* 61:27–36.

Redman, C.W.G., McMichael, A.J., Stirrat, G.M., Sunderland, C.A., Ting, A. (1984). Class I MHC antigens on human extravillous trophoblast. *Immunology* 52:457–468.

Reimers, T., Ullmann, M., Hansel, W. (1985). Progesterone and prostanoid production by bovine binucleate trophoblastic cells. *Biology of Reproduction* 33:1227–1236.

Riley, P., Anson-Cartwright, L., Cross, J.C. (1998). The Hand1 bHLH transcription factor is essential for placentation and cardiac morphogenesis. *Nat Genet* 18:271–275.

Roberts, C.T. and Breed, W.G. (1994). Placentation in the dasyurid marsupial, *Sminthopsis crassicaudata*, the fat-tailed dunnart, and notes on placentation of the didelphid, *Monodelphis domestica*. *J Reprod Fertil* 100:105–113.

Roberts, R. and Bazer, F. (1988). The functions of uterine secretions. *J Reprod Fertil* 82:875–892.

Roberts, R.M. and Bazer, F.W. (1980). In: Beato, M. (ed) *Steroid-Induced Uterine Proteins*, New York: Elsevier/North Holland Press, pp. 133–149.

Roberts, R.M., Ealy, A.D., Alexenko, A.P., Han, C.S., Ezashi, T. (1999). Trophoblast interferons. *Placenta* 20:259–264.

Roberts, R.M., Liu, L., Alexenko, A. (1997). New and atypical families of type I interferons in mammals: comparative functions, structures and evolutionary relationships. *Prog Nucleic Acid Res Mol Biol* 56:287–325.

Rosen, S.D. (2004). Ligands for L-selectin: homing, inflammation, and beyond. *Annual Review of Immunology* 22:129–156.

Rossant, J. and Cross, J.C. (2001). Placental development: Lessons from mouse mutants. *Nat Rev Genet* 2:538–548.

Rouas-Freiss, N., Marchal, R.E., Kirszenbaum, M., Dausset, J., Carosella, E.D. (1997). The alpha 1 domain of HLA-G1 and HLA-G2 inhibits cytotoxicity induced by natural killer cells: Is HLA-G the public ligand for natural killer cell inhibitory receptors? *PNAS* 94:5249–5254.

Rowson, L.E. and Moor, R.M. (1966). Development of the sheep conceptus during the first fourteen days. *J Anat* 100:777–785.

Sadler, T.W. (2000). *Langman's Medical Embryology*. Philadelphia: Lippincott Williams and Wilkins.

Sale, J.B. (1965). Gestation period and neonatal weight of the hyrax. *Nature* 205:1240–1241.

Samuel, C.A. (1971). The development of pig trophoblasts in ectopic sites. *J Reprod Fertil* 27:494–495.

Samuel, C.A., Allen, W.R., Steven, D.H. (1974). Studies on the equine placenta. I. Development of the microcotyledons. *J Reprod Fertil* 41:441–445.

Samuel, C.A., Jack, P.M.B., Nathanielz, P.W. (1975). Ultrastructural studies of the rabbit placenta in the last third of gestation. *J Reprod Fertil* 45:9–14.

Samuel, C.A. and Perry, J.S. (1972). The ultrastructure of pig trophoblast transplanted to an ectopic site in the uterine wall. *J Anat* 113:139–149.

Scanlon, P.F. (1972). Frequency of transuterine migration of embryos in ewes and cows. *J Anim Sci* 34:791–794.

Schlafke, S., Welsh, A.O., Enders, A.C. (1985). Penetration of the basal lamina of the uterine luminal epithelium during implantation in the rat. *Anat Rec* 212:47–56.

Schreiber, J., Riethmacher-Sonnenberg, E., Riethmacher, D., Tuerk, E.E., Enderich, J., Bosl, M.R., Wegner, M. (2000). Placental failure in mice lacking the mammalian homolog of glial cells missing GCMa. *Mol Cell Biol* 20:2466–2474.

Semoff, S., Hogan, B.L.M., Hopkins, C.R. (1982). Localisation of fibronectin, laminin and entactin in Reichert's membrane by immunoelectron microscopy. *EMBO J* 1:1171–1175.

Senger, P.L. (2003). *Pathways to Pregnancy and Parturition.* Pullman, WA: Current Conceptions, Inc.

Sherman, G.B., Wolfe, M.W., Farmerie, T.A., Clay, C.M., Threadgill, D.S., Sharp, D.C., Nilson, J.H. (1992). A single gene encodes the beta-subunits of equine luteinizing hormone and chorionic gonadotropin. *Mol Endocrinol* 6:951–959.

Skidmore, J.A., Wooding, F.B.P., Allen, W.R. (1996). Implantation and early placentation in the one-humped camel (*Camelus dromedarius*). *Placenta* 17:253–262.

Slukvin, I.I., Lunn, D.P., Watkins, D.I., Golos, T.G. (2000). Placental expression of the nonclassical MHC class I molecule Mamu-AG at implantation in the rhesus monkey. *Proc Natl Acad Sci USA* 97:9104–9109.

Smith, K.K. and Strickland, S. (1981). Structural components and characteristics of Reichert's membrane, an extraembryonic basement membrane. *J Biol Chem* 256:4654–4661.

Snow, M.H.L. (1977). Gastrulation in the mouse: Growth and reorganalization of the epiblast. *J Embryol Exp Morphol* 42:293–303.

Soares, M.J. (2004). The prolactin and growth hormone families: Pregnancy-specific hormones/cytokines at the maternal-fetal interface. *Reproductive Biology and Endocrinology* 2:51.

Sol-Church, K., Picerno, G.N., Stabley, D.L., Frenck, J., Xing, S., Bertenshaw, G.P., Mason, R.W. (2002). Evolution of placentally expressed cathepsins. *Biochem Biophys Res Commun* 293:23–29.

Spencer, T.E., Johnson, G.A., Bazer, F.W., Burghardt, R.C. (2004). Implantation mechanisms: insights from the sheep. *Reproduction* 128:657–668.

Steven, D.H. (1982). Placentation in the mare. *J Reprod Fertil* Suppl. 31:41–55.

Steven, D.H. (1983). Interspecies differences in the structure and function of trophoblast. In: Loke, C. and Whyte, A. (eds) *Biology of Trophoblast*, Amsterdam: Elsevier, pp. 111–136.

Steven, D.H. and Morris, G. (1975). Development of the foetal membranes. In: Steven, D.H. (ed) *Comparative Placentation*, New York: Academic Press, pp. 214–267.

Stoye, J.P. and Coffin, J.M. (2000). A provirus put to work. *Nature* 403:715–717.

Sturgess, I. (1948). The early embryology and placentation of *Procavia capensis*. *Acta Zoo* 29:393–479.

Sumar, J.B. (1999). Reproduction in female South American domestic camelids. *J Rep Fert* Suppl 54:169–178.

Tanaka, S., Kunath, T., Hadjantonakis, A.K., Nagy, A., Rossant, J. (1998). Promotion of trophoblast stem cell proliferation by FGF4. *Science* 282:2072–2075.

Thathiah, A. and Carson, D.D. (2002). Mucins and blastocyst attachment. *Reviews in Endocrine and Metabolic Disorders* 3:87–96.

Tibary, A. (1997). *Theriogenology in Camelidae. Anatomy, Physiology, Pathology and Artificial breeding.* Abu Dhabi, UAE: Abu Dhabi Printing and Publishing Company.

Turkewitz, A.P. and Harrison, S.C. (1989). Concentration of transferrin receptor in human placental coated vesicles. *J Cell Biol* 108:2127–2135.

Urwin, V.E. and Allen, W.R. (1982). Pituitary and chorionic gonadotrophic control of ovarian function during early pregnancy in equids. *J Reprod Fertil* Suppl 32:371–381.

van Lennep, E.W. (1963). The histology of the placenta of the one humped camel (*Camelus dromedarius*) during the second half of pregnancy. *Acta Morphologica Neerlandica Scandinavica* 6:373–379.

van Niekerk, C.H. and Allen, W.R. (1975). Early embryonic development in the horse. *J Reprod Fertil* suppl 23:495–498.

Varmuza, S., Prideaux, V., Kothary, R., Rossant, J. (1988). Polytene chromosomes in mouse trophoblast giant cells. *Development* 102:127–134.

Villarreal, L.P. (1997). On viruses, sex, and motherhood. *J Virol* 71.

Vogel, P. (2005). The current molecular phylogeny of eutherian mammals challenges previous interpretations of placental evolution. *Placenta* 26:591–596.

Wada, H.G., Hass, P.E., Sussman, H.H. (1979). Transferrin receptor in human placental brush border membranes. *J Biol Chem* 254:12629–12635.

Wales, R.G. and Cuneo, C.L. (1989). Morphological and chemical analysis of the sheep conceptus from the 13th to the 19th day of pregnancy. *Reprod Fertil Dev* 1:31–39.

Wang, J., Mayernik, L., Schultz, J.F., Armant, D.R. (2000). Acceleration of trophoblast differentiation by heparin-binding EGF-like growth factor is dependent on the stage-specific activation of calcium influx by ErbB receptors in developing mouse blastocysts. *Development* 127:33–44.

Wango, E.O., Wooding, F.B.P., Heap, R.B. (1990b). The role of trophoblastic cells in implantation in the goat: a quantitative study. *Placenta* 11:381–394.

Wartiovaara, J., Leivo, I., Vaheri, A. (1979). Expression of the cell surface-associated glycoprotein, fibronectin, in the early mouse embryo. *Dev Biol* 69:247–257.

Wathes, D.C. and Wooding, F.B.P. (1980). An electron microscopic study of implantation in the cow. *Am J Anat* 159: 285–306.

Wells, M. and Bulmer, J.N. (1988). The human placental bed: histology, immunohistochemistry and pathology. *Histopathology* 13:483–498.

Welsh, A.O. and Enders, A.C. (1983). Occlusion and reformation of the rat uterine lumen during pregnancy. *Am J Anat* 167:463–477.

Welsh, A.O. and Enders, A.C. (1991b). Chorioallantoic placenta formation in the rat: II. Angiogenesis and maternal blood circulation in the mesometrial region of the implantation chamber prior to placenta formation. *Am J Anat* 192:347–365.

West, J.D., Flockhart, J.H., Keighren, M. (1995). Biochemical evidence for cell fusion in placentas of mouse aggregation chimeras. *Dev Biol* 168:76–85.

Whyte, A. (1980). Lectin binding by microvillous membranes and coated-pit regions of human syncytial trophoblast. *Histochem J* 12:599–607.

Wigmore, P.M.C. and Strickland, N.C. (1985). Placental growth in the pig. *Anat Embryol (Berl)* 173:263–268.

Wildman, D.E., Chen, C., Erez, O., Grossman, L.I., Goodman, M., Romero, R. (2006). Evolution of the mammalian placenta revealed by phylogenetic analysis. *PNAS* 103:3203–3208.

Wilmsatt, W.A. (1950). New histological observations on the placenta of the sheep. *Am J Anat* 87:391–457.

Wilmsatt, W.A. (1962). Some aspects of the comparative anatomy of the mammalian placenta. *Am J Obstet Gynecol* 84:1568–1594.

Wimsatt, W.A. (1975). Some comparative aspects of implantation. *Biol Reprod* 12:1–40.

Wintenberger-Torres, S. and Flechon, J. (1974). Ultrastructural evolution of the trophoblastic cells in the preimplantation sheep blastocyst from day 8 to day 18. *J Anat* 118:143–153.

Wislocki, G.B. and Van der Westhuysen, O.P. (1940). The placentation of *Procavia capensis*, with a discussion of the placental affinities of the hyracoidea. *Contr Embryol Carnegie Instn* 28:67–88.

Wooding, F.B.P. (1982a). Structure and function of placental binucleate (giant) cells. *Bibl Anat* 22:134–139.

Wooding, F.B.P. (1982b). The role of binucleate cell in ruminant placental structure. *Reprod Fertil* Suppl 31:31–39.

Wooding, F.B.P. (1983). Frequency and localization of binucleate cells in the placentomes of ruminants. *Placenta* 4:527–540.

Wooding, F.B.P. (1984). Role of binucleate cells in fetomaternal cell fusion at implantation in the sheep. *Am J Anat* 170:233–250.

Wooding, F.B.P. (1987). Ultrastructural evidence for placental lactogen transport and secretion in ruminants. *J Physiol* 386:26p.

Wooding, F.B.P. (1992). Current topic: the synepitheliochorial placenta of ruminants: binucleate cell fusions and hormone production. *Placenta* 13:101–113.

Wooding, F.B.P. and Flint, A.P.F. (1994). Placentation. In: Lamming, G.E. (ed) *Marshall's Physiology of Reproduction*, London: Chapman and Hall, pp. 233–460.

Wooding, F.B.P., Flint, A.P.F., Heap, R.B., Hobbs, T. (1981). Autoradiographic evidence for migration and fusion of cells in the sheep placenta; resolution of a problem in placental classification. *Cell Biology International Reports* 5:821–827.

Wooding, F.B.P., Flint, A.P.F., Heap, R.B., Morgan, G., Buttle, H.L., Young, I.R. (1986). Control of binucleate cell migration in the placenta of ruminants. *J Rep Fert* 76:499–512.

Wooding, F.B.P., Hobbs, T., Morgan, G., Heap, R.B., Flint, A.P.F. (1993). Cellular dynamics of growth in sheep and goat synepitheliochorial placentomes: An autoradiographic study. *J Reprod Fertil* 98:275–283.

Wooding, F.B.P., Morgan, G., Adam, C.L. (1997). Structure and function in the ruminant synepitheliochorial placenta: central role of the trophoblast binucleate cell in deer. *Microsc Res Tech* 38:88–99.

Wooding, F.B.P., Roberts, R.M., Green, J.A. (2005). Light and electron microscope immunocytochemical studies of the distribution of pregnancy-associated glycoproteins (PAGs) throughout pregnancy in the cow: possible functional implications. *Placenta* 26:807–827.

Wooding, F.B.P. and Staples, L.D. (1981). Functions of trophoblast papillae and binucleate cells in implantation in sheep. *J Anat* 133:110–112.

Wooding, F.B.P., Staples, L.D., Peacock, M.A.P. (1982). Structure of trophoblast papillae on the sheep conceptus at implantation. *J Anat* 134:507–516.

Wooding, F.B.P. and Wathes, D.C. (1980). Binucleate cell migration in the bovine placentome. *J Reprod Fertil* 59:425–430.

Wynn, R.M. (1971). Immunological implication of comparative placental ultrastructure. In: Blandau, R.J. (ed) *The Biology of the Blastocyst*, Chicago: The University of Chicago Press, pp. 495–514.

Wynn, R.M. and Byorkman, N. (1968). Ultrastructure of the feline placental membrane. *Am J Obstet Gynecol* 102:34–43.

Wynn, R.M., Hoschner, J.A., Oduor-Okelo, D. (1990). The interhemal membrane of the spotted hyena: an immunohistological reappraisal. *Placenta* 11:215–221.

Xie, S.C., Low, B.G., Nagel, R.J., Kramer, K.K., Anthony, R.V., Zoli, A.P., Beckers, J.F., Roberts, R.M. (1991). Identification of the major pregnancy-specific antigens of cattle and sheep as inactive members of the aspartic proteinase family. *Proc Natl Acad Sci USA* 88:10247–10251.

Zybina, E.V. and Zybina, T.G. (1996). Polytene chromosomes in mammalian cells. *Int Rev Cytol* 165:53–119.

Chapter 13

Pregnancy Diagnosis in Domestic Animals

Clifford F. Shipley, chapter editor

Part 13.1
Pregnancy Diagnosis in the Mare

Clifford F. Shipley

Pregnancy diagnosis in the mare is important for proper management of the pregnancy itself. It also allows the non-pregnant mare to be identified early so that intervention and breeding management will permit her a better chance to become pregnant early in the breeding season. Pregnancy can be affected by a variety of factors, including early embryonic death (EED), uterine infections, genetic abnormalities, and hormonal imbalances; therefore pregnancy should be monitored to assure that it is progressing normally. Monitoring progress also helps in identifying those mares that become pregnant yet cannot maintain pregnancy to term.

This section discusses the methods of confirming pregnancy, as well as their pros and cons. The preferred pregnancy diagnostic test depends on a number of factors, such as cost, skill of the personnel doing the test, lab availability, restraint, tractability of the mare, intensity of management, equipment availability, facilities, value of the mare, etc.

Non-return to Estrus

Mares that have been bred and fail to return to estrus by 16 to 19 days after the last estrus may be pregnant. However, there are other reasons for non-return to estrus during this time, such as EED, silent estrus, lactational anestrous, and prolonged maintenance of the corpus luteum (Ginther, 1992). Some mares that have foals at side, or shy or maiden mares, also may not show estrus. Therefore, it is often best to definitively diagnosis pregnancy by some other means to actually ensure that the mare is, in fact, pregnant. Furthermore, some pregnant mares show estrus even though pregnant (VanNiekirk, 1965).

Palpation per Rectum

At approximately 15 to 18 days of pregnancy, the mare's uterus and cervix start to acquire pronounced tone (VanNiekirk, 1965). This tone is usually much more pronounced than the tone of mid-diestrus. The embryonic vesicle is usually palpable by a skilled palpator by day 18 to day 20, when it reaches a size of approximately 30 to 40 mm in diameter (Zemjanis, 1961; Ginther, 1979; McKinnon and Voss, 1993). This is usually felt as a ventral bulge near the base of the gravid horn. As the pregnancy progresses, the bulge increases in size to 40 to 50 mm by day 30, 65 mm by day 40, and approximately 80 mm by day 50.

At day 60, the fetus and vesicle have taken up much of the gravid horn and are starting to enter the uterine body. There is still good tone to the non-gravid horn and the tip of the gravid horn (see Figure 13.1). From approximately day 65 to day 100, the uterus is pulled further ventral and the ovaries are pulled medially by the weight of the pregnant uterus.

At this time, it is usually difficult to palpate the fetus and a pyometra may be mistaken for a pregnancy. A pyometra usually has a doughier feel to the uterus and less tone. With care and experience, one may be able to differentiate the conditions.

The fetus can usually be palpated after day 100, but there are occasions where it is difficult; repeated exams over time may be required to finally ballot the fetus. If one can readily identify a body part and measure it, one may be able to determine gestational age (Bergin et al., 1967). The fetus may be palpated easily and body parts identified with some degree of accuracy as pregnancy progresses to term. However, one may encounter mares that are intractable, or the necessary facilities or personnel to restrain the mare during rectal exam may not be available.

Vaginal Examination

Examination of the cervix and vagina for pregnancy diagnosis is not definitive and should only be used as an adjunct to one of the other methods. It is also an avenue for

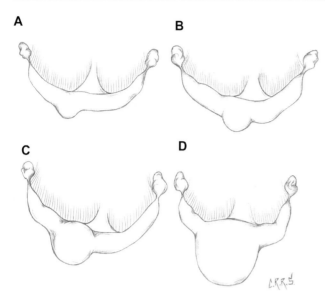

A **B**

C **D**

Figure 13.1. Uterus of the mare at various stages of pregnancy. **A:** uterus at approximately 20 days of pregnancy; **B:** uterus at approximately 30 days of pregnancy; **C:** uterus at approximately 40 days of pregnancy; **D:** uterus at approximately 60 days of pregnancy.

introduction of bacteria into the anterior vagina, which may lead to an ascending cervicitis and placentitis, which may ultimately lead to an abortion.

Vaginal mucus is stickier in the pregnant mare than that in a non-pregnant mare (Zemjanis, 1962). The cervix is usually very toned and elongated by day 15 to day 17. By day 30, the cervix is usually very pale and tight and may be pulled to one side of the anterior vagina (McKinnon et al., 1988). Examination may be undertaken in late pregnancy to determine fetal limb position as well as cervical integrity.

During late gestation it is imperative that care be taken to not stimulate the cervix and precipitate labor.

Ultrasound Examination

Examination of uterus with real-time ultrasound is currently the gold standard of pregnancy determination in the mare. Using either a 5- or 7.5-MHz linear transducer, pregnancy may be diagnosed as early as day 9, but is typically not done until day 12 to day 16. The 7.5-MHz head does not penetrate as deeply as the 5-MHz head, but usually gives better resolution. A 3.5-MHz sector scan head may be useful in late pregnancy trans-abdominally to help diagnose problems in fetal development and placentation or help to determine fetal viability.

Pregnancy may be picked up at the early stage with excellent equipment and skill, but caution must be exercised because pregnancies in the early stages are most prone to EED and the vesicle may be confused with an endometrial cyst.

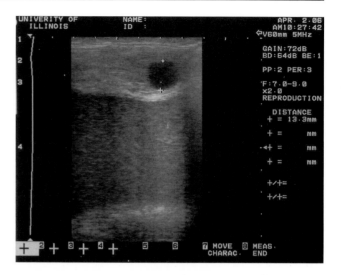

Figure 13.2. Mare uterus with approximately 14-day embryonic vesicle.

It is important to do a thorough scan of the uterus (both horns and uterine body) so that the embryonic vesicle (which is mobile until day 16) is not missed (see Figures 13.2 and 13.3) (Ginther, 1983a, 1983b).

From day 11 to day 16 the embryo grows at a rate of approximately 3.4 mm per day. This growth rate plateaus around day 25, when growth continues at a rate of approximately 1.8 mm per day until approximately day 50 (Ginther, 1986). The growth rate for embryos is nearly the same for all breeds and classes of horses for the first month or so of gestation, at which time draft breed embryos tend to be 1 to 4 mm larger than light breed embryos (Chevalier and Palmer, 1982).

The embryo takes on a guitar pick shape at about 17 to 18 days of pregnancy and will keep this shape until day 21 or so. Starting at day 21 or day 22, the conceptus may be

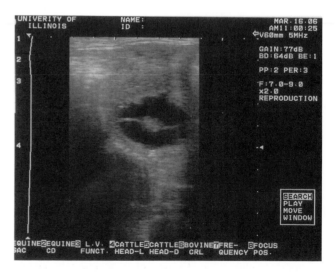

Figure 13.3. Equine uterus with 28-day embryo.

located at the ventral portion of the embryonic sac and a heartbeat may be found if an ultrasound of very high quality or a 7.5-MHz head is used. Usually the heartbeat is found more easily at days 24 to 25 (Allen and Goddard, 1984). It is important to note that lack of heartbeat or proper size for age of the developing embryo may help to determine that the embryo itself is dead or undergoing developmental problems that will ultimately lead to its demise (Ginther et al., 1985). Repeated examinations on those embryos will lead to earlier intervention and a return of mares with EED to the breeding shed.

Ultrasonography is also used to diagnose twins and to help reduce twins to avoid problems late in gestation. The mare will continue cycling the rest of the season if twin reduction is completed before endometrial cup formation at approximately day 35 and if she loses both pregnancies (Roberts, 1982). Manual reduction of one of the twins can be attempted as early as day 14. The earlier the twins are identified and reduced, the more time can be saved in the breeding season for those mares that are prone to twinning.

Mares should be monitored post-embryo reduction for confirmation of reduction and to monitor the remaining pregnancy. Techniques such as ultrasound-assisted embryo reduction using needle aspiration or injection into the fetus are being used with greater success in cases in which twins are not reduced by day 30 to day 35.

The dorsal yolk sac contracts and the allantois grows ventrally from approximately day 22 to day 40. By day 40, the yolk sac is gone and the fetus appears to be suspended by the umbilicus from the dorsal aspect of the vesicle where it lies on its back from day 50 onward. The fetus may be sexed by ultrasound from approximately day 55 until day 80, when it becomes more difficult to reach the fetus and manipulate the probe (Curran and Ginther, 1989).

Other Diagnostic Tests for Pregnancy Determination

Progesterone determination is not a determination of pregnancy. Rather, it merely measures progesterone production. Mares that are in diestrus and those with prolonged maintenance of the corpus luteum, EED, etc. may all have levels of progesterone consistent with pregnancy, yet the mare is open.

Progesterone determination, when used as an adjunct to other methods of pregnancy determination, may yield useful information about the maintenance and viability of the pregnancy. Levels usually rise to above 4 ng/ml five days post-ovulation (Hughes et al., 1972; Ganjam and Kenney, 1975) and continue to rise until day 20. Levels then decline slightly until day 40, rise from day 45 to day 60, decline again by day 90, and then become neglibible by day 150 to 180. Progestagens produced by the fetal-placental unit are also responsible for maintenance of pregnancy but are usually not measured by tests that detect only progesterone.

These progestagens increase in concentration until parturition (Holtan et al., 1975).

Tests for the hormone equine chorionic gonadotropin (eCG) are accurate from approximately day 40 to day 110 (McKinnon and Voss, 1993), but they may be positive if the fetus dies after the endometrial cups are formed. Furthermore, mares carrying a mule fetus produce lower amounts of ECG and the amounts decrease earlier than if carrying a horse fetus (Taylor and Honey, 1980).

Tests for an early conception factor- (ECF) type protein so far have proven to be poor (Parker et al., 2005). There is hope for a test to determine pregnancy early (prior to embryo flush) or to avoid ultrasound or rectal palpation in intractable mares or those that are too small to easily examine per rectum.

Estrogen is produced by the embryo as early as day 12, but measurable amounts are usually not present until after day 35 or so. Concentrations of estrone sulfate are indicative of pregnancy and may be used as a pregnancy test or as a test of fetal viability (Henderson and Eayrs, 2004). Significant amounts are of estrogen are present by day 60 (Cole and Saunders, 1935; Terqui and Palmer, 1979) and may be found in the urine, feces, blood, and milk (Cox, 1934).

Summary

The most commonly used methods for pregnancy diagnosis in the mare are rectal palpation and ultrasound. When done by skilled personnel they are highly accurate and can give the brood mare owner much information about the stage and development of the pregnancy.

References

Allen, W.E. and Goddard, P.J. (1984). Serial investigations of early pregnancy in pony mares using real-time ultrasound scanning. *Equine Vet J* 16(6): 509–14.

Bergin, W.C., Gier, H.T. et al. (1967). Developmental horizons and measurements useful for age determination of equine embryos and fetuses. *Proc Am Assoc Equine Pract* 179–96.

Chevalier, F. and Palmer, E. (1982). Ultrasonic echography in the mare. *J Reprod Fertil Suppl* 32: 423–30.

Cole, H.H. and Saunders, F.J. (1935). The concentration of gonad stimulating hormone in blood serum and of oestrin in the urine throughout pregnancy in the mare. *Endocrinology* 19: 199–208.

Cox, J.E. (1934). Urine tests for pregnancy diagnosis test for mares. *Clin Vet* 57: 85.

Curran, S. and Ginther, O.J. (1989). Ultrasonic diagnosis of equine fetal sex by location of the genital tubercle. *J Equine Vet Sci* 9: 77.

Ganjam, V.K. and Kenney, R.M. (1975). Peripheral blood plasma levels and some unique metabolic aspects of progesterone in pregnant and non-pregnant mares. *Proc Am Assoc Equine Pract*: 264–276.

Ginther, O.J. (1979). *Maternal Aspects of Pregnancy.* Ann Arbor, MI: McNaughton and Gunn, Inc.

Ginther, O.J. (1983a). Fixation and orientation of the early equine conceptus. *Theriogenology* 19(4): 613–23.

Ginther, O.J. (1983b). Mobility of the early equine conceptus. *Theriogenology* 19(4): 603–11.

Ginther, O.J. (1986). *Ultrasonic Imaging and Reproductive Events in the Mare.* Cross Plains, WI: Equiservices.

Ginther, O.J. (1992). *Reproductive Biology of the Mare: Basic and Applied Aspects.* Cross Plains, Wis., USA: Equiservices.

Ginther, O.J., Bergfelt, D.R. et al. (1985). Embryonic loss in mares: Incidence and ultrasonic morphology. *Theriogenology* 24(1): 73–86.

Henderson, K.M. and Eayrs, K. (2004). Pregnancy status determination in mares using a rapid lateral flow test for measuring serum oestrone sulphate. *N Z Vet J* 52(4): 193–6.

Holtan, D.W., Nett, T.M. et al. (1975). Plasma progestins in pregnant, postpartum and cycling mares. *J Anim Sci* 40(2): 251–60.

Hughes, J.P., Stabenfeldt, G.H. et al. (1972). Clinical and endocrine aspects of the estrous cycle of the mare. *Proc Am Assoc Equine Pract* 119–51.

McKinnon, A.O., Squires, E.L. et al. (1988). Ovariectomized steroid-treated mares as embryo transfer recipients and as a model to study the role of progestins in pregnancy maintenance. *Theriogenology* 29(5): 1055–63.

McKinnon, A.O. and Voss, J.L. (1993). *Equine Reproduction.* Philadelphia: Lea and Febiger.

Parker, E., Tibary, A. et al. (2005). Evaluation of a new early pregnancy test in mares. *J Equine Sci* 25(2): 66–9.

Roberts, C.J. (1982). Termination of twin gestation by blastocyst crush in the broodmare. *J Reprod Fertil Suppl* 32: 447–9.

Taylor, T.S. and Honey, P.G. (1980). Use of immunological pregnancy testing in mares carrying mule fetuses. *Equine Pract* 2: 25–8.

Terqui, M. and Palmer, E. (1979). Oestrogen pattern during early pregnancy in the mare. *J Reprod Fertil Suppl*(27): 441–6.

VanNiekirk, C. (1965). Early clinical diagnosis of pregnancy in mares. *J S Afr Vet Med Assoc* 36: 56.

Zemjanis, R. (1961). Pregnancy diagnosis in the mare. *J Am Vet Med Assoc* 139: 543–7.

Zemjanis, R. (1962). *Diagnostic and Therapeutic Techniques in Animal Reproduction.* Baltimore: Williams and Wilkins.

Part 13.2
Bovine Pregnancy Diagnosis

Herris Maxwell

Efficient management of cattle often requires identification and separation of pregnant and non-pregnant animals. Such identification is useful for managing nutritional programs, making culling decisions, and planning for adequate personnel to be available to assist during calving.

To provide the maximum amount of useful information, identification methods should allow accurate identification of status (i.e. pregnant or non-pregnant), be reasonably accurate in assessing the stage of gestation, offer some information about fetal health, and in no way harm the developing fetus or disrupt the normal progression of pregnancy. Although newer methods of pregnancy detection are emerging, the diagnosis and assessment of pregnancy by physical examination can satisfy most of these requirements and will likely continue to be an important skill for stockmen and veterinarians. The following section discusses the methods of pregnancy detection.

Observation for Signs of Estrus

Perhaps the oldest method to determine pregnancy is by observation to detect the signs of estrus. The nonseasonal, polyestrus breeding pattern of cattle results in displays of estrus at approximately 21-day intervals. After an animal becomes pregnant the cycle ceases until sometime following parturition. Astute herdsmen may assume that a cow has become pregnant when that animal fails to return to estrus at the predicted time. Failure to return to estrus, when coupled with known service dates, can be useful in predicting calving dates.

Similarly, after observation of a group of cattle for a period greater than three weeks, those cattle not showing signs of estrus could be assumed to be pregnant (Youngquist, 1997).

This method is time consuming, and can prove to be inaccurate for a variety of reasons. Pregnant animals occasionally exhibit signs of estrus, and a number of physiologic and pathologic conditions can result in animals not cycling or cycling abnormally. It is widely accepted that the efficiency of estrus detection is less than ideal (Heersche and Nebel, 1994), and an unobserved or unrecorded estrus will lead to erroneously high estimates of pregnancy rates.

Visual Appraisal

A number of physical changes may be observed in the later stages of pregnancy, including distension of the abdomen, enlargement of the mammary glands, and loosening of the perivulvar tissues with a distinctive appearance known to cattlemen as "springing."

While none of these signs are specific for pregnancy, they can be helpful to an experienced observer when evaluating late-gestation animals. External signs of pregnancy are not readily detectable in the early stages of pregnancy.

External Ballotment

External ballotment is a commonly used technique that can be valuable when performed by an experienced operator in late pregnancy. To perform the technique, the operator places his or her fist on the lower right abdomen, cranial to the udder and caudal to the last rib. Keeping the fist in contact with the skin at all times, the operator makes a series of jabbing motions on the abdominal wall in a dorsal medial direction to stimulate a wave of motion within the abdomen. The jabbing is discontinued suddenly, with the fist held tightly into the abdomen. The calf can be felt through the abdominal wall as the induced wave returns (Roberts, 1986).

Although many operators feel they are highly accurate, the stage of gestation suitable for "bumping a calf" is generally no earlier than six months, and probably later in most cows. Those with excessive body condition and large cows may be particularly difficult to evaluate with this technique.

Ballotment is commonly carried out by dairy herdsmen as a method to detect or confirm pregnancy prior to drying a cow off.

Transrectal Palpation

Palpation per rectum has been the method of choice for detecting pregnancy in the bovine for well over 50 years. Although more technologically advanced methods are available, it is likely that the skills necessary for accurate evaluation of the reproductive tract of the female bovine will remain necessary to maximize reproductive management. Many of the skills necessary to evaluate the tubular reproductive tract are necessary to master other technologically advanced assisted reproductive techniques such as embryo transfer and transvaginal oocyte aspiration.

Rectal palpation is low cost, rapid, and accurate when carried out by an experienced individual. With practice it can be a very sensitive test for pregnancy from 30 days post-breeding until term. While widely regarded as safe for both the cow and the developing fetus, reports of fetal loss associated with the technique emphasize the necessity for reasonable care during the procedure (Abbitt et al., 1978).

Inherent in the successful mastery of the technique is an appreciation for the normal anatomy of the non-pregnant reproductive tract and the findings associated with the pregnant tract. The ability to confidently evaluate the entire length of both uterine horns is necessary to accurately identify the non-gravid state.

Reproductive tracts obtained from slaughter house samples are quite likely the best materials for training, but are not always available. Although preserved reproductive tracts and plastic models available from commercial sources are useful, they are inferior to fresh tracts or frozen-thawed tracts derived from cadaver cows. Anatomic illustrations detailing the relationships of the vagina, vestibule, cer-vix, uterine body, uterine horns, uterine tubes, ovaries, and products of conception can serve well for general orientation.

To effectively diagnose early pregnancy, it is imperative that the operator be skilled enough to thoroughly and successfully evaluate the cervix, uterine body, and uterine horns. After orientation on cadaver-derived tracts, the student may progress to palpation of live cattle, with the initial goal of gaining the skill necessary to palpate all the applicable structures in non-pregnant cows. After that skill level is obtained, identification of the positive signs of pregnancy and the supportive signs of pregnancy will follow. The palpator should also strive to identify the structures necessary to accurately assess the stage of gestation.

Appropriate restraint of the cow prior to examination is essential for a thorough exam, to provide for operator safety, and to allow the operator to perform the procedure in an ergonomically proper and efficient manner. Facilities that are both operator friendly and cow friendly make it possible to examine large numbers of cattle efficiently and quickly. In some instances, examinations can be done at a rate of 50 or more per hour.

Adequate restraint is dictated by the class of animal being examined. Dairy cattle may work well in stanchion lockups or behind a management rail. Beef cattle are generally handled in corrals with a narrow chute and head restraint. Occasionally, restraint with a halter may be acceptable. In any case, the operator should avoid situations which could result in a cow causing harm to anyone involved in the procedure.

While beyond the scope of this discussion, there are reports of repetitive motion injuries in people who repeatedly perform large numbers of rectal palpations. Efforts to avoid strain and trauma to the elbow, shoulder, and neck should be part of the process of learning rectal palpation (Ailsby, 1996).

In most instances, the accuracy of diagnosis increases as the stage of gestation progresses (Roberts, 1986). Conversely, the accuracy of estimation of gestational age is often much better when examinations are undertaken early in gestation. While accurate diagnosis of pregnancy can be obtained by experienced palpators as soon as 30 days after insemination, less experienced operators often misidentify pregnant cows as non-pregnant at this stage. The ability to accurately identify an animal as non-pregnant assumes increased importance when pharmacologic agents which may interrupt pregnancy are being administered to animals identified as nonpregnant (Youngquist, 1997).

The cow should be visually appraised prior to or simultaneously with palpation. Assessment of body condition score gives the observer an indication of the nutritional or health status of the cow. In addition, the presence of rub marks over the pin bones or tail head may indicate that the cow was recently in heat. Abnormalities of the external genitalia such as scars and tumors should be noted at the same time.

Following adequate restraint, the operator should put on a shoulder-length, disposable plastic sleeve, and apply an adequate amount of a non-irritating lubricant in preparation for palpating the cow. The fingers of the palpating hand should be formed into a cone, and the rectum entered as gently as possible. Fecal material should be removed from the rectum using a raking motion to force the feces from the rectum without removing the hand, and thereby avoiding the introduction of air.

The operator should examine the tract in an orderly and systematic manner (Roberts, 1986). Although not always available, accurate insemination or breeding dates are very useful. In bull-bred herds, the dates of the introduction and removal of the bulls from the herd should be available.

The cervix provides the best and most consistent landmark for proper orientation in the non-pregnant cow. The cervix is easily recognizable due to its firm consistency and tubular shape. The difference in texture makes the cervix easily discernable and relatively easy to locate on the floor or brim of the pelvis. After placing the hand in the rectum, the operator uses his fingers to explore the floor of the pelvis and the pelvic brim to locate the cervix. Although the cervix drops deeper into the abdominal cavity as pregnancy advances, the cervix may be located cranial to the pelvic brim in many older non-pregnant cattle. Thus, cervical location alone is insufficient to diagnose pregnancy.

Following identification and evaluation of the size, consistency, and location of the cervix, the uterus should be palpated by moving the hand forward and using the thumb and fingers to locate the uterus and broad ligament. When the uterus is hanging over the pelvic brim, it may be necessary to apply traction to the cervix, uterus, broad ligament or intercornual ligaments to bring the remainder of the tract within reach.

The bovine uterus branches into two uterine horns a few centimeters cranial to the cervix. After identifying the uterine bifurcation, the operator should attempt to explore the entire length of each uterine horn in a systematic manner to detect signs of pregnancy.

The sequence used by the author is to identify the cervix, proceed to the uterine body, palpate the left uterine horn to its tip, follow the left uterine horn back to the uterine bifurcation, and then palpate the right uterine horn to its tip. The right uterine horn is then followed back to the bifurcation. With this system each uterine horn is palpated twice, allowing for an increase in confidence and accuracy. The normal non-pregnant uterus should contain no fluid, and the uterine surface should be smooth. The palpator should gain an appreciation of the thickness of the uterine wall, because thinning of the uterine wall is one of the earlier indications of pregnancy.

Diagnosis of Pregnancy

The diagnosis of pregnancy should be based only on finding one or more of the four positive (or cardinal) signs of pregnancy (which are further discussed below):

1. Palpation of the chorio-allantoic membrane by the "membrane slip" technique
2. Palpation of the amnionic vesicle
3. Palpation of the fetus
4. Palpation of the placentomes

The following additional findings may support pregnancy and may be useful in estimating gestational age, but cannot be used alone to diagnose pregnancy:

1. Location of the uterus and cervix
2. Thinning of the uterine wall
3. Size of the uterine horn
4. Presence of fluid in the uterus
5. Discrepancy in size of the uterine horns
6. Palpation of the "pulse of pregnancy" in the middle uterine artery

Membrane Slip

Detection of the chorioallantoic membrane is indicative of pregnancy. This technique is most useful from 30 to 90 days of gestation, although it is probably possible to detect the membranes at later stages of pregnancy. The technique consists of grasping the uterine horn between the thumb and forefinger, and slowly allowing the tissue to slip away. The unattached portions of the fetal membranes can be felt as they slip through the fingers in advance of the uterine wall. Detection of this subtle event requires skill and practice, but is very useful in early pregnancy diagnosis (Morrow, 1980).

Amnionic Vesicle

The amnionic vesicle contains the developing fetus and the fluids immediately surrounding it. In early pregnancy, this structure is much more turgid than the surrounding allantoic fluid, and is found in the mid-portion of the uterine horn. Initially spherical in shape, it becomes increasingly oval after 40 days of gestation. To detect the amnionic vesicle, the uterine horn is confined between the thumb and fingers, and the hand is gently advanced along the length of the horn. The vesicle can be felt as a relatively incompressible mass as it slips between the digits. The vesicle gradually loses its tone as pregnancy progresses, and after day 70 palpation of the fetus itself is more likely than palpation of the amnionic vesicle (Morrow, 1980).

Palpation of the Fetus

The fetus becomes palpable at 60 to 70 days (Morrow, 1980), as the amnionic vesicle becomes less turgid. In most cases the fetus can be easily palpated or balloted until three to four months of gestation. Palpation of the fetus becomes more difficult from four to seven months as the pregnant uterus assumes a location deeper in the abdominal cavity. After seven months, the increase in fetal size once again brings the fetus into reach, and detection of fetal parts from that time until term becomes increasingly less difficult (Roberts, 1986).

Palpation of Plancentomes

Placentomes, the areas where the fetal cotyledons and maternal caruncles join, are distinct round to oval structures palpable in the uterine wall of pregnant cattle from approximately day 75 of gestation (Morrow, 1980). They are considered to be a cardinal sign of pregnancy, although they may be palpable for a relatively short period of time in the post-partum cow. The size of the placentomes increases with gestational age until the last third of gestation, which makes placentome size a useful criteria for estimating stage of gestation. It should be noted that all placentomes are not equal in size, and that those in the horn containing the pregnancy tend to be larger than those in the horn contralateral to the pregnancy. Gestational staging using placentome size is most accurate and consistent when the placentomes at the base of the uterine horn, just cranial to the cervix, are used for estimating gestational age (Morrow, 1980; Youngquist, 1997).

Findings in the Non-pregnant Cow

Palpation of the uterine horns fails to reveal any of the cardinal signs of pregnancy (membrane slip, amnionic vesicle, placentomes, or fetus) in the normal non-pregnant cow or heifer. There is no fluid in the uterus, and the uterus is located within the pelvis or easily retracted into the pelvis (Morrow, 1980). The uterine horns vary in diameter from 1.25 cm in some heifers up to 6 cm in some older pluriparous cows. Although the uterus increases in size with pregnancy, the wide variations found within non-pregnant cows make uterine size alone unreliable for pregnancy diagnosis. Similarly, although the horn containing a pregnancy is larger than the contralateral horn, in many instances the horns never achieve equal size following a pregnancy.

Findings 30 to 45 Days After Insemination

Beginning around 30 days after breeding, the uterine wall in the horn containing the pregnancy will be distended by the accumulating fetal fluids, fetal membranes, and fetus. The uterus may remain in the pelvic cavity, or be cranial to the brim of the pelvis. Retraction of the uterus into the pelvis is usually easily accomplished at this stage, and allows for palpation of the length of the uterine horns. The uterine wall will have become thinner and begin to bulge on the dorsal surface. The fluid within the uterine horn results in a palpable fluctuance of the horn (Morrow, 1980). At this stage of gestation, the membrane slip can be felt, and the amnionic vesicle is palpable. The amnionic vesicle provides the most reliable gauge for estimation of gestational age, growing from approximately 1 cm at 30 days to 5 cm by 60 days of gestation (Morrow, 1986).

Findings 45 to 90 Days of Gestation

As pregnancy advances, the uterus begins to descend further past the pelvic brim, and it enlarges. At 45 days, the entire uterus can usually be retracted into the pelvis, and both uterine horns palpated for their entire length. As the uterus enlarges and descends deeper into the pelvis with advancing pregnancy, it becomes increasingly difficult to palpate the entire length of the uterine horns. The fetal membrane slip is readily detectable at 45 days, and while still detectable at 90 days, is rarely needed for pregnancy diagnosis. The amnionic vesicle will have assumed an oval shape by 45 days, but will remain readily palpable. As the pregnancy progresses, the vesicle becomes less turgid, and this loss of tone allows palpation of the fetus proper (Youngquist, 1997). Generally, by 60 to 70 days palpation of the fetus is more likely than palpation of the amnionic vesicle.

Palpation of the fetus becomes possible as the fetus grows and the amnion becomes less turgid. Fetal size provides a method to estimate gestational age, and can be quite accurate in early pregnancy (Morrow, 1986).

The placentomes, the area in which the fetal membranes attach to the uterus, are composed of the fetal cotyledon and the maternal caruncle. They become palpable as oval thickenings in the uterine wall, and may be detected by experienced palpators as early as 75 days and by most palpators by 90 days. The size of the placentomes can be used to estimate gestational age (Roberts, 1986).

Palpation of the "pulse of pregnancy" becomes possible at about 90 days of gestation. The middle uterine artery is located in the broad ligament, and is therefore relatively freely movable as it is palpated. Any condition which increases blood flow to the uterus may result in a detectable middle uterine artery, so this finding alone is not sufficient for pregnancy diagnosis. When positive signs of pregnancy

are present, the size of the middle uterine artery is useful in estimating the fetal age (Roberts, 1986).

Findings From 90 Days Until Term

After 90 days gestation the uterus is located well over the pelvic brim, and it is not possible to palpate the entire uterus. The fetus may be balloted or palpated directly. The gestational age may be estimated by assessing the total fetal size or the size of a palpable fetal part such as the head or a hoof. In some instances, the abdominal location of the uterus makes direct palpation of the fetus difficult or impossible. In such cases, palpation of placentomes may provide the only positive method for diagnosing pregnancy. Placentomes remain palpable throughout the remainder of gestation, but as previously mentioned become less reliable as an indicator of fetal age as pregnancy progresses (Roberts, 1986). Fetal movement may be detected during palpation late in pregnancy.

Other Methods of Pregnancy Diagnosis

A variety of methods other than physical findings are available to diagnose pregnancy and others will likely become available.

Progesterone Analysis of Milk or Serum

Progesterone has been used as a test for pregnancy or non-pregnancy in the cow (Zaied et al., 1979). Because progesterone is necessary for maintaining pregnancy in the cow, a finding of low progesterone indicates non-pregnancy. While finding a relatively high progesterone concentration 18 to 24 days post-insemination is consistent with pregnancy, high progesterone concentrations alone are not sufficient for positive diagnosis.

Ultrasonsography

Real-time, B-mode ultrasonography can detect pregnancy earlier than transrectal palpation, allows for more accurate assessment of ovarian structures, is an effective diagnosis of twins, and allows for monitoring of fetal viability by detection of fetal heartbeat (Curran et al., 1986). The equipment has been relatively expensive, but prices have fallen in recent years. The use of ultrasonography to diagnose and monitor pregnancy continues to increase as the equipment becomes more available.

Pregnancy-associated Proteins

A variety of products produced by the conceptus have been detected in the maternal circulation, and several may have applications in pregnancy diagnosis. The pregnancy-specific protein B (PspB) assay is currently available from commercial sources. It is reported to accurately identify pregnancy from 30 days until term, and return to baseline by 80 days after term. Other pregnancy-specific markers have been identified, but none are currently commercially available.

Summary

Although other modalities of pregnancy diagnosis are available, the ability to diagnose pregnancy by physical means, particularly by rectal palpation, remains a valuable skill. Knowledge of the anatomy and mastery of the tactile skills necessary to assess the tubular reproductive tract are essential to accurate and efficient pregnancy diagnosis and gestational staging.

References

Abbitt, B., Ball, L., et al. (1978). Effect of three methods of palpation for pregnancy diagnosis per rectum on embryonic and fetal attrition in cows. *J Am Vet Med Assoc* 173(8): 973–7.

Ailsby, R.L. (1996). Occupational arm, shoulder, and neck syndrome affecting large animal practitioners. *Can Vet J* 37(7): 411.

Curran, S., Pierson, R.A., et al. (1986). Ultrasonographic appearance of the bovine conceptus from days 20 through 60. *J Am Vet Med Assoc* 189(10): 1295–302.

Heersche, G., Jr. and Nebel, R.L. (1994). Measuring efficiency and accuracy of detection of estrus. *J Dairy Sci* 77(9): 2754–61.

Morrow, D.A. (1980). *Current Therapy in Theriogenology: Diagnosis, Treatment, and Prevention of Reproductive Diseases in Animals*. Philadelphia: Saunders.

Morrow, D.A. (1986). *Current Therapy in Theriogenology 2: Diagnosis, Treatment, and Prevention of Reproductive Diseases in Small and Large Animals*. Philadelphia: Saunders.

Roberts, S.J. (1986). *Veterinary Obstetrics and Genital diseases (Theriogenology)*. Published by the author, Woodstock, Vt., distributed by David and Charles, Inc., North Pomfret, VT.

Youngquist, R.S. (1997). *Pregnancy Diagnosis. Current Therapy in Large Animal Theriogenology*. Philadelphia, London, Toronto, Montreal, Sydney, Tokyo: W.B. Saunders, 295–303.

Zaied, A.A., Bierschwal, C.J., et al. (1979). Concentrations of progesterone in milk as a monitor of early pregnancy diagnosis in dairy cows. *Theriogenology* 12(1): 3–11.

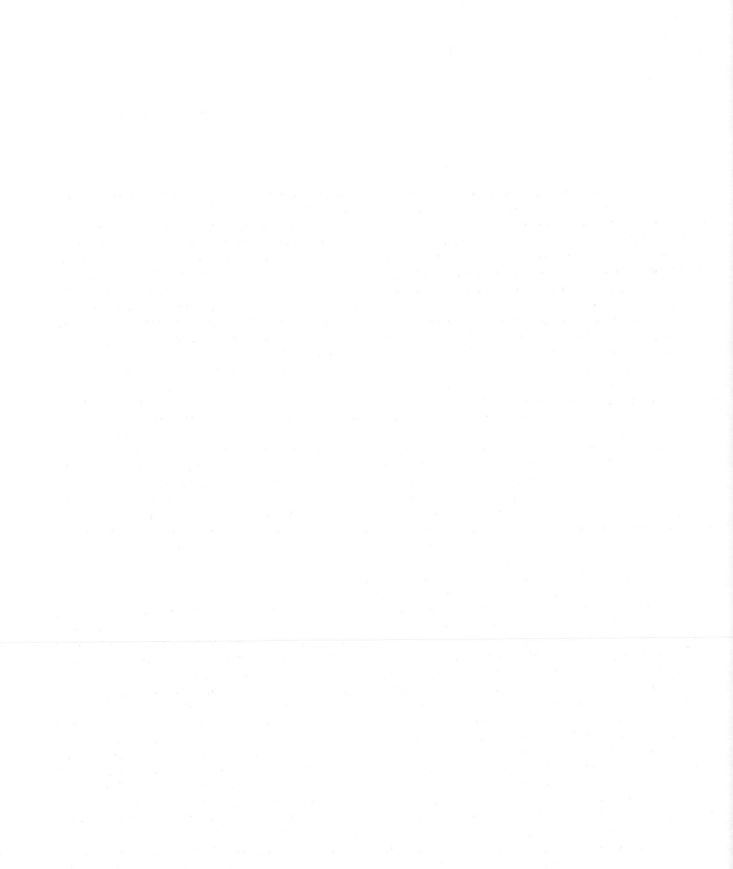

Part 13.3
Pregnancy Diagnosis in Swine

Ross P. Cowart

Commercial swine production is highly dependent on the ability of breeding animals to successfully reproduce. The measure of successful reproduction is, of course, the birth of live baby piglets. However, the knowledge of which females are pregnant and can be expected to give birth gives the manager valuable advance information and can be used to assess the success of breeding management and suggest changes when needed.

The interest in and desire for methods to detect pregnancy in swine is evident by the large array of methods that have been developed over the years. The choice of a specific method of pregnancy diagnosis is influenced by a number of factors. The accuracy, cost, and ease of performance are major factors. The time during pregnancy in which the test can be applied and the timeliness of results are also considerations.

Obviously, the more accurate or trustworthy a test is, the better. However, because no test for pregnancy is perfectly accurate, knowledge of the likelihood and possible reasons for mistaken diagnoses for a particular test can be useful. For example, if one wants to be certain that all pregnant animals in a tested group are diagnosed as pregnant, one would choose a test with a high sensitivity. Sensitivity is mathematically defined as the number of true positives divided by the sum of the true positives and the false negatives. A highly sensitive test minimizes the number of false negatives (animals which are actually pregnant but test as non-pregnant). However, highly sensitive tests may have a higher rate of false positive diagnoses.

Alternatively, if one wants to be certain that all non-pregnant animals in a tested group are diagnosed as non-pregnant, one would choose a test with a high specificity. Specificity is mathematically defined as the number of true negatives divided by the sum of the true negatives and the false positives. A highly specific test minimizes the number of false positives (animals which are actually non-pregnant but test as pregnant). However, highly specific tests may have a higher rate of false negative diagnoses.

How one intends to use the results of a test may influence whether high sensitivity or high specificity is preferred. For example, if one intends to identify the animals that test negative for pregnancy so that they may be observed more closely for signs of estrus and rebred, then a highly specific test would be preferred. The non-pregnant animals would be identified. If a pregnant animal was incorrectly diag-

nosed as non-pregnant (false negative) then she would be unnecessarily subjected to increased scrutiny for signs of estrus, but her pregnancy would eventually become apparent as parturition drew closer. However, if one intends to identify the animals that test negative for pregnancy so that they may be culled for slaughter, then a highly sensitive test would be preferred. The pregnant animals would be identified. In this case, incorrectly diagnosing a pregnant animal as non-pregnant would be a costly and wasteful mistake; therefore the minimal false negative tests of a highly sensitive test would be beneficial.

Means of diagnosing pregnancy in swine generally involve either evaluating the behavior and/or physical appearance of the animal (return to estrus, visual inspection), evaluating the visual or tactile morphology of certain tissues of the animal (vaginal biopsy, laparoscopy, rectal palpation), measuring hormones or other chemical substances (estrone sulfate, prostaglandin $F_{2\alpha}$, progesterone, early pregnancy factor), or using imaging technologies (radiography, ultrasound). The principles and procedures for each method are discussed below; however, the greatest emphasis is on the more commonly used methods of observing return to estrus as well as ultrasound.

Return to Estrus

The most common and time-honored means of diagnosing pregnancy in swine is observing signs of estrus. Sexually mature, non-pregnant sows and gilts normally complete an estrous cycle every 18 to 24 days with an average of 21 days. Estrus (the time of sexual receptivity) is characterized by a standing reflex posture of the female in the presence of a boar and will last for approximately 60 hours. Pregnancy interrupts the estrous cycle. Pregnant sows and gilts fail to return to estrus for the duration of their pregnancies.

Most swine breeding managers closely observe females for physical and behavioral signs of estrus 18 to 24 days after breeding. Failure to return to estrus provides circumstantial evidence that the previous service resulted in pregnancy. Signs of estrus suggest that the previous service did not result in pregnancy.

The degree to which observation for physical and behavioral signs of estrus predicts pregnancy status is very much related to the breeding manager's ability to recognize those signs. Although this fact is intuitively obvious, adequate skills at heat detection cannot be assumed. On many farms, inadequate heat detection limits both the accurate diagnosis of pregnancy and the pregnancy rates associated with controlled boar matings or artificial insemination.

Perhaps the most important factor in good heat detection is boar exposure. The presence of a mature, sexually aggressive boar will enhance typical estrus behaviors in the sow. Furthermore, intermittent or novel boar exposure may be more effective in stimulating estrus behavior than continuous boar exposure. The sow in heat usually moves toward the boar, particularly if the boar is in an adjacent pen. The most consistent indicator of estrus in the sow is a standing reflex posture in the presence of a boar. This posture is manifest by the sow's standing still to allow the boar to mount. It can also be elicited by a human applying pressure to the back of the sow and observing that the sow assumes a rigid, "sawhorse" stance. Other less consistent indicators of estrus include slight swelling and redness of the vulva and an increase in the quantity and thickness of vaginal mucus.

Estrus behavior in pregnant sows is extremely rare. Therefore, the observation of estrus provides an almost certain diagnosis of non-pregnancy. Although a lack of estrus behavior is consistent with pregnancy, a number of other conditions can also cause a sow to fail to return to estrus, including pseudopregnancy; cystic ovarian degeneration; or inactive, acyclic ovaries. Sows may experience physiological estrus but not show recognizable behavioral signs if housed in large groups or in groups with dominant sows, or if boar exposure is inadequate (Almond and Dial, 1987).

Diligent efforts by the manager to detect estrus can be quite accurate in diagnosing pregnancy. In one study, daily exposure to mature, sexually aggressive boars and observation for signs of estrus was 98 percent accurate in predicting farrowing. This was more accurate than measurement of estrone sulfate or progesterone in the blood and evaluation using Doppler or amplitude-depth ultrasound (Almond and Dial, 1986). In addition to its high level of accuracy, observation for signs of estrus is a routine and necessary task for swine units practicing controlled matings or artificial insemination. As a result, this method adds minimal labor or expense for these units. Observation of return to estrus also corresponds with the earliest opportunity to mate these females again if the manager chooses to do so.

Visual Inspection

Many females display external physical signs of pregnancy between 60 and 90 days of pregnancy. Signs may include abdominal distension, udder enlargement, and enlargement of the vulva (Meredith, 1990). These signs are useful in confirming an presumed pregnancy. However, it is preferable to diagnose non-pregnancy sooner after mating. In most units, a female that is initially discovered to be non-pregnant at 60 to 90 days post-breeding is considered to

have used space, feed, and other resources for no productive purpose. The earlier an animal's non-pregnant status can be detected, the sooner steps can be taken to either impregnate her or remove her from the herd.

Vaginal Biopsy

The sow's vaginal mucosa is lined with nonkeratinized stratified sqaumous epithelium. This mucosa has characteristic histologic features associated with various stages of the estrous cycle and pregnancy. Under the influence of estrogen, the thickness of the stratified layer increases to as many as 15 to 20 cell layers and the border between the epithelial and subepithelial layers becomes irregular. This appearance of the vaginal mucosa is consistent with estrus and inconsistent with pregnancy, except in the very late stages of pregnancy when parturition is eminent. In the absence of estrogenic influence, the epithelial layer is thinner (two to four cell layers) and the subepithelial border is smooth and regular. This appearance is consistent with pregnancy but may also be seen in cycling sows during diestrus or in anestrous sows due to cystic or static ovaries (Mather et al. 1970).

The craniodorsal vaginal wall is the recommended site for biopsy. Instruments designed for uterine biopsy in the mare or rectal biopsy in humans may be used. The biopsy specimen can be fixed in formalin or Bouin solution or examined as a frozen section. The specimen is processed for routine histologic examination. A diagnosis of pregnancy is made when the epithelium is thin and regular; a diagnosis of non-pregnancy is made when the epithelium is thick and irregular.

Because estrogenic influence is rare during pregnancy (except immediately prior to parturition), a diagnosis of non-pregnancy by vaginal biopsy is usually accurate. However, false positive pregnancy diagnoses by vaginal biopsy can be fairly common depending on the pregnancy rate in the tested population and the time when the biopsy is obtained. The accuracy of a positive diagnosis may be greater if the biopsy is taken at 18 to 22 days after mating, i.e., when a non-pregnant sow would be expected to return to estrus (Almond and Dial, 1987). The potential for false positives and the expense and time involved in histologic evaluation limits the practical usefulness of vaginal biopsy as a means for routine pregnancy diagnosis.

Laparoscopy

Observation of the ovaries and uterus of the sow by laparoscope can be used to diagnose pregnancy. Differences in color can be noted between gravid and nongravid uteri; this is the result of greater blood flow to the gravid uterus and increased uterine tone in response to hormonal stimulation (Almond and Dial, 1987). This procedure is invasive, time-consuming, and expensive relative to other means of pregnancy diagnosis and is therefore seldom used.

Rectal Palpation

Several structures associated with the female genital tract can be manually palpated through the rectal wall. Cameron (1977) describes the technique and interpretation of rectal palpation in the sow. He reports that the procedure is easily performed on stalled or tethered sows, but gilts are too small to be easily examined. A lubricated, gloved hand and arm are introduced into the rectum and extended forward approximately 30 cm. The cervix and uterine bifurcation can often be palpated ventral to the rectum and along the anterior edge of the pubic symphysis. The uterine horns are usually out of reach. After an evaluation of the size and tone of the cervix and uterine bifurcation, the external iliac and the middle uterine arteries are located. The external iliac artery can be felt along the cranial border of the ilium as it courses ventrally and caudally toward the rear leg along the medial side of the ilium. As the external iliac artery is followed ventrally, the middle uterine artery can be felt crossing it and coursing cranially toward the abdomen.

In the non-pregnant sow, the cervix and uterine bifurcation can be felt distinctly. The size and tone of these structures increase as estrus approaches. The size and pulsations of the middle uterine artery also increase during estrus. In the pregnant sow, the walls of the uterus become thinner and the bifurcation of the uterus can be felt less distinctly. The pulsations of the middle uterine artery become stronger with advancing pregnancy, reaching the point of a continuous fremitus by day 37 of gestation. Cameron was able to correctly diagnose pregnancy 94.3 percent of the time by performing rectal palpation on sows at least 30 days after mating. Accuracy of the technique improved with experience.

Rectal palpation is a relatively quick, economical, and accurate means of pregnancy diagnosis for trained operators, and the results are available immediately. The main limitation of this technique is a lack of trained operators. Rectal palpation in sows is rarely performed or taught, especially in North America. That this procedure is inappropriate for gilts also limits its usefulness.

Estrone Sulfate

The pig embryo begins to synthesize estrogens at approximately 12 days of gestation. The endometrium converts these fetal estrogens into estrone sulfate, which can be detected in maternal serum. Concentrations of estrone sulfate in maternal serum in the pregnant sow begin increasing between days 16 and 20 after mating, peak between days 25 and 30, and decrease to low levels between days 35 and 45. Concentrations rise again at days 70 to 80 and persist until farrowing.

Serum estrone sulfate concentrations greater than 0.5 ng/ml are considered diagnostic of pregnancy. Because viable fetuses are necessary for the production of estrone sulfate, this test may be useful in diagnosing pseudopregnant sows.

The concentration of estrone sulfate is also loosely correlated with litter size, however variability among sows and time of sampling limits its application as a predictor of litter size (Almond and Dial, 1987).

Estrone sulfate may be measured in either plasma or urine (Atkinson and Williamson, 1987). The overall accuracy of this test in diagnosing pregnancy is greater than 80 percent. Accuracy improves when the test is applied between 25 and 30 days post breeding. This test requires that a blood or urine sample be collected. Laboratory support is necessary for analysis; therefore results are not available for hours to days after the sample is collected.

Prostaglandin $F_{2\alpha}$

In the absence of pregnancy, the endometrium normally secretes prostaglandin $F_{2\alpha}$ ($PGF_{2\alpha}$) between days 12 and 15 of the estrous cycle, inducing regression of the corpus luteum and return to estrus. Pregnancy is assumed if serum concentrations of $PGF_{2\alpha}$ are low (less than 200 pg/ml) between days 13 and 15 after mating.

This method has the advantage of detecting pregnancy very early (before the anticipated first return to estrus). The disadvantages are the necessity of blood sampling, narrow window of time in which the test can be accurately applied, and relative lack of laboratories or commercially available assays capable of measuring this hormone (Almond and Dial, 1987).

Progesterone

Progesterone is secreted by the corpus luteum (CL). The ovarian follicle produces estrogen and releases the ova during estrus. After ovulation, the follicle is transformed into a CL. During the diestrual period, the CL produces progesterone which prepares the uterus for a potential pregnancy and inhibits behavioral signs of estrus. If pregnancy is established, the CL persists and continues to secrete progesterone throughout pregnancy. If pregnancy is not established, by day 12 to 15 the endometrium secretes $PGF_{2\alpha}$, which induces lysis of the CL and a decline in progesterone. Another wave of follicles develops and signs of estrus begin by day 18 to 24.

Consequently, high concentrations of progesterone in maternal circulation indicate the presence of corpora lutea and are consistent with either diestrus or pregnancy. If measured at 17 to 24 days after mating, the probability of diestrus is low; therefore a high concentration of progesterone at this time suggests pregnancy. Low concentrations of progesterone in maternal circulation suggest the absence of corpora lutea. This is consistent with proestrus or estrus and therefore is inconsistent with pregnancy.

Various reports suggest that a serum progesterone of greater than 5 ng/ml when measured at 17 to 24 days after mating is greater than 88% accurate in positively diagnosing pregnancy (Almond and Dial, 1987). Possible causes for a false positive test include any condition which causes persistence of the CL, such as pseudopregnancy or pyometra. A serum progesterone of less than 4 ng/ml is nearly 100% accurate in diagnosing non-pregnancy. The advantage of this test is that non-pregnancy can potentially be detected prior to the next estrus. Laboratory support and commercially available test kits for progesterone are readily available. Disadvantages include the necessity to collect blood, the time lag between collecting the sample and receiving results, and the relatively narrow window after mating in which the test can be used to positively diagnose pregnancy.

Early Pregnancy Factor

In sows, as well as in all other species that have been studied, a substance in the serum of pregnant females downregulates certain aspects of immune function. Presumably, this substance, which has been called early pregnancy factor (EPF), prevents the dam from immunologically rejecting the foreign antigens present in her fetuses. The biological assay for EPF relates to its ability to inhibit T-lymphocytes from forming spontaneous rosettes with heterologous red blood cells.

The details of the assay will not be discussed here except to say that the results of the assay can be expressed numerically as the rosette inhibition titer (RIT). A higher value for the RIT indicates the presence of EPF and, by extension, is diagnostic of pregnancy. According to Koch, Morton, and Ellendorff, a cut-off value of 12 was established for the RIT; that is, values below 12 were associated with non-pregnancy and values above 12 were indicative of pregnancy (Koch and Morton et al., 1983). In a small sample (12 sows), all sows which eventually farrowed had an RIT above 12 beginning at 24 hours after mating and persisting throughout pregnancy. Non-pregnant sows and those that had not yet been mated had an RIT below 12. Two sows showed a transient elevation of the RIT into the pregnancy range, which eventually dropped to the non-pregnant range. These two sows eventually returned to estrus and were presumed to have experienced early pregnancy loss.

Assays for EPF are the earliest diagnostic indicator of pregnancy (as early as 24 hours after mating). Unfortunately, the rosette inhibition assay is cumbersome and time consuming and is not well suited to testing large numbers of samples. Few laboratories are equipped to perform this assay; therefore EPF measurement is seldom used as a practical means of pregnancy diagnosis.

Radiography

Pregnancy can be detected by radiography beginning in the sixth week of pregnancy when the fetal skeleton begins to calcify. Expense and radiation safety concerns limit the usefulness of this technique as a routine method of pregnancy diagnosis (Almond and Dial, 1987).

Doppler Ultrasound

Doppler ultrasound devices make use of the Doppler phenomenon. A sound wave of a given frequency, when reflected back from a moving object, changes in frequency relative to the direction of movement and velocity of the object from which it is reflected. Doppler ultrasound devices emit high frequency sound waves and a transducer detects the reflected sound and converts it to sound in the audible frequency range. The audible frequencies are amplified and sent to a speaker or earphones for the operator to hear.

Doppler devices designed for pregnancy diagnosis of sows may have transducer probes designed to be placed either on the external abdomen or inside the rectum. The transducer is placed such that ultrasound waves are directed toward the internal genital tract of the sow. Movements that can be detected and suggest pregnancy include pulsations of the middle uterine artery, umbilical vessels, or fetal heart. Pulsations associated with fetal heartbeat often have a distinctive "clapping" sound at a rate higher than that of the maternal heart. Pulsations associated with uterine circulation are often described as "gushing" or "swishing" sounds at a rate equal to that of the maternal heart. Other movements that can be detected and must be distinguished from the sounds associated with pregnancy include gastrointestinal movement (described as a slow "rolling" sound) and friction between the transducer and the subject (described as a "crushing" sound).

Although some training and interpretation is required in the use of Doppler ultrasound, an accuracy of 85% or greater can be expected when the test is applied to sows 30 days or more after mating. False positives may occur during estrus when blood flow to the genital tract is greater. False positives may also occur in females with active endometritis. False negatives may occur if the test is used too early (before 30 days after mating) or if a noisy environment obscures the sounds of pregnancy (Fraser et al., 1971; Almond and Dial, 1987). The machines are relatively economical and offer immediate results.

Amplitude-depth Ultrasound

Amplitude-depth (or A-mode) ultrasound devices operate on the principle that body tissues vary in acoustic impedance. Areas of highly contrasting acoustic impedance (such as the interface between fluid and tissue) reflect more acoustic energy than areas of more uniform acoustic impedance. Amplitude-depth ultrasound devices emit ultrasound energy as piezoelectric crystals within a probe are stimulated with an electric current. The same probe detects reflected ultrasound waves. The time between the emission of the ultrasound waves and the detection of the reflection (or echo) is directly correlated to the distance between the probe and the reflective surface. On many amplitude-depth ultrasound devices, this is represented graphically as a line tracing on an oscilloscope. The intensity (amplitude) of the echo is represented on the Y axis of the line tracing; the distance (depth) between the probe and the reflective surface is represented on the X axis.

Pregnancy in swine is characterized by an increase in the fluid contained within the amniotic and allantoic membranes between days 23 and 80 of pregnancy. After day 80, the relative amount of fluid decreases as fetal growth increases. When an amplitude-depth ultrasound device is properly applied to the flank of a sow between days 30 and 80 of pregnancy, a characteristic band of echos is noted at a depth of 15 to 20 cm, corresponding to the location of the amniotic and allantoic fluid. Some machines simply activate a tone and/or a light if the characteristic echos are present.

When examining a sow for pregnancy, the probe should be placed on the lower flank of the standing animal, just cranial to the rear leg and lateral to the udder line. An acoustic coupling agent such as oil or ultrasound gel should be used between the probe and the skin. The probe should be pointed toward the uterus, i.e., medially, dorsally, and sometimes cranially. A possible cause for a false positive test is pointing the probe caudally and detecting the fluid interface of a distended urinary bladder. False negative tests may occur in late pregnancy (greater than 80 days) because of the decreased amounts of fluid in the uterus.

The overall accuracy rate of amplitude-depth ultrasound devices is reported to be as high as 95% (Almond and Dial, 1987). There appears to be some variability of the accuracy of different machines on the market. The timing of the test post-mating and the experience of the operator may also affect accuracy. Causes of false positive tests include the detection of a distended urinary bladder, excessive fluid in the uterus due to pyometra, and endometrial edema from zearalenone intoxication. Causes of false negative tests include improper timing (less than 30 days or more than 80 days after mating) or poor coupling of the probe with the skin. Machines are readily available, relatively economical (especially machines which just activate a tone or light in response to a positive test), and provide immediate results.

Real-time Ultrasound

Real-time (or B-mode) ultrasound is similar to amplitude-depth ultrasound in that it is based on the principle that body tissues vary in acoustic impedance or "echogenicity." However, with real-time ultrasound, a greater number of ultrasound pulses are emitted and echos received in a given period of time. In addition, the pulses and echos are spread over a larger area of tissue. The impulses from the echos are resolved relative to the direction of the pulse and the depth of the echo into a two-dimensional image which is displayed on a screen.

Commercially available real-time ultrasound machines are available with transducer probes which produce varying frequencies of ultrasound waves. Commonly available

transducer probes are available at 3.5 MHz, 5 MHz, or 7.5 MHz. In general, the lower the frequency of the probe, the deeper the ultrasound waves penetrate the tissues. However, the resultant image is of lower resolution. Higher frequency probes do not penetrate as deeply but produce higher image resolution.

Probes may also vary in the arrangement of the ultrasound-emitting crystals. If the ultrasound pulses originate from a narrow source and project outward in a widening path (sector-scan), the resulting image is pie-shaped (narrower near the probe and wider farther away from the probe). If the ultrasound pulses originate from a wider linear array of crystals projecting straight into the tissue (linear scan), the resulting image is rectangular. Each arrangement has found use in diagnosing pregnancy in swine.

Ultrasound probes may be directed toward the reproductive tract of the sow either through the skin and body wall of the flank (similar to amplitude-depth ultrasound) or through the rectal wall. Transrectal ultrasound with a 7.5-MHz linear probe allows a closer approach to the uterus and a higher resolution image. Transabdominal ultrasound is more often performed with a 3.5-MHz or 5-MHz probe to allow for deeper penetration of tissues.

Early pregnancy is positively diagnosed when fluids associated with the embryonic vesicles are identified as dark, anechoic areas within the uterus. As pregnancy advances, the fetus can be visualized within the pocket of fluid. In advanced pregnancies, parts of the fetus such as skeleton or heart may be visualized.

Numerous studies have validated the accuracy of real-time ultrasound in diagnosing of pregnancy. Pregnancies have been detected as early as day 16 post-mating with transrectal ultrasound using a 7.5-MHz linear probe (Knox and Althouse, 1999), although this method is not consistently accurate until days 20 to 22 post-mating. Transabdominal ultrasound using a 3.5-MHz probe is as accurate as transrectal ultrasound (95 percent) by 24 days post-mating (Miller et al., 2003).

Compared to other ultrasound technologies such as Doppler and amplitude-depth, real-time ultrasound offers the advantage of earlier and more accurate diagnosis of pregnancy. It is consistently accurate by day 24 post-mating; Doppler and amplitude-depth ultrasound reach their peak accuracy by day 30 to day 35. A full urinary bladder, which may cause a false positive on amplitude-depth ultrasound, can be clearly discerned from a pregnancy with real-time ultrasound.

Other conditions which may yield false positive results on either Doppler or amplitude-depth ultrasound, such as increased blood flow during estrus, endometritis, pyometra, endometrial edema, and pseudopregnancy, can be more clearly recognized and distinguished from pregnancy with real-time ultrasound. The primary disadvantage of real-time ultrasound is the cost of the equipment. Currently, these machines cost approximately four to 10 times more than Doppler and amplitude-depth machines. Fortunately, real-time machines have decreased remarkably in price in the last 15 years and are currently being adapted and targeted for the swine reproductive diagnostics market. The machines and support for them are readily available.

References

Almond, G.W. and Dial, G.D. (1986). Pregnancy diagnosis in swine: a comparison of the accuracies of mechanical and endocrine tests with return to estrus. *J Am Vet Med Assoc* 189(12): 1567–71.

Almond, G.W. and Dial, G.D. (1987). Pregnancy diagnosis in swine: principles, applications, and accuracy of available techniques. *J Am Vet Med Assoc* 191(7): 858–70.

Atkinson, S. and Williamson, P. (1987). Measurement of urinary and plasma estrone sulphate concentrations from pregnant sows. *Domest Anim Endocrinol* 4(2): 133–8.

Cameron, R.D. (1977). Pregnancy diagnosis in the sow by rectal examination. *Aust Vet J* 53(9): 432–5.

Fraser, A.F., Nagaratnam, V. et al. (1971). The comprehensive use of doppler ultra-sound in farm animal reproduction. *Vet Rec* 88(8): 202–5.

Knox, R. and Althouse, G. (1999). Visualizing the reproductive tract of the female pig using real-time ultrasonography. *Swine Health and Production* 7(5): 207–215.

Koch, E., Morton, H. et al. (1983). Early pregnancy factor: biology and practical application. *Br Vet J* 139(1): 52–8.

Mather, E.C., Diehl, J.R. et al. (1970). Pregnancy diagnosis in swine utilizing the vaginal biopsy technique. *J Am Vet Med Assoc* 157(11): 1522–7.

Meredith, M. (1990). Pregnancy diagnosis in pigs. *Veterinary Annual* 30: 107–12.

Miller, G., Breen, S. et al. (2003). Characterization of image and labor requirements for positive pregnancy diagnosis in swine using two methods of real-time ultrasound. *Journal of Swine Health and Production* 11(5): 233–9.

Part 13.4
Pregnancy Diagnosis in the Ewe

Manoel Tamassia

Introduction

Techniques for diagnosing pregnant ewes have been available for many years; however, one of the major limitations to progress in sheep farming has been the inability to know in advance how many lambs each ewe is carrying. This is not due to the lack of interest or research on the subject; rather, most methods of early pregnancy detection have not satisfied one or more of the following desired criteria: sensitivity, accuracy, speed, safety, or low cost.

Pregnancy diagnosis is an essential management tool for the sheep producer. Early detection allows better management of the animals and farm resources. The development of a method to accurately estimate the stage of pregnancy when precise breeding dates are not available would assist management in maximizing the survival rate of offspring. Separation of the ewes into pregnant and open groups can reduce production and reproduction losses, allowing earlier identification of reproductive waste and the selection of animals with increased fecundity.

Flock Management and Available Techniques

Before deciding to identify pregnant ewes, the cost and benefits of pregnancy diagnosis must be assessed. The benefits from the procedure take different forms:

- Pasture/feeding management—pregnant ewes can be placed in better pastures and rations can be adjusted to gestation status and number of fetuses
- Flock managemen—open and pregnant ewes can be separated; pregnant ewes can be separated into early or late lambing groups which allows better management and monitoring of ewes near term
- Better culling/selection based on production
- Diagnosis to determine the causes of abortion, stillbirths, and other reproductive problems
- Separation of ewes that lambed and lost their lambs from those that failed to conceive
- Prediction of the number of fetuses to make nutritional adjustments and avoid pregnancy toxemia, optimize birth and weaning weights, and increase fetal survivability
- Creation of better marketing plans for lambs
- Possible creation of an off-season breeding flock

Several methods of pregnancy diagnosis are used in sheep. The choice of technique depends on the experience of the operator, length of pregnancy, and the available facilities and equipment. Most techniques require appropriate training and continual practice to master accurate diagnosis. The gestation length may limit when a particular technique can be used; mastering more than one technique can be beneficial. The cost and facilities available can limit the use of a particular technique, as is the case for pregnancy diagnoses that require blood sampling. In this section we first discuss pregnancy diagnosis methods that do not require special equipment, and then those that require equipment or shipping of samples.

Independent of the technique used, the information generated can only be used to its full potential with the use of individual animal identification.

Non-return to Estrus

Non-return to heat has been widely used as an indication of early pregnancy. This technique has better results and is easier to accomplish when a short breeding season (less than 60 days) is allowed. Teaser animals (vasectomized or epididymectomized rams or androgenized ewes) fitted with marking harnesses are introduced with the ewes after all breeding rams have been removed. The teaser animals mount and mark the ewes that come into heat (not pregnant). Occasionally a teaser ram will mount (mark) a female that is pregnant; this occurs mainly if the ewes are confined to a tight pen.

Teaser rams should be used to the harness—rams should be harnessed at least one week before being introduced with the ewes. This allows enough time for the harness to settle and be adjusted while the ram gets used to it. It is extremely important that the mark left from the harness last for at least 3 weeks. There are a variety of colors of crayon on the market and they should be changed regularly on a timely schedule (e.g. weekly or every three weeks).

This method is cheap and it allows early non-pregnancy diagnosis. Its accuracy is high (±90 percent); however, it does not detect the ewes that are not cycling (anestrous) or those that have pathological conditions such as pyometra and hydrometra.

Transrectal Palpation

The internal reproductive organs of the ewe can be digitally palpated by rectum using a two-hand technique (Kutty,

1999). This technique can be used to palpate the vagina, cervix, uterine horns, and ovaries, allowing for early pregnancy diagnosis and assessment of the stage of gestation. A few precautions taken before examination increase the success rate: examining animals before feeding and watering, fasting fat animals for 12 hours, removing all the fecal material from the rectum, and emptying the urinary bladder.

The technique requires the use of both hands. The index finger of the gloved palpation hand is inserted in the rectum while the other hand is held vertically with the finger tips touching the ventral floor of the posterior abdomen; this hand is lifted upward to move abdominal organs forward. Then, using manual manipulation of the abdomen, the reproductive tract within the pelvic cavity can be identified and palpated.

At 30 days of gestation the uterus and the cervix are located in the pelvic cavity and there is clear asymmetry between horns. At 45 days the uterus has fallen in to the abdomen but can be pushed back over the pelvic brim; the uterus is softer in consistency compared to day 30. At 60 days the uterus is distended and it is in the abdominal cavity, the uterine horns are indistinguishable, the cervix is soft and slightly hypertrophied, and the vaginal wall is distended. At 90 days placentomes and the fetus can be palpated, the vagina is stretched, and the cervix is soft and hypertrophied. At 120 days of gestation the cervix is large, soft, and difficult to palpate; the fetus and large placentomes are palpable.

This method is described as simple and effective; however, like any of the pregnancy diagnoses described in this review, training is necessary.

Rectal Abdominal Palpation

This is a simple, cheap, and quick technique to diagnose pregnant ewes. It consists of inserting a lubricated rod into the rectum of a ewe that is lying on its back. One hand is placed on the abdomen of the ewe while the other hand manipulates the rod toward the hand that is over the abdomen. The technique is not indicated for early pregnancy diagnosis because the sensitivity is reportedly low (59 percent sensitivity between days 21 to 55) (White et al., 1984). With the advance of gestation, at 85 to 109 days after breeding, it has a reported accuracy of 100 percent (Hulet, 1972; Turner and Hindson, 1975; Plant, 1980; Ott et al., 1981; Trapp and Slyter, 1983). However, some authors haven't had the same success rate, indicating that operator experience with this technique is very important.

A serious disadvantage of the technique is the risk of rectal injury to the ewe and the induction of abortion (Turner and Hindson, 1975; Trapp and Slyter, 1983).

Transabdominal Palpation

The presence of a fetus is detected by manual palpation of the ewe's abdomen. This is more easily accomplished with the ewe in the seated position. The operator's hands are placed on both sides of the abdomen. With one hand pressing on one side of the abdomen, the fingers of the other hand palpate the abdomen in search of fetuses. The presence of lambs is felt as a free floating mass that bounces against the operator's fingers.

Although simple and inexpensive, the technique requires training and is limited to the last two months of gestation. The accuracy of the technique varies with the experience of the operator, starting at 80 percent and reaching 90 percent in thin ewes that have been recently shorn. The accuracy can be increased if the method is used in association with other techniques such as udder examination.

Udder Examination (Wet and Dry Techniques)

This is an indirect method of detecting pregnancy in ewes. It can be performed during late gestation and can have a high accuracy rate if associated with other techniques such as abdominal enlargement and transabdominal palpation. It is best performed during the last month of gestation when ewes start their udder development. This technique also yields the best results if the breeding (lambing) season is short; otherwise the udder inspection needs to be performed twice with a three-to-four-week interval. At this stage the udder is firm and enlarged and feels warm. Colostrum can be milked at this stage to confirm pregnancy and differentiate from mastitis or fat open ewes that have been fed estrogenic rich clover. These animals have an enlarged udder that is soft and cold to the touch and their secretions can vary from a watery fluid to thick white milk. In contrast, colostrum should be thick and cream-colored or it can be thick and yellow with a honey appearance.

At this stage, ewes identified as pregnant can be separated from the flock for adequate management. It is advisable to do a final check within the last week of the lambing season to identify/cull the ewes that did not conceive during the breeding season. This technique does not allow the determination of the lambing date or the number of fetuses.

Radiography

This is a technique that, despite its high accuracy in detection of pregnancy and number of fetuses, has seen limited use. This is mainly due to the high cost of the equipment and the potential health hazards to the operator. By using video-fluoroscopy systems the speed of pregnancy diagnosis is greatly increased and problems associated with film development are eliminated. Four hundred to 600 ewes per day may be checked under farm conditions with an accuracy rate of 94 percent to 100 percent (Ford et al., 1963; Grace et al., 1989).

Biochemical Tests

Several biochemical tests can diagnose pregnancy in the ewe. Despite their high accuracy, these methods present some major disadvantages when compared to other methods. There is the need to collect samples (blood, serum, urine, or feces), the results are not available immediately, and they usually have a higher cost. The tests can measure progesterone, estrone sulphate, ovine chorionic somatomammotrophin, pregnancy-specific protein B (PSPB), and ovine pregnancy-associated glycoproteins. The specificity and sensitivity of these tests can be quite high. Nevertheless, no single early pregnancy diagnosis can guarantee the birth of a live lamb. Two or more tests (e.g. progesterone and estrone sulphate) at the same time can provide complementary information and increase.

Estrone Sulphate

The presence of estrone sulphate in serum is an indicator of a viable fetal-placental unit. It can be measured from 30 days of gestation and it increases steadily until parturition (Tsang, 1974; Tsang and Hackett, 1979). The reported accuracy for this test was of 44 percent for non-pregnancy and 88 percent for pregnancy (Worsfold et al., 1986). Estrone sulphate concentration is correlated with the number of fetuses; however, its use as a predictor of fetal numbers is limited due to the high variation between animals of the hormone in the serum.

Progesterone

Several progesterone tests have been developed that use either radioimmunoassay (RIA) or enzyme immunoassay (EIA). Early in gestation progesterone is produced only by the *corpus luteum* (CL) with placental production starting at 50 days. Measurement of high progesterone early in gestation is an indication that a ewe has functional CL. Progesterone levels above 2.5 ng/ml (determined by EIA) on day 18 post-breeding are a reasonably reliable, indirect method to detect pregnancy with high accuracy (88 percent to 100 percent) (McPhee and Tiberghien, 1987; Boscos et al., 2003). Accuracy of nearly 100 percent was reported for both ewe lambs and mature ewes at 100 to 110 days post-breeding (Schneider and Hallford, 1996).

However, there is conflicting information in the literature concerning the diagnosis of non-pregnancy (60 percent to 100 percent). The measurement of high progesterone in blood during the non-breeding season suggests pregnancy. The major suspects of the low accuracy are associated with embryonic death, pseudopregnancy, hydrometra, pyometra, ovarian pathology, or measuring progesterone during diestrus.

The conclusion is that progesterone measurement associated with accurate reproductive data (estrus detection, dates of breeding/AI) is highly accurate in detecting pregnant and open ewes. It should be emphasized that any early pregnancy diagnosis test has an inherent inaccuracy (Karen et al., 2003). Presence of an embryo at the time of testing cannot assure the birth of live young.

The progesterone metabolite iPdG (immunoreactive Pregnendiol-3-Glucuronide) is secreted in feces and has been used to diagnose pregnancy in sheep with 100 percent accuracy from 60 days of gestation (Borjesson and Boyce et al., 1996).

During early pregnancy there is a positive correlation between the number of CLs, progesterone levels, and the number of fetuses; however, this relationship is not a simple linear function (Quirke and Manrahan et al., 1979; Quirke and Jennings et al., 1979). Although progesterone levels can be higher in ewes carrying twins and triplets, it is a poor predictor of fetal number.

Ovine Pregnancy-associated Glycoprotein

Ovine pregnancy-associated glycoproteins are secreted by binucleated placental thophectodermic cells and increase steadily from week three until parturition. They can be measured in the maternal serum. The accuracy of this technique for pregnancy diagnosis is lacking (Humblot, 1988; Karen et al., 2003; Spencer et al., 2004; Karen et al., 2005).

Pregnancy-specific Protein B

PSPB, or pregnancy-specific associated protein B, is secreted by binucleated placental cells and has been 100 percent accurate in diagnosing pregnancy and 83 percent accurate in diagnosing non-pregnancy (Humblot, 1988; Karen et al., 2003). Because the test was developed to detect the hormone in cows and there is limited cross reaction with ovine serum, it cannot be used to quantitatively measure fetal numbers (Humblot, 1988).

Ultrasound

None of the above-mentioned methods of early gestation pregnancy diagnosis in ewes have satisfied the criteria of sensitivity, accuracy, speed, safety, and low cost. One technique that does meet most of those criteria is real-time ultrasonography, and the techonology has been rapidly adopted where it is available. In addition to diagnosing pregnancy, real-time ultrasound has been widely used to determine the size of the litters (Trapp and Slyter, 1983; Karen et al., 2005).

The earliest techniques to detect pregnancy used A-mode ultrasound, or amplitude-depth ultrasonography (Meredith and Madani, 1980; Madel, 1983). This is a probe equipped with a single piezoelectric crystal that, when electrically stimulated, converts electrical energy in sound. As the sound waves travel through the tissues some waves are reflected and captured by the same crystals that generated the sound. The crystals can then reconvert the sound into electric impulses. Sound waves are reflected differently according to the tissue density; fluid-filled structures reflect fewer sound waves. These reflected sound waves are in the range of 1 to 10 MHz, above the human hearing capacity (20,000 Hz).

Pregnancy diagnosis using A-mode ultrasonography is performed by placing the probe in the lower flank and pointing it toward the uterus. A-mode ultrasound uses a single crystal to emit sound that penetrates the tissues and recaptures the wave. The return signal is processed (as audible sound or peaks on an oscilloscope with a horizontal scale representing the depth of the tissue) to reveal the presence of tissue interfaces of different densities (fluid-filled uterus). The reported accuracy, starting at 60 days, varies widely (80 percent to 96 percent) with specificity varying from 69 percent to 87.5 percent (Lane and Lewis, 1981; Madel, 1983). This is a quick, simple, safe, cheap technique; however, it cannot detect fetal viability and fetal numbers.

Doppler ultrasound uses the Doppler shift principle to detect sound reflection from moving tissues such as blood (fremitus of the uterine artery) or fetal heartbeat. Doppler utrasonography can be performed with an abdominal transducer or intra-rectal transducer. The accuracy with the intrarectal transducer increases with gestation length, in the neighborhood of 85 percent. The accuracy for non-pregnancy is higher, varying from 91 percent at 41 to 60 days of gestation to 94 percent after day 71. The transabdonimal transducer is similarly accurate (Ott et al., 1981; Galan et al., 1999).

The disadvantage of these machines is their inability to diagnose gestation age. It can however, be used to diagnose multiple pregnancies when in the hands of a skilled operator (Fukui et al., 1984).

Real-time or B-mode Utrasonography

Real-time ultrasonography displays the return echo information in a monitor. The pattern and frequency of intermittent crystal excitation allow the monitor to be updated continuously at a rate that produces an apparently moving image.

The configuration of the crystals in the probe head determines the shape of the image in the monitor. They are generally linear or sector. Linear probes have the crystals arranged in line and emit parallel sound beams. The resulting image is rectangular. Sector probes emit sound from a rotating group of crystals through a sound transparent scan-head generating a pie-shaped image.

The uterus is examined rectally (with the linear probe) during early gestation, or by transabdominal (linear or sector probes) later in gestation. The wool-free area in the right lower flank is best suited for the placement of the probe. The area must be cleaned or shaved to allow the probe to touch the skin in good apposition. The use of contact gel assures acoustic coupling with the skin; any other obstetric lubricant can be used with the same efficacy.

Pregnancy diagnosis can be performed as early as day 13 after breeding with a linear (7.5 MHz) probe placed into the rectum (Gonzalez et al., 1998). Using a 5 MHz transrectal probe, the uterus can be seen as dark anechoic areas dorso-cranial to the bladder on day 17 to 19 after breeding. The embryo can be visualized after day 25 (Kaulfuss and Uhlich et al., 1996; Kaulfuss and Zipper et al., 1996).

Transabdominal ultrasonography can be performed with a linear 5 MHz probe at day ±25 after breeding with lower sensitivity and specificity (Kaulfuss et al., 1996). The success rate increase to near 100 percent from days 46 to 106. In pregnant ewes the fluid-filled uterus can first be seen at day 21, and the embryo and heartbeat can be seen at day 25 (Medan et al., 2004).

The images consistent with pregnancy include multiple fluid-filled uterine sections, placentomes, and the fetus (see Figures 13.4 and 13.5). Their presence can be used to diagnose gestation. Pregnancy length can be accurately estimated with the measurement of fetal structures (Greenwood et al. 2002). Gestation length (y) can be estimated by measuring the distance from the crown to the rump of the fetus (x): $y = 14.05 + 1.16x - 0.012x^2$ (Schrick and Inskeep, 1993). These changes are described in Table 13.1.

Real-time ultrasonography for the diagnosis of gestation in sheep is accurate, sensitive, rapid, and safe, fulfilling most of the prerequisites of the producer. It has the advan-

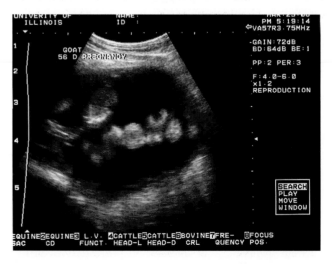

Figure 13.4. Caprine pregnant uterus, approximately 56 days. Note the cotyledons (round, doughnut and "C" shapes) and uterine fluid (black).

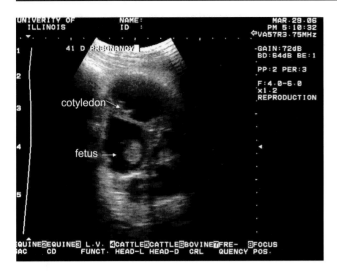

Figure 13.5. Caprine pregnant uterus, 41 days. Note the different sections of the uterus, developing cotyledons, and fetus.

tage of determining fetal numbers and estimating fetal age and fetal health (White et al., 1984).

Conclusion

Pregnancy detection has economical benefits for the producer. To provide benefits to the producer, the diagnostic method should be accurate, fast, and inexpensive. The operator should be trained to use the technique and all equipment must be checked in advance. Among the techniques discussed, transabdominal B-mode ultrasound appears to be the most advantageous, despite its high cost. It accurately diagnoses pregnancy rate, fetal numbers, and fetal viability. Regardless of the technique used, this information can only bring benefits if the data generated is accurately recorded and used to improve flock management.

Table 13.1. Diagnosis of gestation in sheep and goats by ultrasonography.

Gestation age (days)	Uterine findings	Probe placement (probe MHz)
13	Uterine fluid	Transrectal (7.5)
19 to 25	First visualization fetus	Transrectal (7.5)
25 to 30	Multiple luminal sections filled with fluid	Transabdominal (5)
>40	Placentome and fetus	Transabdominal (5)
46 to 100	Determination of fetal number	Transabdominal (5)

References

Borjesson, D.L., Boyce, W.M. et al. (1996). Pregnancy detection in bighorn sheep (*Ovis canadensis*) using a fecal-based enzyme immunoassay. *J Wildl Dis* 32(1): 67–74.

Boscos, C.M., Samartzi, F.C. et al. (2003). Assessment of progesterone concentration using enzymeimmunoassay, for early pregnancy diagnosis in sheep and goats. *Reprod Domest Anim* 38(3): 170–4.

Ford, E.J.H., Clark, J.W. et al. (1963). The detection of fetal numbers in sheep by means of X-rays. *Veterinary Record* 75: 958–960.

Fukui, Y., Kimura, T. et al. (1984). Multiple pregnancy diagnosis in sheep using an ultrasonic Doppler method. *Vet Rec* 114(6): 145.

Galan, H.L., Jozwik, M. et al. (1999). Umbilical vein blood flow determination in the ovine fetus: comparison of Doppler ultrasonographic and steady-state diffusion techniques. *Am J Obstet Gynecol* 181(5 Pt 1): 1149–53.

Gonzalez, B.A., Santiago, M.J. et al. (1998). Estimation of fetal development on Manchega dairy ewes by transrectal ultrasonography measurements. *Small Ruminat Research* (27): 243–50.

Grace, N.D., Beach, A.D. et al. (1989). Multiple pregnancy diagnosis using real-time ultrasonic bocy scanner and video-fluoroscopy systems. *Proc N Z Soc Anim Prod* 49: 107–11.

Greenwood, P.L., Slepetis, R.M. et al. (2002). Prediction of stage of pregnancy in prolific sheep using ultrasound measurement of fetal bones. *Reprod Fertil Dev* 14(1–2): 7–13.

Hulet, C. V. (1972). A rectal-abdominal palpation technique for diagnosing pregnancy in the ewe. *J Anim Sci* 35(4): 814–9.

Humblot, P. (1988). Proteins specific for pregnancy in ruminants. *Reprod Nutr Dev* 28(6B): 1753–61.

Karen, A., Amiri, B.E. et al. (2005). Comparison of accuracy of transabdominal ultrasonography, progesterone and pregnancy-associated glycoproteins tests for discrimination between single and multiple pregnancy in sheep. *Theriogenology* 66(2): 314–22.

Karen, A., Beckers, J.F. et al. (2003). Early pregnancy diagnosis in sheep by progesterone and pregnancy-associated glycoprotein tests. *Theriogenology* 59(9): 1941–8.

Kaulfuss, K.H., Uhlich, K. et al. (1996). Real-time ultrasonic pregnancy diagnosis (B-mode) in sheep. 1. Frequent examinations during the first month of pregnancy. *Tierarztl Prax* 24(5): 443–52.

Kaulfuss, K.H., Zipper, N. et al. (1996). Ultrasonic pregnancy diagnosis (B-mode) in sheep. 2. Comparative studies using transcutaneous and transrectal pregnancy diagnosis. *Tierarztl Prax* 24(6): 559–66.

Kutty, C.I. (1999). Gynecological examination and pregnancy diagnosis in small ruminants using bimanual palpation technique: a review. *Theriogenology* 51(8): 1555–64.

Lane, S.F. and Lewis, P.E. (1981). Detection of pregnancy in ewes with the ultrasonic scanopreg. *J Anim Sci* 52(3): 463–7.

Madel, A.J. (1983). Detection of pregnancy in ewe lambs by A-mode ultrasound. *Vet Rec* 112(1): 11–2.

McPhee, I.M. and Tiberghien, M.P. (1987). Assessment of pregnancy in sheep by analysis of plasma progesterone using an amplified enzyme immunoassay technique. *Vet Rec* 121(3): 63–5.

Medan, M., Watanabe, G. et al. (2004). Early pregnancy diagnosis by means of ultrasonography as a method of improving reproductive efficiency in goats. *J Reprod Dev* 50(4): 391–7.

Meredith, M.J. and Madani, M.O. (1980). The detection of pregnancy in sheep by a-mode ultrasound. *Br Vet J* 136(4): 325–30.

Ott, R.S., Braun, W.F. et al. (1981). A comparison of intrarectal Doppler and rectal abdominal palpation for pregnancy testing in goats. *J Am Vet Med Assoc* 178(7): 730–1.

Plant, J.W. (1980). Pregnancy diagnosis in sheep using a rectal probe. *Vet Rec* 106(14): 305–6.

Quirke, J.F., Hanrahan, J.P. et al. (1979). Plasma progesterone levels throughout the oestrous cycle and release of LH at oestrus in sheep with different ovulation rates. *J Reprod Fertil* 55(1): 37–44.

Quirke, J.F., Jennings, J.J. et al. (1979). Oestrus, time of ovulation, ovulation rate and conception rate in progestagen-treated ewes given Gn-RH, Gn-TH analogues and gonadotrophins. *J Reprod Fertil* 56(2): 479–88.

Schneider, F.A. and Hallford, C.M. (1996). Use of rapid progesterone radioimmunoassay to predict pregnancy and fetal numbers in sheep. *Sheep and Goat Research Journal* 12: 33–8.

Schrick, F.N. and Inskeep, E.K. (1993). Determination of early pregnancy in ewes utilizing transrectal ultrasonography. *Theriogenology* 40: 295–306.

Spencer, T.E., Johnson, G.A. et al. (2004). Implantation mechanisms: insights from the sheep. *Reproduction* 128(6):657–68.

Trapp, M.J. and Slyter, A.L. (1983). Pregnancy diagnosis in the ewe. *J Anim Sci* 57(1): 1–5.

Tsang, C.P. (1974). Changes in plasma levels of estrone sulfate and estrone in the pregnant ewe around parturition. *Steroids* 23(6): 855–68.

Tsang, C.P. and Hackett, A.J. (1979). Metabolism of progesterone in the pregnant sheep near term: identification of 3 beta-hydroxy-5 alpha-pregnan-20-one 3-sulfate as a major metabolite. *Steroids* 33(5): 577–88.

Turner, C.B. and Hindson, J.C. (1975). An assessment of a method of manual pregnancy diagnosis in the ewe. *Vet Rec* 96(3): 56–8.

White, I.R., Russel, A.J. et al. (1984). Real-time ultrasonic scanning in the diagnosis of pregnancy and the determination of fetal numbers in sheep. *Vet Rec* 115(7): 140–3.

Worsfold, A.I., Chamings, R.J. et al. (1986). Measurement of oestrone sulphate in sheep plasma as a possible indicator of pregnancy and the number of viable fetuses present. *Br Vet J* 142(2): 195–7.

Part 13.5
Canine and Feline Pregnancy Diagnois

Suzanne Whitaker and Richard Meadows

The goal of this section is to familiarize the reader with the different ways in which canine pregnancy can be timed and the techniques for diagnosing pregnancy in the bitch. A few pertinent items about pregnancy diagnosis in the queen are also included.

For many years seasoned practitioners primarily used abdominal palpation to diagnose pregnancy in the bitch and queen. Unfortunately, this technique is only accurate between days 20 and 35 or during the last seven to 10 days of the dog's pregnancy. Pregnancy can be palpated in the queen as early as days 14 to 20 after breeding (Tibary and Memon, 2003).

Many clients are anxious to know whether breeding was successful or if they should hormonally end diestrus and breed the bitch again. Other clients are anxious to know if a mis-mating took place. This desire for an earlier, reliable pregnancy diagnosis has led researchers to search for a pregnancy hormone similar to human chorionic gonadotropin (HCG) in humans and equine chorionic gonadotropin (ECG) in horses. No such hormone exists in the bitch. With the exception of modern, real-time (B-mode), ultrasound imaging, the quest to diagnose pregnancy earlier has not significantly advanced.

As is the case in human medicine, real-time ultrasonography is now the gold standard of pregnancy diagnosis in both canines and felines. It has improved in quality and availability and has allowed practitioners to estimate the stage of pregnancy, assess fetal viability, and detect fetal distress much earlier. Accurately determining litter size in large litters, while better than palpation, remains problematic in veterinary theriogenology.

Timing of Pregnancy

Canine and feline pregnancies have been stated as lasting an average of 63 and 65 days, respectively. However, counting from the first breeding date, a normal canine gestation has been reported to vary by as much as eighteen days, from 54 to 72 days (Krzyzanowski et al., 1975; Barr, 1988) although 57 to 72 days is a more frequently quoted range (Tibary and Memon, 2003; Feldman and Nelson, 2004; Johnston et al., 2001). This large variation depends upon what event the breeder or clinician calls day 0.

The wide range in gestational length can be eliminated when the timing of the pregnancy begins with the pre-ovulatory surge in luteinizing hormone (LH). If one uses the LH surge as day 0, the average gestational length in the bitch is 64 to 66 days (Barr, 1988; Feldman and Nelson, 2004; Johnston et al., 2001). This elevation of LH is transient, typically lasting approximately 24 hours, and it precedes ovulation by two to three days. If the timing of the LH surge is known, the timing of the events that occur during pregnancy become highly predictable. In fact, when timed correctly, the events of canine pregnancy have been found to be consistent and predictable across repeated studies (Concannon, 2000). Therefore, all of the discussions in this section that refer to a specific date during pregnancy are based on the LH surge timetable. However, we will briefly discuss the other gestational timetables in the event that the LH surge is not known for a particular patient.

Timing of events that allow for such a variable gestation length in the dog include the time between onset of "standing" estrus (i.e., female receptivity) and mating and the time between mating (e.g., forced early mating from aggressive males) and ovulation. The unique physiology of the bitch also compounds the variability of gestation length. Canine oocytes are ovulated in an immature state and require two to three days after ovulation to mature. In addition, the tubo-uterine junction, which allows for the passage of the blastocyst(s) into the uterus, does not open until approximately eight days after ovulation (Gradil et al., 2000). Dog sperm can survive seven to nine days in the uterus. This potential longevity of sperm in the unique canine female reproductive tract means that fertile matings can occur as early as five days before ovulation or as late as seven days after ovulation (Gradil et al., 2000).

A 15- to 18-day window for timing of parturition is not clinically useful for parturition management, especially in brachycephalic canine breeds. In these breeds spontaneous parturition might not occur safely and cesearan sections need to be precisely timed to maximize survival of the puppies and the bitch. The LH peak allows for precise timing, and can be detected by serial testing directly for increased LH blood or urine levels and/or indirectly by assays for the beginning of increased progesterone blood levels. These assays are available through commercial laboratories or as in-house kits which can be purchased by the general public.

Various other methods used to calculate gestation length, listed from most precise to least precise, include (Tibary and Memon, 2003; Concannon, 2000):

- estimating the day of ovulation by ultrasound
- observing end-of-estrus (metestrus or diestrus) changes in vaginal cytology
- observing changes in the vaginoscopic appearance of the vaginal mucosa
- timing the pre-ovulatory softening of the vulva and perineum

Repeated ultrasound exams might be required to image recent ovulation and, as a result, this technique is not practical in many clinical cases. Counting from diestrus day 1, approximately 80 percent of the bitches whelp at diestrus day 57. Most can be expected to whelp 57 (± three) days after diestrus day 1 (Gradil et al., 2000). Calculating gestation length based on the changes in gross appearance of the vaginal mucosa, vulva, and perineum is not recommended.

How this consistent 65-day (± one day) gestation length remains reliable in late- or early-bred bitches is only partly understood. There are three, and perhaps four, likely reasons for this consistency (Concannon, 2000). First, as previously noted, dog sperm can live seven to nine days in the bitch's reproductive tract. Second, eggs fertilized after maturation appear to divide slightly faster than those penetrated by sperm before maturation. Third, there is a very narrow window of time in which the uterus is receptive for implantation. The receptivity of the uterus to implantation is influenced by changes in serum concentrations of estrogen and progesterone. The changes in these two hormones are not affected by the timing of mating, fertilization, or early embryo cleavage rate. Fourth, anecdotal reports indicate that the fetal signal for parturition is weak in small litters, and parturition may be delayed for one to two days (Concannon, 2000).

For a timetable of events during a canine pregnancy, see Table 13.2.

Palpation

Palpation is still commonly used to diagnose pregnancy in the bitch. This technique is inexpensive and simple, but success depends on various factors including the stage of pregnancy, number of fetuses, size and body condition of the bitch or queen (the small uterine enlargements are more difficult to detect in large breed dogs), temperament of the bitch or queen, and skill of the palpator.

Uterine swellings are readily palpable for only 10 to 15 days (typically days 20 to 35 of the pregnancy). The pregnancy can potentially be palpated as early as day 19 post-LH surge (Johnston et al., 2001). During this early stage of pregnancy the uterus is firm and the ovoid, 1 to 2 cm diameter chorioallantoic swellings are separated from each other and easily palpated. The most caudal swellings are the easiest to palpate but must be differentiated from firm fecal deposits, particularly in cats.

The thumb and fingers of the palpator's most sensitive hand (not necessarily the dominant hand) should be used to

Table 13.2. A timetable of events during a canine pregnancy, timed from the luteinizing hormone (LH) surge as day 0.

Method of pregnancy detection	Day post-LH surge
Palpation gestational sacs	22–30
Radiography fetal mineralization	42–45
Ultrasound (B-mode) gestational sacs beating heart visible fetal movement	19–25 22–29 28–39
Cytologic diestrus to whelping	54–60
Breeding date gestational sacs on palpation gestational sacs on ultrasound mineralization of fetuses on radiographs	26–28 30 42–52
C-reactive protein increases*	30–50
Fibrinogen increases*	21–50
Hematocrit decreases due to hemodilution*	20
Relaxin concentration first detectable relaxin concentration peaks	25 40–50

*Denotes methods that are not recommended for pregnancy diagnosis or determination of whelping date.

locate the body of the uterus first. The uterine body is found between the bladder and rectum, immediately cranial to the cervix in the caudodorsal abdominal cavity. In some instances, raising the forequarters of the bitch or queen allows the uterine horns to fall ventrally and caudally, thus facilitating palpation of any swellings in the cranial sections of the uterine horns that were perhaps lying under the ribs.

As a rule, palpation for pregnancy should be scheduled for three to four weeks after the first breeding if more precise timing criteria are not known. If pregnancy is not detected, the palpation should be repeated one week later. After day 30 of gestation, the uterus enlarges rapidly and uniformly and occupies a more cranioventral position in the abdominal cavity. The conceptuses lose their firm, distinct bulges in the more uniformly enlarged uterus and palpation becomes much more difficult. The individual fetuses again become easily palpable after days 45 to 50. Movement of puppies may occasionally be detected in the last seven to 10 days of pregnancy.

False positive results may be due to pyometra, particularly forms that present sacculations similar to those palpated in normal pregnancies (Gradil et al., 2000).

Some bitches are intolerant of abdominal palpation due to nervousness, aggression, or obesity, and an alternate method of pregnancy diagnosis must be performed. Among those that allow palpation, this diagnostic technique is relatively accurate (87 percent to 88 percent positive predictive value and 73 percent negative predictive value in the second trimester of pregnancy) (Allen and Meredith, 1981; Toal et al., 1986). Palpation has been reported to be only 12 percent accurate in assessment of litter size, in part because the most cranial conceptuses are most often missed due to their proximity to the rib cage (Toal et al., 1986).

Pregnancy palpation should be done with safety of the conceptuses in mind. Studies evaluating the safety of repeated palpation or use of excessive force have not been reported, to the author's knowledge. However, there have been anecdotal reports of increased fetal resorption in a kennel setting due to repeated palpation, with subsequent decreased resorption once palpating was discontinued (Johnston et al., 2001). Another drawback to abdominal palpation is that it does provide any way to assess fetal viability of all fetuses, even if movement is detected in one or more of them. The practitioner must always caution the client that fetal resorption can occur at any time during the pregnancy.

Radiography

Radiography is another readily available and relatively inexpensive way to diagnose pregnancy. However, due to potential ionizing effects on organogenesis, radiography is not recommended early in pregnancy (Miles, 1995). The most common indications for abdominal radiographs are for pre-partum determination of litter size or post-partum determination that all pups have been whelped.

Pregnancy can be detected as uterine enlargement as early as 21 to 28 days (Barr, 1988; Gradil et al., 2000) This enlargement may be quite subtle, especially in the presence of a full colon. The enlargement is frequently indistinguishable from a pyometra. Fetal skeletons have been reported to be mineralized by day 42 to day 45 or day 44 to day 47; however, most practitioners wait to radiograph until day 45 to day 50 to allow adequate mineralization for visualization and to ensure a more accurate fetal count (Miles, 1995; Concannon and Rendano, 1983).

The fetal vertebral column is the first identifiable mineralization, closely followed by the head, ribs, and pelvis (Johnston et al., 2001). Fetal teeth, if ever visualized, become detectable only in the last week of pregnancy (days 58 to 63).

Abdominal radiographs remain the gold standard for assessing litter size. Counting fetal heads and vertebral columns is the most reliable method for estimating litter size, but in large litters in which fetuses overlap and other intestinal contents impede the clinician's view, an accurate fetal count can be more difficult. Typically one can state a minimum number of fetuses more accurately than a total number.

Radiography does not allow for evaluation of fetal distress or for timely assessment of fetal viability. It can take 24 to 48 hours for radiographic evidence of fetal death to appear (Johnston et al., 2001; Root Kustritz, 2005). Reported signs of fetal death include evidence of depression

of the frontal bones of the fetus, abnormal angulations of the spine, or presence of intra- or extra-uterine gas (Root Kustritz, 2005). Because the fetal skull is pliable and compressible and the pelvis is distensible, using radiography to determine fetal-pelvic incompatibility is of questionable use for prediction of dystocia, even when there are only one or two large fetuses (Tibary and Memon, 2003; Feldman and Nelson, 2004; Johnston et al., 2001).

Radiography is very commonly used when there is a dystocia or the bitch seems to stall during labor. In those cases the radiograph simply determines if any fetuses remain. Radiography remains very useful for detection of retained fetuses at the apparent conclusion of parturition.

Ultrasonography

The gold standard of pregnancy diagnosis and monitoring is now considered to be real-time ultrasonographic evaluation. Ultrasound technology is now readily available to the average practitioner and the patient at a reasonable cost. A skilled ultrasonographer with quality equipment can diagnose pregnancy in the bitch (by the presence of fetal vesicles) as early as 18 to 20 days of gestation or 19 to 21 days post-LH surge (Tibary and Memon, 2003; Feldman and Nelson, 2004; England et al., 2003). Ultrasonography in the queen can detect pregnancy as early as 13 to 15 days post-mating, with fetal heartbeats detectable by 16 to 25 days post-mating (Tibary and Memon, 2003).

Most ultrasonographers prefer to wait at least until 21 to 25 days post-LH surge in canines to have a more accurate diagnosis. (Tibary and Memon, 2003; Root Kustritz, 2005). While ultrasound diagnosis of pregnancy is not accurately performed much earlier than a diagnosis of pregnancy by an experienced palpator, it does offer more information than palpation alone.

The main advantage to ultrasound pregnancy diagnosis and monitoring is that fetal viability can be monitored throughout pregnancy if needed. Fetal heartbeats can be detected as early as days 22–29 of gestation (England et al., 2003). The typical fetal heart rate should be 200 to 255 beats per minute (Verstegen et al., 1993). Fetal movement is typically detected between days 28 and 36 (Tibary and Memon, 2003; Yeager et al., 1992). There is quite a wide time frame for the detection of fetal movement, and clinical skill with ultrasound plays quite an important role in determining when a pregnancy can be diagnosed and fetal heartbeats and fetal movement can first be detected. Due to a wide range in ultrasonographer skill, these numbers should be used as guidelines only.

Fetal distress in high-risk pregnancies or during difficult whelpings can be evaluated by monitoring for decreased fetal movement and heart rate (Barr, 1988; Poffenbarger and Feeney, 1986). A fetal heart rate less than 180 beats per minute indicates fetal distress (England et al., 2003). Fetal death can be easily determined by the absence of a fetal heartbeat.

Alternatively, a simple, hand-held, Doppler ultrasound unit can be used to monitor fetal heart rate as an indicator of distress. These simple Doppler units may be used to initially detect whelps around day 30 to day 35 of gestation, with a "fairly accurate" litter count detectable around 45 days of gestation (www.Whelpwise.com, 2005). The ultrasound Doppler is also very helpful during a whelp, because distressed puppies can be detected early, giving the owner time to intervene before pups are lost (www.Whelpwise. com, 2005).

Researchers constantly evaluate new formulas to determine more information from the pregnancy ultrasound (Yeager et al., 1992; England et al., 1990). Many formulas try to determine gestational age of the fetus based on ultrasonographic measurements. The only area in which radiography is still considered to be a better diagnostic tool is fetal counts. Because ultrasound waves only see limited parts and planes of the abdomen at the same time, and due to acoustic artifact when fetuses overlap, it is difficult to accurately assess litter size. At its best, ultrasound has been shown to be only 38 percent accurate in assessing litter size (Tibary and Memon, 2003; Toal et al., 1986; England et al., 1990; Bondestam et al., 1984). Other studies have shown that ultrasound is more accurate in assessing litter size in smaller litters, and that accuracy decreases as litter size increases (Tibary and Memon, 2003; Gradil et al., 2000; Bondestam et al., 1984).

The main drawbacks to ultrasonography are the cost of the machine and the amount of skill that is required. Most practitioners who are not confident in their ultrasound skills can refer clients to specialist; however, some clients may be deterred by the increased expense and traveling to the specialist.

Not all pregnant bitches are good candidates for ultrasonographic evaluation. Those that are nervous or aggressive are unlikely to be willing to lay in dorsal recumbency for an extended period of time, and many practitioners are nervous about sedating these patients. Some patients may be examined while standing, if the clinician prefers, or if the patient is more compliant in that position (Tibary and Memon, 2003). As a result, some of these patients continue to be monitored through palpation and a quick radiograph unless assessment of fetal viability is absolutely necessary.

For the general practitioner a 5 MHz probe is considered to be an all purpose pregnancy detection probe (Gradil et al., 2000). A 7.5 MHz probe is recommended for earlier detection of pregnancy and for smaller dogs or cats (Gradil et al., 2000). Shaving the abdomen is recommended, but is not necessary in all patients for general evaluations. Shaving may be necessary in more advanced studies to determine fetal viability.

Blood and Urine Tests

Diagnosing pregnancy with a simple in-house or send-out blood or urine test (or tests), while appealing in concept, is unlikely to ever yield information regarding fetal number, viability, stress, or death. These tests could have a place in confirming or refuting the presence of pregnancy but will not supplant the need for evaluation with ultrasonography and/or radiography.

Relaxin

Relaxin is a peptide that was first identified in serum from pregnant guinea pigs (Hisaw, 1926). It has become a molecule of interest in human medicine because it is a pleiotropic hormone with potential for therapeutic uses above and beyond pregnancy. A concise review of relaxin's pleiotropic actions has been published recently (Jae-Il et al., 2005). In humans, seven peptides are known to belong to the relaxin family. As an oversimplified statement it might be said that regulation of connective tissue turnover, through the activation of different proteases important in extracellular matrix degradation and tissue remodeling in a variety of organs, is the major function of relaxin.

Relaxin also appears to promote wound healing by increasing the expression of the vascular endothelial growth factor (VEGF) and inducing vasodilation in the ovaries, heart, kidney, and liver tissues (if not more) through a nitric oxide mediated mechanism (Jae-Il et al., 2005). Specific reproductive actions of relaxin molecules in various animals and humans that have been reported include implantation, regulation of uterine contraction and parturition, widening of the birth canal, softening and lengthening of the inter-public ligament, promotion of growth and softening of the uterine cervix, development of the mammary gland parenchyma in general and the nipples in particular, and lactation. Additional general actions reported for relaxin include cardiovascular homeostasis, positive effects in wound healing, and inhibition of tissue fibrosis in the lung, kidneys, and liver (Jae-Il et al., 2005).

In humans, relaxin is present in the circulation during the menstrual cycle, at elevated levels upon luteal rescue and throughout pregnancy (Jae-Il et al., 2005). In contrast, relaxin is a hormone produced primarily by the canine placenta from implantation until whelping, and is, therefore, the nearest thing to a pregnancy-specific hormone known in the dog (Steinetz et al., 2000; Steinetz et al., 1989; Steinetz et al., 1990; Steinetz et al., 1987; Kuniyuki and Hughes, 1992; Tsutsui and Stewart, 1991). Relaxin is typically not detectable in non-pregnant or pseudopregnant bitches (Steinetz et al., 2000).

Serum relaxin concentrations in pregnant dogs rise significantly compared to non-pregnant dogs, beginning at 20 to 30 days of gestation, and peak at mid-gestation (Steinetz et al., 2000). Using relaxin levels, pregnancy may be diagnosed as early as 21 days post-breeding. Negative test results at 21 days should be rechecked one week later (Root Kustritz, 2005; Steinetz et al., 2000).

These test kits are highly sensitive (i.e., few false negatives) in dogs and cats from mid-gestation on. They are also highly specific (i.e., few false positives) in dogs but cystic ovaries in cats may result in a positive test in a non-pregnant queen. The tests remain positive for an undetermined amount of time after pregnancy loss occurs. Relaxin assays are of no value in estimating litter size.

In-house assays for canine relaxin are commercially available. Evaluation by researchers at several veterinary medicine colleges of the performance characteristics of these test kits in dogs and cats is available on several Web sites (www.synbiotics.com/cgi, 2005; www.synbiotics.com/Products, 2005; www.megacor, 2005).

Other Blood Tests

Many metabolic changes occur during pregnancy, and many of these are predictable and overall significantly different than values in non-pregnant bitches. Some of the metabolic changes investigated include decreased creatinine, decreased immunoglobulin G (IgG), decreased antithrombin III, and development of a normocytic, normochromic anemia (Root Kustritz, 2005; Fisher and Fisher, 1981). However, overlap in absolute values between pregnant and non pregnant bitches precludes use of these assays as routine pregnancy tests.

A number of acute phase proteins (haptoglobin, ceruloplasmin, alpha-globulin, C-reactive protein, and fibrinogen) are released in pregnancy (Root Kustritz, 2005; Kuniyuki and Hughes, 1992). The usefulness of assaying these proteins as a marker of pregnancy is severely limited by the fact that they are also elevated in the presence of inflammatory conditions.

However, unlike the other acute phase proteins, assaying serum fibrinogen appears to be useful in diagnosing pregnancy in the bitch. Fibrinogen concentrations have been shown to rise to more than 250 mg/dL by days 21 to 30 of gestation (Gunzel-Apel et al., 1997; Concannon, 1997; Concannon et al., 1996; Eckersall et al., 1993; Vannucchi et al., 2002; Smith, 1993; Concannon et al., 1989; Hart, 1997). In one study of serum fibrinogen concentrations as a pregnancy test, nearly 100 percent accuracy was achieved with a cut-off value of greater than 300 mg/dL (Hart, 1997). In that small study, samples were analyzed with an in-house hematology analyzer (QBC AutoRead™ and the fibrin precipitator from IDEXX Laboratories, Westbrook, ME, USA). They also described enhanced accuracy of samples drawn 28 days post-breeding compared to those drawn pre-breeding. The only commercially available send-in assay for fibrinogen has been withdrawn from the market. It was reported to be 93 percent accurate (Root Kustritz, 2005; Fisher and Fisher, 1981).

Other Hormonal Assays

Many hormones, including progesterone, estrogen, prolactin, follicle stimulating hormone, and C peptide have been evaluated in dogs and cats for their use as a marker of pregnancy (Root Kustritz, 2005). Progesterone is not useful because its level is elevated similarly in females dogs post-estrus, regardless of their pregnancy status. One study reported that serum prolactin concentrations were significantly higher in pregnant dogs stimulated with naloxone than in similarly treated, non-bred bitches, five to eight days post-breeding (Smith, 1993). C-peptide is a portion of the prohormone for canine relaxin, and is detectable in urine as relaxin is formed and degraded in the second and third trimesters of pregnancy (Kuniyuki and Hughes, 1992). Concentrations of follicle stimulating hormone (FSH) decline to less than 150 ng/mL post-implantation (after 17 days of gestation) in non-pregnant dogs and remain above 150 ng/mL in pregnant dogs (www.synbiotics.com/Products, 2005). Total estrogen concentrations in urine have been reported to be increased 21 days post-mating in pregnant dogs compared to non-pregnant dogs (Concannon et al., 1989).

Unfortunately, no assays for canine prolactin, C peptide, FSH, or estrogen are commercially available at this time, although perfection of in-house assays for any or all of these could be marketable and useful (Root Kustritz, 2005).

Bibliography

Allen, W.E. and Meredith, M.J. (1981). Detection of pregnancy in the bitch: a study of abdominal palpation, A-mode ultrasound and Doppler ultrasound techniques. *J Small Anim Pract*; 22:609–22.

Barr, F.J. (1988). Pregnancy diagnosis and assessment of fetal viability in the dog: A review. *J Small Anim Pract* 29. pp 647–56.

Bondestam, S., Karkkainen, M., Alitalo, L., Forss, M. (1984). Evaluating the accuracy of canine pregnancy diagnosis and litter size using real-time ultrasound. *Acta Vet Scand*; 25:327–32.

Bystead, B.V. et al. (2000). Embryonic development stages in relation to the LH peak in the bitch. In: Farsted, W., Steel, C. (eds.) *Proceedings, the Fourth International Symposium on Canine and Feline Reproduction*, Oslo, Norway.

Concannon, P.W. (1997). A review for breeding management and artificial insemination with chilled or frozen semen. *Proceedings of the Canine Male Reproduction Symposium.* Montreal, Quebec, Canada: Society for Theriogenology; pp 1–17.

Concannon, P.W. (2000). Canine Pregnancy: Predicting Parturition and Timing Events of Gestation In: Concannon, P.W., England, G., Verstegen III, J. and Linde-Forsberg, C. (eds.) *Recent Advances in Small Animal Reproduction*, Ithaca, NY: International Veterinary Information Service, (www.ivis.org); A1202.0500.

Concannon, P.W., Gimpel, T., Newton, L., Castracane, V.D. (1996). Postimplantation increase in plasma fibrinogen concentration with increase in relaxin concentration in pregnant dogs. *Am J Vet Res*; 57:1382–5.

Concannon, P.W., McCann, J.P., Temple, M. (1989). Biology and endocrinology of ovulation, pregnancy and parturition in the dog. *J Reprod Fertil* Suppl; 39:3–25.

Concannon, P.W. and Rendano, V. (1983). Radiographic diagnosis of canine pregnancy: onset of fetal skeletal radiography in relation to times of breeding, preovulatory luteinizing hormone release, and parturition. *Am J Vet Res*; 44:1506–11.

Eckersall, P.D., Harvey, M.F.A., Ferguson, J.M., et al. (1993). Acute phase proteins in canine pregnancy (*Canis familiaris*). *J Reprod Fertil* Suppl; 47:159–64.

England, G.C.W., Allen, W.E., Porter, D.J. (1990). Studies on canine pregnancy using B-mode ultrasound. Development of the conceptus and determination of gestational age. *J Small Anim Pract*; 31:324–9.

England, G., Yeager, A., Concannon, P.W. (2003). Ultrasound imaging of the reproductive tract of the bitch. In: Concannon, P.W., England, G., Verstegen III, J. and Linde-Forsberg C. (eds.) *Recent Advances in Small Animal Reproduction*, Ithaca, NY: International Veterinary Information Service, (www.ivis.org); A1203.0703.

Feldman, E.C. and Nelson, R.W. (2004). Breeding, pregnancy and parturition. In: *Canine and Feline Endocrinology and Reproduction. Third Edition.* St. Louis, MO: Saunders pp 775–807.

Fisher, T.M. and Fisher, D.R. (1981). Serum assay for canine pregnancy testing. *Mod Vet Pract*; 62:466.

Gradil, C.M., Yeager, A.E. Concannon, P.W. (2000). Pregnancy diagnosis in the bitch, In: Bonagura, J.D. (ed) *Kirk's Current Veterinary Therapy XIII Small Animal Practice.* Philadelphia, PA: WB Saunders, pp 918–23.

Gunzel-Apel, A.-R, Hayer, M., Mischke, R., et al. (1997). Dynamics of haemostasis during the oestrus cycle and pregnancy in bitches. *J Reprod Fertil* Suppl; 51:185–93.

Hart, A.H. (1997). A rapid, accurate in-house pregnancy test for dogs. *Vet Forum*; 14:40–3.

Hisaw, F.L. (1926). Experimental relaxation of the pubic ligment of the guinea pig. *Proc Soc Exp Bio Med*; 23:661–3.

Jae-Il, P., Chia Lin, C. Sheau, Y.T.H. (2005). New insights into biological roles of relaxin and relaxin-related peptides. *Reviews in Endocrine and Metabolic Disorders*; 6:291–6.

Johnston, S.D., Root Kustritz, M.V. Olson, P.N.S. (2001). Canine Pregnancy in Canine and Feline Theriogenology. Philadelphia, PA: WB Saunders, pp 66–104.

Krzyzanowski, J., Malinowsky, E. Studnicki, W. (1975) Studies on the Duration of Pregnancy in Some Breeds of Dogs in Poland. *Medycyna Weterynaryjna*.31. pp 371–4.

Kuniyuki, A.H. and Hughes, M.J. (1992). Pregnancy diagnosis by biochemical assay. *Prob Vet Med*; 4:505–30.

Miles, K. (1995). Imaging pregnant dogs and cats. *Comp Cont Ed*; 17:1217–26.

Poffenbarger, E.M. and Feeney, D.A. (1986). Use of gray scale ultrasonography in the diagnosis of reproductive disease in the bitch. *J Am Vet Med Assoc*, vol 189. pp 90–5.

Root Kustritz, M.V. (2005). Pregancy diagnosis and abnormalities of pregnancy in the dog. *Theriogenology*; 64:755–65.

Smith, F.O. (1993). Pregnancy diagnosis in the canine. *Proceedings of the Society for Theriogenology Short Course.* Jacksonville, Florida: Society for Theriogenology; p 76.

Steinetz, B.G., Goldsmith, L.T., Brown, M.C., Lust, G. (2000). Use of Serum Relaxin For Pregnancy Diagnosis in the Bitch, In: Bonagura, J.D. (ed) *Kirk's Current Veterinary Therapy XIII Small Animal Practice.* Philadelphia, PA: WB Saunders, pp 924–5.

Steinetz, B.G., Goldsmith, L.T., Harvey, H.J., et al. (1989). Serum relaxin and progesterone concentrations in pregnant, pseudopregnant, and ovariectomized, progestin-treated pregnant bitches: Detection of relaxin as a marker of pregnancy. *Am J Vet Res*; 50:68.

Steinetz, B.G., Goldsmith, L., Hasan, S., et al. (1990). Diurnal variation of serum progesterone, but not relaxin, prolactin, or estradiol-1713 in the pregnant bitch. *Endocrinology*; 127:1057.

Steinetz, B.G., Goldsmith, L.T., Lust, G.: (1987). Plasma relaxin levels in pregnant and lactating dogs. *Bio Reprod*; 37:719.

Tibary, A. and Memon, M. (2003). Pregnancy. In: Root Kustritz, M.V. (ed) *Small Animal Theriogenology.* St. Louis, MO: Butterworth Heinemann, pp 207–40.

Toal, R.L., Walker, M.A., Henry, G.A. (1986). A comparison of real-time ultrasound, palpation and radiography in pregnancy detection and litter size determination in the bitch. *Vet Rad*; 27:102–8.

Tsutsui, T. and Stewart, D.R. (1991). Determination of the source of relaxin immunoreactivity during pregnancy in the dog. *J Vet Med Sci*; 53:1025–9.

Vannucchi, C.I, Mirandola, R.M., Oliveira, C.M. (2002). Acute-phase protein profile during gestation and diestrous: proposal for an early pregnancy test in bitches. *Anim Reprod Sci*; 74:87–99.

Verstegen, J.P., Silva, L.D.M., Onclin, K., et al. (1993). Echocardiographic study of heart rate in dog and cat fetuses in utero. *J Reprod Fertil*; 47:175.

www.megacor.at/news/news_full.php?id=52 accessed 12/02/2005.

www.megacor.at/products/product_detail.php?name=FASTest%26reg%3B%20RELAXIN accessed 12/02/2005.

www.synbiotics.com/cgi-bin/Products.pl?cgifunction=Search&Product%20Code=96-0303 accessed 12/04/2005.

www.synbiotics.com/Products/PDF_lib/96-0303b.pdf accessed 12/04/2005.

www.whelpwise.com/ accessed 12/04/2005. (Web site for Veterinary Perinatal Specialties Inc. Wheat Ridge, Colorado 80033)

Yeager, A.E., Hussni, H.O., Meyers-Wallen, V., Vannerson, L., Concannon, P.W. (1992). Ultrasonic appearance of the uterus, placenta, fetus, ad fetal membranes throughout accurately timed pregnancy in beagles. *Am J Vet Res*; vol 53, No. 3, March. pp 342–51.

Chapter 14

Ultrasonography in Small Ruminant Reproduction

Sabine Meinecke-Tillmann and Burkhard Meinecke

Introduction

Ultrasonography is an excellent tool for collecting information on morphological aspects of the female and male genital tracts in small ruminants. Previously, the internal reproductive organs of sheep and goats were only accessible following their excision or during surgery (laparotomy, laparoscopy). Transrectal as well as transcutaneous imaging gives scientists and clinicians a noninvasive and nondisruptive technique to visualize the reproductive tract in situ, and, even more important, a way to follow the dynamic processes in the course of physiological and pathological events.

Research and clinical data on ultrasonic imaging of reproductive organs and events in small ruminants are predominantly scattered in the literature. This chapter aims to systematically review the knowledge about this topic.

Examination Techniques

Examinations of the non-gravid genital tract and those performed during early pregnancy are predominantly performed transrectally. However, as gestation proceeds or during the first days post-partum, transabdominal visualization of the uterus and its contents is indicated. Scanning should be done with a suitable transducer (3.5 to 7.5 MHz) and depth setting, depending on the purpose of ultrasonic investigation. Transvaginal as well as laparoscopic ultrasound are of minor importance in small ruminants.

For imaging of the reproductive tract, animals are presented in a standing position and restrained in a cradle or other suitable device, against a fence or wall (Haibel, 1986; Russel, 1989; Riesenberg et al., 1995, 2001a,b; Kaulfuss, et al., 1996b; Martínez et al., 1998; Viñoles et al., 2004), in dorsal recumbency (Schrick and Inskeep, 1993; Schrick et al., 1993; Kaulfuss et al., 1995, 2003a,b; González de Bulnes et al., 1998, 2000; Romano et al., 1998a,b,c; Strmšq nik et al., 2002), and sometimes sitting or restrained on their side (Davey, 1986; Russel, 1989; Tainturier, 1992).

Some authors recommend that the animals be kept from feed or feed and water for at least 12 hours (Buckrell et al., 1988; Kähn, 1991; Romano et al., 1998a; Karen et al., 2004) or 24 hours before scanning (Lastovica, 1990) because feces or accumulated gas can interfere with the visualiza-

tion of the reproductive tract (Gearhart et al., 1988; Bretzlaff et al., 1993). It should be noted that this might result in a slightly elevated embryonic mortality rate in pregnant animals (Bretzlaff, 1993). Furthermore, starvation of ewes carrying multiplets can induce pregnancy ketosis (Ford et al., 1983; Henze et al., 1998).

Transabdominal scanning can be done in goats sheared in the inguinal region just lateral to the mammary gland and in a more cranioventral area later in pregnancy. If scanning is attempted without clipping, the hair is parted and coupling gel is applied copiously to obtain some images. However, no detailed analysis is possible in this case. In sheep, the fleece-less inguinal region serves as a window, and shearing is not necessary unless the number or sex of fetuses must be determined during pregnancy. The size of the clipped area in both species should be based on the stage of gestation and enlarged as needed to include the entire uterus and all fetuses. Ultrasonic imaging is preferably done from the right side of the animals; otherwise, the large rumen may interfere with a proper examination.

A thorough cleaning of the skin prior to the application of the ultrasonic coupling gel is helpful. Commercial coupling gels are most widely used, although the use of vegetable oil for transabdominal scanning (Watt et al., 1984; White et al., 1984) or lubrication with surgical soap during transrectal ultrasonography (Tainturier, 1992) has been reported. When scanning is performed transvaginally it should be noted that coupling gels can be toxic for spermatozoa (Shimonovitz et al., 1994). For transrectal investigations a lubricant gel is introduced into the rectum. A preceding removal of feces is usually not necessary. Additionally, the transducer is coated with the lubricant before insertion into the rectum. The ultrasound transducer should be covered with a plastic sleeve for hygiene reasons.

When sheep and goats are scanned transrectally it is necessary to use rigid transducers (for example, as used for prostate scanning in men) or adapters strengthening the probe with conducting cable to allow management from outside the body and permit the rotation of the transducer to both sides of the body line. Fingertip probes are more comfortable for the animals because of their smaller diameter, and are better tolerated than other transducers.

To avoid traumata of the rectum and perform a safe and thorough examination, the animals should be restrained properly and the hand holding the transducer should react elastically to movements of the animals or peristalsis of the intestine. The probe should not be forced into position but gently inserted and carefully moved forward until the urinary bladder is recognized. The bladder is imaged as a fluid-filled non-echogenic area with a distinct wall. Wall thickness depends on the filling grade. The uterine horns are usually observed cranial to the bladder and the probe is then oriented laterally to both sides to visualize the ovaries. Lifting of the abdomen might be necessary to reach the regions of interest in standing animals during transrectal examination (Tajik et al., 2001; Karen et al., 2004). It should be noted that in pluriparous animals the uterus might descend earlier during pregnancy than in young individuals, which results in difficulties in visualizing the reproductive tract during transrectal scanning.

When transcutaneous investigations are performed the transducer is brought into contact with the animal's inguinal region and is directed dorsocaudally/caudomedially to visualize bladder and uterus. Again, the latter can usually be found in the area of the cranial bladder pole. During pregnancy the uterus is more and more distended and finally lies in contact with the ventral body wall.

After examination the animals should be wiped clean of ultrasonic lubricant and/or feces.

Female Reproductive System

The female reproductive system includes ovaries, oviducts, uterus, cervix, vagina, and external genitals. The inner reproductive tract is located beneath the rectum and is separated from it by the recto-genital pouch. The rectum of ewes and goats is too small to allow a palpation of the internal female organs by an inserted human arm or hand. As a result, examinations of the ovaries and uterus in these species were restricted to noninvasive, indirect (vaginoscopy, behavior) or invasive, direct (laparoscopy or laparotomy) examination techniques. A new field of systematic studies was opened when real-time, non-invasive ultrasonography was introduced in small ruminants for visualization of internal structures and contents of the reproductive organs. This added the dimension of dynamics to our understanding of reproductive functions.

Ovary

Ultrasonography has become a routine procedure for ovary visualization in small ruminants (Dorn et al., 1989; Kähn, 1991; Bor et al., 1992; Popovski et al., 1992; Schrick et al., 1993; Ravindra et al., 1994; Kaulfuss et al., 1995; Riesenberg et al., 1995, 2001a,b; Souza et al., 1997a,b) and contributes to the increase of knowledge in reproductive physiology. Transrectal ultrasonic examinations help monitor Graafian follicle and corpus luteum (CL) morphology and development and assess numbers of follicles or CL under physiological or experimental situations, in embryo donors, or when identifying fertile genotypes. It is possible to follow follicle turnover during the season, transitional period, or anestrus; during puberty, maturity or aging; during early pregnancy, the post-partum period, and lactation; during and after estrus induction, estrus synchronization, and induction of polyovulations or superovulation; and when comparing individuals or breeds. The technique also can be used for diagnosis and follow-up during and after treatment of pathological ovarian processes, and to visualize ovaries for OPU or before embryo transfer to select suitable recipients.

This section exclusively reviews studies which used ultrasonic techniques to follow the fate of ovarian follicles and CL.

The main advantage of ultrasonic investigation is that it is non-invasive, but major limitations in small ruminants concern the small size of ovaries and their functional structures. In adult animals they are located deep in the abdomen/pelvis and out of reach for transcutaneous investigations, so there is an inability to manipulate the reproductive tract and the rectal probes used in larger species are obstructive.

Detection of normal ovarian structures in small ruminants is influenced by the experience of the operator, ultrasonic device and type of probe used, species, breed, size, age, state of nutrition, and presentation of the animals.

In contrast to earlier invasive or postmortem studies or indirect analyses on the basis of hormone profiles, ultrasonography enables continuous non-invasive investigations of visible ovarian events. Because follicles cannot be marked and ovaries left in situ cannot be fixed in a reproducible fashion, frequent scanning combined with the preparation of ovarian maps helps to identify larger individual antral follicles and follow their fate.

Most investigators use transducers with a frequency of 7.5 MHz. Presentation of animals in dorsal recumbency normally allows better visualization of the ovaries, because together with the uterus they are shifted from their normal position into closer contact with the ultrasonic transducer. Aspects of animal welfare must be considered: dorsal recumbency is not so well tolerated in small ruminants, particularly goats. This is especially true in frequently repeated investigations.

When ewes were restrained in dorsal recumbency it was possible to scan both ovaries in 90 percent of superovulated animals during estrus and in 60 percent on day 8 of the cycle (Kaulfuss et al., 1995). Kühholzer et al. (1998: animals standing and, if necessary, in dorsal recumbency) visualized 83.3 percent and Riesenberg (1997) and Riesenberg et al. (2001a) visualized 70 to 74.2 percent of all ovaries in superovulated sheep during estrus and interestrus. Both ovaries were located in 80 percent (Dorn et al., 1989: scanning method not described) or 98.6 percent (Riesenberg, 2001b) of superovulated goats and in 99.5 percent (Ginther and Kot, 1994) or 25 percent (McBride Johnson et al., 1994) of normally cycling does scanned in a standing position during interovulatory intervals, respectively.

Ultrasonography is an accurate method for estimating size and number of follicles larger than 3 mm as well as CL, although it has been postulated that fluid accumulations in the uterus during estrus obscure ovarian follicles, which results in their suboptimal detectability (Ślósarz et al., 2003). Eighty percent to 94 percent of corpora lutea were detected when animals were presented in dorsal recumbency (Schrick et al., 1993; Ślósarz et al., 2003), while during scanning of standing animals 38 percent (Dickie et al., 1999: 5 MHz) or 100 percent of the CL were visualized (Viñoles et al., 2004). Follicle detection rates of about 80 percent were reported for follicles greater than 5 mm (Ślósarz et al., 2003: dorsal recumbency), and 62 percent, 95 percent, 90 percent, and 90 percent for follicles that were 2 mm, 3 mm, 4 mm and larger than 5 mm, respectively (Viñoles et al 2004: standing position). Simões et al. (2005) investigated the accuracy of ultrasonic follicle and CL detection in goats. They noticed no significant differences between the average numbers of CL identified per ovary by ultrasonography, laparoscopy, or laparotomy and slicing, but the number of follicles (especially those less than 2 mm) was underestimated during ultrasonic scanning.

Standard equipment is suitable for identifying follicles greater than or equal to 2 mm. However, newer high resolution ultrasonography allowed identification of follicles greater than or equal to 0.4 mm, and all antral follicles greater than or equal to 1 mm could be quantified (Duggavathi et al., 2003a).

Follicles

Follicles within the ovary are well-defined anechogenic spherical structures. In contrast to other large follicles, pre-ovulatory goat follicles have irregular outlines and a heterogeneously hypoechogenic antrum (Gonzalez-Bulnes et al., 2004b). Ovarian cysts can be easily diagnosed because of their size (Christman et al., 2000; Medan et al., 2004b). The understanding of follicle dynamics in cycling animals as well as during anestrus is of principle importance in reproductive physiology.

During the cycle the development of three to six large antral follicles was documented (Schrick et al., 1993; Ginther and Kot, 1994; Ravindra et al., 1994; Ginther et al., 1995). They grew at a rate of 0.7 to 1.5 mm per day in sheep (Ravindra et al., 1994; Ravindra and Rawlings, 1997; Bartlewski et al., 1999a; Gibbons et al., 1999) and 0.8 to 1.2 mm in goats (Ginther and Kot, 1994; Gonzalez-Bulnes et al., 1999; Schwarz and Wierzchos, 2000).

Caprine ovulatory follicles attain a size of approximately 7 to 8.7 mm in diameter (Ginther and Kot, 1995; Schwarz and Wierzchos, 2000; Gonzalez-Bulnes et al., 2004b), while the size of the largest follicles in non-ovulatory waves reached 6.2 to 7.2 mm (Ginther and Kot, 1994; Schwarz and Wierzchos, 2000). Depending on the breed, ovulatory follicle diameters between greater than 4 mm to 7.7 mm were recognized in sheep (Schrick et al., 1993; Ravindra et al., 1994; Ravindra and Rawlings, 1997; Bartlewski et al.,

1999a, 2000c; Gibbons et al., 1999; Cline et al., 2001). More prolific ewes showed smaller sized ovulatory follicles than ewes with a lower ovulation rate (Souza et al., 1997b; Bartlewski et al., 1999a; Gibbons et al., 1999; Campbell et al., 2003).

Growth of visible antral follicles follows a wave pattern in cycling small ruminants, although in some ultrasonic studies (Schrick et al., 1993; Ravindra et al., 1994; Landau et al., 1996; Lopez-Sebastian et al., 1997) random emergence instead of wave pattern was reported.

Follicular waves are defined as one or more follicles growing from 2 or 3 mm to more than 5 mm in diameter (Ginther and Kot, 1994; Ginther et al., 1995; Bartlewski et al., 1999a; Gibbons et al., 1999; Duggavathi et al., 2003a; Medan et al., 2003a) before they ovulate or regress. Individual follicles emerging within a time period of more than one day (Ginther and Kot, 1994; Gibbons et al., 1999) or less than 48 hours (Bartlewski et al., 1998) were grouped to the same follicular wave. But it was shown by using high resolution ultrasonography that all follicles of a wave emerged within a 24-hour period (Dugghavathi et al., 2003a).

Ovine ovarian follicular waves emerge every three to five days (Zieba et al., 2002; Duggavathi et al., 2003a, 2004). A mean duration of these waves of about four to five days (Ginther et al., 1995; Bartlewski et al., 1998, 1999a, 2000c) was recognized in sheep of different breeds, while in goats 4.8 or 5.6 days were reported (Lassala et al., 2004).

In sheep, the following numbers of follicular waves were described: two (Ravindra et al., 1994), two or three (Leyva et al., 1998b; Evans et al., 2000), two to four (Gibbons et al., 1999; Duggavathi et al., 2003a), three (Souza et al., 1998), three or four (Bartlewski et al., 1999a), five (Zieba et al., 2002), or three to six (Ginther et al., 1995). In goats, the following numbers of waves were described: two to four (De Castro et al., 1998), three to four (Menchaca and Rubianes, 2002; Medan et al., 2003a; Lassala et al., 2004), four (Ginther and Kot, 1994), or a mean of five (Schwarz and Wierzchos 2000).

The days of wave emergence were influenced by the breed of ewes; detailed data for each wave are presented in the literature (sheep: Ginther et al., 1995; Bartlewski et al., 1999a; Zieba et al., 2002; Duggavathi et al., 2003a; goats: Ginther and Kot, 1994; De Casto et al., 1998; Medan et al., 2003a; Lassala et al., 2004). In summary, the first follicular wave starts around the time of estrus, and the last wave emerges approximately at the beginning of luteal regression. The waves in between commence about day 5 to day 6 and day 9 to day 10. Fewer waves were associated with shorter interovulatory intervals (Ginther et al., 1995).

Waves are preceded by a peak in follicle stimulating hormone (FSH) secretion (Ginther et al., 1995; Bartlewski et al., 1998, 1999a, 2000a,b; Gibbons et al., 1999; Evans et al., 2002; Zieba et al., 2004; Duggavathi et al., 2004), and are related to the plasma estradiol profile (Bartlewski et al., 1999a; De Castro et al., 1999; Duggavathi et al., 2004). After ablation of all follicles on day 4.5 of the cycle, the next FSH peak is advanced and the number of small follicles associated with the development of the second follicular wave is greater (Evans et al., 2002). Prolactin may influence the viability of gonadotrophin-responsive follicles shortly after luteolysis but does not modify the total number or the number of newly detected 4 to 5 mm follicles during the cycle, the number of follicles larger than 5 mm, or the ovulation rate (Picazo et al., 2000).

During transition to anestrus a more variable number of follicular waves was noticed in goats (Ginther and Kot, 1994).

Antral follicle dynamics are continued during seasonal anestrus. In a 17-day scanning period a mean of four follicular waves occurred in Finn sheep (Bartlewski et al., 2000c), whereas in Western white-faced ewes three waves emerged (Bartlewski et al., 1998). It was noted that Finn ewes entering anestrus later than others developed higher numbers of large follicles with a larger maximum diameter (Bartlewski et al., 2000c).

During anestrus the size range and numbers of ovarian antral follicles were similar to those seen during the breeding season. However, numbers of small antral follicles (2 to 3 mm in diameter) decreased during late anestrus, and maximum follicle diameters increased just before the short period of progesterone secretion preceding the first observed ovulation (Ravindra and Rawlings, 1997). These elevated progesterone concentrations seem to be essential for the prevention of premature luteolysis during the ensuing luteal phase (Bartlewski et al., 1999a). Ram induction during anestrus induced follicular development and ovulation in ewe lambs (Knights et al., 2002), but Ungerfeld et al. (2002) reported variable ovarian responses of anestrous ewes to the ram effect.

The development of non-ovulatory follicles during the season or follicles during anestrus is characterized by a growing phase, followed by a static and a regressing phase. Again, the duration is influenced by the breed of sheep and was reported to be about 1.6 to 3.3, 1.2 to 2.1, and 2.1 to 3.9 days, respectively (Ravindra et al., 1994; Bartlewski et al., 1998, 1999a, 2000c). Follicular growth rates of approximately 1 mm per day (Bartlewski et al., 2000c) increase significantly from early to late anestrus (1 mm vs. 1.5 mm; Bartlewski et al., 1998).

In goats, three to six follicles with diameters between 1 and 7 mm were seen ultrasonically throughout the estrus cycle (Orita et al., 2000), while an average of 4.5 new follicles per ewe were detected on each day (Lopez-Sebastian et al., 1997). The relationship between each day of the cycle and follicle emergence was investigated in other studies, too, but results differed between the reports (Ravindra et al., 1994; Ravindra and Rawlings, 1997; Bartlewski et al., 1999a; Zieba et al., 2002; Duggavathi et al., 2003a). Increasing numbers of follicles with a diameter of 2 to 3 mm were

realized at the time of follicle recruitment (Schrick et al., 1993; Viñoles et al., 1999; Evans et al., 2000), although this was not the case in other studies (Ginther et al., 1995; Bartlewski et al., 1999a). Interestingly, at the time of wave emergence, no increase in numbers of small or medium follicles was noted in a study using high resolution ultrasonography, and only the one to three follicles in the 2 to 3 mm range that grew to 5 mm or larger commenced growth during the successive follicular waves from a stable small follicle pool (Duggavathi et al., 2003a).

Ovulatory follicles emerged coincidentally with the beginning of CL regression in Shiba goats (Orita et al., 2000) or on day 10 to day 12 of the cycle in domestic sheep (Ravindra et al., 1994; Bartlewski et al., 1999a). But some differences in the origin of the ovulatory follicle are evident between breeds. While ovulatory follicles were derived from the last follicular wave in Finnish landrace as well as Western white-faced ewes, a high percentage of follicles out of the preceding follicular wave ovulated in Finn sheep, too. This phenomenon finds its origins in the extended life span of these large follicles in Finn sheep and their later emergence compared with non-ovulatory follicles of the same wave (Bartlewski et al., 1999a). In the strictly monovular Mouflon, the ovulating follicle was the largest one present at the time of luteolysis (González-Bulnes et al., 2001). Similarly, ovulatory follicles of prolific Olkuska ewes originated from the large follicles present at the time of luteal regression (Zieba et al., 2002). The latter was also true for most of the ovulatory follicles in Saanen goats (Ginther and Kot, 1994; De Castro et al., 1999).

The possible dominance of large ovarian follicles inhibiting the growth of subordinate ones has been the subject of controversial discussions in small ruminants, and ultrasonography has proven to be helpful in taking a critical look at this problem. However, at least in sheep, it must be recognized that follicle size alone is not an adequate parameter for dominance—this must be taken into account when studying the dynamics of follicle growth (Souza et al., 1996).

When a follicle attains dominance the divergence of growth within the follicular wave occurs: dominant follicles become disproportionately larger in comparison with the subordinate ones (Ginther and Kot, 1994). The total number of small follicles decreases in correlation with the growth of the largest follicle in wave 1 (Menchaca et al., 2002). Ablation of the largest follicle results in an increased life span of the second largest, indicating a regulatory role of dominant follicles over smaller subordinate follicles (Evans et al., 2002). González-Bulnes et al. (2004c) recognized that in the presence of dominant follicles the inhibition of the others was most obvious in the ovary ipsilateral to the dominant follicle. They postulated that in addition to systemic factors, local inhibitors were also acting. Besides that of the ovulatory follicle, the expression of dominance was also reported for the largest follicle of wave 1 (Viñoles et al., 1999), and Ginther and Kot (1994) stated that follicular dominance in goats was more common during waves 1 and 4, compared with waves 2 and 3.

Follicular dominance in sheep was questioned in other ultrasonic studies (Duggavathi et al., 2003a, 2004), especially because after exogenous FSH treatment during the growth phase of a follicular wave, the emergence of an additional follicular wave during the regular interwave interval was induced, but the emergence of the second regular wave was not delayed by this intervention. Schwarz and Wierzchos (2000) mentioned that the occurrence of dominance is doubtful in goats, as well. A lack of dominance was also noticed during the luteal phase of the cycle in a monovular breed of ewes (Lopez-Sebastian et al., 1997).

Local effects of luteal structures on follicle turnover were recognized in unilaterally ovulating ewes during the cycle (Bartlewski et al., 2001b). Inhibiting local effects in the CL-bearing ovary were evident during early pregnancy (Beard et al., 1995; Bartlewski et al., 2000b) and during the postpartum period too, although the action was ascribed at least in part or primarily to the developing conceptus (Beard et al., 1995; Bartlewski et al., 2000b). Following parturition follicles larger than 3 mm were not seen before day 21 to day 25 postpartum (Bartlewski et al., 2000b).

The stage of breeding season, age, weight, and body condition are determining factors for the transrectally detected ovulation rate (Kaulfuss et al., 2003b). Ovulation is recognized ultrasonically by the disappearance of the previously identified preovulatory follicles (Schrick et al., 1993; Ginther and Kot, 1994; Ravindra et al., 1994; Riesenberg et al., 2001a,b; Duggavathi et al., 2003b; Gonzalez-Bulnes et al., 2004b).

Corpus Luteum

In the corpus hemorrhagicum the echotexture is hypoechogenic with echogenic freckling, but its identification is difficult. High resolution ultrasonography is helpful in identifying these structures (Duggavathi et al., 2003b). In goats, corpora hemorrhagica with a diameter of approximately 8.6 mm was measured (Gonzalez-Bulnes et al., 2004b).

Luteal tissue is homogenously echogenic, hypoechoic compared with the ovarian stroma, and well separated from the latter. Corpora lutea attain their maximal diameter of about 8 to 12 mm approximately between day 5 and day 11 after ovulation (Ravindra et al., 1994; Orita et al., 2000; Kaulfuss et al., 2003a; Medan et al., 2003a), while their regression starts in non-pregnant sheep about four days before a new estrus (Kaulfuss et al., 2003a). The maximum diameter (8.1 mm) of goat CL remains constant until day 14 and diminishes rapidly to about 5.2 mm on the day of the next ovulation (Orita et al., 2000).

Using standard equipment, first ultrasonic diagnosis of developing CL depends on their size and is related to the number of ovulating follicles. In sheep with higher ovulation rates the CL were detectable one to two days later than in animals with only one or two ovulations (Kaulfuss et al., 2003a). Luteal tissue was identified when its diameter reached more than 6 mm (Kaulfuss et al., 2003a), when progesterone concentrations increased above the basal level (Bartlewski et al., 1999b), at about day 3 (Orita et al., 2000; González de Bulnes et al., 2000; Kaulfuss et al., 2003a; Medan et al., 2003a), between day 4 and day 5 (Schrick et al., 1993; Kaulfuss et al., 1995; Ravindra and Rawlings, 1997; Bartlewski et al., 1999b; Dickie et al., 1999); or between day 5 and day 7 after ovulation (Johnson et al., 1996); or on day 2 to day 3 or day 1 to day 3 after superovulation (Riesenberg et al., 1995, 2001a,c; Kühholzer et al., 1998). The accuracy of detection might decrease when CL numbers are increasing (Dickie et al., 1999) because physiological or induced higher ovulation rates result in an accumulation of smaller CL (Riesenberg et al., 1995, 2001a; Kaulfuss et al., 2003a).

Corpora lutea occur in two forms: compact and those that initially contain a central anechoic cavity which disappears later during the cycle. The latter are reported to occur in a range of 12 percent to 68 percent (Schrick et al., 1993; Dickie et al., 1999; González de Bulnes et al., 2000; Kaulfuss et al., 2003a). Corpora lutea that contain a large cavity are difficult to distinguish from large luteinized follicles. These follicles are known to occur frequently after equine chorionic gonadotrophin (eCG) treatment, and are also seen during unstimulated estrus cycles. González-Bulnes et al. (1999) suggested distinguishing luteinized follicles and corpora lutea on the basis of the ratio between cavity diameter and total luteal tissue diameter.

Regressing corpora lutea are hyperechogenic (González de Bulnes et al., 2000). Corpora albicantia may be realized as hypoechogenic structures with indistinct boundaries until the beginning of the new cycle (Kaulfuss et al., 2003a).

Ovulatory-sized antral follicles can give rise to either normal or inadequate CL (Bartlewski et al., 2001a). Short-lived CL or luteinized follicles can occur together with normal CL without disruption of the cycle (Bartlewski et al., 1999b), and are also observed ultrasonically after superovulation (Riesenberg 2001a,b).

Although corpora lutea in sheep are not necessary for maintaining gestation from day 50 of pregnancy—in contrast to goats—the structures are preserved in this species because of the missing uterine prostaglandin production. The ovaries can only be visualized ultrasonically during early pregnancy.

There is a close association between hormone profiles and CL development (Ginther et al., 1995; Souza et al., 1997a,b; Bartlewski et al., 1998, 1999a, 2000a; Medan et al., 2003a). Plasma progesterone concentrations correspond well to the CL area in monovular ewes (Gonzalez de Bulnes et al., 2000), to the total volume of luteal tissue in sheep with single or multiple ovulations (Kaulfuss et al., 2003a), or to the mean of total large diameters of corpora lutea in goats (Orita et al., 2000), with the exception of the

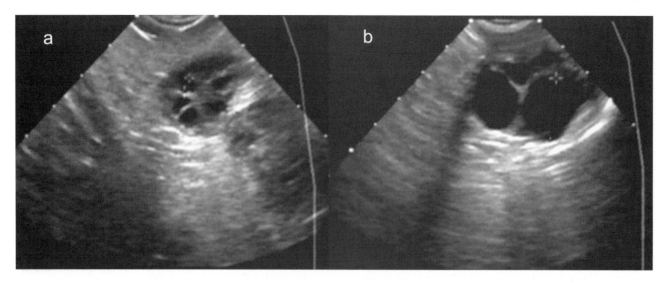

Figure 14.1. Transrectal ultrasonography, 7.5-MHz. **(a):** goat ovary with multiple medium-sized follicles, early estrus; **(b):** sheep ovary with large unovulated follicles, day 4 after estrus.

late luteal phase when progesterone levels decreased more rapidly than the diameter of the ovarian structures (Orita et al., 2000).

Reproductive Biotechnologies

Ultrasonic investigations of the ovary have proven to be useful during embryo transfer and associated biotechnologies (see Figures 14.1 and 14.2).

The time of ovulation and the origin of ovulatory follicles following estrus synchronization are recorded to optimize fertility (Cardwell et al., 1998; Viñoles and Rubianes, 1998; Evans et al., 2001; Viñoles et al., 2001). Lassala et al. (2004) noted that follicle turnover and subsequent fertility

were not affected by the presence or absence of a CL during estrus synchronization in goats. However, changes in follicle turnover were seen in other investigations. Treatment with medroxy progesterone acetate (MAP) in the absence of luteal progesterone increased ovulation rates by approximately 50 percent in Western white-faced sheep (Bartlewski et al., 2003), and following application of a standard dose of eCG (500 IU) at the end of MAP treatment during seasonal anestrus, animals ovulated follicles from several follicular waves in contrast to ovulations from the final wave in untreated control animals (Barrett et al., 2004). Synchronization of sheep with a single progestagen-impregnated intravaginal sponge in the absence of a CL resulted in the

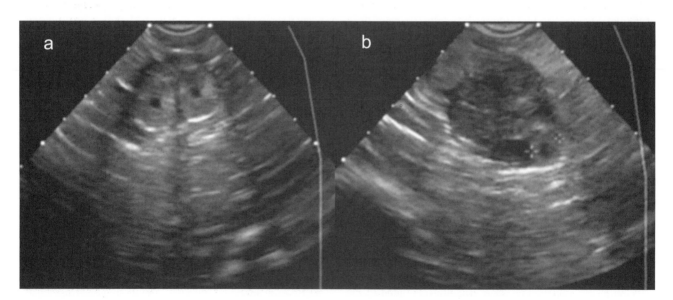

Figure 14.2. Transrectal ultrasonography, 7.5-MHz, of goat. **(a):** ovary with two corpora lutea with cavities, mid-cycle; **(b):** ovary with multiple corpora lutea following superovulation, day 6 after estrus.

ovulation of a persistent follicle showing prolonged growth before ovulation (Flynn et al., 2000), but oocytes from follicles of this age had a normal developmental competence (Evans et al., 2001). Progesterone exposure early in the ovulatory cycle caused short or shortened cycles in goats. When progesterone treatment was begun on day 0 the ovulatory follicle arose from wave 1, but it arose from wave 2 when progesterone treatment started on day 3 (Menchaca and Rubianes, 2001).

Ultrasonic scanning of the ovaries is part of embryo transfer programs. It is helpful in verifying the success of superovulatory treatments and selecting well-responding animals on the basis of CL (Dorn et al., 1989; Kähn 1991; Kaulfuss et al., 1995; Kühholzer et al., 1998), or omitting flushing of overstimulated ewes or does. However, it must be recognized that CL numbers are often underestimated in well-responding superovulated animals (Gonzalez de Bulnes et al., 1999; Riesenberg et al., 2001a).

Ovarian reaction to superovulation depends on variations in the number of responsive follicles present on the ovarian surface at the start of gonadotrophin application and the number of ovulations is associated with the number of larger follicles at the time of estrus (Kühholzer et al., 1998; Riesenberg et al., 2001a; Gonzales-Bulnes et al., 2002c). Therefore, it is possible to some extent to preselect potential embryo donors. Additionally, a relationship between follicles (2 to 4 mm, ewes; larger than 4 mm, goats) at the beginning of FSH treatment and the number of viable embryos was demonstrated (González-Bulnes et al., 2003a, 2004d).

Administration of ovine FSH (oFSH), porcine FSH (pFSH), human menopausal gonadotrophin (hMG), or eCG induced a significant rise in the number of follicles greater than or equal to 4 mm, an increase in the number of newly detected follicles, and a decrease in follicular regression rate (Riesenberg et al., 2001a; Gonzalez-Bulnes et al., 2002b). Crowded follicles often have a polygonal appearance following superovulation (Riesenberg, 1997).

The presence of a dominant follicle at the time of superovulation had negative effects on follicle recruitment and the ovulatory response in goats (Menchaca et al., 2002) or ewes (Rubianes et al., 1997; Gonzalez-Bulnes et al., 2002a), and was associated with a lower number of transferable embryos in sheep (Rubianes et al., 1997; Gonzales-Bulnes et al., 2002c, 2003b). Therefore, it is recommended that superovulatory treatment is started soon after ovulation (Menchaca et al., 2002) or during the early luteal phase in the presence of a CL but the absence of a large follicle (González-Bulnes et al., 2002a), although it was realized that a CL had an inhibiting effect on the activity of large follicles in progestagen-treated ewes (Rubianes et al., 1996).

Kähn (1991) stated that following superovulation with eCG or FSH, follicles with a diameter of 5 to 6 mm were seen on the first day after prostaglandin injection, and with a diameter of 6 to 8 mm on the day of ovulation. But in small ruminants synchronized with FGA-impregnated intravaginal sponges and superovulated with pFSH, eCG or hMG corpora lutea correlated mainly with medium-sized follicles (3.1 to 4.5 mm), indicating that the majority of ovulating follicles in superovulated German Merino ewes and in goats is smaller than 4.5 mm (Riesenberg et al., 2001a,b).

Ultrasonography does not allow the differentiation between CL, which will develop normally or will undergo premature regression (Riesenberg et al., 2001a,b).

The success of new superovulation methods was controlled ultrasonically in small ruminants. It has been shown in several species that the application of GnRH antagonists induces reduced FSH and LH plasma levels and affects follicle turnover. This is true in sheep and goats too. Treatment with these antagonists resulted in a significant decrease in the number follicles beyond 3 mm in sheep and goats (Campbell et al., 1998; Gonzalez-Bulnes et al., 2004e), but a significant increase in small follicles in goats (Gonzalez-Bulnes et al., 2004e). It favored a greater superovulatory response in sheep because ovulatory follicles were recruited from a wider range of follicular size classes (Dufour et al., 2000). In GnRH-suppressed ewes FSH alone was sufficient to induce the development of ovulatory-sized follicles, but LH was found to be necessary for normal steroidogenesis (Campbell et al., 1998). After immunization against inhibin or estradiol, follicular turnover was also altered (Mann et al., 1993; Medan et al., 2003b), and passive immunization against inhibin resulted in a significantly higher ovulation rate (Medan et al., 2003b).

As in cattle, ultrasonography was used during ovum pick-up in goats. The technique was difficult to learn and only feasible in small does, although the percentage of oocytes recovered was comparable to that obtained by laparoscopy (Graff et al., 1999). In larger goats and sheep the attachment of ovaries to the vaginal wall together with transvaginal ultrasonography might be used for ovum pick-up, similar to the technique reported for the evaluation of follicle turnover in red deer (Asher et al., 1997).

Uterus

Ultrasonic monitoring of uterine contents is particularly important to observe physiological (pregnancy) and/or pathological (embryonic/fetal death, accumulation of fluids) conditions. Early pregnancy diagnosis allows accurately timed management of the pregnant animals in a flock as well as a proper supervision of parturition. The detection of fluid accumulation in the uterus or in the oviduct, on the other hand, permits early therapeutic intervention or helps to exclude individual animals from the breeding program.

Uterus and Oviducts

The non-pregnant uterus with its coiled horns is imaged as a homogenously echogenic structure in cross- or

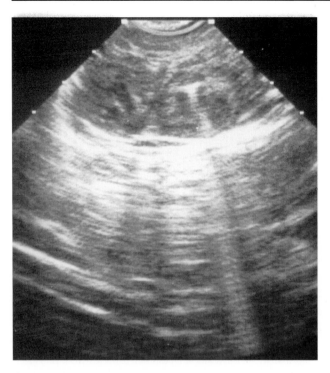

Figure 14.3. Transcervical embryo collection from a sheep using transrectal ultrasonography, 7.5-MHz. Transverse sections of both uterine horns are visualized during flushing. The catheter is imaged within the lumen of the right uterine horn.

longitudinal sections. It can easily be distinguished from other tissues, especially during estrus, because of its altered echogenic properties.

Ultrasonic imaging of the uterus is helpful during transcervical embryo collection (Göbel et al., 1995). Particularly in large ewes, the proper digital control of the flushing catheter position is not possible. Transverse imaging of the organ with a sector scanner allows the visualization of the catheter with mandrin within the left or right uterine horn, since strongly reflecting substances such as metal create a comet-tail effect due to reverberations (see Figure 14.3). A change of the catheter position from one horn to the other is performed during imaging of the corpus uteri. The latter is identified ultrasonically as the site where the twin-tube-like cross-sections of both uterine horns unify to a single structure. The procedure ensures the flushing of both uterine horns. It may be used during non-surgical intrauterine embryo transfer to deposit the embryo into the side ipsilateral to the corpus luteum (Meinecke-Tillmann, 1995, unpublished results). Small fluid-filled anechoic vesicles with a diameter of about 2 mm are sometimes seen on the outer surface of the uterus as an after-effect of surgical embryo collection.

Normal oviducts are not visible ultrasonically, but may occasionally be imaged after embryo collection procedures or during pathological processes, e.g. the rare condition of a hydrosalpinx. Sometimes cysts originating from remnants of the mesonephric or paramesonephric ducts are present

and intimately associated with the ovary. If large enough, they may be mistaken for follicles. A differentiation might be possible by repeated observations, because the structures retain their size.

Pyometra is a rare event in small ruminants with characteristic snowstorm-like imaging of the uterine contents.

Pregnancy

Following syngamy (fusion of the male and female pronucleus), the zygote becomes an embryo. Because the embryo has not acquired the typical anatomical form of a specific species, the term embryo entitles an organism during the early stages of development. A fetus is defined as a potential offspring that is still within the uterus, but is generally recognizable as a member of the given species. In ewes and goats, embryos enter the uterus three to four days following ovulation. The embryos must signal their presence in the uterus to the dam by day 13 to 14 post-ovulation to ensure maternal recognition of pregnancy. If an adequate signal is not delivered in a timely manner, the dam will experience luteolysis. In this case the early pregnancy will be terminated and the dam will return to estrus. On the other hand, if maternal recognition of pregnancy occurs and the embryo is lost afterward, then the dam may not return to estrus during the season (pseudopregnacy). Therefore, it is important to determine the presence of the early embryo within the uterus to discriminate between pregnant and pseudo-pregnant animals.

Pregnancy Diagnosis

Early pregnancy detection, identification of pregnant or non-pregnant animals, knowledge about the stage of gestation or fetal and placental development, estimation of fetal health, prediction of sex of the lambs or kids, and evaluation of embryonic and fetal mortality and puerperal changes is of clinical, economic, and scientific value in small ruminants. Barren animals can be bred again or marketed; animals carrying fetuses of undesired sex can be sold; slaughter of pregnant animals can be avoided; unwanted pregnancies can be terminated early; and pregnant and non-pregnant animals can be housed, fed, and handled separately.

The prediction of fetal numbers/diagnosis of multiple pregnancies allows optimal feeding and precautions to prevent pregnancy-associated diseases or progeny loss. Placing animals carrying singletons, twins, or more than two fetuses in separate pens is another management tool, as is dividing a flock according to early or late lambing/kidding and barren animals. Additionally, the flock fertility can be increased by selecting replacement animals from those pregnant with the desired number of fetuses, and sire fertility can be evaluated.

Pregnancy diagnosis in small ruminants with high-frequency ultrasound was first reported in the 1960s (Lindahl, 1966, 1969a,b). Since that time three different ultrasonic systems have been used for routine diagnosis:

- A-mode (Wroth, 1979; BonDurant, 1980; Meredith and Madani, 1980; Madel, 1983; Langford et al., 1984; Watt et al., 1984; Jardon, 1988): a simple method without the possibility of predicting fetal age, numbers, viability, or sex, or evaluating the placenta
- Doppler ultrasound (Fraser and Robertson, 1967; Hulet, 1969; Bosc, 1971; Lindahl, 1971; Fortmeyer et al., 1972; Richardson, 1972; Weiss, 1975; Aswad et al., 1976; Royal and Tainturier, 1976; Schweizer, 1976; Deas, 1977; Rüsch et al., 1981; Trapp and Slyter, 1983; Fukui et al., 1986; Russel and Goddard, 1995): a method inappropriate for predicting fetal sex and with controversial results concerning the prediction of fetal age
- Real-time B-mode (Stouffer et al., 1969; Lindahl, 1976; Fowler and Wilkins, 1984; White et al., 1984; Taverne et al., 1985; Buckrell et al., 1986; Scheibe et al., 1986; Buckrell, 1988; Gearhart et al., 1988; Kaspar, 1989; Schrick and Inskeep, 1993; Wani et al., 1998; Medan et al., 2004a): the method that is suitable in every respect

Accuracy of early pregnancy detection in small ruminants is influenced by the experience of the operator as well as the ultrasonic device and type of probe used, the species, breed, size, age, state of nutrition and presentation of the animals, and the number of days post-breeding or insemination.

Ultrasonic images typical for pregnancy are multiple anechoic luminal sections of the uterus, the presence of anechoic fluid and C- or O-shaped placentomes, and, most important, the embryo or the fetus (see Figure 14.4). Signs of a beginning gestation can be recognized as small and later extending anechoic areas within the uterus quite early after fertilization. As development continues endometrial folds protrude into the fluid-filled lumen and the complete uterus appears to be divided into a number of chambers.

Using transrectal real-time ultrasound, embryonic vesicles were first identified in the uterine lumen of sheep on day 12 (González de Bulnes et al., 1998); day 13 to day 21 (Kaulfuss, 1996a); day 14 to day 19 (Buckrell 1988); day 16 to day 20 (Romano et al., 1998b); or day 17 to day 19 (Tainturier, 1992; Garcia et al., 1993; Doize et al., 1997) after mating; while the first recognition of the embryo proper on the floor of the embryonic vesicle was reported on day 16 (Strmšnik et al., 2002); day 17 (Romano et al., 1998b); day 17 to day 20.5 (Kaulfuss et al., 1996a); day 19

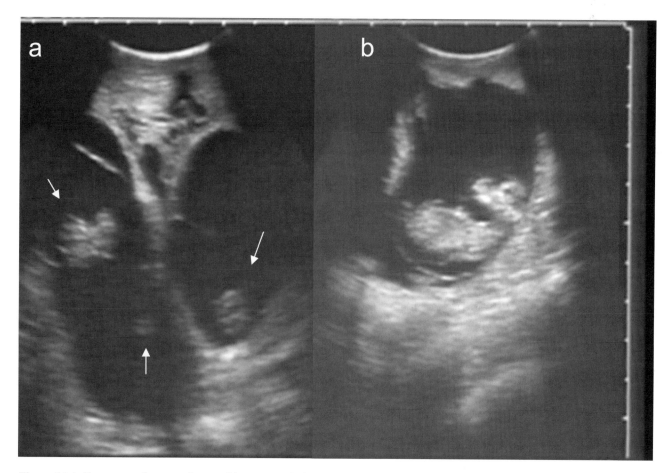

Figure 14.4. Pregnancy of a goat, shown with transrectal ultrasonography, 5-MHz. (**a**): **arrows** point to triplet fetuses on day 40. (**b**): the head and trunk of the fetus on day 44.

(González de Bulnes et al., 1998); day 20 (Tainturier, 1992; Schrick and Inskeep, 1993); or day 25 (Buckrell et al., 1986).

Following transabdominal scanning, pregnancies were first diagnosed on day 17 (Kaulfuss et al., 1996b), day 25 (Gearhart et al., 1988), or day 30 (Bretzlaff et al., 1993).

Anechoic areas in the uterus indicating a gestation in goats were reported from about day 13 (Parraguez et al., 1999), day 20 (Medan et al., 2004a) or day 22 (Hesselink and Taverne, 1994); and amniotic vesicles from day 20 (Botero-Herrera et al., 1984). Embryos or fetuses in transrectally scanned goats were identified frequently on day 24 or day 25, in most cases until day 30, and always after day 30 (Baronet and Vaillancourt, 1989; Kaspar, 1989; Kähn et al., 1990; Bretzlaff et al., 1993; Hesselink and Taverne, 1994; Medan et al., 2004a).

Although the embryo can be detected very early, it is most practical to scan the females that are expected to have embryos greater than 30 days of age. Only the definite detection of an embryo proper can be used as a reliable criterion of gestation. The latter is especially true in goats because of the possibility of a developing hydrometra (White and Russell, 1993; Hesselink and Taverne, 1994).

The diagnostic accuracy, sensitivity, specificity, and predictive values of real-time ultrasonography were investigated to evaluate this method's reliability in pregnancy detection (see Table 14.1). Ultrasonic diagnostic accuracy refers to the percentage of correct diagnoses in relation to the total number of ultrasound examinations. Sensitivity describes the percentage of animals realized to be pregnant compared to the total number of pregnant animals. Specificity is the percentage of animals found by ultrasound to be not pregnant and confirmed as non-pregnant. The positive predictive value is the percentage of animals correctly classified as pregnant in relation to the total number of positive pregnancy diagnoses, whereas the negative predictive

Table 14.1. Pregnancy diagnosis in small ruminants. Diagnostic accuracy, sensitivity, specificity, and positive and negative predictive values of transrectal or transabdominal ultrasonography (given percentages summarize data of the different authors).

Scan	Days of pregnancy	% Accuracy	% Sensitivity	% Specificity	% Positive predictive value	% Negative predictive value	Authors
tr	≤25 (26)	52–100	11–100	40–100	67–100	50–93	Gearhart et al., 1988; Garcia et al., 1993; Kaulfuss et al., 1996b; Romano et al., 1998b; Karen et al., 2003, 2004; González et al., 2004
tr	≤50 (60)	62–100	32–100	78–100	43–100	64–100	Buckrell et al., 1986; Gearhart et al., 1988; Garcia et al., 1993; Kähn et al., 1993; Schrick and Inskeep, 1993; Kaulfuss et al., 1996b; Karen et al., 2003, 2004
tr	61–90	100	100	100	100	100	Kähn et al., 1993
tr	91–120	94	94	88	98	70	Kähn et al., 1993
tr	121–147	75	75	—	100		Kähn et al., 1993
ta	<24	32–67	0–65	80–100	96–100	25	Kaulfuss et al., 1996b
ta	25–29 (22)	78	77	88	98	32	Kaulfuss et al., 1996b
ta	30–60	30–95	60–> 97	36–90	88–100	0–80	Kähn et al., 1993; Kaulfuss et al., 1994, 1996b
ta	60–>89 (>120)	94–100	95–100	89–100	93–100	67–100	Kähn et al., 1993; Kaulfuss et al., 1994, 1996b
ta	different time periods between 29–106	95–100	99–100	87–100	99–100	8–100	Fowler and Wilkins, 1984; White et al., 1984; Taverne et al., 1985; Davey, 1986; Logue et al., 1987; Gearhart, 1988; Lavoir and Taverne, 1989

tr: transrectal ultrasonography.
ta: transabdominal ultrasonography.
(): 1 reference only.

value describes the percentage of correctly classified negative animals in relation to the total number of sheep or goats diagnosed to be non-pregnant (Buckrell et al., 1986; Kähn et al., 1993). It is obvious that success rates varied in the first weeks of pregnancy, but later became consistent.

Better diagnostic results are obtained with the transrectal method during early gestation. Later, equivalent success rates are reached with transrectal or transcutaneous imaging, but after day 70 of pregnancy transabdominal scanning proved to be superior (Kähn 1991).

In routine settings it is possible to perform an ultrasonic pregnancy diagnosis in the following number of ewes per hour: 50 to 100 (Levy et al., 1990), about 100 (De Bois and Taverne, 1984), 150 (Davey, 1986), 150 to 200 (Kaulfuss et al., 1994), 200 to 250 (Kaulfuss et al., 1996b), and 250 to 375 (Lastovica, 1990). A rate of 1,450 animals per day has been reported (Davey 1986).

Determination of Fetal Numbers
Transrectal ultrasonography can determine embryo or fetal numbers as early as day 19 (González de Bulnes et al., 1998) or day 23 to 26 (Tainturier, 1992; Schrick and Inkeep, 1993; Kaulfuss et al., 1996a). Using this technique, optimal results are obtained until day 40 of pregnancy, but in the field transabdominal scanning is preferred. From day 40 until about day 100 transabdominal counting is practical because the fetuses are well separated from each other. Later in pregnancy they are in close contact and too large to distinguish multiple conceptuses without any problems. Localization of the different fetal heads is helpful for identification of individuals. In small ruminants carrying multiplets there is a tendency to underestimate fetal numbers (Rawlings et al., 1983; Logue et al., 1987; White and Russel, 1987; Gearhart et al., 1988; Bürstel, 2002; Bürstel et al., 2002).

Diagnostic accuracy, sensitivity, specificity, and positive and negative predictive values were reported for the determination of fetal numbers in small ruminants. Transrectal diagnosis between days 26 and 50 and days 51 and 71 resulted in a sensitivity of 5 percent and 97 percent and a specificity of 80 percent and 100 percent in sheep (Gearhart et al., 1988). Taverne et al. (1985) determined fetal numbers transabdominally with an accuracy of 93 percent, a sensitivity of 93 percent, a specificity of 91 percent, a positive predictive value of 97 percent, and a negative predictive value of 84 percent after scanning ewes on day 45 to day 47. Between day 50 and day 100 of gestation singleton and twin pregnancies were predicted in about 97 percent to 100 percent of the cases; however, it was more difficult to detect triplets (82 percent predicted reliably) (Fowler and Wilkins, 1984; White et al., 1984; Jardon, 1988). Sensitivities and specificities between 94 percent and 99 percent and 94 percent and 100 percent, respectively, and high positive (between 95 percent and 99 percent) and negative predictive values (between 84 percent and 99 percent) were reached after transabdominal scanning (Fowler and

Wilkins, 1984; White et al., 1984; Davey et al., 1986; Logue et al., 1987).

The best period for counting fetal numbers in goats is between days 40 and 70 (Lavoir and Taverne, 1989). An accuracy of 92 percent on day 60 compared to 67 percent on day 40 or 84 percent on day 50 was reported (Medan et al., 2004a). Five weeks after breeding singletons, twins and triplets were predicted in goats with an accuracy of 44 percent, 73 percent, and 67 percent, respectively, compared with 83 percent, 89 percent, and 100 percent at 7 weeks of gestation (Dawson et al., 1994).

Transabdominal scanning takes about one to two minutes per animal. Scanning 100 to 150 animals per hour was possible when testing for the presence of multiple fetuses (Lastovica, 1990). Davey (1986) estimated 10 seconds are needed to diagnose a single pregnancy at commercial speed between day 50 to 100, and 20 to 30 seconds are needed to detect non-pregnant ewes or to confirm diagnosis when twins are suspected. It has been stated that a greater volume of intrauterine fluid is present in animals carrying twins compared with those pregnant with singletons, and that this difference might be the only parameter for diagnosing twins at commercial speed (Davey, 1986).

Estimation of Gestational Age
When the date of breeding is unknown, gestational age can be estimated by monitoring embryonic or fetal parameters (see Table 14.2 and Figure 14.5). These parameters include

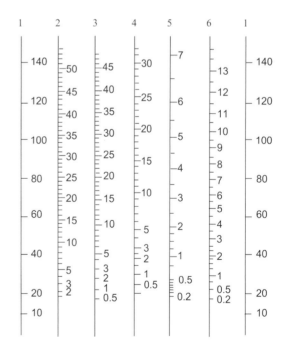

Figure 14.5. Parameters to determine the fetal age of sheep (Merino) from one or more dimensions. Column 1 = age in days, column 2 = curved crown rump length (cm), column 3 = straight crown rump length (cm), column 4 = length of trunk (cm), column 5 = width of head (cm), column 5 = length of head (cm). Modified from Cloete, 1939.

Table 14.2. Estimation of gestational age in small ruminants—correlation between some embryonic/fetal parameters and gestational age.

Parameter	Days of gestation[1]	Correlation (r) between parameter and gestational age	Authors
Embryonic vesicle	8–65 (s) until 45 (g)	0.76–0.91 0.89	Kähn et al., 1992; González-Bulnes et al., 1998; Parraguez et al., 1999
Total embryo/ fetal length	20–45 (g)	0.82	Parraguez et al., 1999
Crown rump length (CRL)	16–50 (s), 19–50 (g) 26–65 (s), 35–56 (g)	0.90–0.99 0.87–0.89	González-Bulnes et al., 1998; Martínez et al., 1998; Romano et al., 1998c; Kaulfuss et al., 1999b; Souza, 2000; Kähn et al., 1992
Trunk diameter	26–111	0.98	Kähn et al., 1992
Abdominal diameter and/or circumference	mating or day 90—lambing (s) 41–130 (g)	0.95–0.96 0.89–0.93	Chavez-Moreno et al., 1996; Noia et al., 2002; Souza, 2000
Thoracic diameter, thorax height	23–119 (s) repeatedly (g)	0.95–0.96 0.72	Sergeev et al., 1990; González-Bulnes et al., 1998; Parraguez et al., 1999
Biparietal diameter of the head (BPD)	32–123 (s) 41–133 (g) 44–lambing (s) 54–123 (s), 27–45 (g)	0.90–0.98 0.88–0.95 0.87 0.66–0.76	Haibel, 1988; Haibel and Perkins, 1989;Kelly and Newnham, 1989; Sergeev et al., 1990; González-Bulnes et al., 1998; Greenwood et al., 2002; Souza, 2000; Aiumlamai et al., 1992; Kähn et al., 1992; Parraguez et al., 1999
Fetal head length	38–91 (s) mating–lambing (s)	0.95 0.89	González-Bulnes et al., 1998; Noia et al., 2002
Orbita	36–128 (s)	0.89–0.92	Kähn et al., 1992; González-Bulnes et al., 1998
Cervical vertebrae	50–91 (s)	0.71	González-Bulnes et al., 1998
Thoracic vertebrae	50–90 (s)	0.79	González-Bulnes et al., 1998
Lumbar vertebrae	50–90 (s)	0.90	González-Bulnes et al., 1998
Coccygeal vertebrae	57–90 (s)	0.96	González-Bulnes et al., 1998
Ribs	52–116 (s)	0.77–0.82	Kähn et al., 1992; González-Bulnes et al., 1998
Humerus length	mating–lambing (s)	0.94	Noia et al., 2002
Femur length	61–90 (s), 49–126 (g) mating–lambing (s)	0.78–0.83 0.95	González-Bulnes et al., 1998; Souza, 2000; Noia et al., 2002
Metacarpus length	60–120 (s)	0.95	Greenwood et al., 2002

[1]Days of gestation: the range of days given covers all different time periods investigated by different authors.
s: sheep, g: goats.
Vertebrae = vertebrae width: measurement of 3 vertebrae with their intervertebral spaces.
Ribs: width of one rib with intercostal space (Kähn et al., 1992) or of three ribs with intercostal spaces (González-Bulnes et al., 1998).

size of embryonic vesicles (González de Bulnes et al., 1998); crown-rump length (Schrick and Inskeep, 1993; Chavez Moreno et al., 1996; González de Bulnes et al., 1998); head diameters as the biparietal diameter, fetal head length, orbita diameter or inter-eye distance (Haibel, 1988; Russel, 1989; Haibel and Perkins, 1989; Haibel et al., 1989, 1990; Kelly and Newnham, 1989; Reichle and Haibel, 1991; Sergeev et al., 1990; Aiumlamai et al., 1992; Barbera et al., 1995; Chavez Moreno et al., 1996; González de Bulnes et al., 1998; Greenwood et al., 2002; Noia et al., 2002); thoracic diameter (Kleemann et al., 1987; Sergeev et al.,

1990; Chavez Moreno et al., 1996; González de Bulnes et al., 1998); trunk diameter (Russel, 1989; Aiumlamai et al., 1992); abdominal diameter and circumference (Barbera et al., 1995; Chavez Moreno et al., 1996; Noia et al., 2002); vertebrae width and umbilical cord diameter (González de Bulnes et al., 1998); and femur, tibia, humerus or metacarpus length (Barbera et al., 1995; González de Bulnes et al., 1998; Greenwood et al., 2002; Noia et al., 2002); as well as the fetal heart rate (Aiumlamai et al., 1992; Garcia et al., 1993; Schrick and Inskeep, 1993; Chavez Moreno et al., 1996). Additionally, placentome size was correlated to the gestational age (Buckrell et al., 1986; Kelly et al., 1987; Doize et al., 1997; González de Bulnes et al., 1998; Kaulfuss et al., 1998). Mathematical descriptions of the different growth curves can be found in the individual publications.

Two parameters are relatively easy to measure and are therefore frequently used: crown-rump length (CRL), which increases about 1.6 to 2 mm per day, and the biparietal diameter of the head (BPD), which increases about 0.6 mm per day.

The CRL reaches 2.4 mm on day 16, 5.7 to 6 mm on day 20, about 10 to 11 mm on day 25, 16 to 20 mm on day 30, 21 to 25 mm on day 35, 29 to 40 mm on day 40, 49 mm on day 45, and 57 to 70 mm on day 50 of pregnancy (Schrick and Inskeep, 1993; Kaulfuss et al., 1996a, 1999; González de Bulnes et al., 1998; Martínez et al., 1998; Romano et al., 1998c). Interpretation of data from the literature can be difficult because often neither the definition of CRL, nor the number of observations for each pregnancy interval, nor the breed of animals investigated is reported (Romano et al., 1998c). Instead of CRL, the maximal embryo length might have been used, resulting in an overestimation of size.

The BPD reaches 6 mm at week 4.5, 10 to 12 mm at week 5, 16 to 18 mm at week 7, 28 to 30 mm at week 10, 36 to 40 mm at week 12, 48 to 50 mm at week 15, 55 mm at week 18, and 70 mm at week 20 during pregnancy (Kelly and Newnham, 1989; Aiumlamai et al., 1992; González de Bulnes et al., 1998; Tajik et al., 2001). Later than day 100 it becomes increasingly difficult to measure the BPD because of the variability of fetal location (Haibel, 1988).

The time between day 40 and day 80 allows the most accurate prediction of gestational age in ewes bearing singletons or twins from measurements of the skull (Kelly and Newnham, 1989). These parameters become increasingly unreliable after day 80.

Early in development, heartbeat is imaged as a fluttering movement within the echogenic embryo proper. Fetal heart rates are related to gestational age and fetal activity and are important indicators of fetal well-being. But the rapid movements of the normal conceptus often make it difficult to obtain exact measurements.

Heart pulsation is first observed in sheep on days 18 to 19 (Schrick and Inskeep, 1993) or days 21 to 23 (Garcia et al., 1993; Kaulfuss et al., 1996a; Strmšnik et al., 2002) after breeding; and in goats on days 19 to 23 (Martínez et al., 1998). In the latter species a decrease in the heartbeat rate was observed during the embryonic period until the early fetal period, from 168.3 plus or minus 2.8 beats per minute (day 21) to 158.3 plus or minus 2 beats per minute (day 40). Seven weeks before birth, sheep fetal heart rate reached a plateau (167 plus or minus 1.5 beats per minute), but then decreased at three weeks before parturition (139 plus or minus 15.7 beats per minute) until birth (117 plus or minus 9.2 bpm) (Aiumlamai et al., 1992). This plateau was not observed by Chavez Moreno et al., (1996).

Because of the fetal size a 5 MHz transducer is preferred for scanning until day 60 to 100. Later, good results can be obtained with a 3-MHz to 3.5 MHz transducer (Kähn, 1991).

Embryonic and early fetal growth was found to be quite uniform, well correlated with gestational age and with only small differences during the first half of pregnancy concerning breed, sex, or litter size, although differences in fetal growth in goats were more striking (Haibel et al., 1989; Reichle and Haibel, 1991; González de Bulnes et al., 1998; Noia et al., 2002). It has been suggested that differences between breeds and developmental stage of the conceptuses can be neglected until day 80 of pregnancy (Haibel and Perkins, 1989), but other authors described significant breed differences from day 39 post-coitum (Kaulfuss et al., 1999b). Triplet fetuses differed from those of singletons and twins (measurements between days 49 and 91, Sergeev et al., 1990), and in twin pregnancies one fetus grew faster than the other (measurements before day 50, Kaulfuss et al., 1999b).

The investigation of embryo or fetal movements is important for clinical and scientific purposes. They were studied in sheep and goats (Natale et al., 1981; Scheerboom and Taverne, 1985; Fraser and Broom, 1990; Romano et al., 1998c). Changes of fetal position depend primarily on active movements, but passive displacement during uterine contractures was also observed (Scheerboom and Taverne, 1985). Romano et al. (1998) observed fewer movements in embryos sooner than day 30 and vigorous movements in fetuses after day 30. Fetal movements occur up to day 70 to 75 of pregnancy (Lastovica, 1990), with a decreasing trend toward parturition (Fraser and Broom, 1990). They are related to gestational age and can be divided, for example, into general movements, fetal rotation, head movements, forelimb or hindlimb movements, and kicking or chewing. The effect of poisonous plants on the developing fetus has been investigated. A significant reduction in fetal movements was ultrasonically observed in sheep following ingestion of plants containing piperidine alkaloid (Bunch et al., 1992).

Fetal Membranes and Placenta

In addition to the conceptus, fetal membranes and placenta are ultrasonically imaged during pregnancy.

The amnion can be recognized for the first time between day 25 and day 30 as an echogenic line surrounding the embryo in a distance of about 1 to 2 mm (Kähn, 1991).

Sheep placentomes are identified transrectally as small echogenic areas or swellings on the endometrial surface from day 25 (Kähn, 1991; Tainturier, 1992), day 28 (Kaulfuss et al., 1996a; Buckrell et al., 1988), day 30 (Buckrell et al., 1986), or day 32 (Doize et al., 1997). The typical cup-shaped form is present on day 42 and maximal placentome size is reached by day 74 (Doize et al., 1997) or day 75 to 80 (Kaulfuss et al., 1998: about 35 mm diameter). After a plateau phase between day 115 and 130 of pregnancy, the placentome diameter starts to slowly shrink.

In goats, placentomes are visualized from day 28 (Baronet and Vaillancourt, 1989) or about day 35 (Medan et al., 2004a), and the typical semilunar or circular structures with echo-free centers are observed from about day 38 of pregnancy (Hesselink and Taverne, 1994).

During gestation placentomes of variable size are observed in sheep, whereas a more uniform size predominates in goats.

Determination of Fetal Sex

Identification of the genital tubercle, prepuce/penis, or scrotum allows the diagnosis of fetal sex in sheep and goats (Coubrough and Castell, 1998: days 60 to 69 of gestation, single pregnancies; Bürstel et al., 2001, 2002: days 50 to 75, single and multiple pregnancies; Nan et al., 2001: days 50 to 130, single pregnancies; Reichenbach et al., 2004: days 50 to 75, single and multiple pregnancies; 5 MHz, respectively). The umbilicus serves as the checkpoint for the determination of the presence or absence of a penis or scrotum (see Figure 14.6). The prepuce is often imaged as a bilobulated echogenic structure close to the umbilical

cord, whereas the scrotum appears as a triangular structure between the hind limbs (Bürstel et al., 2001, 2002). In female fetuses the genital tubercle is identified in the area of the tail (Coubrough and Castell, 1998; Reichenbach et al., 2004), but it remains predominantly unobserved because the region is obscured by the tail basis (Bürstel et al., 2001, 2002; Nan et al., 2001). Successful ultrasonic scanning for sex determination is done transrectally (animals fasted and standing or in dorsal recumbency: Coubrough and Castell, 1998) or transcutaneously (Bürstel et al., 2001, 2002; Nan et al., 2001). It requires a skilled examiner.

Embryonic and Fetal Mortality

Embryonic mortality (EM) and fetal mortality (FM) can be estimated by using ultrasonography. EM losses of up to 25 percent can occur until day 30, but there are significant differences between. FM is not so pronounced in small ruminants.

Wilkins et al. (1982) reported a low level of fetal loss in mid- to late gestation (days 60 to 90), whereas Kaulfuss et al. (1996a) observed the loss of some or all embryos before day 30 and an EM in relation to the ovulation rate of about 37 percent before day 31 of gestation in 25 percent of sheep

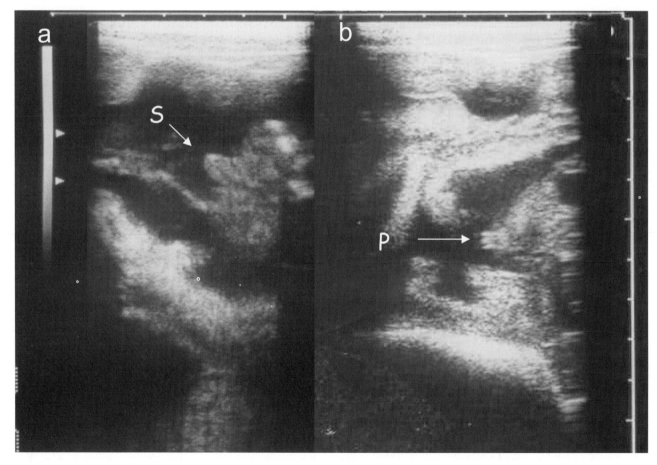

Figure 14.6. Fetal sex determination in a goat using transabdominal ultrasonography, 5-MHz. **(a)**: **S-arrow** points to triangular scrotum; **(b)**: **P-arrow** points to penis/prepuce.

(Kaulfuss et al., 1997). Kilgour (1992) estimated after ultrasonic investigations that Merino sheep in New South Wales achieve only two-thirds of their reproductive potential.

Signs of EM include disappearing embryonic vesicles, smaller embryos compared to the healthy ones, or missing heart pulsations (Kaulfuss et al., 1997). The embryo may show distorted outlines.

The absence of fetal movements and heartbeats are the first ultrasonic signs of fetal death. Subsequently, the conceptus looses its clear contours, but fetal membranes may stay intact for some time. Normally plenty of anechoic fluid surrounds the fetuses, but missing or cloudy fetal fluids as well as placentomes which cannot be clearly imaged suggest fetal disease and death. Finally, images identical to a pyometra are possible. FM in later stages of gestation may result in echogenic/hyperechoic structures in the uterus, representing bony remnants of fetuses (Kaulfuss et al., 1999a) or mummification (Hesselink and Taverne, 1994). In these cases, although uncommon findings in small ruminants, placentomes and fetal fluid are absent. Other fetuses of the same pregnancy may also be in the process of mummification, or they may be viable (Haibel, 1990). When partial fetal death occurs relatively early during gestation but after placentation, in addition to pictures of a normal pregnancy a distended fluid-filled uterine horn is imaged on the contralateral side. It may contain floating echogenic particles without the presence of placentomes or a fetus (Haibel, 1990).

It has been shown that nutritional restriction during mid-pregnancy (day 30 to day 95) may have a significant effect on fetal mortality in this period (Kelly et al., 1989). This must be considered when ultrasonography is used to predict the number of lambs that will be born (Wilkins et al., 1982; Kelly et al., 1989).

Following abortion, an extended fluid-filled uterus with prominent caruncles and, occasionally, remnants of fetal membranes is observed. Later, pictures similar to puerperal changes occur (Kaulfuss et al., 1999).

Anomalies of Pregnancy and Puerperium

Application of ultrasonography is a clinical aid in sheep and goats with obstetrical and gynecological problems (Buckrell et al., 1988; Morin and Badertscher, 1990; Scott and Gessert, 1998, 2000; Scott et al., 2001).

Ultrasonography has been used to diagnose anomalies of pregnancy or puerperium, e.g. hydrometra in goats (Pieterse and Taverne, 1986; Buckrell et al., 1988; Haibel, 1990; White and Russel, 1993; Wittek et al., 1998) and sheep (Bretzlaff, 1993; Kaulfuss et al., 1999), and uterine torsion intra-partum (Wehrend et al., 2002), as well as retained fetal membranes and lochiometra in sheep (Hauser, 2000). Retained fetal membranes may be recognized floating in the uterine lumen or surrounding the caruncles, while the lochiometra has been described as a hypoechoic fluid accumulation including echointensive particles within an extended uterus. The ultrasonic image of a hydrometra is a

large thin-walled uterus containing anechoic or slightly turbid fluid. The lumen is transversed by straight echogenic lines representing folds of the uterine wall.

Moreover, the technique has enabled studies on pathological processes that occur in the fetus or placenta after experimental infection with Chlamydia psittaci, Listeria monocytogenes, or Toxoplasma gondii, or after feeding poisonous plants such as Tetrapterys multiglandulosa, ergot of rye, or Nicotiana glauca (Panter and Keeler, 1992; Ortego-Pacheco, 1993, cited from Jonker, 2004; Engeland et al., 1996, 1998; Zarrouk et al., 1999; Melo et al., 2001).

Puerperium

During the puerperal period, progressive changes of the uterine horn, uterine lumen, or caruncle diameters have been described in sheep (Hauser, 2000; Hauser and Bostedt, 2002) and goats (Wustmann and Bernhard, 1994) to evaluate uterine involution. Differences following spontaneous parturition, assisted lambing, or caesarian section were evident in these parameters when animals were controlled continuously between days 1 and 30 post-partum (Hauser, 2000; Hauser and Bostedt, 2002). These differences were most distinct during the early puerperium. Ram exposure did not hasten the ultrasonically observed uterine involution (Godfrey et al., 1998).

Monitoring Pregnancies in Biotechnological or Experimental Projects

Pregnancy monitoring is also of interest after estrus synchronization, insemination, embryo transfer, *in vitro* fertilization, intracytoplasmatic sperm injection, cryoconservation of embryos, cloning, sexing, or other embryo-transfer-associated techniques to evaluate fertility following the procedure, as well as the size of embryos or fetuses, size of placentomes, time of embryonic/fetal mortality, development of fetal hydrops, etc. (e.g. Schiewe et al., 1984; Udy, 1987; Ritar et al., 1990; Gustafson et al., 1993; MacLaren et al., 1993; Jones and Fecteau, 1995; Thompson et al., 1995; Holm et al., 1996; Gomez et al., 1998; Beckett et al., 1999; White et al., 1999; Samake et al., 2000; Drion et al., 2001; Oppenheim et al., 2001; Viñoles et al., 2001).

Furthermore, ultrasonography use during small ruminant pregnancy has turned out to be a valuable tool for animal models in human medicine; e.g. ultrasound-guided procedures were developed to deliver a DNA label (Greenwood et al., 1999) or hematopoietic stem cells (Lovell et al., 2001) into the peritoneal cavity of fetal sheep, or to inject corticosteroids (Quinlivan et al., 2001) or adenoviral vectors encoding the beta-galactosidase and human factor IX genes (David et al., 2003a).

Ultrasound-guided transcutaneous fetal liver stem cell sampling from the early ovine fetus for prenatal *ex vivo* gene therapy was performed at about day 57 of gestation, and it was stated that the number of collectable fetal liver cells is large enough for autologous transplantation and engraftment of transfected stem cells (Surbek et al., 2002).

The transabdominal ultrasonic visualization and measurement of the tracheal diameter in sheep fetuses was performed (Kalache et al., 2001), and percutaneous ultrasound-guided injections into the trachea of fetal sheep were used to target the fetal airways (David et al., 2003b). Changes in fetal urinary tract appearance were detected using serial ultrasound examinations in an ovine model of fetal bladder outflow obstruction (Duncomb et al., 2002), and the fetal urinary bladder volume was estimated (Fagerquist et al., 2002).

Circulation of fetuses, umbilical blood flow, or placental circulation during acute hypoxemia of fetal lambs; nicotine treatment; and maternal oxygen administration were studied ultrasonically in pregnant sheep used as animal models for human gestation (Irion and Clark, 1990; Van Huisseling et al., 1991; Arabeille et al., 1994; Sonesson et al., 1994; Schmidt et al., 1996).

The well-being of the conceptus can also be investigated, for example, after fetal surgery in sheep models for human gestation.

Mammary Gland

Ultrasound is suitable for the evaluation of udder morphology, certain aspects of milk production, and pathological changes of the mammary gland (Ruberte et al., 1994).

For ultrasonic examinations of the udder it is essential not to deform the tissue during scanning. Therefore, the teats or whole glands are immersed in a hand-warm water bath (Fahr et al., 2001; Franz et al., 2003). As an alternative, Bruckmaier and Blum (1992) and Bruckmaier et al. (1997) placed goats and/or sheep into warm water reaching to the level of the animals' ventral abdomen. Only degassed water should be used to avoid disturbances originating from small air bubbles. This was achieved by filling the container with hot water (about 80°C) some hours before scanning and allowing it to cool to body temperature. Dipping into cold water resulted in teat contractions. In other investigations the transducer was placed into direct contact with the udder after applying acoustic coupling gel (Ruberte et al., 1994; Franz et al., 2003; Mavrogianni et al., 2004). Measurements of mammary cistern size in small ruminants using a simple ultrasonic technique were reported by Nudda et al. (2000) and Wójtowski et al. (2002).

For ultrasonic imaging of cistern areas and glandular parenchyma, a 5 MHz (Bruckmaier and Blum, 1992; Ruberte et al., 1994) or 8.5 MHz linear array probe (Franz et al., 2003) was successfully used. The glandular parenchyma in lactating ewes was found to be echogenic with a mean gray-scale value of 219, and the fine hypoechoic spotting corresponded to the milk-filled mammary ducts (Ruberte et al., 1994). Franz et al. (2003) described the appearance of the gland tissue at the end of lactation in 68 percent and 60 percent of the animals as homogenous and/or hypoechoic, respectively, while in 40 percent and 32 percent a hyperechoic and/or non-homogenous image was realized.

Undisturbed milk in the cistern appeared anechoic, but during milk ejection whirling of gray particles from the tissue border into the gland cistern occurred. This was accompanied by an area increase reaching its maximum after about 30 seconds (Bruckmaier and Blum, 1992).

During ultrasonic measurements of the cisternal and alveolar udder compartments in lactating goats it was recognized that goats possess large cisterns (Bruckmaier and Blum, 1992; Salama et al., 2004). While in mammary glands of cattle most of the milk is stored in the gland tissue, the contrary was observed in goats. In this species the cisternal fraction of total milk is much higher than the alveolar fraction (Bruckmaier and Blum, 1992).

The ultrasonically measured cisternal area increased linearly after milking, which indicated continuous milk storage in the cisterns at any filling degree of the alveoli. From the results after an oxytocin challenge at different milking intervals it was stated that no milk return from cistern to alveoli is expected in goats if milking is delayed after milk letdown (Salama et al., 2004). Phenylephrine or oxytocin administration caused rapid changes of the cistern volume (Bruckmaier and Blum, 1992; Bruckmaier et al., 1997). Breed variations must be considered when investigations of cistern volumes are performed (Bruckmaier et al., 1997).

Further investigations with 5 MHz or 8.5 MHz transducers were unsatisfactory in small ruminants because the teat canal was either not able to be distinguished or not clearly imaged, and the triple-layered structure of isolated teats from freshly removed sheep udders was not visible (Bruckmaier and Blum, 1992; Franz et al., 2001). In contrast, a 12 MHz linear array transducer proved to be suitable in this respect, and the hyperechoic mucosal membrane, the less echoic homogenously appearing muscle/connective tissue layer as well as the hyperechoic skin, were clearly recognized. The hyperechoic Fuerstenberg's rosette and the teat canal could also be visualized under these experimental conditions. The rosette forms a distinct border between the lumen of the teat cistern and the distally located teat canal. The latter appears ultrasonically as a white line bordered by parallel thick hypoechogenic bands (Franz et al., 2001).

In a later report Franz et al. (2003) were able to recognize the teat canal in about 50 percent of the investigated ewes as well as the triple-layered teat wall in nearly all ewes with the 8.5 MHz probe. The animals were scanned at the end of lactation, and a mean teat canal length and width of 8.6 mm and 2.3 mm was measured, respectively. Mavrogianni et al. (2004) described only two ultrasonically distinct layers of normal teats visualized with a 6 MHz sector scanner. The skin was represented as a thin bright echoic line, and the underlying tissue as a thicker homogenous and less echoic layer with unechoic cavities.

Fahr et al. (2001) performed detailed studies in dairy goats on the alterations caused by machine milking. After repeated ultrasonic measurements (10 MHz) of several teat parameters before and after machine milking they realized significant changes of the teat thickness and the length of the teat canal for a period of at least 1 hour. It was stated that these changes might be a result of haemostasis and tissue edema.

The ultrasound Doppler principle was used to perform mammary blood flow measurements in lactating goats (Christensen et al., 1989) and to compare changes during lactation in animals with high or low milk yield (Nielsen et al., 1990). Relationships between milk yield and milk vein blood velocity were realized. During pulsed wave-Doppler ultrasonic examinations in ewes significant differences between morning and afternoon blood flow values were realized in machine-milked animals. This was not the case in sheep with suckling lambs stimulating the udder constantly (Piccione et al., 2004).

Teat stenosis was experimentally induced in lactating ewes (Mavrogianni et al., 2004). Four days after intracisternal inoculation of an ovine mastitis strain (Staphylococcus chromogenes), the first ultrasonic changes occurred in comparison to normal teats. Ultrasonography was used to describe the image of a clinical mastitis in one ewe (Franz et al., 2003) and a mammary fibroepithelial hyperplasia in one goat (Andreasen et al., 1993).

Additionally, sheep mammary glands have served as breast models in human medicine, and continuous ultrasonic scannings were performed after cryosurgery (Rabin et al., 1999).

Male Reproductive System

Ultrasonography allows visualization of normal and abnormal testicular and epididymal features as well as analysis of accessory sex glands, thus complementing the clinical fertility evaluation of rams and bucks. However, despite its informational value, there are few data published that deal with the use of ultrasonography to evaluate small ruminant male reproductive organs.

Ultrasonic imaging was achieved by using devices fitted with 6 MHz sector or 7.5 MHz linear-array transducers. Animals were restrained in a standing position for scanning, and the scrotal hair was trimmed and the testicles were gently pulled downwards within the scrotum and maintained in this position (Ahmad et al., 1991; Gouletsou et al., 2003).

Ovine and caprine testicular parenchyma appears homogenous and moderately echogenic. When imaged in the longitudinal plane the mediastinum testis is visualized as a centrally located hyperechogenic line or as a nearly circular echogenic area in the transverse plane (Ahmad et al., 1991). This was recognized in 87 percent of the animals, and in 69 percent of the rams it was detected in both testicles, but the presence or absence of a visible mediastinum testis should not be evaluated as an observation of clinical significance (Gouletsou et al., 2003). The echogenicity score of the mediastinum testis increased with the age of the rams (younger or older than 13 months).

No relationships between the ultrasonic appearance of the testis and semen parameters were noticeable (Cartee et al., 1990).

Of the three segments of the epididymis, the body cannot be imaged in situ (Ahmad et al., 1991; Gouletsou et al., 2003). The epididymal head as well as the tail appear less echoic than the testis itself. Large parts of the caput epididymis are clearly detectable with a sector scanner, whereas the structures cannot be imaged regularly by using a linear probe because they are masked by the pampiniform plexus.

The pampiniform plexus is identified as a cone-shaped structure and appears less echoic than the testicular parenchyma. Numerous convoluted anechoic tubular structures represent the small spermatic veins (Gouletsou et al., 2003). Ultrasonically, the testicular tunica and capsule are realized as a distinct hyperechoic contour encircling the testicular parenchyma. A thin anechoic line, due to a small amount of extra-testicular fluid between the parietal and visceral layers of the tunica vaginalis, is seen in almost all of the goats and rams (Ahmad et al., 1991). This liquid is normal peritoneal fluid.

The testicular and epididymal tissue appear slightly more echogenic out of the reproductive period than during the season (Ahmad et al., 1991; Gouletsou et al., 2003).

Ahmad et al. (1991) recognized no differences in testicular or epididymal ultrasonic images in rams investigated continuously in 14-day intervals from the age of 15 to 40 weeks. In goats, however, significant changes were recorded when the animals passed puberty. The prepuberal testis turned out to be less echogenic than the testis of mature bucks. Furthermore, the tail of the epididymis was either completely anechoic or could not be imaged in bucks that were about 15 weeks of age. Both structures attained normal echogenicity within four to six weeks and remained unchanged until the end of the study when the goats were 37 weeks of age.

Ultrasonic appearance of testes, prostate, and vesicular glands has been documented in GnRH-treated lambs and their controls from two to 26 weeks of age (Chandolia et al., 1997). Image analyses revealed that numerical pixel values of testes decreased from two to eight weeks, increased to 22 weeks, and then remained on a plateau. Prostate width increased from four to 26 weeks and its pixel values declined from four to eight weeks. In contrast, the length and width of the vesicular glands increased slowly to eight weeks, more rapidly to 18 weeks, and then plateaued. Pixel values of these structures declined from four to 10 weeks, after which the values increased to 12 weeks, decreased to a nadir at 18 weeks, and then increased slowly to 26 weeks.

Spontaneous sperm granulomas in the epididymal body and tail, respectively, of two rams appeared as anechoic areas with indistinct walls (Ahmad et al., 2000), whereas Buckrell et al. (1988) and Karaca et al. (1999) described granulomas in caput and tail as anechoic or hyperechoic regions with a distinct margin and with or without a hyperechoic capsule. Granulomas located in the caput epididymis were associated with an enlargement of the mediastinum testis. Areas of testicular degeneration imaged as numerous hyperechogenic foci within the heterogeneous testicular parenchyma. They were associated with granulomas within the epididymis or testis. However, testicular granulomas could not be identified ultrasonically (Karaca et al., 1999).

After unilateral vasectomy of goats and rams, the epididymal tail lost its characteristic heterogeneous echotexture and enlarged. Anechoic masses representing sperm granulomas were visible within the epididymal tail of rams, the epididymal head of one buck, and at the cut end of the vas deferens in another goat. These alterations were observed as early as four to six weeks after surgery (Ahmad and Noakes, 1995a).

Testicular degeneration in two infertile goats was accompanied by the ultrasonically uncharacteristic heterogeneity of the testicular parenchyma and dense hyperechoic areas caused by foci of mineralization (Ahmad and Noakes 1995b). Such hyperechoic zones indicating fibrosis or calcification were also seen after scrotal myiasis (Cisale et al., 1999). In contrast, necrotic areas were initially visualized as regions of decreased echogenicity after induction of ischemic necrosis of the testis by unilateral testicular artery ligation in bucks (Eilts et al., 1989). Later, the granulation tissue was difficult to ultrasonically differentiate from normal testicular parenchyma.

Sequential ultrasonic changes in the testis and the epididymis were monitored after unilateral intra-testicular and intra-epididymal tail injection of chlorhexidine gluconate solution (a chemical used as substitute for vasectomy in cats, dogs, and bulls) in three bucks and a ram (Ahmad and Noakes, 1995c). Within 24 hours hyperechogenic areas were imaged corresponding to the sites of injection. During the following 16 weeks of observation the lesions decreased in echogenicity and showed acoustic shadowing. They were surrounded by a distinct hyperechogenic border. The epididymal tail showed an increased echogenicity and anechoic lesions with ill-defined borders within 24 hours after injection. A hyperechogenic margin was subsequently observed around the lesions.

In a ram suffering from a unilateral scrotal hernia the ultrasonic image of the testis was covered by a hyperechogenic area representing omental fat within the hernial sac (Ahmad et al., 2000).

References

Ahmad, N., England, G.C.W., Noakes, D.E. (2000). Ultrasonography of spontaneous lesions of the genital system of three rams, and their influence on semen quality. *Vet. Rec.* 146:10–15.

Ahmad, N., Noakes, D.E. (1995a). A clinical and ultrasonographic study of the testes and related structures of goats and rams after unilateral vasectomy. *Vet. Rec.* 137:112–117.

Ahmad, N., Noakes, D.E. (1995b). Ultrasound imaging in determining the presence of testicular degeneration in two male goats. *British Vet. J.* 151:101–110.

Ahmad, N., Noakes, D.E. (1995c). A clinical and ultrasonographic study of induced testicular and epididymal lesions in goats and a ram. *Anim. Reprod. Sci.* 39:35–49.

Ahmad, N., Noakes, D.E., Subandrio, A.L. (1991). B-mode real time ultrasonographic imaging of the testis and epididymis of sheep and goats. *Vet. Rec.* 128:491–496.

Aiumlamai, S., Fredericksson, G., Nilsfors, L. (1992). Real-time ultrasonography for determining the gestational age of ewes. *Vet. Rec.* 131:560–562.

Andreasen, C.B., Huber, M.J., Mattoon, J.S. (1993). Unilateral hyperplasia of the mammary gland in a goat. *J. Am. Vet. Assoc.* 202:1279–1280.

Arbeille, B., Fignon, A., Bosc, M., Bodart, S. (1994). Modifications des circulations utéro-placentaire et cérébrale foetales induites par la nicotine chez le fetus ovin. *J. Gynecol, Obstet. Biol. Reprod.,* Paris 23:51–56.

Asher, G.W., Scott, I.C., O'Neill, K.T., Smith, J.F., Inskeep, E.K., Townsend, E.C. (1997). Ultrasonographic monitoring of antral follicle development in red deer (*Cervus elaphus*). *J. Reprod. Fertil.* 11:91–99.

Aswad, A., Abdou, M.S.S., Al-Bayatty, F., El-Sawaf, S.A. (1976). The validity of the "ultra-sonic method" for pregnancy diagnosis in ewes and goats. *Zbl. Vet. Med.* A 23:467–474.

Barbera, A., Jones, O.W., Zerbe, G.O., Hobbins, J.C., Battaglia, F.C., Meschia, G. (1995). Ultrasonographic assessment of fetal growth: Comparison between human and ovine fetus. *Am. J. Obstet. Gynec.* 173:1765–1769.

Baronet, D., Vaillancourt, D. (1989). Diagnostic de gestation par echotomographie chez la chèvre. *Méd. Vet.* Quebec 19:67–73.

Barrett, D.M., Bartlewski, P.M., Batista-Arteaga, M., Symington, A., Rawlings, N.C. (2004). Ultrasound and endocrine evaluation of the ovarian response to a single dose of 500 IU of eCG following a 12-day treatment with progestogen-releasing intravaginal sponges in the breeding and nonbreeding seasons in ewes. *Theriogenology* 61:311–327.

Bartlewski, P.M., Beard, A.P., Chapman, C.L., Nelson, M.L., Palmer, B., Aravindakshan, J., Cook, S.J., Rawlings, N.C. (2001a). Ovarian response in gonadotrophin-releasing hormone-treated anoestrous ewes: follicular and endocrine correlates with luteal outcome. *Reprod. Fert. Dev.* 13:133–142.

Bartlewski, P.M., Beard, A.P., Cook, S.J., Chandolia, R.K., Honaramooz, A., Rawlings, N.C. (1999a). Ovarian antral follicular dynamics and their relationships with endocrine variables throughout the oestrous cycle in breeds of sheep differing in prolificacy. *J. Reprod. Fertil.* 115:111–124.

Bartlewski, P.M., Beard, A.P., Cook, S.J., Rawlings, N.C. (1998). Ovarian follicular dynamics during anoestrus in ewes. *J. Reprod. Fertil.* 113:275–285.

Bartlewski, P.M., Beard, A.P., Rawlings, N.C. (1999b). An ultrasonographic study of luteal function in breeds of sheep with different ovulation rates. *Theriogenology* 52:115–130.

Bartlewski, P.M., Beard, A.P., Rawlings, N.C. (2000a). An ultrasound-aided study of temporal relationships between the patterns of LH/FSH secretion, development of ovulatory-sized antral follicles and formation of corpora lutea in ewes. *Theriogenology* 54:229–245.

Bartlewski, P.M., Beard, A.P., Rawlings, N.C. (2000b). Ultrasonographic study of ovarian function during early pregnancy and after parturition in the ewe. *Theriogenology* 53:673–689.

Bartlewski, P.M., Beard, A.P., Rawlings, N.C. (2001b). Ultrasonographic study of the effects of the corpus luteum on antral follicular development in unilaterally ovulating Western white-faced ewes. *Anim. Reprod. Sci.* 65:231–244.

Bartlewski, P.M., Duggavathi, R., Aravindakshan, J., Barrett, D. M., Cook, S.J., Rawlings, N.C. (2003). Effects of a 6-day treatment with medroxyprogesterone acetate after prostaglandin F2 alpha-induced luteolysis at midcycle on antral follicular development and ovulation rate in nonprolific Western white-faced ewes. *Biol. Reprod.* 68:1403–1412.

Bartlewski, P.M., Vanderpol, J., Beard, A.P., Cook, S.J., Rawlings, N.C. (2000c). Ovarian antral follicular dynamics and their association with peripheral concentrations of gonadotropins and ovarian steroids in aneoestrous Finnish Landrace ewes. *Anim. Reprod. Sci.* 58:273–291.

Beard, A.P., Bartlewski, P.M., Rawlings, N.C. (1995). Ovarian follicular development during early pregnancy in the ewe. *J. Reprod. Fert. No. 15, Ann. Conf. Soc. Study Fert., Dublin, Abstract Series, No. 191.*

Beckett, D.M., Oppenheim, S.M., Moyer, A.L., BonDurant, R.H., Rowe, J.D., Anderson, G.B. (1999). Progestin implants can rescue demi-embryo pregnancies in goats: a case study. *Theriogenology* 51:1505–1511.

BonDurant, R.H. (1980). Pregnancy diagnosis in sheep and goats: field tests with an ultrasound unit. *California Veterinarian* 34:26–28.

Bor, A., Braw-Tal, R., Gootwine, W. (1992). Monitoring ovarian response of Booroola Assaf ewe lambs to PMSG, using ultrasonography and serum estradiol. *Theriogenology* 38:645–652.

Bosc, M.J. (1971). Etude d'un diagnostic de gestation par ultrasons et effet Doppler chez la brebis. *Ann. Zootech.* 20:107–110.

Botero-Herrera, O., González-Stagnaro, C., Poulin, N., Cognié, Y. (1984). Early pregnancy diagnosis in goats and sheep using transrectal ultrasonography. *Proc. 10th Int. Congr. Anim. Reprod. A. I.* I:79, (abstr.).

Bretzlaff, K.N. (1993). Development of hydrometra in a ewe flock after ultrasonography for determination of pregnancy. *J. Am. Vet. Med. Assoc.* 203:122–125.

Bretzlaff, K., Edwards, J., Forrest, D., Nuti, L. (1993). Ultrasonographic determination of pregnancy in small ruminants. *Vet. Med.* 88:12–24.

Bruckmaier, R.M., Blum, J.W. (1992). B-mode ultrasonography of mammary glands of cows, goats and sheep during α- and β-adrenergic agonist and oxytocin administration. *J. Dairy Res.* 59:151–159.

Bruckmaier, R.M., Paul, G., Mayer, H., Schams, D. (1997). Machine milking of Ostfriesian and Lacaune dairy sheep: udder anatomy, milk ejection and milking characteristics. *J. Dairy Res.* 64:163–172.

Buckrell. B.C. (1988). Applications of ultrasonography in reproduction in sheep and goats. *Theriogenology* 29:71–84.

Buckrell, B.C., Bonnett, B.N., Johnson, W.H. (1986). The use of real-time ultrasound rectally for early pregnancy diagnosis in sheep. *Theriogenology* 25:665–673.

Bürstel, D. (2002). Untersuchungen zur intrauterinen Geschlechtsfeststellung bei Feten kleiner Wiederkäuer mittels Ultrasonographie. (Determination of fetal sex in small ruminants using ultrasonography). Dissertation. Hannover, University of Veterinary Medicine.

Bürstel, D., Meinecke-Tillmann, S., Meinecke, B. (2001). Ultrasonographic determination of fetal sex in small ruminants. Proc. 5th Ann. Conf. European Society for Domestic Animal Reproduction. Vienna, Sept 13 –15, *ESDAR Newsletter* 6:53–54 (abstr).

Bürstel, D., Meinecke-Tillmann, S., Meinecke, B. (2002). Ultrasonographic diagnosis of fetal sex in small ruminants bearing multiple fetuses. *Vet. Rec.* 151:635–636.

Bunch, T.D., Panter, K.E, James, L.F. (1992). Ultrasound studies on the effects of certain poisonous plants on uterine function and fetal development in livestock. *J. Anim. Sci.* 70:1639–1643.

Campbell, B.K., Baird, D.T., Souza, C.J.H., Webb, R. (2003). The FecB (Booroola) gene acts at the ovary: in vivo evidence. *Reproduction* 126:101–111.

Campbell, B.K., Dobson, H., Scaramuzzi, R.J. (1998). Ovarian function in ewes made hypogonadal with GnRH antagonist and stimulated with FSH in the presence or absence of low amplitude LH pulses. *J. Endocrinol.* 156:213–222.

Cardwell, B.E., Fitch, G.Q., Geisert, R.D. (1998). Ultrasonic evaluation for the time of ovulation in ewes treated with norgestomet and norgestomet followed by pregnant mare's serum gonadotropin. *J. Anim. Sci.* 76:2235–2238.

Cartee, R.E., Rumph, P.F., Abuzaid, S., Carson, R. (1990). Ultrasonographic examination and measurement of ram testicles. *Theriogenology* 33:867–887.

Chandolia, R.K., Bartlewski, P.M., Omeke, B.C., Beard, A.P., Rawlings, N.C., Pierson, R.A. (1997). Ultrasonography of the developing reproductive tract in ram lambs: effects of a GnRH agonist. *Theriogenology* 48:99–117.

Chavez Moreno, J., Steinmann Chavez, C., Bickardt, K. (1996). Fetale Herzfrequenzmessung und sonographische Fetometrie zur Bestimmung des Trächtigkeitsstadiums beim Schaf. (Fetal heart measurement and sonographic fetometry for determination of fetal age in sheep). *Dtsch. Tierärztl. Wschr.* 103: 478–480.

Christensen, K., Nielsen, M.O., Bauer, R., Hilden, K. (1989). Evaluation of mammary blood flow measurements in lactating goats using the ultrasound Doppler principle. *Comp. Biochem. Physiol.* 92:385–392.

Christman, S.A., Bailey, M.T., Head, W.A., Wheaton, J.E. (2000). Induction of ovarian cystic follicles in sheep. *Domest. Anim. Endocrinol.* 19:133–146.

Cisale, H.O., Rivolta, M.A., Fernandez, H.A. (1999). Semen characteristics of rams after scrotal myiasis. *Vet. Rec.* 145: 642–643.

Cline, M.A., Ralston, J.N., Seals, R.C., Lewis, G.S. (2001). Intervals from norgestomet withdrawal and injection of equine chorionic gonadotropin or P.G. 600 to estrus and ovulation in ewes. *J. Anim. Sci.* 79:589–594.

Cloete, J.H.L. (1939). Prenatal growth in the Merino sheep. *Onderstepoort Vet. Sci. Anim. Ind.* 13:417–458.

Coubrough, C.A., Castell, M.C. (1998). Fetal sex determination by ultrasonically locating the genital tubercle in ewes. *Theriogenology* 50:263–267.

Davey, C.G. (1986). An evaluation of pregnancy testing in sheep using a real-time ultrasound scanner. *Aust. Vet. J.* 63:347–348.

David, A., Cook, T., Waddington, S., Peebles, D., Nivsarkar, M., Knapton, H., Miah, M., Dahse, T., Noakes, D., Schneider, H., Rodeck, C., Coutelle, C., Themis, M. (2003a). Ultrasound-guided percutaneous delivery of adenoviral vectors encoding the beta-galactosidase and human factor IX genes to early gestation fetal sheep in utero. *Hum. Gene Ther.* 14:353–364.

David, A.L., Peebles, D.M., Gregory, L., Themis, M., Cook, T., Coutelle, C., Rodecke, C.H. (2003b). Percutaneous ultrasound-guided injection of the trachea in fetal sheep: a novel technique to target the fetal airways. *Fetal Diagn. Ther.* 18:385–390.

Dawson, L.J., Sahlu, T., Hart, S.P., Detweiler, G., Gipson, T.A., Teh, T.H., Henry, G.A., Bahr, R.J. (1994). Determination of fetal numbers in Alpine does by real-time ultrasonography. *Small Ruminant Res.* 14:225–231.

Deas, D.W. (1977). Pregnancy diagnosis in the ewe by an ultrasonic rectal probe. *Vet. Rec.* 101:113–115.

De Castro, T., Rubianes, E., Menchaca, A., Rivero, A. (1998). Ultrasonic study of follicular dynamics during the estrous cycle in goats. *Theriogenology* 49:399 (abstr.).

De Bois, C.H.W., Taverne, M.A.M. (1984). Drachtigheitsonderzoek bij het schaap D. M. V. twee-dimensionele echografie. *Vlaams diergeneek. Tidjdschr.* 53:240–252.

Dickie, A.M., Paterson, C., Anderson, J.L.M., Boyd, J.S. (1999). Determination of corpora lutea numbers in Booroola-Texel ewes using transrectal ultrasound. *Theriogenology* 51:1209–1224.

Doize, F., Vaillancourt, D., Carabin, H., Belanger, D. (1997). Determination of gestational age in sheep and goats using transrectal ultrasonographic measurements of placentomes. *Theriogenology* 48:449–460.

Dorn, C.G., Wolfe, B.A., Bessoudo, E., Kraemer, D.C. (1989). Follicular detection in goats by ultrasonography. *Theriogenology* 31:185 (abstr.).

Drion, P.V., Furtoss, V., Baril, G., Manfredi, E., Bouvier, F., Pougnard, J.L., Bernelas, D., Caugnon, P., McNamara, E.M., Remy, B., Sulon, J., Beckers, J.F., Bodin, L., Leboeuf, B. (2001). Four years of induction/synchronization of oestrus in dairy goats: effect on the evolution of eCG binding rate in relation with the parameters of reproduction. *Reprod. Nutr. Dev.* 41:401–412.

Dufour, J.J., Cognié, Y., Mermillod, P., Mariana, J.C., Romain, R.F. (2000). Effects of the Booroola Fec gene on ovarian follicular populations in superovulated Romanov ewes pretreated with a GnRH antagonist. *J. Reprod. Fertil.* 118:85–94.

Duggavathi, R., Bartlewski, P.M., Barrett, D.M.W., Gratton, C., Bagu, E.T., Rawlings, N.C. (2004). Patterns of antral follicular wave dynamics and accompanying endocrine changes in cyclic and seasonally anestrous ewes treated with exogenous ovine follicle-stimulating hormone during the inter-wave interval. *Biol. Reprod.* 70:821–827.

Duggavathi, R., Bartlewski, P.M., Barrett, D.M., Rawlings, N.C. (2003a). Use of high-resolution transrectal ultrasonography to assess changes in numbers of small ovarian antral follicles and their relationships to the emergence of follicular waves in cyclic ewes. *Theriogenology* 60:495–510.

Duggavathi, R., Bartlewski, P.M., Pierson, R.A., Rawlings, N.C. (2003b). Luteogenesis in cyclic ewes: echotextural, histological, and functional correlates. *Biol. Reprod.* 69: 634–639.

Duncomb, G.J., Barker, A.P., Moss, T.J., Gurrin, L.C., Charles, A.K., Smith, N.M., Newnham, J.P. (2002). The effects of overcoming experimental bladder outflow obstruction in fetal sheep. *J. Matern. Fetal. Neonatal. Med.* 11:130–137.

Eilts, B.E. (1992). Testicular ultrasonography in ruminants. *Proc. Ann. Meet. Soc. Theriogenol.,* Aug. 14–15, San Antonio, Texas:37–40.

Eilts, B.E., Pechman, R.D., Taylor, H.W., Usenik E.A. (1989). Ultrasonographic evaluation of induced testicular lesions in male goats. *Am. J. Vet. Res.* 50:1361–1364.

Engeland, I.V., Andresen, O., Ropstad, E., Kindahl, H., Waldeland, H., Daskin, A., Eik, L.O. (1998). Effect of fungal alkaloids on the development of pregnancy and endocrine foetal-placental function in the goat. *Anim. Reprod. Sci.* 52:289–302.

Engeland, I.V., Waldeland, H., Kindahl, H., Ropstad, E., Andresen, O. (1996). Effect of Toxoplasma gondii infection on the development of pregnancy and on endocrine foetal-placental function in the goat. *Vet. Parasitol.* 67:61–74.

Evans, A.C.O., Duffy, P., Hynes, N., Boland, M.P. (2000). Waves of follicle development during the estrous cycle in sheep. *Theriogenology* 53:699–715.

Evans, A.C.O., Flynn, J.D., Quinn, K.M., Duffy, P., Quinn, P., Madgwick, S., Crosby, T.F., Boland, M.P., Beard, A.P. (2001). Ovulation of aged follicles does not affect embryo quality or fertility after a 14-day progestagen estrus synchronization protocol in ewes. *Theriogenology* 56:923–936.

Evans, A.C., Flynn, J.D., Duffy, P., Knight, P.G., Boland, M.P. (2002). Effects of ovarian follicle ablation on FSH, oestradiol and inhibin A concentrations and growth of other follicles in sheep. *Reproduction* 123:59–66.

Fagerquist, M., Fagerquist, U., Steyskal, H., Oden, A., Blomber, S.G. (2002). Accuracy in estimating fetal urinary bladder volume using a modified ultrasound technique. *Ultrasound Obstet. Gynecol.* 19:371–379.

Fahr, R.D., Schulz, J., Rosner, F. (2001). Melkbedingte Veränderungen an der Zitzenspitze der Ziege. (Milking associated changes of the teat end in goats). *Tierärztliche Prax.* 29(G):151–156.

Flynn, J.D., Duffy, P., Boland, M.P., Evans, A.C. (2000). Progestagen synchronization in the absence of a corpus luteum results in the ovulation of a persistent follicle in cyclic ewe lambs. *Anim. Reprod. Sci.* 62:285–296.

Ford, E.J.H. (1983). Pregnancy toxemia. In: Martin, W.B., Aitken, I.D. (eds), *Diseases of Sheep*, London: Blackwell Scientific Publications, pp 147–151.

Fortmeyer, H.P., Berg, D., Bonath, K., Kirschner, A. (1972). Bunstsynchronisation und Trächtigkeitsdiagnose bei Schafen. *Dtsch. Tierärztl. Wschr.* 79:51–55.

Fowler, D.G., Wilkins, J.F. (1980). The identification of single and multiple bearing ewes by ultrasonic imaging. *Proc. Aust. Soc. Anim. Prod.* 13:492 (abstr.).

Fowler, D.G., Wilkins, J.F. (1984). Diagnosis of pregnancy and number of foetuses in sheep by real-time ultrasonic imaging. 1. Effects of number of foetuses, stage of gestation, operator and breed of ewe on accuracy of diagnosis. *Livest. Prod. Sci.* 11:437–450.

Franz, S., Hofman-Parisot, M., Baumgartner, W., Windischbauer, G., Suchy, A., Bauder, B. (2001). Ultrasonography of the teat canal in cows and sheep. *Vet. Rec.* 149:109–112.

Franz, S., Hofman-Parisot, M., Gütler, S., Baumgartner, W. (2003). Clinical and ultrasonographic findings in the mammary gland of sheep. *New Zeal. J. Vet. J.* 51:238–243.

Fraser, A.F., Broom, D.M. (1990). Farm Animal Behaviour and Welfare 3rd ed., Ballière Tindall, 198–207.

Fraser, A.F., Robertson, J.G. (1967). The detection of fetal life in ewes and sows. *Vet. Rec.* 80:528–529.

Fukui, Y., Kobayashi, M., Tsubaki, M., Tetsuka, K., Shimoda, K., Ono, H. (1986). Comparison of two ultrasonic methods for multiple pregnancy diagnosis in sheep and indicators of multiple pregnant ewes in the blood. *Anim. Reprod. Sci.* 11:25–33.

Garcia, A., Neary, M.K., Kelly, G.R., Pierson, R.A. (1993). Accuracy of ultrasonography in early pregnancy diagnosis in the ewe. *Theriogenology* 39:847–861.

Gearhart, M.A., Wingfield, W.E., Knight, A.P., Smith, J.A., Dargatz, D.A., Boon, J.A., Stokes, C.A. (1988). Real-time ultrasonography for determining pregnancy status and viable fetal numbers in ewes. *Theriogenology* 30:323–337.

Gibbons, J.R., Kot, K., Thomas, D.L., Wiltbank, M.C., Ginther, O.J. (1999). Follicular and FSH dynamics in ewes with a history of high and low ovulation rates. *Theriogenology* 52:1004–1020.

Ginther, O.J., Kot, K. (1994). Follicular dynamics during the ovulatory season in goats. *Theriogenology* 42:987–1001.

Ginther, O.J., Kot, K., Wiltbank, M.C. (1995). Associations between emergence of follicular waves and fluctuations in FSH concentrations during the estrus cycle in ewes. *Theriogenology* 43:689–703.

Göbel, W., Meinecke-Tillmann, S., Meinecke, B. (1995). Transcervical embryo collection in small ruminants controlled by transrectal ultrasonography—preliminary results. *Proc. 11th Scientific Meeting of the European Embryo Transfer Association (A.E.T.E.)*, Hannover 8–9 September 1995. Edition Fondation Marcel Mérieux. 178 (abstr.).

Godfrey, R.W., Gray, M.L., Collins, J.R. (1998). The effect of ram exposure on uterine involution and luteal function during the postpartum period of hair sheep ewes in the tropics. *J. Anim. Sci.* 76:3090–3094.

Gomez, M.C., Catt, J.W., Evans, G., Maxwell, W.M. (1998). Cleavage, development and competence of sheep embryos fertilized by intracytoplasmic sperm injection and in vitro fertilization. *Theriogenology* 49:1143–1154.

González, F., Cabrera, F., Batista, M., Rodríguez, N., Álamo, D., Sulon, J., Beckers, J.-F., Gracia, A. (2004a). A comparison of diagnosis of pregnancy in the goat via transrectal ultrasound scanning, progesterone, and pregnancy-associated glycoprotein assays. *Theriogenology* 62:1108–1115.

González-Bulnes, A., Diaz-Delfa, C., Urrutia, B., Carrizosa, J.A., Lopez-Sebastian, A. (2004b). Ultrasonographic screening of the ovulatory process in goats. *Small Ruminant Res.* 52:165–168.

González-Bulnes, A., Garcia-Garcia, R.M., Carrizosa, J.A., Urrutia, B., Souza, C.J.H., Cocero, M.J., Lopez-Sebastian, A., McNeilly, A.S. (2004d). Plasma inhibin A determination at start of superovulatory treatments is predictive for embryo outcome in goats. *Dom. Anim. Endocrinol.* 26:259–266.

González-Bulnes, A., Garcia-Garcia, R.M., Castellanos, V., Santiago-Moreno, J., Ariznaverrata, C., Domínguez, V., López-Sebastián, A., Tresguerres, J., Cocero, M.J. (2003a). Influence of maternal environment on the number of transferable embryos obtained in response to superovulatory FSH treatments in ewes. *Reprod. Nutr. Dev.* 43:17–28.

González-Bulnes, A., Garcia-Garcia, R.M., Santiago-Moreno, J., López-Sebastián, A., Cocero, M.J. (2002a). Effect of follicular status on superovulatory response in ewes is influenced by presence of corpus luteum at first FSH dose. *Theriogenology* 58:1607–1614.

González-Bulnes, A., Garcia-Garcia, R.M., Santiago-Moreno, J., Dominguez, V., Lopez-Sebastian, C., Cocero, M.J. (2003b). Reproductive season affects inhibitory effects from large follicles on the response to superovulatory FSH treatments in ewes. *Theriogenology* 60:281–288.

González-Bulnes, A., Garcia-Garcia, R.M., Souza, C.J., Santiago-Moreno, J., Lopez-Sebastian, A., Cocero, M.J., Baird, D.T. (2002b). Patterns of follicular growth in superovulated sheep and influence on endocrine and ovarian response. *Reprod. Domest. Anim.* 37:357–361.

González-Bulnes, A., Souza, C.J., Campbell, B.K., Baird, D.T. (2004c). Systemic and intraovarian effects of dominant follicles on ovine follicular growth. *Anim. Reprod. Sci.* 84:107–119.

Gonzalez-Bulnes, A., Santiago-Moreno, J., Cocero, M.J., Souza, C.J.H., Groome, N.P., Garcia-Garcia, R.M., Lopez-Sebastian, A., Baird, D.T. (2002c). Measurement of inhibin A and follicular status predicts the response of ewes to superovulatory FSH treatments. *Theriogenology* 57:1363–1372.

Gonzalez-Bulnes, A., Santiago-Moreno, J., Garcia-Garcia, R.M., del Campo, A., Gomez-Brunet, A., Lopez-Sebastian, A. (2001). Origin of the preovulatory follicle in Mouflon sheep (*Ovis gmelini musimon*) and effect on growth of remaining follicles during the follicular phase of oestrous cycle. *Anim. Reprod. Sci.* 65:265–272.

Gonzalez-Bulnes, A., Santiago-Moreno, J., Garcia-Garcia, R.M., Souza, C.J., Lopez-Sebastian, A., McNeilly, A.S. (2004e). Effect of GnRH antagonists treatment on gonadotrophin secretion, follicular development and inhibin A secretion in goats. *Theriogenology* 61:977–985.

González de Bulnes, A., Santiago Moreno, J., Gomez Brunet, A., López Sebastián, A. (2000). Relationship between ultrasonographic assessment of the corpus luteum and plasma progesterone concentration during the oestrous cycle in monovular ewes. *Reprod. Dom. Anim.* 35:65–68.

González de Bulnes, A., Santiago Moreno, J., López Sebastián, A. (1998). Estimation of fetal development in Manchega ewes by transrectal ultrasonographic measurements. *Small Ruminant Res.* 127:243–250.

González de Bulnes, A., Osoro, K., Sebastian, A.L. (1999). Ultrasonographic assessment of the ovarian response in eCG-treated goats. *Small Ruminant Res.* 34:65–69.

Gouletsou, P.G., Amiridis, G.S., Cripps, P.J., Lainas, T., Deligiannis, K., Saratsis, P., Fthenakis, G.C. (2003). Ultrasonographic appearance of clinically healthy testicles and epididymis of rams. *Theriogenology* 59:1959–1972.

Graff, K.J., Meintjes, M., Dyer, V.W., Paul, J.B., Denniston, R.S., Ziomek, C., Godke, R.A. (1999). Transvaginal ultrasound-guided oocyte retrieval following FSH stimulation of domestic goats. *Theriogenology* 51:1099–1119.

Greenwood, P.L., Slepetis, R.M., Hermanson, J.W., Bell, A.W. (1999). An ultrasound-guided procedure to administer a label of DNA synthesis into fetal sheep. *Reprod. Fertil. Dev.* 11:303–307.

Greenwood, P.L., Slepetis, R.M., McPhee, M.J., Bell, A.W. (2002). Prediction of stage of pregnancy in prolific sheep using ultrasound measurement of fetal bones. *Reprod. Fertil. Dev.* 14:7–13.

Gustafson, R.A., Anderson, G.B., BonDurant, R.H., Sasser, G.R. (1993). Failure of sheep-goat hybrid conceptuses to develop to term in sheep-goat chimeras. *J. Reprod. Fertil.* 99:267–273.

Haibel, G.K. (1986). Real-time ultrasonic assessment of the uterus and fetus in small ruminants. *Proc. Ann. Meet. Soc. Theriogenol.* Sept 17–19, Rochester, NY, 275–277.

Haibel, G.K. (1988). Real-time ultrasonic fetal head measurement and gestational age in dairy goats. *Theriogenology* 30:1053–1057.

Haibel, G.K. (1990). Use of ultrasonography in reproductive management of sheep and goat herds. *Vet. Clinics North America: Food Anim. Pract.* 6:597–613.

Haibel, G.K., Perkins, N.R. (1989). Real-time ultrasonic biparietal diameter of second trimester Suffolk and Finn sheep fetuses and prediction of gestational age. *Theriogenology* 32:863–869.

Haibel, G.K., Perkins, N.R., Lidl, G.M. (1989). Breed differences in biparietal diameter of second trimester Toggenburg, Nubian and Angora goat fetuses. *Theriogenology* 32:827–834.

Haibel, G.K., Perkins, N.R., Reichle, J.K., Fung, E.D., Lidl, G.M. (1990). Real-time ultrasonic measurement of fetal biparietal diameter (BPD) for the prediction of gestational age (GA) in

small domestic ungulates. *Ann. Conf. Soc. Theriogenol. Toronto Soc. Theriogenology Newsletter* 13, No. 5 (abstr.).

Hauser, B. (2000). Ultrasonographische Untersuchung der postpartalen Uterusinvolution beim Schaf unter besonderer Berücksichtigung des Geburtsverlaufs. Dissertation Giessen, Justus-Liebig-Universität Giessen.

Hauser, B., Bostedt, H. (2002). Ultrasonographic observations of the uterine regression in the ewe under different obstetrical conditions. *J. Vet. Med.* A 49:511–516.

Henze, P., Bickhardt, K., Fuhrmann, H., Sallmann, H.P. (1998). Spontaneous pregnancy toxaemia (ketosis) in sheep and the role of insulin. *J. Vet. Med.* A 45:255–266.

Hesselink, J.W., Taverne, M.A.M. (1994). Ultrasonography of the uterus of the goat. *Vet. Quarterly* 16:41–45.

Holm, P., Walker, S.K., Seamark, R.F. (1996). Embryo viability, duration of gestation and birth weight in sheep after transfer of in vitro matured and in vitro fertilized zygotes cultured in vitro or in vivo. *J. Reprod. Fertil.* 107:175–181.

Hulet, C.V. (1969). Pregnancy diagnosis in the ewe using an ultrasonic Doppler instrument. *J. Anim. Sci.* 28:44–47.

Irion, G.L., Clark, K.-E. (1990). Direct determination of the ovine fetal umbilical artery blood flow waveform. *Am. J. Obstet. Gynec.* 162:541–549.

Jardon, C. (1988). Utilisation actuelle du diagnostic de gestation, en élevage, chez la brebis. *Rec. Méd. Vét.* 164:135–140.

Johnson, S.K., Dailey, R.A., Inskeep, E.K., Lewis, P.E. (1996). Effects of peripheral concentrations of progesterone on follicular growth and fertility in ewes. *Dom. Anim. Endocrinol.* 13:69–79.

Jones, S.L., Fecteau, G. (1995). Hydrops uteri in a caprine doe pregnant with a goat-sheep hybrid fetus. *J. Am. Vet. Med. Assoc.* 206:1920–1922.

Kähn, W. (1991). Atlas und Lehrbuch der Ultraschalldiagnostik, pp. 187–210. Hannover: *Schlütersche Verlagsgesellschaft.*

Kähn, W., Fraunholtz, J., Kaspar, B., Pyczak, T. (1990). Die Frühträchtigkeitsdiagnose bei Pferd, Rind, Schaf, Ziege, Schwein, Hund und Katze-Richtwerte und Grenzen. *Berl. Münch. Tierärztl. Wschr.* 103:206–211.

Kähn, W., Kähn, B., Richter, A., Schulz, J., Wolf, M. (1992). Zur Sonographie der Gravidität bei Schafen. I. Fetometrie zur Bestimmung des Gestationsstadiums und Vorhersage des Geburtszeitpunktes. *Dtsch. Tierärztl. Wschr.* 99:449–452.

Kähn, W., Achtzehn, J., Kähn, B., Richter, A., Schulz, J., Wolf, M. (1993). Zur Sonographie der Gravidität bei Schafen. II. Genauigkeit der transrektalen und der transkutanen Trächtigkeitsdiagnose. *Dtsch. Tierärztl. Wschr.* 100:29–31.

Kalache, K.D., Nishina, H., Ojutiku, D., Hanson, M.A. (2001). Visualisation and measurement of tracheal diameter in the sheep fetus: an ultrasound study with stereomicroscopic correlation. *Fetal Diagn. Ther.* 16:342–345.

Karaca, F., Aksoy, M., Kaya, A., Ataman, M.B., Tekeli, T. (1999). Spermatic granuloma in the ram: diagnosis by ultrasonography and semen characteristics. *Vet. Radiol. Ultrasound.* 40:402–406.

Karen, A., Beckers, J.-F., Sulon, J., El Amiri, B., Szabados, K., Ismail, S., Reiczigel, J., Szenci, O. (2003). Evaluation of false transrectal ultrasonographic pregnancy diagnoses in sheep by measuring the plasma level of pregnancy-associated glycoproteins. *Reprod. Nutr. Dev.* 43:577–586.

Karen, A., Szabados, K., Reiczigel, J., Beckers, J.F., Szenci, O. (2004). Accuracy of transrectal ultrasonography for determination of pregnancy in sheep: effect of fasting and handling of the animals. *Theriogenology* 61:1291–1298.

Kaspar, B. (1989). Ultraschalluntersuchungen bei Ziegen: Eine zuverlässige Methode zur Trächtigkeitsfeststellung. Ziegenzüchter 5:8–12.

Kaulfuss, K.-H., Brabant, S., Blume, K., May, J. (1995). Die Optimierung von Embryotransferprogrammen beim Schaf durch die transrektale ultrasonographische Ovardiagnostik (B-Mode) bei superovulierten Tieren. (The improvement of embryo transfer programmes by examination of the ovary response in superovulated donor ewes by transrectal real-time ultrasound). Dtsch. Tierärztl. Wschr. 102:208–212.

Kaulfuss, K.-H., Giucci, E., May, J. (2003b). Einflussfaktoren auf die Höhe der Ovulationsraten beim Schaf innerhalb der Hauptzuchtsaison—eine ultrasonographische Studie. (Influencing factors on the level of the ovulation rate in sheep during the main breeding season—an ultrasonographic study). Dtsch. Tierärztl. Wschr. 110:445–450.

Kaulfuss, K.-H., May, J., Süss, R., Moog, U. (1997). In vivo diagnosis of embryo mortality in sheep by real-time ultrasound. *Small Ruminant Res.* 24:141–145.

Kaulfuss, K.-H., Moritz, S., Giucci, E. (2003a). The influence of the ovulation rate on ultrasonically determined ovine corpus luteum morphometry and progesterone concentrations in cyclic and early pregnant sheep. Dtsch. Tierärztl. Wschr. 110:249–254.

Kaulfuss, K.-H., Süss, R., Schenk, P. (1999a). Die ultrasonographische Trächtigkeitsdiagnostik (B-mode) beim Schaf. Teil 4: Ergebnisse einer Feldstudie in Deutschland. (Real-time ultrasonographic pregnancy diagnosis in sheep. Part 4: Results of a field study in Germany). Tierärztl. Prax. 27(G): 74–82.

Kaulfuss, K.-H., Uhlich, K., Brabant, S., Blume, K., Strittmatter, K. (1996a). Die ultrasonographische Trächtigkeitsdiagnostik (B-mode) beim Schaf. Teil 1: Verlaufsuntersuchungen im ersten Trächtigkeitsmonat. (Real-time ultrasonic pregnancy diagnosis (B-mode) in sheep. Part 1: Frequent examinations during the first month of pregnancy). Tierärztl. Prax 24:443–452.

Kaulfuss, K.-H., Uhlich, K., Gille, U. (1998). Ultrasonographische Untersuchungen zum Plazentomwachstum beim trächtigen Schaf. (Ultrasonic examination of the placentome development in sheep). Dtsch. Tierärztl. Wschr. 105:137–172.

Kaulfuss, K.-H., Uhlich, K., Gille, U. (1999b). Ultrasonographische Messungen zum fetalen Wachstum des Schafes zwischen dem 20. und 50. Trächtigkeitstag. (Ultrasonographic examinations of the ovine fetal growth from day 20 to 50 after mating). Dtsch. Tierärztl. Wschr. 106:433–438.

Kaulfuss, K.-H., Zipper, N., May, J., Müller, S. (1994). Ergebnisse der ultrasonographischen transcutanen Trächtigkeitsdiagnostik (B-mode) beim Merinofleischschaf ab dem 20. Tag post

conceptionem unter Praxisbedingungen. (Results of transcutaneous pregnancy diagnosis in Merino-mutton sheep by real-time ultrasound under field conditions from day 20 post conception). 27. Jahrestagung über Physiologie und Pathologie der Fortpflanzung, Febr., Berlin. *Reprod. Dom. Anim.* 29:270 (abstr.).

Kaulfuss, K.-H., Zipper, N., May, J., Süss, R. (1996b). Die ultrasonographische Trächtigkeitsdiagnostik (B-mode) beim Schaf. Teil 2: Vergleichende Untersuchungen zur transkutanen und transrektalen Trächtigkeitsdiagnostik. (Real time ultrasonic pregnancy diagnosis in sheep. Part 2: Comparison of transrectal versus transcutaneous pregnancy diagnosis). Tierärztl. Prax. 24:559–566.

Keane, M.G. (1969). Pregnancy diagnosis in sheep by an ultrasonic method. *Irish Vet. J.* 23:194–196.

Kelly, R.W., Newnham, J.P. (1989). Estimation of gestational age in Merino ewes by ultrasound measurements of fetal head size. *Aust. J. Agric. Res.* 40:1293–1299.

Kelly, R.W., Newnham, J.P., Johnson, T., Speijers, E.J. (1987). An ultrasound technique to measure placental growth in ewes. *Aust. J. Agric. Res.* 38:757–764.

Kelly, R.W., Wilkins, J.F., Newnham, J.P. (1989). Fetal mortality from day 30 of pregnancy in Merino ewes offered different levels of nutrition. *Australian J. Exp. Agric.* 29:339–342.

Kilgourm, R.J. (1992). Lambing potential and mortality in Merino sheep as ascertained by ultrasonography. *Australian J. Exp. Agric.* 29:311–313.

Kleemann, D.O., Smith, D.H., Walker, S.K., Seamark, R.F. (1987). A study of real-time ultrasonography for predicting ovine foetal growth under field conditions. *Australian Vet. J.* 64:352–353.

Knights, M., Baptiste, Q.S., Lewis, P.E. (2002). Ability of ram introduction to induce LH secretion, estrus and ovulation in fall-born ewe lambs during anestrus. *Anim. Reprod. Sci.* 69:199–209.

Kühholzer, B., Schmoll, F., Besenfelder, U., Möstl, E., Krüger, E., Brem, G., Schellander, K. (1995). Examination of the ovarian follicular- and corpus luteum-development in superovulated ewes by ultrasonography. *Proc. 11th Scientific Meeting of the European Embryo Transfer Association* (A.E.T.E.), Hannover 8–9 September 1995. *Edition Fondation Marcel Mérieux.* 198 (abstr.).

Kühholzer, B., Schmoll, F., Besenfelder, U., Möstl, E., Krüger, E., Brem, G., Schellander, K. (1998). Ultrasonographic examination of ovarian structure dynamics in superovulated ewes. *Reprod. Dom. Anim.* 33:343–346.

Landau, S., Houghton, J.A.S., Mawhinney, J.R., Inskeep, E.K. (1996). Protein sources affect follicular dynamics in ewes near the onset of the breeding season. *Reprod. Fertil. Dev.* 8:1021–1028.

Langford, G.A., Shresta, J.N., Fiser, P.S., Ainsworth, L., Heaney, D.P., Marcus, G.J. (1984). Improved diagnostic accuracy by repetitive ultrasonic pregnancy testing in sheep. *Theriogenology* 21:691–698.

Lassala, A., Hernández-Cerón, J., Rodríguez-Maltos, R., Gutierrez, C.G. (2004). The influence of the corpus luteum on ovarian follicular dynamics during estrous synchronization in goats. *Anim. Reprod. Sci.* 84:369–375.

Lastovica, R.L. (1990). Ultrasound pregnancy diagnosis in sheep and goats. *Soc. Theriogenology , Newsletter* 13, No. 2.

Lavoir, M.C., Taverne, M.A.M. (1989). The diagnosis of pregnancy and pseudopregnancy, and the determination of fetal numbers in goats, by means of real-time ultrasound scanning. In: Taverne, M.A.M., Willemse, A.H. (eds), *Diagnostic Ultrasound and Animal Reproduction*, Dordrecht: Kluwer Acad. Publ. pp. 89–96.

Levy, I., Emery, P., Mialot, J.P. (1990). Echographie et gestion des troupeaux ovins. *Rec. Méd. Vét.* 166:751–764.

Leyva, V., Buckrell, B.C., Walton, J.S. (1998). Regulation of follicular activity and ovulation in ewes by exogenous progestagen. *Theriogenology* 50:395–416.

Lindahl, I.L. (1966). Detection of pregnancy in sheep by means of ultrasound. *Nature* 212:642–243.

Lindahl, I.L. (1969a). Comparison of ultrasonic techniques for the detection of pregnancy in ewes. *J. Reprod. Fertil.* 18:117–120.

Lindahl, I.L. (1969b). Pregnancy diagnosis in dairy goats using ultrasonic Doppler instrument. *J. Dairy Sci.* 52:529–530.

Lindahl, I.L. (1971). Pregnancy diagnosis in the ewe by intrarectal Doppler. *J. Anim. Sci.* 32:922–925.

Lindahl, I.L. (1976). Pregnancy diagnosis in ewes by ultrasonic scanning. *J. Anim. Sci.* 43:1135–1140.

Logue, N.D., Hall, J.T., McRoberts, S., Waterhouse, H. (1987). Real-time ultrasound scanning in sheep: The results of first year of its application on farms in South-West Scotland. *Vet. Rec.* 121:146–149.

Lopez-Sebastian, A., Gonzales de Bulnes, A., Santiago Moreno, J., Gomez-Brunet, A., Townsend, E.C., Inskeep, E.K. (1997). Patterns of follicular development during the oestrous cycle in monovular Merino des Pais ewes. *Anim. Reprod. Sci.* 48:279–291.

Lovell, K.L., Kraemer, S.A., Leipprandt, J.R., Sprecher, D.J., Ames, N.K., Nichols-Torrez, J., Carter, K.D., Rahmani, D.K., Jones, M.Z. (2001). In utero hematopoietic stem cell transplantation: a caprine model for prenatal therapy in inherited metabolic diseases. *Fetal. Diagn. Ther.* 16:13–17.

MacLaren, L.A., Anderson, G.B., BonDurant, R.H., Edmondson, A.J. (1993). Reproductive cycles and pregnancy in interspecific sheep ↔ goat chimaeras. *Reprod. Fertil. Dev.* 5:261–270.

Madel, A.J. (1983). Detection of pregnancy in ewe lambs by A-mode ultrasound. *Vet. Rec.* 112:11–12.

Mann, G., Campbell, B.K., McNeilly, A.S., Baird, D.T. (1993). Follicular development and ovarian hormone secretion following passive immunization of ewes against inhibin or oestradiol. *J. Endocrinol.* 136:225–233.

Martínez, M.F., Bosch, P., Bosch, R.A. (1998). Determination of early pregnancy and embryonic growth in goats by transrectal ultrasound scanning. *Theriogenology* 49:1555–1565.

Mavrogianni, V.S., Fthenakis, G.C., Burriel, A.R., Gouletsou, P., Papaioannou, N., Taitzoglou, I.A. (2004). Experimentally induced teat stenosis in dairy ewes: clinical, pathological and ultrasonographic features. *J. Comp. Pathol.* 130:70–74.

McBride Johnson, B., Nuti, L.C., Wiltz, D. (1994). Ultrasonographic examination of the caprine ovary. *Vet. Med.* 89:477–480.

Medan, M., Watanabe, G., Absy, G., Sasaki, K., Sharawy, S., Groome, N.P., Taya, K. (2003a). Ovarian dynamics and their associations with peripheral concentrations of gonadotropins, ovarian steroids, and inhibin during the estrous cycle in goats. *Biol. Reprod.* 69:57–63.

Medan, M., Watanabe, G., Absy, G., Sasaki, K., Sharawy, S., Taya, K. (2004a). Early pregnancy diagnosis by means of ultrasonography as a method of improving reproductive efficiency in goats. *J. Reprod. Dev.* 50:391–397.

Medan, M.S., Watanabe, G., Sasaki, K., Nagura, Y., Sakaime, H., Fujita, M., Sharawy, S., Taya, K. (2003b). Effects of passive immunization of goats against inhibin on follicular development, hormone profile and ovulation rate. *Reproduction* 125:751–757.

Medan, M.S., Watanabe, G., Sasaki, K., Taya, K. (2004b). Transrectal ultrasonic diagnosis of ovarian follicular cysts in goats and treatment with GnRH. *Domest. Anim. Endocrinol.* 27:115–124.

Melo, M.M., Vasconcelos, A.C., Dantas, G.C., Serakides, R., Alzamora-Filho, F. (2001). Experimental intoxication of pregnant goats with Tetrapterys multiglandulosa A. Juss (Malpghiaceae). *Arch. Brasil. Med. Vet. Zootec.* 53:58–65.

Menchaca, A., Pinczak, A., Rubianes, E. (2002). Follicular recruitment and ovulatory response to FSH treatment initiated on Day 0 or Day 3 post-ovulation in goats. *Theriogenology* 58:1713–1721.

Menchaca, A., Rubianes, E. (2001). Effect of high progesterone concentrations during the early luteal phase on the length of the ovulatory cycle of goats. *Anim. Reprod. Sci.* 68:69–76.

Menchaca, A., Rubianes, E. (2002). Relation between progesterone concentrations during the early luteal phase and follicular dynamics in goats. *Theriogenology* 57:1411–1419.

Meredith, M.J., Madani, M.O.K. (1980). The detection of pregnancy in sheep by A-mode ultrasound. *Br. Vet. J.* 136:325–330.

Morin, D.E., Badertscher, R.R. (1990). Ultrasonographic diagnosis of obstructive uropathy in a caprine doe. *J. Am. Vet. Med. Assos.* 197:378–380.

Nan, D., van Oord, H.A., Taverne, M.A.M. (2001). Determination of foetal gender in sheep by transabdominal ultrasonographic scanning. *Proc. 5th Ann. Conf. European Society for Domestic Animal Reproduction. Vienna, Sept 13–15. ESDAR Newsletter* 6:70 (abstr.).

Natale, R., Clewlow, F., Dawes, G.S. (1981). Measurement of fetal forelimb movements in the lamb in utero. *Am. J. Obstetr. Gynecol.* 140:545–551.

Nielsen, M.O., Jakobsen, K., Jorgensen, J.N. (1990). Changes in mammary blood flow during the lactation period in goats measured by the ultrasound Doppler principle. *Comp. Biochem. Physiol.* 97:519–524.

Noia, G., Romano, D., Terzano, G.M., De Santis, M., Di Domenico, M., Cavaliere, A., Ligato, M.S., Petrone, A., Fortunato, G., Filippetti, F., Caruso, A., Mancuso, S. (2002). Ovine fetal growth curves in twin pregnancy: ultrasonographic assessment. *Clin. Exp. Obstet. Gynecol.* 29:251–256.

Nudda, A., Pulina, G., Vallebella, R., Bencini, R., Enne, G. (2000). Ultrasound technique for measuring mammary cistern size of dairy ewes. *J. Dairy Res.* 67:101–106.

Oppenheim, S.M., Moyer, A.L., BonDurant, R.H., Rowe, J.D., Anderson, G.B. (2001). Evidence against humoral immune attack as the cause of sheep-goat interspecies and hybrid pregnancy failure in the doe. *Theriogenology* 55:1567–1581.

Orita, J., Tanaka, T., Kamomae, H., Kaneda, Y. (2000). Ultrasonographic observation of follicular and luteal dynamics during the estrous cycle in Shiba goats. *J. Reprod. Dev.* 46:31–37.

Ortego-Pacheco, A. (1993). Endocrine and ultrasonic studies of infectious fetal losses in sheep. Thesis, Master of Veterinary Science. University of Liverpool, UK, cited from: Jonker, F. H.: Fetal death: comparative aspects in large domestic animals. *Anim. Reprod. Sci.* 2004, 82–83:415–430.

Panter, K.E., Keeler, R.F. (1992). Induction of cleft palate in goats by Nicotiana glauca during a narrow gestational period and the relation to reduction in fetal movement. *J. Nat. Toxins* 1:25–32.

Parraguez, V.H.G., Gallegos, J.L.M., Raggi, L.A.S., Manterola, H.B., Muñoz, B.M. (1999). Diagnóstico precoz de gestación y determinación del número de embriones por ecografía transrectal en la cabra criolla chilena (Early pregnancy diagnosis and determination of embryo number by transrectal echography in Chilean creole goats). *Arch. Zootec.* 48:261–271.

Picazo, R.A., Gonzalez de Bulnes, A., Gomez Brunet, A., del Campo, A., Granados, B., Tresguerres, J., Lopez Sebastian, A. (2000). Effects of bromocriptine administration during the follicular phase of the oestrous cycle on prolactin and gonadotrophin secretion and follicular dynamics in Merino monovular ewes. *J. Reprod. Fertil.* 120:177–186.

Piccione, G., Arcigli, A., Assenza, A., Percipalle, M., Caola, G. (2004). Pulsed wave-Doppler ultrasonographic evaluation of the mammary blood flow in the ewe. *Acta Vet.* Brno 73:23–27.

Pieterse, M.C., Taverne, M.A.M. (1986). Hydrometra in goats: Diagnosis with real-time ultrasound and treatment with prostaglandins. *Theriogenology* 26:813–821.

Popovski, K., Kocoski, L.J., Trojacanec, O., Dovenski, T., Petkov, V., Veselinovic, S., Georgievski, B., Mickovski, G., Adamov, M. (1992). Ultrasonic examination of the ovarian response in donor ewes. *Proc. 8th Meeting A.E.T.E., 11–12. Sept. Lyon. Edition Fondation Marcel Merieux.* 200 (abstr.).

Quinlivan, J.A., Beazley, L.D., Braekevelt, C.R., Evans, S.F., Newnham, J.P., Dunlop, S.A. (2001). Repeated ultrasound guided fetal injections of corticosteroid alter nervous system maturation in the ovine fetus. *J. Perinat. Med.* 29:112–127.

Rabin, Y., Julian, T.B., Olson, P., Taylor, M.J., Wolmark, N. (1999). Long-term follow-up post-cryosurgery in a sheep breast model. *Cryobiol.* 39:29–46.

Rawlings, N.C., Jeffcoate, I.A., Savage, N.C. (1983). Pregnancy diagnosis and assessment of fetal numbers in the ewe in a commercial setting. *Theriogenology* 19:655.

Ravindra, J.P., Rawlings, N.C. (1997). Ovarian follicular dynamics in ewes during the transition from anoestrus to the breeding season. *J. Reprod. Fertil.* 110:279–289.

Ravindra, J.P., Rawlings, N.A., Evans, A.C.O., Adams, G.P. (1994). Ultrasonographic study of ovarian follicular dynamics in ewes during the oestrous cycle. *J. Reprod. Fertil.* 101:501–509.

Reichenbach, H.-D., Santos, M.H.B., Oliveira, M.A.L., Bürstel, D., Meinecke-Tillmann, S. (2004). Sexagem fetal na cabra e na ovelha por ultra-sonografia. In: *Diagnóstico de gestação na cabra e na ovelha.* Santos, M.H.B., Oliveira, M.A.L., Lima, P.F. (eds). São Paulo: Varela Editora e Livraria Ltda., pp 117–136.

Reichle, J.K., Haibel, G.K. (1991). Ultrasonic biparietal diameter of second trimester Pygmy goat fetuses. *Theriogenology* 35:689–694.

Richardson, C. (1972). Pregnancy diagnosis in the ewe. A review. *Vet. Rec.* 90:264–275.

Riesenberg, S. (1997). Ultrasonographische Dokumentation der Wachstumsdynamik ovarieller Funktionskörper unter Einbeziehung der östradiol-17β- und Progesteronplasmakonzentrationen während vier verschiedener Superovulationsmethoden bei kleinen Wiederkäuern. (Ultrasonographic documentation of the growth dynamics of ovarian follicles and corpora lutea in small ruminants with regard to the estradiol-17ß and progesterone plasma concentrations following four different superovulatory treatments). Dissertation, Hannover. School of Veterinary Medicine Hannover.

Riesenberg, S., Lewalski, H., Meinecke-Tillmann, S., Meinecke, B. (1996). Ultrasonic documentation of follicular dynamics following different superovulatory regimens in small ruminants—preliminary results. 29th Conference on Physiology and Pathology of Reproduction, Leipzig 1996. *Reprod. Dom. Anim.* 30:339 (abstr.).

Riesenberg, S., Meinecke-Tillmann, S., Meinecke, B. (2001a). Ultrasonic study of follicular dynamics following superovulation in German Merino ewes. *Theriogenology* 55:847–65.

Riesenberg, S., Meinecke-Tillmann, S., Meinecke, B. (2001b). Ultrasonic survey of follicular development following superovulation with a single application of pFSH, eCG or hMG in goats. *Small Ruminant Res.* 40:83–93.

Riesenberg, S., Meinecke-Tillmann, S., Meinecke, B. (2001c). Estradiol-17ß and progesterone in the peripheral blood plasma of goats following superovulation with a single dose of pFSH, hMG or eCG. *Small Ruminant Res.* 40:73–82.

Ritar, A.J., Ball, P.D., O'May, P.J. (1990). Artificial insemination of cashmere goats: effects on fertility and fecundity of intravaginal treatment, method and time of insemination, semen freezing process, number of motile spermatozoa and age of females. *Reprod. Fertil. Dev.* 2:377–384.

Romano, J.E., Christians, C.J., Crabo, B.G. (1998a). Application of transrectal ultrasonography in ewe reproduction. *Minnesota Sheep Research Report.* Dpt. Anim. Sci. and Univ. Minnesota Ext. Service and Agric. Exp. Station, Univ. Minnesota, 81–82.

Romano, J.E., Christians, C.J., Crabo, B.G. (1998b). Early pregnancy detection by transrectal ultrasonography in Suffolk ewes. *Minnesota Sheep Research Report*. Dpt. Anim Sci. and Univ. Minnesota Ext. Service and Agric. Exp. Station, Univ. Minnesota, 83–86.

Romano, J.E., Christians, C.J., Crabo, B.G. (1998c). Embryo development from day 15 to 40 of pregnancy in Suffolk ewes determined by transrectal ultrasonography. *Minnesota Sheep Research Report*. Dpt. Anim Sci. and Univ. Minnesota Ext. Service and Agric. Exp. Station, Univ. Minnesota, 87–90.

Royal, L., Tainturier, D. (1976). Mise au point sur les procédés modernes de diagnostic de gestation chez la brebis. *Rev. Méd. Vét.* 127:1009–1034.

Ruberte, J., Carretero, A., Fernández, M., Navarro, M., Caja, G., Kirchner, F., Such, X. (1994). Ultrasound mammography in the lactating ewe and its correspondence to anatomical sections. *Small Ruminant Res.* 13:199–204.

Rubianes, E., De Castro, T., Carjaval, B. (1996). Effect of high progesterone levels during the growing phase of the dominant follicle of wave 1 in ultrasonographically monitored ewes. *Can. J. Anim. Sci.* 76:473–475.

Rubianes, E., Ungerfeld, R., Viñoles, C., Rivero, A., Adams, G.P. (1997). Ovarian response to gonadotropin treatment initiated relative to wave emergence in ultrasonographically monitored ewes. *Theriogenology* 47:1479–1488.

Rüsch, P., Berchtold, M., Egger, L. (1981). Das Echolotverfahren zum Trächtigkeitsnachweis beim Schaf im Vergleich zur Ultraschall-Doppler-Technik.(The echo-sound method of pregnancy diagnosis in sheep compared with the ultrasonic Doppler technique). *Tierärztl. Umschau* 36:180–188.

Russel, A.J.F. (1989). The application of real-time ultrasonic scanning in commercial sheep, goats and cattle production enterprises. In: Taverne, M.M., Willemse, A.H. (eds) *Current Topics in Veterinary Medicine and Animal Science, Vol. 51: Diagnostic Ultrasound and Animal Reproduction*. Dordrecht: Kluwer Academic Publishers, pp 73–87.

Russel, A.J.F., Goddard, P.J. (1995). Small ruminant reproductive ultrasonography. In: Goddard, P.G. (eds) *Veterinary Ultrasonography*. Wallingford, UK: CAB International, pp 257–274.

Salama, A.A.K., Caja, G., Such, X., Peris, S., Sorensen, A., Knight, C.H. (2004). Changes in cisternal udder compartment induced by milking interval in dairy goats milked once or twice daily. *J. Dairy Sci.* 87:1181–1187.

Samake, S., Amoah, E.A., Mobini, S., Gazal, O., Gelaye, S. (2000). In vitro fertilization of goat oocytes during the non-breeding season. *Small Ruminant Res.* 35:49–54.

Scheerboom, J.E., Taverne, M.A. (1985). A study of the pregnant uterus of the ewe and the goat using real-time ultrasound and electromyelography. *Vet. Res. Commun.* 9:45–56.

Scheibe, K.M., Emeling, G., Marshall, L. (1986). Vergleichende Untersuchungen zur Trächtigkeitsdiagnose beim Schaf. Mh. *Vet. Med.* 41:158–164.

Schiewe, M.C., Bush, M., Stuart, L.S., Wildt, D.E. (1984). Laparoscopic embryo transfer in domestic sheep: a preliminary study. *Theriogenology* 22:675–682.

Schmidt, K.G., Silverman, N.H., Rudolph, A.M. (1996). Assessment of flow events at the ductus venosus-inferior vena cava junction and at the foramen ovale in fetal sheep by use of multimodal ultrasound. *Circulation* 93:826–833.

Schrick, F.N., Inskeep, E.K. (1993). Determination of early pregnancy in ewes utilizing transrectal ultrasonography. *Theriogenology* 40:295–306.

Schrick, F.N., Surface, R.A., Pritchard, J.Y., Dailey, R.A., Townsend, E.C., Inskeep, E.K. (1993). Ovarian structures during the oestrous cycle and early pregnancy in ewes. *Biol. Reprod.* 49:1133–1140.

Schwarz, T., Wierzchos, E. (2000). Wzrost pecherzykow jajnikowych w cyklu rujowym koz. (Growth of the ovary follicles in the oestrus cycle in goats). Medycyna Weterynaryjna 56:194–197.

Schweizer, F. (1976). Trächtigkeitsdiagnose beim Schaf unter Praxisverhältnissen mit Hilfe der Ultraschall-Doppler-Technik. (Pregnancy diagnosis in sheep under field conditions using a Doppler ultrasonic instrument). Tierärztl. Umschau 31:452–454.

Scott, P.R., Gessert, M.E. (1998). Ultrasonographic examination of 12 ovine vaginal prolapses. *Vet. J.* 155:323–324.

Scott, P.R., Gessert, M.E. (2000). Application of ultrasonographic examination of the ovine fetus in normal sheep and those presenting with obstetrical problems. *Vet. J.* 159:291–292.

Scott, P.R., Sargison, N.D., Wilson, D. (2001). Ultrasonographic findings of urinary retention caused by a vaginal stricture following dystocia in a ewe. *Vet. Rec.* 148:315–316.

Sergeev, L., Kleemann, D.O., Walker, S.K., Smith, D.H., Grosser, T.I., Mann, T., Seamark, R.F. (1990). Real-time ultrasound imaging for predicting ovine fetal age. *Theriogenology* 34:593–601.

Shimonovitz, S., Yagel, S., Zacut, D., Ben Chetrit, A., Ever-Hadani, P., Har-Nir, R., Ron, M. (1994). Ultrasound transmission gel in the vagina can impair sperm motility. *Hum. Reprod.* 9:482–483.

Simões, J., Potes, J., Azevedo, J., Almeida, J.C., Fontes, P., Baril, G., Mascarenhas, R. (2005). Morphometry of ovarian structures by transrectal ultrasonography in Serrana goats. *Anim. Reprod. Sci.* 85:263–273.

Ślósarz, P., Frankowska, A., Miś, M. (2003). Transrectal ultrasonography in diagnosing ovulation rate in sheep. *Anim. Sci. Papers and Reports* 3:183–189.

Sonesson, S.E., Fouron, J.C., Teyssier, G., Bonnin, P. (1994). Doppler echographic assessment of changes in the central circulation of the fetal sheep induced by maternal oxygen administration. *Acta Pediatr.* 83:1007–1011.

Souza, C.J.H., Campbell, B.K., Baird, D.T. (1996). Follicular dynamics and ovarian steroid secretion in sheep during anoestrus. *J. Reprod. Fertil.* 108:101–106.

Souza, C.J.H., Campbell, B.K., Baird, D.T. (1997a). Follicular dynamics and ovarian steroid secretion in sheep during the follicular and early luteal phases of the estrous cycle. *Biol. Reprod.* 56:483–488.

Souza, C.J.H., Campbell, B.K., Baird, D.T. (1998). Follicular waves and concentrations of steroids and inhibin A in ovarian venous blood during the luteal phase of the oestrous cycle in ewes with an ovarian autotransplant. *J. Endocrinol.* 156: 563–572.

Souza, C.J.H., Campbell, B.K., Webb, R., Baird, D.T. (1997b). Secretion of inhibin A and follicular dynamics throughout the estrous cycle in the sheep with and without Booroola gene (Fec-B). *Endocrinology* 138:5333–5340.

Souza, D.M.B. (2004). Avaliação ultra-sonográfica do crescimento fetal em caprinos. Recife, 2000. Dissertação, Faculdade de Medicina Veterinária, Universidade Federal Rural de Pernambuco. Cited from: Messias, J.B., Souza D.M.B., Santos, M.H.B, Moraes, É.P.B.X. Estimativa da idade e do peso embrioário e fetal através da ultra-sonografia. In: Diagnóstico de gestação na cabra e na ovelha. Santos, M.H B., Oliveira, M.A.L., Lima, P.F. (eds) Varela Editora e Livraria Ltda., São Paulo, pp 149–157.

Stouffer, J.R., White, W., Hogue, D.E., Hunt, G.L. (1969). Ultrasonic scanner for detection of single or multiple pregnancy in sheep. *J. Anim. Sci.* 29:104.

Strmšnik, L., Pogačnik, M., Čebulj Kadunc, N., Kosec, M. (2002). Examination of oestrus cycle and early pregnancy in sheep using transrectal ultrasonography. *Slov. Vet. Res.* 39:47–58.

Surbek, D.V., Young, A., Danzer, E., Schoeberlein, A., Dudler, L., Holzgreve, W. (2002). Ultrasound-guided stem cell sampling from the early ovine fetus for prenatal ex vivo gene therapy. *Am. J. Obstet. Gynecol.* 187:960–963.

Tainturier, D. (1992). Diagnostic de gestation chez la brebis par echotomographie transrectale. Rencontre Franco-Allemande Nantes Giessen, 2 Octobre 1992. Actualités veterinaries dans la gestion de la reproduction des animaux de rente.

Tajik, P., Abbas, V., Sarang, S. (2001). Measurement of different parts in Chall fetuses to determine pregnancy age. *Proc 5th Int Sheep Vet Conf, Univ. Stellenbosch, South Africa.*

Taverne, M.A.M., Lavoir, M.C., van Oord, R., van der Weyden, G.C. (1985). Accuracy of pregnancy diagnosis and prediction of fetal numbers in sheep with linear-array real-time ultrasound scanning. *Vet. Quart.* 7:256–263.

Thompson, J.G., Gardner, D.K., Pugh, P.A., McMillan, W.H., Tervit, H.R. (1995). Lamb birth weight is affected by culture system utilized during in vitro pre-elongation development of ovine embryos. *Biol. Reprod.* 53:1385–1391.

Trapp, M.J., Slyter, A.L. (1983). Pregnancy diagnosis in the ewe. *J. Anim. Sci.* 57:1–5.

Udy, G.B. (1987). Commercial splitting of goat embryos. *Theriogenology* 28:837–847.

Ungerfeld, R., Pinczak, A., Forsberg, M., Rubianes, E. (2002). Ovarian responses of anestrous ewes to the "ram effect." *Can. J. Anim. Sci.* 82:599–602.

Van Huisseling, H., Hasaart, T.H.M., Muijseres, G.J.I.M., Dehaan, J. (1991). Umbilical artery pulsatility index and placental vascular resistance during acute hypoxemia in fetal lambs. *Gyn. Obstet. Invest.* 3:61–66.

Viñoles, C., Forsberg, M., Banchero, G., Rubianes, E. (2001). Effect of long-term and short-term progestagen treatment on follicular development and pregnancy rate in cyclic ewes. *Theriogenology* 55:993–1004.

Viñoles, C., Meikle, A., Forsberg, M. (2004). Accuracy of evaluation of ovarian structures by transrectal ultrasonography in ewes. *Anim. Reprod. Sci.* 80:69–79.

Viñoles, C., Meikle, A., Forsberg, M., Rubianes, E. (1999). The effect of subluteal levels of exogenous progesterone on follicular dynamics and endocrine patterns during the early luteal phase of the ewe. *Theriogenology* 51:1351–1361.

Viñoles, C., Rubianes, E. (1998). Origin of the preovulatory follicle after induced luteolysis during the early luteal phase in ewes. *Can. J. Anim. Sci.* 78:429–443.

Wani, N.A., Wani, G.M., Mufti, A.M., Khan, M.Z. (1998). Ultrasonic pregnancy diagnosis in Gaddi goats. *Small Ruminant Res.* 29:239–240.

Watt, B.R., Anderson, G.A., Campbell, I.P. (1984). A comparison of six methods used for detecting pregnancy in sheep. *Aust. Vet. J.* 61:377–382.

Wehrend, A., Bostedt, H., Burkhardt, E. (2002). The use of transabdominal B mode ultrasonography to diagnose intra-partum uterine torsion in the ewe. *Vet. J.* 164:69–70.

Weiss, G. (1975). Möglichkeiten und Grenzen der Graviditätsdiagnose bei Haustieren mit Hilfe der Ultraschall-Doppler-Technik. (Possibilities and limitations in the use of the ultrasonic Doppler technique for pregnancy diagnosis in domestic livestock). Schweiz. Arch. Tierh. 117:123–134.

White, I.R., Russel, A.J.F. (1993). Incidence of hydrometra in goats. *Vet. Rec.* 132:110–112.

White, I.R., Russel, A.J.F., Fowler, D.G. (1984). Real-time ultrasonic scanning in the diagnosis of pregnancy and the determination of fetal numbers in sheep. *Vet. Rec.* 115:140–143.

White, K.L., Bunch, T.D., Mitalipov, S., Reed, W.A. (1999). Establishment of pregnancy after the transfer of nuclear transfer embryos produced from the fusion of Argali (ovis ammon) nuclei into domestic sheep (Ovis aries) enucleated oocytes. *Cloning* 1:47–54.

Wilkins, J.F., Fowler, D.G., Piper, L.R., Bindon, B.M. (1982). Observations on litter-size and reproductive wastage using ultrasonic scanning. *Proc. Austr. Soc. Anim. Prod.* 14:637 (abstr.).

Wittek, T., Erices, J., Elze, K. (1998). Histology of the endometrium, clinical-chemical parameters of the uterine fluid and blood plasma concentrations of progesterone, estradiol-17beta and prolactin during hydrometra in goats. *Small Ruminant Res.* 30:105–112.

Wójtowski, J., Ślósarz, P., Malecha W., Danków, R. (2002). Ultrasonograficzne pomiary zatoki mlekonośnej wymienia kóz podczas laktacji. (Ultrasound measurements of goat's mammary gland cisterns during lactation). *Medycyna Wet.* 58:977–980.

Wroth, R.H., McCallum, M.J. (1979). Diagnosing pregnancy in sheep—the "Scanopreg." *J. Agric.* (Western Australia) 20:85.

Wustmann, T., Bernhard, A. (1994). Klinische und sonographische Untersuchungen zum physiologischen Puerperalverlauf bei der Ziege. (Clinical and sonographical examinations of the physiological puerperal period in goats). *Reprod. Dom. Anim.* 29:265.

Zarrouk, A., Engeland, I.V., Sulon, J., Beckers, J.F. (1999). Pregnancy-associated glycoprotein levels in pregnant goats inoculated with Toxoplasma gondii or Listeria monocytogenes: a retrospective study. *Theriogenology* 52:1095–1104.

Zieba, D.A., Murawski, M., Schwarz, T., Wierzchos, E. (2002). Pattern of follicular development in high fecundity Olkuska ewes during the estrous cycle. *Reprod. Biol.* 2:39–58.

Index

Page references in *italics* denote figures. References followed by t denote tables.